Medical Radiology

Radiation Oncology

Series editors
Luther W. Brady
Jiade J. Lu

Honorary editors
Hans-Peter Heilmann
Michael Molls

For further volumes:
http://www.springer.com/series/4353

Mark Trombetta • Jean-Philippe Pignol
Paolo Montemaggi • Luther W. Brady
Editors

Alternate Fractionation in Radiotherapy

Paradigm Change

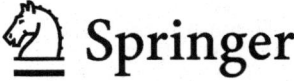

Editors
Mark Trombetta
Allegheny General Hospital
Allegheny Health Network Cancer
Institute
Drexel University College of Medicine
Pittsburgh, PA
USA

Paolo Montemaggi
Allegheny Health Network
Temple University School of Medicine
Pittsburgh Campus
Pittsburgh, PA
USA

Jean-Philippe Pignol
Radiation Oncology Department
Erasmus University Medical Center
Rotterdam
The Netherlands

Luther W. Brady
Hylda Cohn/American Cancer Society
Drexel University College of Medicine
Philadelphia, PA
USA

ISSN 0942-5373   ISSN 2197-4187   (electronic)
Medical Radiology
ISBN 978-3-030-09596-3   ISBN 978-3-319-42617-4   (eBook)
https://doi.org/10.1007/978-3-319-42617-4

This Springer imprint is published by the registered company Springer Nature Switzerland AG
The registered company address is: Gewerbestrasse 11, 6330 Cham, Switzerland

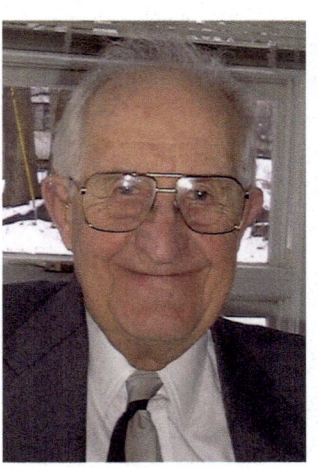

John F. (Jack) Fowler
DSc, PhD, MD (Hon), FIPEM, FInstP, FRCR, FACR, FASTRO, FAAPM

The authors of this book have dedicated it to Dr. Jack Fowler, an incredibly internationally renowned radiation biologist, radiation therapy physicist, as well as a major and significant supporter of all of the research efforts in radiation oncology. Dr. Fowler was renowned for his leadership at the Gray Laboratory in London and, upon his retirement, spent 7 years as professor at the University of Wisconsin, in Madison. His work in biology, particularly in reference to altered fractionation technologies and the designation of alpha beta ratios of normal tissues and tumor tissues, was critically important in the evolution and development of stereotactic body radiosurgery. It was his groundbreaking contributions that led to the justification of altering fractionation technologies, which had not changed significantly since 1921. He pointed out that with the appropriate use of alpha beta ratios one could alter the fractionation and protraction techniques to shorter periods with larger doses without compromising normal tissue toxicities, but with improved outcome relative to management when compared with other technologies in radiation therapy. Stereotactic body radiosurgery upon this foundation is now being employed in the treatment of tumors in all locations in the body from primary and secondary brain tumors, to head and neck tumors, to lung tumors, gastrointestinal tumors, pelvic tumors, bladder and prostate tumors. His contributions have been revolutionary in character substantiated by firm foundations in data to support the concept.

It is upon Dr. Fowler's basic scientific work that the present programs allow for altered fractionation technology with excellent results and without significant increase in complications.

To Dr. Fowler, we owe a great debt of gratitude for his wise counsel, his innovative leadership, and his significant contributions to the field of radiation oncology.

Luther W. Brady, MD
Mark Trombetta, MD
Jean-Philippe Pignol, MD, PhD
Paolo Montemaggi, MD

Contents

Contributors

Sara Alcorn The Johns Hopkins Hospital, Baltimore, MD, USA

Sushil Beriwal Department of Radiation Oncology, University of Pittsburgh Cancer Institute, Pittsburgh, PA, USA

Gerrit J. Blom Department of Radiation Oncology, VU University Medical Center, Amsterdam, The Netherlands

Luther Brady Hylda Cohn/American Cancer Society, Drexel University College of Medicine, Philadelphia, PA, USA

Thomas B. Brunner Freiburg University Medical Center, Freiburg, Germany

Krzysztof Bujko The Maria Sklodowska-Curie Memorial Cancer Centre and Institute of Oncology, Warsaw, Poland

Eric Chang University of Southern California, Los Angeles, CA, USA

Linda Chen Department of Radiation Oncology, Johns Hopkins University School of Medicine, Baltimore, MD, USA

Edward Chow University of Toronto, Toronto, ON, Canada

Christopher Crane Memorial Sloan Kettering Cancer Center, New York, NY, USA

Slobodan Devic McGill University, Montreal, QC, Canada

Olgun Elicin Department of Radiation Oncology, Inselspital, University Hospital of Bern, University of Bern, Bern, Switzerland

John C. Flickinger University of Pittsburgh, Pittsburgh, PA, USA

James Fontanesi William Beaumont Health Systems, Farmington Hills, Cancer Center, Oakland University School of Medicine, Rochester, MI, USA

Matthew Foote Department of Radiation Oncology, Princess Alexandra Hospital, Brisbane, Queensland, Australia

University of Queensland, Brisbane, Queensland, Australia

Olivier Gayou John D Cronin Cancer Center, Lexington, KY, USA

Brian J. Gebhardt Department of Radiation Oncology, University of Pittsburgh Cancer Institute, Pittsburgh, PA, USA

Matthias Guckenberger Department of Radiation Oncology, University Hospital Zurich (USZ), Zurich, Switzerland

Patrizia Guerrieri Department of Radiation Oncology, Allegheny Health Network Cancer Institute, Pittsburgh, PA, USA

Shaakir Hasan Department of Radiation Oncology, Allegheny Health Network Cancer Institute, Pittsburgh, PA, USA

Ben J.M. Heijmen Erasmus Medical Center, Rotterdam, The Netherlands

Joseph M. Herman Department of Radiation Oncology, University of Texas MD Anderson Cancer Center, Houston, TX, USA

Richard P. Hill Princess Margaret Cancer Centre, Toronto, ON, Canada

Nienke Hoekstra Department of Radiation Oncology, Erasmus University Medical Center, Rotterdam, The Netherlands

Zachary D. Horne Department of Radiation Oncology, University of Pittsburgh Cancer Institute, Pittsburgh, PA, USA

Geoffrey S. Ibbott Department of Radiation Physics, UT MD Anderson Cancer Center, Houston, TX, USA

Luca Incrocci Erasmus Medical Center, Rotterdam, The Netherlands

Joanne Jang Beth Israel Deaconess Medical Center, Boston, MA, USA

Joshua Jones University of Pennsylvania, Philadelphia, PA, USA

Irene Karam Department of Radiation Oncology, University of Toronto, Sunnybrook Health Sciences Centre, Toronto, ON, Canada

Alexander V. Kirichenko Department of Radiation Oncology, Allegheny Health Network Cancer Institute, Pittsburgh, PA, USA

Eugene J. Koay MD Anderson Cancer Center, Houston, TX, USA

Brian Kopitzki Clarkston Dermatology, Clarkston, MI, USA

Gargi Kothari The Royal Marsden Hospital NHS Foundation Trust, London, UK

Yun Liang Department of Radiation Oncology, Allegheny Health Network Cancer Institute, Pittsburgh, PA, USA

Michael Lock Division of Radiation Oncology, London Health Science Centre, London, ON, Canada

Department of Oncology, Western University Radiation, London, ON, Canada

Department of Medical Biophysics, Western University Radiation, London, ON, Canada

Lawson Health Research Institute, London, ON, Canada

London Regional Cancer Program, London, ON, Canada

Schulich School of Medicine and Dentistry, University of Western Ontario, London, ON, Canada

Natalie Logie University of Alberta, Edmonton, AB, Canada

Mauro Loi Erasmus Medical Center, Rotterdam, The Netherlands

Simon S. Lo Department of Radiation Oncology, University of Washington School of Medicine, Seattle, WA, USA

Steven Lutz Blanchard Valley Health System, Findlay, OH, USA

E. Mahmut Ozsahin Department of Radiation Oncology, Lausanne University Hospital, University of Lausanne, Lausanne, Switzerland

Fernand Missohou Division of Radiation Oncology, Institut de Cancérologie de Libreville (ICL), Libreville, Gabon

Paolo Montemaggi Allegheny Health Network, Temple University School of Medicine, Pittsburgh Campus, Pittsburgh, PA, USA

Alan E. Nahum Physics Department, University of Liverpool, Liverpool, UK

J.J. Nuyttens Erasmus Medical Center, Rotterdam, The Netherlands

Nathan Ogden Department of Radiology, Allegheny Health Network Cancer Institute, Pittsburgh, PA, USA

Jean-Philippe Pignol Radiation Oncology Department, Erasmus University Medical Center, Rotterdam, The Netherlands

Srinivas Raman University of Toronto, Toronto, ON, Canada

Alejandra Méndez Romero Erasmus Medical Center, Rotterdam, The Netherlands

Lauren M. Rosati Department of Radiation Oncology, Johns Hopkins University School of Medicine, Baltimore, MD, USA

Arjun Sahgal Department of Radiation Oncology, University of Toronto, Sunnybrook Health Sciences Centre, Toronto, ON, Canada

Shankar Siva Division of Radiation Oncology and Cancer Imaging, Peter MacCallum Cancer Centre, Melbourne, VC, Australia

Janusz Skowronek Brachytherapy Department, Greater Poland Cancer Centre, Poznań, Poland

Electroradiology Department (Secondary), Poznan University of Medical Science, Poznań, Poland

Ben J. Slotman Department of Radiation Oncology, VU University Medical Centre, Amsterdam, The Netherlands

Stephanie Terezakis The Johns Hopkins Hospital, Baltimore, MD, USA

Wolfgang A. Tomé Albert Einstein College of Medicine, Montefiore Medical Center, Bronx, New York, NY, USA

Mark Trombetta Allegheny General Hospital, Allegheny Health Network Cancer Institute, Drexel University College of Medicine, Pittsburgh, PA, USA

Akila N. Viswanathan Sidney Kimmel Comprehensive Cancer Center, Johns-Hopkins University, Baltimore, MD, USA

Te Vuong McGill University, Montreal, QC, Canada

Ruud C. Wortel Erasmus Medical Center, Rotterdam, The Netherlands

Theodore E. Yaeger Drexel University School of Medicine, Pittsburgh, PA, USA

University of North Carolina at Chapel Hill, Wake Forest University School of Medicine, Winston-Salem, NC, USA

Richard Zekman Oakland Medical Oncology, Michigan Healthcare Professionals, MI, USA

Introduction

Theodore E. Yaeger, Paolo Montemaggi,
Mark Trombetta, Jean-Philippe Pignol,
and Luther Brady

Contents

T.E. Yaeger, M.D., F.A.C.R.
Distinguished Alumnus, Drexel University School of
Medicine, Professor of Radiation Oncology (ret.),
University of North Carolina at Chapel Hill, Wake
Forest University School of Medicine,
Winston-Salem, North Carolina, USA

P. Montemaggi, M.D.
Allegheny Health Network, Professor of Radiation
Oncology (Emeritus), Temple University School of
Medicine, Pittsburgh Campus, Pittsburgh,
Pennsylvania, USA

M. Trombetta, M.D., F.A.C.R., F.A.C.R.O. (✉)
Allegheny General Hospital, Allegheny Health
Network Cancer Institute, Professor of Radiation
Oncology, Drexel University College of Medicine,
Pittsburgh, Pennsylvania, USA
e-mail: mtrombet@wpahs.org

J.-P. Pignol, M.D., Ph.D.
Professor and Chair, Radiation Oncology Department,
Erasmus University Medical Center,
Rotterdam, The Netherlands

L. Brady, M.D.
Distinguished University Professor,
Hylda Cohn/American Cancer Society, Professor of
Clinical Oncology, Professor of Radiation Oncology,
Drexel University College of Medicine, Philadelphia,
Pennsylvania, USA

1 Introduction

The near-miraculous discovery of the X-ray by Wilhelm Roentgen in 1895 (University of Wurzburg-Bavaris 1901) was coincidentally coupled with the most recent developments in rapid long-distance communication abilities. Those simultaneous discoveries made it possible to quickly to propel forth a new discipline of research into the possible applications of this new radiation breakthrough. From the outset, radiation was thought to be not only an important diagnostic tool—evaluating fractures without the then standard-of-care painful manipulations—but also as a possible therapeutic option, especially for cancer. Following Emil Grubbe's discovery that radiation exposure adversely affected cancerous growths (Grubbe 1903), the medical world became almost immediately excited that a new therapy option could become a surgical accessory, if not an alternative, for the treatment of cancers. There were big questions to answer: What to treat, who to treat, and how to treat? The intent of this book focuses on the latter question since- at this point within the modern era of radiation therapy there is little doubt in the therapeutic advantages of radiation, especially for the curative and conservation techniques (Chou et al. 2001).

In just the last two decades radiation therapy has vastly improved. It has been a wondrous journey that radiation oncologists did not go through alone. The modern vision of radiation oncology

Med Radiol Radiat Oncol (2017)
DOI 10.1007/174_2017_92, © Springer International Publishing AG
Published Online: 27 July 2017

and its role in the more and more complex scenario of integrated therapies for cancer treatment derive from the continuous interaction between biology, physics, medical imaging, translational research, and technical evolution in medicine. This may seem a new approach, but in reality it has been like this since the beginning. As usual, it would be useful and educational going briefly over the steps that have led the field to its present challenges.

The delivery of modern external beam radiotherapy is now a computer-controlled, multiple-layered safety mechanism modality. It is also visually confirmed daily for treatment setup with precise dose delivery and accurate documentation of all calculations leading to implementation of treatment (American College Radiology Practice Standards 2014). Patients for treatment are identified daily, treatment sites are computer and visually confirmed, and "time-out" procedures are strictly enforced. Any deviation (no matter how small) is registered and remedied as quickly as possible or practicable. Any major deviation of dose, treatment site, or excessive reaction/complication is reported to appropriate oversight or controlling agencies for investigation or reporting as needed/required. Over a century of refinement has resulted in a maximally safe and well-documented effective treatment, mostly for cancers and some limited benign conditions (Brady and Seegenschmiedt 1987). Lately there has developed a somewhat contrary disincentive to continued treatment refinement, perhaps less due to therapy failures, but more so from the successes of uniformly accepted treatment and well-researched protocols.

Incidentally, the declining rates of organized patient research protocol participation (Ulrich et al. 2010) may actually be the result of decreasing interest to question the "status quo" among other limiting factors such as manpower and financial support.

As such, it can be recognized that modern radiotherapy application has become an entrenched treatment with standard (universally accepted) regimens and has simply developed an everyday expectation of success, even if mediocre, in some instances. Rather than reconsidering

alternatives to the usual radiotherapy applications, more recent approaches have, more or less, focused on combining radiation with other therapeutic modalities. A mainstream cancer treatment investigation typically includes chemotherapy, biologics, sensitizers, and/or radio-protectants to traditional radiotherapy regimens (Conroy et al. 1976; Damsker et al. 1978; Brady 1975). In these cases, the dose of medications and/or radiation may be slightly modified, usually based on concerns about excessive toxicities. For the most part the radiation aspects remain with little change with regard to the overall length of the treatment course as different combinations, timing, or dosing techniques of the various medical agents are investigated. The common effort is usually trying to improve outcomes, enhance treatment tolerance, or modify excessive toxicities (Bower et al. 2011). Still, this begs the question of what role "traditional" radiotherapy could offer in this modern era that might become an improvement *in itself*. It seems that now is the perfect time radiation oncologists should not dismiss such matters and rather cultivate a curiosity to consider alternatives to the time-honored and generally accepted protracted-fractionated radiation schema (Cooper 1990; Yang et al. 2011).

Many professional radiation-based organizations have embraced a newer concept of improving the "now" standards of precise radiation delivery. There is emphasis on reducing dose whenever possible or practicable, investigating emerging treatment techniques, enhancing patient tolerance, and reducing lasting side effects while maintaining treatment effectiveness (American Society of Therapeutic Radiation Oncology (ASTRO) 2016). To this noble quest, the concept of investigating truly different approaches of radiation delivery has returned to the front line including reconsidering fractionation. But the concept of altering fractionation schemes in radiotherapy is not really that new at all. Historically, ***altered fractionation*** techniques have been studied since the beginnings of the broader application of external beam radiation therapy. In the early part of the twentieth century there was a desire for treating physicians to find the "ideal" dose (even a single dose) of radiation exposure that would cure cancer (Brady and Levitt 1999). And why not consider some "magical" X-ray dose when brachytherapy (radiation implants of nuclear sources) was considered essentially a single large fraction of radiation at that time? In retrospect, it is probable that some of these research interventions led to the realization of the actual dangers of radiation to patients (and the treating physicians) (Brady and Yaeger 2013). Fundamentally, much of the large-fraction dosing trials were abandoned when Coutard reported acceptable tolerance and good success in treating carcinoma of the larynx for conservation using multiple small daily doses of X-rays delivered over several successive weeks.

That outcome was an awakening that broadly laid the foundation for protracted courses of external beam regimens—widely applied to cancer sites—for the many decades that have followed, including the decades of this "modern" era (Chamberlain and Young 1937).

It is assumed that, post-World War II, there became a recognition that a divergence occurred to define palliative versus curative radiotherapy interventions. This was particularly important for the appreciation of the appropriateness of shorter versus longer radiation courses, respectively. Nevertheless, the latter has arguably remained little changed, if perhaps just tweaked incrementally. So enter now the premise of this book. There has been increasing evidence during the recent years that traditional fractionation techniques are certainly effective. But there is a growing appreciation of potentially unacceptable toxicities (especially when used with combined medical therapies) or that long regimens are simply patient unfriendly causing poorer compliance to the prescription (Curran et al. 2011). Additionally, oncology in general has entered the era of resource and cost containment. In summation, newer treatment options such as altering (shortening) the fraction schedules/courses and modified dosing are being reported as correspondingly effective, similar or less toxic, cost containing, and with improved patient compliance/tolerance (Whelan et al. 2010). These aspirations are not exactly like searching for some "Holy Grail" of an ideal treatment. The newer concepts about fractionation

variations are better described as "thinking inside the *alpha-beta* box" (Yang 2011) for more than just innovative treatment refinements. Likewise this is not a history-repeating-itself story because modern radiotherapy is no longer some crude application of a hopeful X-ray based on limited biologic understanding and application capabilities. These new therapy models are building upon the sophisticated technologies that exist today … and into the nearer future. Intensity-modulated, image-guided, radiosurgery-capable treatment machines coupled with multi-modality-based treatment plans are now opening up new possibilities for radiation treatment administration (Brady et al. 2006).

This is the first book of its kind in the modern era of radiotherapy. The author's intentions are to begin the consolidation of the newest but somewhat scattered research and reports of the concepts of possible treatment alternatives, concentrating on altered fractionation formats. The emphasis is to begin an earnest conversation on evaluating how traditional regimens could be altered without deleterious effects, with dependable (improved?) tolerance and acceptable outcomes. The following chapters will cover many treatment sites and compare innovative regimens. Each section represents the latest in thinking about exploring the frontiers of alternatives to traditional fractionation in the treatment of cancer in the words of the defined experts of the modern era. We wish this book to be a touchstone to rekindle interest in the development of a new paradigm in radiotherapy … ***altered fractionation***.

References

American College Radiology Practice Standards; Resolution 39 (Amended 2014): https://www.acr.org/~/media/AF1480B0F95842E7B163F09F1CE00977.pdf

American Society of Therapeutic Radiation Oncology (ASTRO) (2016) Choosing Wisely; recommendations. http://www.choosingwisely.org/societies/american-society-for-radiation-oncology/

Bower JE, Ganz PE, Irwin MR et al (2011) Inflammation and behavioral symptoms after breast cancer treatment. J Clin Oncol 29(26):3517–3522

Brady LW (1975) Combined modality therapy of gynecologic cancer. Cancer 35:76–83

Brady LW, Levitt SH (1999) The American Radium Society. Radiation oncology in the 3rd millennium. Radiology 209(3):593–596

Brady LW, Seegenschmiedt HM (1987) Radiation therapy. JAMA 258(16):2285–2287

Brady LW, Yaeger TE (eds) (2013) Encyclopedia of radiation oncology. History of radiation oncology. Springer, New York

Brady LW, Markoe A, Micaily B et al (2006) Innovative techniques in radiation oncology. Clinical research programs to improve local and regional control in cancer. Cancer 65(53):610–624

Chamberlain WE, Young BR (1937) Should the method of Coutard be applied in all cases of cancer treated by Roentgen rays? Radiology 29(2):186–187

Chou RH, Wilder RB, Wong MS et al (2001) Recent advances in radiotherapy for head and neck cancer. Ear Nose Throat J 80(10):704–707

Conroy JF, Lewis GC, Brady LW et al (1976) Low dose Bleomycin and Methotrexate in cervical cancer. Cancer 37:660–664

Cooper JS (1990) Will altered fraction schemes alter the future? Int J Radiat Oncol Biol Phys 19(6):1621–1622

Curran WJ, Paulus R, Langer CJ et al (2011) Sequential vs. concurrent chemoradiation for stage III non-small cell lung cancer: randomized phase III trial RTOG 9410. J Natl Cancer Inst 103(19):1452–1460

Damsker JI, Macklis R, Brady LW (1978) Radiosensitization of malignant melanoma. The effect of 7-hydroxychlorpromazine on the in vivo radiation response of Fortner's melanoma. Int J Radiat Oncol Biol Phys 4(9–10):821–824

Grubbe E (1903) High frequency electric current in medicine. Am Electro-Therapy X-Ray Era iii:427–433

Ulrich CM, James JL, Walker EM et al (2010) RTOG physician and research associate attitudes, beliefs and practices regarding clinical trials: implications for improving patient recruitment. Contemp Clin Trials 32(3):221–228

University of Wurzburg-Bavaris (n.d.) https://www.uni-wuerzburg.de/en/ueber/university/roentgenring_science_mile/nobel_laureates/wilhelm_conrad_roentgen_1901/

Whelan T, Pignol JP, Levine M et al (2010) Long-term result of hypofractionated radiation therapy for breast cancer. N Engl J Med 362(6):513–520

Yang J (2011) Radiation dose, fractionation, and alpha/beta effects on red shell volume using the linear quadratic model (Abstract). Proceedings of the 2011 CyberKnife® Robotic Radiosurgery Summit, San Francisco, CA

Yang J, Lamond J, Rowler R et al (2011) Fractionation effect on SBRT treatments using the red shell concept and the linear quadratic model. Int J Radiat Oncol Biol Phys 82(2):5864

The Radiobiological Aspects of Altered Fractionation

Alan E. Nahum and Richard P. Hill

Contents

The original version of this chapter was revised. The erratum to this chapter is available online at DOI 10.1007/174_2018_174

A. E. Nahum (✉)
Physics Department, University of Liverpool, Liverpool, UK
e-mail: alan_e_nahum@yahoo.co.uk

R. P. Hill
Princess Margaret Cancer Centre, Toronto, Ontario, Canada

1 Introduction

Fractionation is central to the clinical effectiveness of external beam radiotherapy (EBRT). An understanding of the effect of splitting a total dose into a number of small *fractions* involves virtually all of the so-called 5 Rs of radiobiology: *repair, repopulation, reassortment, reoxygenation,* and *radiosensitivity* (Steel 2007a). Small fraction sizes had been originally established empirically (Coutard 1929)—this yielded the best *therapeutic ratio* (loosely defined as 'the probability of local tumor control for a given, acceptably low complication probability'). Around the early 1980s significant advances were made in *theoretical* radiobiology, focused around the linear quadratic (LQ) model and the associated α/β ratio (e.g., Williams et al. 1985; Fowler 1989); it was believed that α/β was generally high (~10 Gy) for tumor clonogens and low (~3 Gy) for dose-limiting 'late' normal tissue complications (e.g., Steel 2002a, 2007b; Brown et al. 2014). Until relatively recently, fraction sizes of around 2 Gy were the 'gold standard' in EBRT and a modest increase in fraction size (to ~3 Gy) was termed *hypo*-fractionation.

Significant advances in 3D imaging of tumors and surrounding organs (e.g., De Los Santos et al. 2013), paralleled by developments in 3D planning and delivery of EBRT (e.g., Nahum and Uzan 2012), principally the shaping of beams through devices such as multileaf collimators and the *modulation* of beam intensity (IMRT), are now commonplace in radiotherapy departments. Thus today we have an array of tools and techniques enabling ever tighter 'conformation' of the high-dose volume to the tumor/target volume, thereby further improving normal tissue sparing.

Radiobiological modelling has also moved significantly beyond the LQ-based computation of *iso-effective* fractionation schemes (Withers et al. 1983). Around the early 1990s moderately sophisticated *macroscopic* radiobiological models were developed for predicting tumor control probability (TCP) and normal-tissue complication probability (NTCP). The more mechanistic of these models take account of how cell killing depends on total dose, fraction size, inter-fraction interval, dose-rate, cell cycle, hypoxic status, and other factors (Nahum and Kutcher 2007; Uzan and Nahum 2012; Chapman and Nahum 2015; Jones and Dale 2007). Of particular relevance are so-called volume effects for (late) complications in various normal tissues (principally lung, liver, heart, parotid glands, rectum), expressed by the value of the parameter *n* in the Lyman–Kutcher–Burman NTCP model (e.g., Nahum and Kutcher 2007) and in the expression for *generalized* equivalent uniform dose (gEUD) (Niemierko 1999); a value of *n* close to zero indicates 'serial' behavior (e.g., spinal cord), and a value close to unity, 'parallel' behavior (Nahum and Kutcher 2007; Marks et al. 2010a). Alternatively, the parameter *s* in the *relative seriality* model (Källman et al. 1992) represents the degree of 'seriality' of the tissue concerned, a very low value indicating 'parallel' behavior. By computing TCP and NTCP from the dose-volume histograms of a treatment plan one can predict how the probability of local control ought to vary with the number of fractions, and hence how fraction number can be *individualized* to yield maximum local control (see later section).

2 Cell Killing and the Linear-Quadratic Model

The linear quadratic (LQ) model (e.g., Williams et al. 1985; Fowler 1989; Chapman 2003, 2014) represented a major step forward in describing

cell killing by ionizing radiation, especially regarding the radiation treatment of cancer. For a population of cells each with identical radiosensitivity, the LQ model predicts that the surviving fraction SF of irradiated cells depends on the dose *d* according to

$$SF = \frac{\overline{N_s}}{N_o} = \exp\left\{-\alpha d - \beta d^2\right\} \qquad (1)$$

where N_o is the initial number of cells (tumor clonogens), and $\overline{N_s}$ the mean number of surviving cells after a radiation dose *d*. The coefficient α describes 'single-hit' (i.e., unrepairable) killing and the coefficient β describes cell killing as a result of the combination of two independent sublethal lesions in close proximity (Chapman 2003; Chapman and Nahum 2015). Both α and β vary according to the phase of the cell cycle; when the LQ model is applied to populations of 'asynchronous' cells, which is the default situation (in living organisms and also in the laboratory), the resulting α and β are necessarily averages over the cell cycle (Chapman and Nahum 2015). It can be noted that the distribution of cells between the different phases (G_0, G_1, G_2, S, and mitosis) may differ between cells in tissue and cells growing in culture.

A key assumption behind Eq. (1) is that the dose *d* is delivered in a time much shorter than the 'repair half-time' of the sublethal lesions (at a high dose rate linear accelerators easily fulfil this condition as the total time to deliver a total dose from beams from many different directions, often intensity modulated, is still generally short compared to the repair half-time of the sublethal lesions). However, if the dose rate is extremely low, as in certain brachytherapy techniques, only single-hit (non-repairable) alpha cell killing takes place, all sublethal lesions being repaired before any of them can combine to form lethal lesions (Steel 2002b). For doses in the 0–0.6 Gy range major deviations from the behavior described by Eq. (1) have been found for certain cell types; this is known as *low-dose hypersensitivity* (Short et al. 1999, 2001); however, this need not concern us further as clinical fraction sizes (see next section) are almost never below ~1.8–2 Gy.

Figure 1a shows survival curves as a function of dose for a number of human tumor cell lines

(Chapman 2003); the logarithmic SF scale should be noted. Though they differ widely in their slopes, all these curves show some degree of curvature or 'bending' with increasing dose, corresponding to the βd^2 term of Eq. (1). A simple transformation of Eq. (1) yields

$$-\left[\ln SF\right]/D = \alpha + \beta D \qquad (2)$$

In Fig. 1b the quantity ln SF/D has been plotted against dose D for the data points of each cell survival curve. Several important features can be observed. Firstly, well-separated straight lines can be drawn through each set of data points, consistent with the functional form of Eq. (2) and therefore of Eq. (1); in other words the *linear quadratic* expression describes these data very well. Secondly the intercepts on the y-axis (corresponding to $D = 0$) yield α for each cell line, and it can be seen that these α vary enormously in magnitude. Thirdly the values of β are given by the gradients of the straight lines; these show only a modest inter-variation.

Chapman (2014) has summarized a vast amount of data on in vitro and in some cases in vivo radiosensitivity for a variety of human tumor cell lines; these radiosensitivities are given in Table 1 and the corresponding α/β ratios have been added. Following Chapman (2014), α and β have been written with a bar to emphasize that they are averages for *asynchronous* cell populations.

It can be seen that the values of $\bar{\alpha}/\bar{\beta}$ vary from 12.6 to 4.5 Gy, and are mostly lower than the generic value of 10 Gy for tumors (see later section). Note further that a standard deviation has been assigned to each mean α value; though the *average* radiosensitivity only differs by mostly a factor 2 (at maximum 3) between each tumor type, within any given type there is a wide range.

Despite strong experimental evidence exemplified by the data of Fig. 1, the validity of the LQ model has been questioned by several investigators, especially at large doses, i.e., large fraction sizes (Wang et al. 2010; Carlone et al. 2005; Kirkpatrick et al. 2009; Sheu et al. 2013) while being robustly

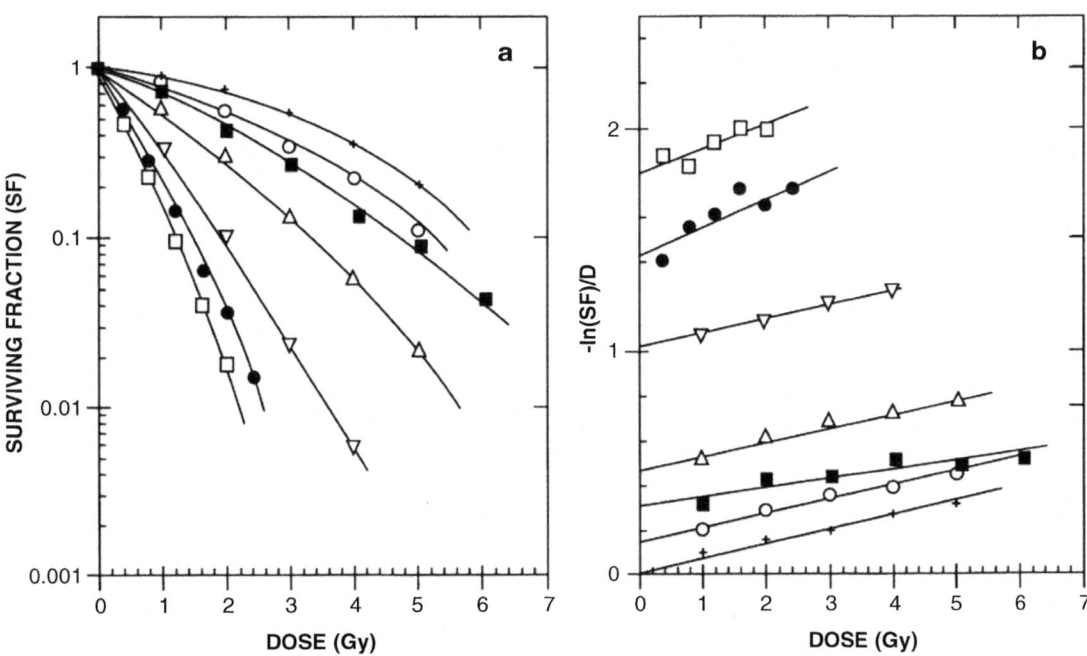

Fig. 1 (**a, b**) Radiation survival curves for *asynchronous* populations of several human tumor lines: HT-29 (+), OVCAR10 (*open circle*), MCF7 (*filled square*), A2780 (*open triangle*), HX142 (*inverted triangle*), HT-144 (*filled circle*), and Mo59J (*open square*); the data for the HX142 cell line are from Deacon et al. (1985). (**b**) The same data are plotted as –ln*SF/D* vs. *D* (from Chapman J.D. *International Journal of Radiation Biology* 79, 71–81, 2003. ©Taylor & Francis www.tandfonline.com. Reproduced with permission)

Table 1 Intrinsic radiosensitivity coefficients for human tumor cell lines irradiated under well-oxygenated conditions (adapted from Chapman 2014)

Tumor histology	$\bar{\alpha}$ -parameter (Gy^{-1})	$\sqrt{\bar{\beta}}$ -parameter (Gy^{-1})	$\bar{\alpha}$ / $\bar{\beta}$ (Gy)
Groups A and B: comprising lymphoma, myeloma, neuroblastoma, medulloblastoma and SSLC	0.73 ± 0.23	0.241	12.6
Groups C and D: comprising breast, bladder, cervical carcinoma, pancreatic, colorectal and squamous lung cancer	0.36 ± 0.25	0.241	6.2
Group E: comprising melanoma, osteosarcoma, glioblastoma, renal carcinoma	0.26 ± 0.17	0.241	4.5
Cervical carcinoma	0.35 ± 0.21	0.241	6.0
Head and neck carcinoma	0.40 ± 0.21	0.241	6.9
Prostate carcinoma	0.26 ± 0.17	0.177	8.3

SSCL small cell lung cancer. Data for Groups A-E from Deacon et al. (1984); data for 'Cervical carcinoma' from West et al. (1993); data for 'Head and neck carcinoma' from Björk-Eriksson et al. (2000); data for 'Prostate carcinoma' from Algan et al. (1996) and Nahum et al. (2003).
The standard deviation on $\bar{\alpha}$ expresses the wide variation in *in vitro* radiosensitivity for a given tumor type.

defended by others (Chapman and Nahum 2015; Brown et al. 2014; Chapman and Gillespie 2012; Brenner et al. 2012). The theoretical case *against* the LQ model for *all* values of the dose, no matter how low or high, was enunciated most clearly by Wang et al. (2010). These authors pointed out that the 'single-hit', unrepairable α mechanism (hence αD) and the 'double-hit', repairable β mechanism (hence βD^2) cannot be *independent of one another*. This is because the 'pool of sublethal lesions' created at the *start* of the duration of a dose fraction will inevitably be *reduced* by α killing occurring at slightly *later* times during the delivery of this same dose fraction. Wang et al. proposed a *generalized LQ model* (gLQ) and showed that this fitted certain cell survival data better than the LQ model, and also yielded different values for α and β. However, as Fig. 1 demonstrates convincingly, the LQ model (Eq. 1) fits (most) experimental surviving fraction, *SF*, vs. dose, *D*, data remarkably well (e.g., Chapman and Nahum 2015). At the present time this *experimental-theoretical discrepancy* is unresolved. From a pragmatic point of view, if the LQ model describes well the *clinical* data on tumor control over a wide range of doses, fraction sizes, and treatment durations (Brown et al. 2014; Brenner et al. 2012), then it is appropriate to employ it to

model and predict radiotherapy outcomes for alternative dose and fractionation regimens.

As we have seen, some workers maintain that the LQ model *over*-estimates cell killing at large fraction sizes (e.g., Wang et al. 2010; Carlone et al. 2005; Kirkpatrick et al. 2009; Sheu et al. 2013), in line with the gLQ model, whereas others consider that the clinical outcomes from extreme hypofractionation (see later section) are consistent with the linear quadratic model (Brown et al. 2014; Mehta et al. 2012). Still others, e.g., Song et al. (2013), claim that the LQ model *under*-predicts the level of reproductive cell death required to achieve the observed tumor control at these very large fraction sizes; this only makes sense if there is significant hypoxia. Song et al. maintain that additional mechanisms are involved, such as indirect/necrotic cell death due to vascular damage.

3　The LQ Model Applied to Fractionation and Iso-effect

Consider now *n* fractions each of dose *d*, assuming full repair of all sublethal lesions in the interval between consecutive fractions (this must be at least 6 h (Steel 2007b); from Eq. (1) the cell surviving fraction after n (dose) fractions will be given by

$$SF = \left[\exp\left(-\alpha d - \beta d^2\right) \right]^n$$
$$= \exp\left(-\alpha n d - \beta n d^2\right) \quad (3)$$

and replacing $n \times d$ by the *total* dose D, Eq. (3) can be rewritten as

$$SF = \exp\left(-\alpha D - \beta dD\right) \quad (4)$$

or alternatively as

$$SF = \exp\left[-\alpha D\left(1 + \frac{d}{\alpha / \beta}\right)\right] \quad (5)$$

The term $D[1 + d/(\alpha/\beta)]$ is known as the *biologically effective dose* (BED); a total dose equal to the BED delivered in an infinite number of vanishingly small fractions is radiobiologically equivalent (i.e., yields the identical surviving fraction) to the regimen under study (n fractions of size d) (Fowler 1989). Equation (5) can therefore be rewritten as $SF = \exp[-\alpha BED]$. The term $[1 + d/(\alpha/\beta)]$ multiplying the total dose D is sometimes known as the *relative effectiveness* (RE) (Steel 2007b); this tends to unity as either

the fraction size d tends to zero or (α/β) tends to infinity, which is consistent with the definition of BED. The BED can be modified to take into account cell proliferation during fractionated radiotherapy:

$$BED = \left[D\left(1 + d / \left(\alpha / \beta\right)\right) - \left[\gamma / \alpha\right]\left(T - T_k\right) \right] \quad (6)$$

where $\gamma = \ln 2/T_d$; T is the overall treatment time, T_k is the time during which no proliferation is assumed to take place, and T_d is the cell-doubling time.

Figure 2a and b shows cell survival curves according to the linear quadratic model (Eq. 1) corresponding to different fraction sizes (2.75 Gy, 11.1 Gy), for (a) $\alpha/\beta = 10$ Gy (generic tumor value) and (b) $\alpha/\beta = 3$ Gy (generic value for late complications). Note that complete repair of sublethal lesions between fractions has been assumed.

The two regimens, 3×11.1 Gy and 20×2.75 Gy, result in identical surviving fractions (aka *iso-effective*) for $\alpha/\beta = 10$ Gy (default tumor value) but the 3×11.1 Gy regimen is considerably more 'toxic' for $\alpha/\beta = 3$ Gy (default late-complication value). The concept of iso-effectivity is discussed in more detail in the next two sections.

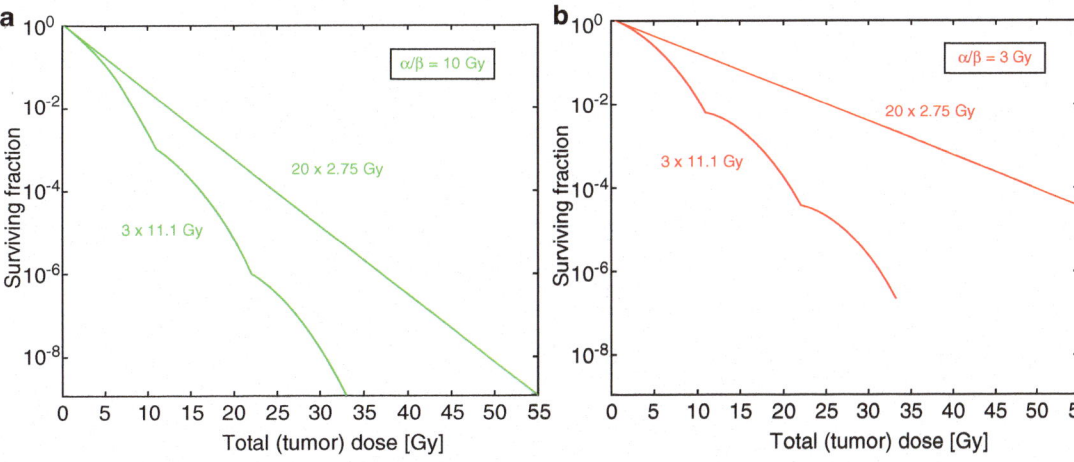

Fig. 2 Surviving fraction as a function of total dose for (**a**) tumor $(\alpha/\beta)^T = 10$ Gy and (**b**) normal tissue $(\alpha/\beta)^{NT} = 3$ Gy under tumor-iso-effective schemes of 20×2.75 Gy and 3×11.1 Gy. Note the difference in surviving fractions for the normal tissue, which is a factor of $\approx 6 \times 10^{-2}$ lower for 3×11.1 Gy than for 20×2.75 Gy (curves constructed for $\alpha_{tumor} = 0.3$ Gy^{-1} and $\alpha_{NT} = 0.1$ Gy^{-1})

The BED concept can be used to show how the *therapeutic ratio* (TR) varies with the number of fractions. For example, one can calculate the value of $BED_{\alpha/\beta=3Gy}$, representing (late) normal tissue effects, for a *constant* of $BED_{\alpha/\beta=10Gy}$, representing constant tumor effect. $BED_{\alpha/\beta=3Gy}$ decreases steadily as the number of fractions increases, thus demonstrating that the highest TR is obtained at small fraction sizes. Here, we prefer to employ the more directly clinically relevant quantities TCP and NTCP to illustrate these inter-relationships (see Fig. 3).

Figure 3 shows how tumor local control (TCP) varies as the number of fractions is changed for different values of tumor α/β. The other parameters in the TCP model have been adjusted such that TCP is always 70% for 35 × 2-Gy fractions—corresponding to a tumor control rate for a patient population. For each number of fractions, the total dose and hence fraction size have been adjusted in order to keep the NTCP value, using $\alpha/\beta = 3$ Gy, constant (i.e., 'isotoxic'). The complication is rectal bleeding which is quasi-serial i.e. it has a *low* value of the volume parameter *n* (the significance of the value of *n* is discussed in the next section). For tumor $\alpha/\beta = 10$ Gy the advantage of a large number of fractions is immediately apparent. If only 5 fractions are used the TCP is reduced to below 40% compared to 70% at 35 fractions.

As the tumor α/β is progressively reduced the disadvantage of a smaller number of fractions is also reduced. When α/β for tumor and critical normal tissues are equal, $\alpha/\beta = 3$ Gy, the dependence of TCP on fraction number disappears. For tumor $\alpha/\beta = 1.5$ Gy, i.e., *lower* than that for the complication, the TCP *increases* with decreasing fraction number, the maximum TCP being achieved with a single fraction. It is important to note, however, that *reoxygenation between fractions*, which would tend to favor a large number of small fractions (Ruggieri et al. 2010, 2017), has not been taken into account; in other words tumor hypoxia has been assumed to be negligible. Further, tumor-clonogen proliferation has also been assumed to be negligible (cf. Eq. 6). Both of these issues are discussed later.

There is now a considerable amount of evidence that α/β may be relatively low for two important tumor types, breast and prostate (Yarnold et al. 2011; Miralbell et al. 2012). For both of these tumors hypofractionated treatment protocols (cf. Fig. 1) are in progress with encouraging results though there is still some controversy about low α/β in the case of prostate tumors (Nahum et al. 2003; Valdagni et al. 2005). It should be borne in mind that hypofractionated regimens are generally derived for *normal tissue* iso-effect (Withers et al. 1983; Hoffmann and Nahum 2013) which requires a value of α/β for the critical normal-tissue

Fig. 3 Tumor control probability (nominally for a prostate tumor) as a function of the number of fractions, for a total dose ensuring a constant NTCP of 4.3%, i.e., 'isotoxic,' for rectal bleeding with $\alpha/\beta = 3$ Gy. *Open circles,* $\alpha/\beta = 10$ Gy; *triangles,* $\alpha/\beta = 5$ Gy; *squares,* $\alpha/\beta = 3$ Gy; *diamonds,* $\alpha/\beta = 1.5$ Gy (from Uzan J. and Nahum A.E. *British Journal of Radiology* 85, 1279–1286, 2012. ©British Institute of Radiology. With permission)

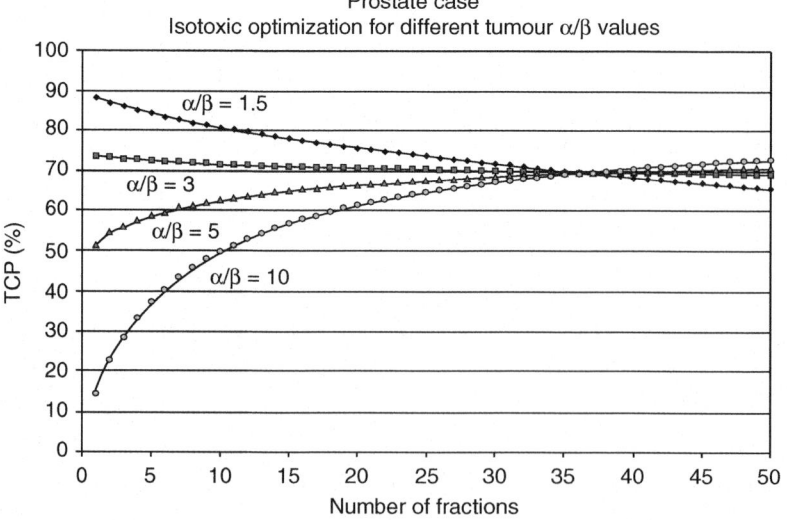

endpoint; Fiorino et al. (2014) found that the very low value of $\alpha/\beta = 0.4$ Gy for bladder yielded a superior fit to data on severe urinary toxicity.

4 Iso-effect, Withers, and the α/β Ratio

If the BEDs of two fractionation regimens are equal, then it follows from Eq. (5) that these regimens achieve identical surviving fractions; two such regimens are said to be *iso-effective*. Thus for the reference regimen with total dose and fraction size (D_{ref}, d_{ref}) and the new regimen (D_{new}, d_{new}), equating their respective BEDs and rearranging, we obtain

$$\frac{D_{new}}{D_{ref}} = \frac{1 + \left[d_{ref} / (\alpha / \beta) \right]}{1 + \left[d_{new} / (\alpha / \beta) \right]} \qquad (7)$$

The value of α/β for the tumor should be used in Eq. (7) if tumor *iso-effectivity* is desired (e.g., 10 Gy). In the more commonly desired case of (late) normal tissue iso-effectivity, $\alpha/\beta = 3$ Gy is usually appropriate. The above expression is the well-known Withers iso-effect formula or WIF (Withers et al. 1983). Referring to Fig. 2a, we see that the two regimens, 20 × 2.75 Gy and 3 × 11.1 Gy, are iso-effective for $\alpha/\beta = 10$ Gy (generic tumor), thereby satisfying Eq. (7) for BED = 70.125 Gy. Assuming now that $\alpha/\beta = 3$ Gy, the generic value for late complications (Fig. 2b), a regimen of 3 × 11.1 Gy (BED = 156.51 Gy) would be more toxic than 20 × 2.75 Gy (in other words a lower SF); for 'normal tissue' iso-effectivity the fraction size should be reduced from 11.1 to 8.88 Gy, thereby yielding a BED of 105.42 Gy for both regimens.

5 Normal Tissues: Volume Effects, Conformality, and the $(\alpha/\beta)_{eff}$ Ratio

Figure 3 can suggest that the optimal fraction size/number depends solely on the relative α/β values of the tumor and critical normal tissue. On this basis it is difficult to understand the current success of the extremely hypofractionated SBRT or SABR regimens for treating non-small-cell lung tumors (NSCLC) (e.g., Fowler et al. 2004; Timmerman 2008; Lagerwaard et al. 2008)—see also later. For these tumors there is no evidence that α/β is lower than or even of the same order as α/β (= 3 Gy) for the principal late complication of radiation pneumonitis (Borst et al. 2009; Marks et al. 2010b). To gain insight into this apparent puzzle we need to examine in detail the assumptions behind the Withers formula.

Several research groups have explored the connection between fractionation, dose distribution in the irradiated normal tissue, and NT volume effect, i.e., the parameter n (Jin et al. 2010; Vogelius et al. 2010; Myerson 2011). Hoffmann and Nahum (2013) pointed out that the 'Withers' LQ-based iso-effect formula (see previous section) implicitly assumes that the critical normal tissue receives the same dose as the tumor (i.e., the prescription dose) and either does so uniformly—which is almost never the case—or its response is solely a function of the *maximum* dose it receives ($\approx$ the tumor dose). The latter is strictly true only for 100% 'serial' organs such as the spinal cord.

Hoffmann and Nahum wanted to retain the simplicity of the WIF (which uses the *tumor* prescription dose) to determine a new iso-effective fractionation regimen while taking full account of i) dose heterogeneity in the normal tissue and ii) the value of the volume-effect parameter n indicating the position of the NT on the 'series-parallel' axis ($n = 0$ to 1): hence their $\left(\alpha / \beta \right)_{eff}^{NT}$ concept. By replacing the *intrinsic* α/β ratio for normal tissue (e.g., 3 Gy for late complications) by $\left(\alpha / \beta \right)_{eff}^{NT}$ in the WIF, i.e., in Eq. (6), one obtains fractionation regimens that are more truly iso-effective for an arbitrary NT dose distribution and arbitrary n varying from zero (100% serial) to unity (100% parallel), in contrast to the unmodified WIF.

For the extremely simple, if 'unclinical', case of the normal tissue receiving a 100% *uniform* dose d^{NT}, where the tumor receives dose d^{T}, Hoffman and Nahum (2013) showed that

$$\left(\alpha/\beta\right)_{\text{eff}}^{\text{NT}} = \frac{d^{\text{T}}}{d^{\text{NT}}}\left(\alpha/\beta\right)_{\text{intr}}^{\text{NT}} \qquad (8)$$

where $\left(\alpha/\beta\right)_{\text{intr}}^{\text{NT}}$ is the *intrinsic* normal tissue α/β (e.g., 3 Gy); for this simple case the volume-effect parameter n doesn't enter into the expression. For the much more clinically realistic situation of a *heterogeneous* dose distribution in a *parallel* normal tissue, with $n = 1$, Hoffmann and Nahum derived

$$\left(\alpha/\beta\right)_{\text{eff}}^{\text{NT}} = \frac{1}{1+\left(\sigma_d^{\text{NT}}/\overline{d^{\text{NT}}}\right)^2}\frac{d^{\text{T}}}{d^{\text{NT}}}\left(\alpha/\beta\right)_{\text{intr}}^{\text{NT}} \qquad (9)$$

where $\overline{d^{\text{NT}}}$ is the mean dose in the normal tissue and σ_d^{NT} is the standard deviation of the NT dose distribution; for $\sigma_d^{\text{NT}} = 0$, i.e., uniform NT dose, Eq. (9) reduces to Eq. (8) as expected. For the case of an arbitrary n the expression is more complex—see Hoffmann and Nahum (2013).

Figure 4 shows how $\left(\alpha/\beta\right)_{\text{eff}}^{\text{NT}}$ varies with n for the critical normal tissue volume in three different IMRT plans. For $n = 0$ (i.e., 100% serial NT) there is essentially no difference between the 'effective' and intrinsic α/β, but as the NT becomes more 'parallel' (i.e., as n approaches unity) $\left(\alpha/\beta\right)_{\text{eff}}^{\text{NT}}$ increases. Additionally, the rate of this increase depends on the degree of conformality of the NT dose-volume histogram. The curve labelled IMRT_3 corresponds to the most conformal plan, i.e., achieves the most lung sparing, whereas IMRT_1 is the least conformal and this is reflected in the respective values of $\left(\alpha/\beta\right)_{\text{eff}}^{\text{NT}}$. The double curves for each treatment plan in Fig. 4 are the envelopes of the values of $\left(\alpha/\beta\right)_{\text{eff}}^{\text{NT}}$, which for $n \neq 0$ or 1 show a slight dependence on the initial and final number of fractions.

Summarizing, the value of $\left(\alpha/\beta\right)_{\text{eff}}^{\text{NT}}$ for the critical normal tissue is a guide to the *hypofractionation potential* of a given treatment plan. For 'serial' organs (low n) the 'intrinsic' α/β and $\left(\alpha/\beta\right)_{\text{eff}}^{\text{NT}}$ will be approximately equal, irrespective of the degree of heterogeneity of the NT dose distribution, as Fig. 4 demonstrates. Conversely, if $\left(\alpha/\beta\right)_{\text{eff}}^{\text{NT}}$ is close to or even higher than the tumor α/β (which, as we have seen above, may be significantly lower than the generic value of

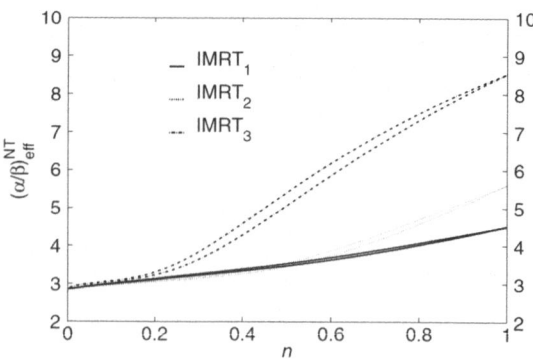

Fig. 4 The variation of $\left(\alpha/\beta\right)_{\text{eff}}^{\text{NT}}$ with the volume-effect parameter n for three IMRT plans, of differing degrees of conformality, assuming an intrinsic $\left(\alpha/\beta\right)^{\text{NT}} = 3$ Gy (from Hoffmann A.L. and Nahum A.E. Fractionation in normal tissues: the $\left(\alpha/\beta\right)_{\text{eff}}$ concept can account for dose heterogeneity and volume effects. *Physics in Medicine and Biology* 58, 6897–6914, 2013. ©Institute of Physics and Engineering in Medicine. Reproduced by permission of IOP Publishing. All right reserved)

10 Gy) then Fig. 3 indicates that a small number of (large) fractions (*hypo*-fractionation) is a viable treatment option.

6 Variation of Tumor Local Control from Conventional to SBRT Fraction Sizes

Extreme hypofractionation is becoming the 'treatment of choice' for early-stage NSC lung tumors, following the pioneering work by Blomgren et al. (1995). A variety of regimens are in use, the most extreme being three fractions of 18–20 Gy, prescribed to the 80% isodose. Such a prescription results in a non-uniform, 'peaked' dose distribution in the target volume; this deliberate dose heterogeneity enables field sizes to be as small as possible, thereby maximizing the sparing of the (uninvolved) lung surrounding the tumor. Much effort is generally expended to avoid 'geographic misses', principally due to respiratory movement (Franks et al. 2015; Selvaraj et al. 2013; Schwarz et al. 2017). These treatments are known as *stereotactic body radiotherapy* (SBRT) or *stereotactic ablative radiotherapy* (SABR). Hoffmann and Nahum (2013) analyzed a number of SABR treatment plans and found values of $\left(\alpha / \beta\right)_{\text{eff}}^{\text{NT}}$ between 7 and 9 Gy for $n = 1$, i.e., values close to the tumor α/β; this is consistent with the safe use of very large fractions.

Figure 5 gathers together on one graph mean clinical local control rates (i.e., TCP values) for a very wide range of fraction sizes/numbers, ranging from conventional fractionation (2–3 Gy fractions) delivered with conventional 3D–CRT techniques through to SBRT/SABR treatments (3–5 fractions) and even a single fraction (Brown et al. 2014). These different prescriptions have been converted to BED using a tumor α/β of 8.6 Gy (Mehta et al. 2012). Both these groups and others claim that the smooth curve of TCP vs. BED through the error bars of the clinical data points (see Fig. 5) demonstrates that the LQ model adequately describes cell killing over this extremely wide range of fraction sizes, despite the counter-claims of Wang et al. (2010) and others (see earlier section).

It can be noted, however, that the analysis represented by the data in Fig. 5 takes no account of the differences in the range of tumor volumes treated by the different techniques. For the same BED the on-the-average larger tumors treated by 3D-CRT would be expected to show a lower TCP than the much smaller ones treated by SBRT (aka SABR). Furthermore, the rate of increase of TCP with BED will be a function of $\bar{\alpha} / \sigma_{\alpha}$ in the 'Marsden' TCP model (Nahum and Sanchez-Nieto 2001).

7 The Individualization of Fraction Size/Number

A dichotomy currently exists between conventional, i.e., small, fraction sizes of 2–3 Gy (aka hyperfrac-tionation) and the very large fraction sizes of 15–20 Gy (extreme hypofractionation) employed to treat early-stage non-small-cell lung tumors (SBRT or SABR). Does this major difference between 'hyper' and 'extreme hypo' represent

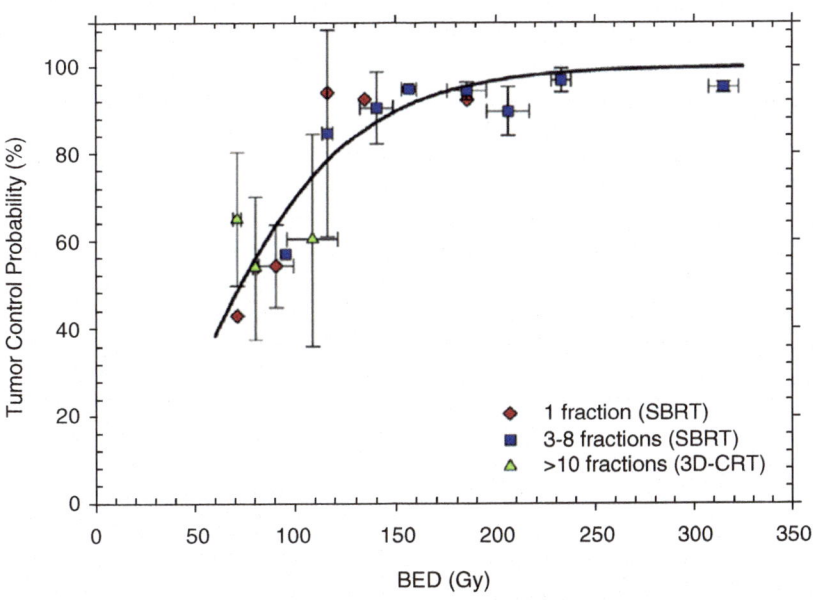

Fig. 5 Tumor control probability (TCP) as a function of biologically effective dose (BED), with $\alpha/\beta = 8.6$ Gy, for stage I non-small-cell lung cancer: mean local control rates (≥ 2 years) from data reported by Mehta et al. (2012), weighted for the different numbers of patients in each study, with symbols distinguishing 3D conformal (3D-CRT) and stereotactic body radiotherapy (SBRT) techniques. The *solid line* shows a linear quadratic based fit to the data, which, according to the authors, given the error bars on the clinical data, demonstrates that single doses, a small number of SBRT fractions, and 3D-CRT radiotherapy produce the same TCP for the same BED. (from Brown J.M., Carlson D.J., Brenner D.J. *Int. J. Radiat. Oncol. Biol. Phys.* 88, 254–262, 2014. ©Elsevier. Reproduced with permission)

optimal radiotherapy? Lung tumors have a wide range of volumes and are located in widely different positions in either lung; this suggests treatment plan-specific *individualization* of fraction number (Nahum 2015). The dose-volume histograms from three NSCLC treatment plans have been analyzed with the *BioSuite* software (Uzan and Nahum 2012). Figure 6 shows, for each case, the variation of TCP with number of fractions under the constraint of a constant NTCP of 11% risk of ≥grade 2 radiation pneumonitis; $\alpha/\beta = 3$ Gy was used in the 'isotoxic' NTCP calculations, as in Fig. 3.

Consider the middle curve of the figure, labelled 'Patient 1'. Several important radiobiological features can be observed. Firstly the steep reduction in TCP as the number of fractions is reduced (for constant normal tissue effect) is the 'classical radiobiology' result (cf. the curve for tumor $\alpha/\beta = 10$ Gy in Fig. 3). The reduction in TCP for fraction numbers greater than around

18–20 is due to clonogen proliferation, which was assumed here to begin after 21 days, i.e., at 15 fractions (5 fractions per week), at which the maximum TCP is obtained. For this particular case the 'standard' prescription of 55 Gy in 20 fractions yielded 30.8% TCP and 8.1% NTCP.

The uppermost curve of Fig. 6, for Patient 2, is very different. In this case, the TCP values are close to 100% over virtually the whole range of fraction numbers. This patient would clearly be a candidate for extreme hypofractionation or SABR (Blomgren et al. 1995; Mehta et al. 2012; Schwarz et al. 2017). Here, significantly higher tumor doses can be delivered for various numbers of fractions before 11% NTCP is reached. This is due to a more favorable dose distribution in the (paired lung—GTV) volume, i.e., the ratio (mean lung dose/tumor dose) is lower, probably due to shorter beam paths through the healthy lung, resulting in a value of $\left(\alpha/\beta\right)^{\mathrm{NT}}_{\mathrm{eff}}$ close to 10 Gy.

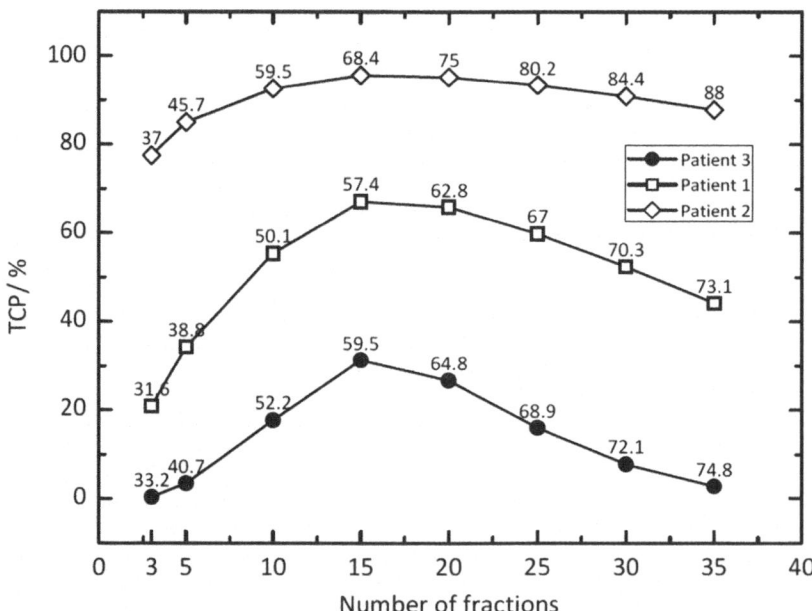

Fig. 6 The variation of tumor control probability (TCP) with the number of fractions (one per weekday) under 11% NTCP (aka isotoxicity) for radiation pneumonitis, for three different non-small-cell lung tumor treatment plans. All results obtained with the *BioSuite* software (Uzan and Nahum 2012). The TCP was computed using the 'Marsden' model (Nahum and Sanchez-Nieto 2001) with parameters $\bar{\alpha} = 0.293$ Gy^{-1}, $\sigma_\alpha = 0.051$ Gy^{-1}, $\alpha/\beta = 10$ Gy, $\rho_{\mathrm{clon}} = 10^7$ cm^{-3}, $T_k = 21$ days, and $T_d = 3.7$ days (Baker et al. 2015); the NTCP was computed using the Lyman–Kutcher–Burman model (Lyman 1985; Kutcher et al. 1991) with parameters TD$_{50} = 29.20$ Gy, $m = 0.45$, $n = 1.0$, and $\alpha/\beta = 3$ Gy (Seppenwoolde et al. 2003). The numbers above each data point are the total doses in Gy achieving NTCP = 11% for that number of fractions

Patient 3 represents the least favorable case (filled circles). TCP peaks fairly sharply at 15 fractions, at close to 30%, with no room for either reducing or increasing the number of fractions. This *BioSuite*-based method of 'isotoxic' treatment-plan analysis strongly suggests that the optimal number of fractions varies from case to case, in contrast to today's rather rigid prescribing policies. The type of computation illustrated in Fig. 6 would be a desirable addition to the capabilities of commercial treatment planning systems (Nahum and Uzan 2012).

8 What Role Might Hypoxia Play?

It has long been established that (α/β) is higher for hypoxic tumor cells (e.g., Williams et al. 1985; Nahum et al. 2003; Chapman and Nahum 2015). Consequently, increasing the fraction size (for a given D_{tot}) will at best only have a small influence on the control of tumors containing significant numbers of *hypoxic clonogens* (any given patient series is likely to contain such a subpopulation). For standard low-dose fraction sizes, hypoxia plays a limited role in tumor response due to the size of the dose fractions and the multiple rounds of reoxygenation

between the treatments. Reducing the number of fractions may compromise this vital process (Carlson et al. 2011). The modelling by Ruggieri and Nahum (2006) and Ruggieri et al. (2010) of the interaction between fraction size and hypoxia showed that reducing the number of fractions, and hence the opportunities for reoxygenation, below around five might compromise tumor control. It is however possible that extreme hypofractionation may *improve* the response of certain hypoxic tumors due to the lack of reoxygenation of *chronically* hypoxic cells, which then die through oxygen starvation. Thus the picture is highly complex.

9 Is a Single Value of α/β for Tumors of a Given Type a Sound Concept for a Patient Population?

Alpha (for asynchronous cell populations) varies across tumor types, as Fig. 1 and Table 1 demonstrate; this population variation explains the relatively shallow TCP vs. dose curves obtained from analyses of clinical outcomes (Bentzen 2002; Nahum and Sanchez-Nieto 2001). In complete contrast, beta (for asynchronous cell populations) varies relatively little across the tumor population

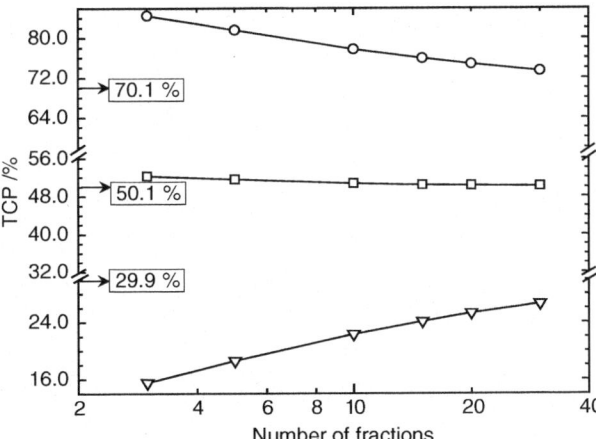

Fig. 7 The effect on tumor control probability of keeping β constant while α varies, with a certain σ_α, for total doses corresponding to tumor iso-effect for *constant* $\alpha/\beta = 10$ Gy as computed from Eq. (6). The computations of TCP with constant β but variable α were made with BioSuite II (Julien Uzan, private communication). The *uppermost curve* corresponds to $\bar{\alpha} = 0.34$ Gy^{-1}, the *middle curve* to $\bar{\alpha} = 0.291$ Gy^{-1}, and the *lowest curve* to $\bar{\alpha} = 0.248$ Gy^{-1}, with $\sigma_\alpha = 0.09$ Gy^{-1} and $\alpha/\beta = 10$ Gy in each case. The TCP values opposite the arrows correspond to assuming a constant α/β.

(Chapman and Nahum 2015 and Table 1). Consequently the (α/β) ratio must vary over a (patient) population of tumors. Radiosensitive (i.e., high α) ones will have a high (α/β) ratio, and radioresistant ones (i.e., low α) will have a low (α/β) ratio. Preliminary indications are that this challenges the whole notion of tumor iso-effect.

Figure 7 shows that the combinations of total dose and fraction size ensuring tumor iso-effectivity (or constant TCP) when the α/β ratio is held constant (at 10 Gy) no longer yield constant TCP when β is held constant, except for the case of TCP $\approx$50%. When TCP $\approx$70% the constant-β TCP *decreases* with increasing numbers of fractions; when TCP $\approx$30% the constant-β TCP *increases* with increasing numbers of fractions.

These results challenge the whole notion of tumor iso-effect and demand further investigation.

10   Concluding Remarks

The principal 'take-home messages' from this review are:

- Despite serious challenges on theoretical-mechanistic grounds, experimental cell survival curves demonstrate the essential correctness of the linear quadratic model of cell killing; LQ remains the bedrock of modelling and predicting clinical responses to changes in fractionation.
- *In vitro* $\bar{\alpha}/\bar{\beta}$ vary between 12.6 (e.g., neuroblastoma) and 4.5 (e.g., glioblastoma) for asynchronous human tumor cell lines (α varies a great deal from cell line to cell line for the same tumor type while β shows very little variation).
- Analyses of radiotherapy outcomes are consistent with relatively low α/β for breast and prostate tumors, supporting the use of larger fraction sizes.
- The Hoffmann–Nahum (α/β)$_{\text{eff}}$ concept takes account of both volume effects *and* the dose distribution in NTs. High values (~8–10 Gy) strongly indicate *hypo*fractionation potential; (α/β)$_{\text{eff}}$ increases with the degree of conformality.
- The large patient-to-patient differences, e.g., for NSCLC plans, in TCP as a function of number of fractions for constant NTCP

(*isotoxicity*) suggest that fraction size could be *individualized* more widely than just the conventional 2–3 Gy vs. the 12–20 Gy of SABR.

- Over a population of tumors of a given type (e.g., lung, prostate), α/β is not constant but will follow the wide variation in α as the population variation in β is small; the established Withers method for deriving alternative tumor iso-effective fractionation regimens may need modification.

11   Summary

Fundamental to understanding and modelling fractionation is the linear quadratic model (LQM) of cell killing. Experimental evidence for LQM is robust despite recent challenges on theoretical grounds at fraction sizes much larger than 2–3 Gy. If α/β is ~3 Gy for 'late' complications but ~10 Gy for tumors, LQM predicts an *increasing* therapeutic ratio as the fraction size *decreases*: hence the typical 2 Gy fraction delivered each weekday. The LQ-based 'Withers' formula is conventionally employed to convert a standard regimen (in terms of total dose and fraction size) to an alternative one that is *iso-effective* for either tumor or normal tissue, by appropriate choice of the α/β ratio. The above can be said to summarize 'classical' radiobiology. Evidence for prostate and breast tumors of α/β ~ 2–4 Gy rather than ~10 Gy suggests that much larger fraction sizes (*hypofractionation*) ought to be clinically effective for these tumors and hypofractionated regimens are currently being tested.

The response of normal tissues is heavily influenced by their *architecture*—'parallel' tissues such as lung respond to *mean* not *maximum* dose (the latter is implicitly assumed by the Withers formula)—hence the clinical success of extremely hypofractionated stereotactic body radiotherapy (SBRT) or stereotactic ablative radiotherapy (SABR) treatments (e.g., 3 × 15–18 Gy) for early-stage lung tumors where small fields lower the mean lung dose. The Hoffmann–Nahum (α/β)$_{\text{eff,NT}}$ concept explicitly accounts for normal tissue (NT) architecture; high (α/β)$_{\text{eff}}$ indicates hypofractionation potential, and the more conformal the treatment plan—e.g., IMRT or proton therapy—the greater is $(\alpha/\beta)_{eff,NT}$. By specifying an acceptable NTCP for the critical normal tissue (aka 'isotoxicity'), the variation of TCP with the number of fractions can be computed pointing to not only to the individualization of prescription dose, but also to *individualization of fraction number*. Finally, a closer look at *in-vitro* α and β values for cell lines of a given tumor type reveals that α varies strongly whereas β is approximately constant. Consequently α/β must vary across a patient population, impacting on *tumor iso-effect* modelling.

Acknowledgements We are very grateful to Dhvanil Karia for providing dose-volume histogram data for the computations of Fig. 6, to Sudhir Kumar for his expertise in creating Figs. 6 and 7, and to Julien Uzan for his help with the BioSuite II software.

References

Algan O, Stobbe CC, Helt AM et al. (1996) Radiation inactivation of human prostate cancer cells: role of apoptosis. Radiat Res 146:267–275

Baker C, Carver A, Nahum A Local control prediction for NSCLC using a common LQ-based TCP model for both SABR and 3D-CRT fractionation. In: Abstract at ESTRO 3rd Forum, Barcelona 24–28 April 2015

Bentzen SM (2002) Dose-response relationships in radiotherapy. In: Steel GG (ed) Basic clinical radiobiology. Arnold, London, pp 94–104

Björk-Eriksson T, West CML, Karlsson et al. (2000) Tumor radiosensitivity (SF2Gy) is a prognostic factor for local control in head and neck cancers. Int J Radiat Oncol Biol Phys 46:13–19

Blomgren H, Lax I, Näslund I et al (1995) Stereotactic high dose fraction radiation therapy of extracranial tumors using an accelerator—clinical experience of the first thirty-one patients. Acta Oncol 34:861–870

Borst GR, Ishikawa M, Nijkamp J et al (2009) Radiation pneumonitis in patients treated for malignant pulmonary lesions with hypofractionated radiation therapy. Radiother Oncol 91:307–313

Brenner DJ, Rainer KS, Peters LJ et al (2012) We forget at our peril the lessons built into the α/β model. Int J Radiat Oncol Biol Phys 82:1312–1314

Brown JM, Carlson DJ, Brenner DJ (2014) The tumor radiobiology of SRS and SBRT: are more than the 5 Rs involved? Int J Radiat Oncol Biol Phys 88:254–262

Carlone M, Wilkins D, Raaphorst P (2005) The modified linear-quadratic model of Guerrero and Li can be derived from a mechanistic basis and exhibits linear-quadratic-linear behaviour. Phys Med Biol 50:L9–L13

Carlson DJ, Keall PJ, Loo BW et al (2011) Hypofractionation results in reduced tumour cell kill compared to conventional fractionation for tumors with regions of hypoxia. Int J Radiat Oncol Biol Phys 79:1188–1195

Chapman JD (2003) Single-hit mechanism of tumour cell killing by radiation. Int J Radiat Biol 79:71 81

Chapman JD (2014) Can the two mechanisms of tumor cell killing by radiation be exploited for therapeutic gain? J Radiat Res 55:2–9. doi:10.1093/jrr/rrt111

Chapman JD, Gillespie CJ (2012) The power of radiation biophysics—let's use it. Int J Radiat Oncol Biol Phys 84:309–311

Chapman JD, Nahum AE (2015) Radiotherapy treatment planning: *linear-quadratic radiobiology*. CRC Press (Taylor & Francis Group), Boca Raton, FL

Coutard H (1929) Die Röntgenbehandlung der epithelialen Krebse der Tonsillengegend. Strahlentherapie 33:249–252

Deacon J, Peckham MJ, Steel GG. (1984) The radioresponsiveness of human tumors and the initial slope of the cell survival curve. Radiother Oncol 2:621–629

Deacon JM, Wilson P, Steel GG (1985) Radiosensitivity of neuroblastoma. Prog Clin Biol Res 175:525–531

De Los SJ, Popple R, Agazaryan N et al (2013) Image guided radiation therapy (IGRT) technologies for radiation therapy localization and delivery. Int J Radiat Oncol Biol Phys 87:33–45

Fiorino C, Cozzarini C, Rancati T et al (2014) Modelling the impact of fractionation on late urinary toxicity after post-prostatectomy radiation therapy. Int J Radiat Oncol Biol Phys 90:1250–1257

Fowler JF (1989) The linear-quadratic formula and progress in fractionated radiotherapy. Br J Radiol 62:679–694

Fowler JF, Tomé WA, Fenwick JD et al (2004) A challenge to traditional radiation oncology. Int J Radiat Oncol Biol Phys 60:1241–1256

Franks KN, Jain P, Snee MP (2015) Stereotactic ablative body radiotherapy for lung cancer. Clin Oncol 27:280–289

Hoffmann AL, Nahum AE (2013) Fractionation in normal tissues: the $(\alpha/\beta)_{eff}$ concept can account for dose heterogeneity and volume effects. Phys Med Biol 58:6897–6914

Jin JY, Kong FM, Chetty IJ et al (2010) Impact of fraction size on lung radiation toxicity: hypofractionation may be beneficial in dose escalation of radiotherapy for lung cancers. Int J Radiat Oncol Biol Phys 76:782–788

Jones B, Dale R (eds) (2007) Radiobiological modelling in radiation oncology. British Institute of Radiology, London

Kirkpatrick JP, Brenner DJ, Orton CG (2009) Point/counterpoint: the linear-quadratic model is inappropriate to model high dose per fraction effects in radiosurgery. Med Phys 36:3381–3384

Kutcher GJ, Burman C, Brewster L et al (1991) Histogram reduction method for calculating complication probabilities for three-dimensional treatment planning evaluations. Int J Radiat Oncol Biol Phys 21:137–146

Källman P, Ågren A, Brahme A (1992) Tumour and normal tissue responses to fractionated non-uniform dose delivery. Int J Radiat Biol Oncol Phys 62:249–262

Lagerwaard FJ, Haasbeek CJ, Smit EF et al (2008) Outcomes of risk-adapted fractionated stereotactic radiotherapy for stage I non-small-cell lung cancer. Int J Radiat Oncol Biol Phys 70:685–692

Lyman JT (1985) Complication probability as assessed from dose–volume histograms. Radiat Res 8:S13–S19

Marks LB, Ten Haken RT, Martel M (eds) (2010a) Quantitative analyses of normal tissue effects in the clinic (QUANTEC). Int J Radiat Oncol Biol Phys 76(Suppl 3):S3–S9

Marks LB, Bentzen SM, Deasy JO et al (2010b) Radiation dose-volume effects in the lung. Int J Radiat Oncol Biol Phys 76(Suppl. 3):S70–S76

Mehta N, King CR, Agazaryan N et al (2012) Stereotactic body radiation therapy and 3-dimensional conformal radiotherapy for stage I non-small cell lung cancer: a pooled analysis of biological equivalent dose and local control. Pract Radiat Oncol 2:288–295

Miralbell R, Roberts SA, Zubizarreta E et al (2012) Dose-fractionation sensitivity of prostate cancer deduced from radiotherapy outcomes of 5,969 patients in seven international institutional datasets: $\alpha/\beta = 1.4$ (0.9–2.2) Gy. Int J Radiat Oncol Biol Phys 82:e17–e24

Myerson RJ (2011) Normal tissue dose conformality measures to guide radiotherapy fractionation decisions. Med Phys 38:1799–1805

Nahum AE (2015) The radiobiology of hypofractionation. Clin Oncol 27:260–269

Nahum A, Kutcher G (2007) Biological evaluation of treatment plans. In: Mayles P, Nahum A, Rosenwald J-C (eds) Handbook of radiotherapy physics—theory and practice. Taylor and Francis, London, pp 731–771

Nahum AE, Sanchez-Nieto B (2001) Tumour control probability modelling: basic principles and applications in treatment planning. Phys Med 17(Suppl. 2):13–23

Nahum AE, Uzan J (2012) (Radio)Biological optimization of external-beam radiotherapy. Computational and mathematical methods in medicine. 2012:Article ID 329214. doi:10.1155/2012/329214

Nahum AE, Movsas B, Horwitz EM et al (2003) Incorporating clinical measurements of hypoxia into tumor local control modeling of prostate cancer: implications for the α/β ratio. Int J Radiat Oncol Biol Phys 57:391–401

Niemierko A (1999) A generalized concept of equivalent uniform dose (EUD). Med Phys 26:1100

Ruggieri R, Nahum AE (2006) The impact of hypofractionation on simultaneous dose-boosting to hypoxic tumor subvolumes. Med Phys 33:4044–4055

Ruggieri R, Naccarato S, Nahum AE (2010) Severe hypofractionation: non-homogeneous tumour dose delivery can counteract tumour hypoxia. Acta Oncol 49:1304–1314

Ruggieri R, Stavrev P, Naccarato S et al (2017) Optimal dose and fraction number in SBRT of lung tumours: a radiobiological analysis. Phys Med. In Press

Schwarz M, Cattaneo GM, Marrazzo L (2017) Geometrical and dosimetrical uncertainties in hypofractionated radiotherapy of the lung: a review. Phys Med 36:126–139

Selvaraj J, Uzan J, Baker C, Nahum A (2013) Loss of local control due to tumour displacement as a function of margin size, dose-response slope and number of fractions. Med Phys 40:041715-1–04171511

Seppenwoolde Y, Lebesque JV, de Jaeger K et al (2003) Comparing different NTCP models that predict the incidence of radiation pneumonitis. Int J Radiat Oncol Biol Phys 55:724–735

Sheu T, Molkentine J, Transtrum MK et al (2013) Use of the LQ model with large fraction sizes results in underestimation of isoeffect doses. Radiother Oncol 109:21–25

Short SC, Mayes C, Woodcock M et al (1999) Low dose hypersensitivity in the T98G human glioblastoma cell line. Int J Radiat Biol 75:847–855

Short SC, Kelly J, Mayes CR et al (2001) Low-dose hypersensitivity after fractionated low-dose irradiation in vitro. Int J Radiat Biol 77:655–664

Song CW, Cho WLC, Yuan J et al (2013) Radiobiology of stereotactic body radiation therapy/stereotactic radiosurgery and the linear-quadratic model. Int J Radiat Oncol Biol Phys 87:18–19

Steel GG (2002a) Cell survival as a determinant of tumour response. In: Steel GG (ed) Basic clinical radiobiology, 3rd edn. Arnold, London, pp 52–63

Steel GG (2002b) The dose rate effect: brachytherapy and targeted radiotherapy. In: Steel GG (ed) Basic clinical radiobiology, 3rd edn. Arnold, London, pp 192–204

Steel GG (2007a) Radiobiology of tumours. In: Mayles P, Nahum AE, Rosenwald J-C (eds) Handbook of radiotherapy physics—theory and practice. Taylor and Francis, London, pp 127–148

Steel GG (2007b) Dose fractionation in radiotherapy. In: Mayles P, Nahum AE, Rosenwald J-C (eds) Handbook of radiotherapy physics—theory and practice. Taylor and Francis, London, pp 163–177

Timmerman RD (2008) An overview of hypofractionation and introduction to this issue of seminars in radiation oncology. Semin Radiat Oncol 18:215–222

Uzan J, Nahum AE (2012) Radiobiologically guided optimization of the prescription dose and fractionation scheme in radiotherapy using BioSuite. Br J Radiol 85:1279–1286

Valdagni R, Italia C, Montanaro P et al (2005) Is the alpha-beta ratio of prostate cancer really low? A prospective non-randomized trial comparing standard and hyperfractionated conformal radiation therapy. Radiother Oncol 75:74–82

Vogelius IS, Westerly DC, Cannon GM et al (2010) Hypofractionation does not increase radiation pneumonitis risk with modern conformal radiation delivery techniques. Acta Oncol 49:1052–1057

Wang JZ, Huang Z, Lo SS et al (2010) A generalized linear-quadratic model for radiosurgery, stereotactic body radiation therapy, and high-dose rate brachytherapy. Sci Transl Med 2:39–48

West DML, Davidson SE, Roberts SA et al. (1993) Intrinsic radiosensitivity and prediction of patient response to radiotherapy of carcinomas of the cervix. Brit J Cancer 68:819–823

Williams MV, Denekamp J, Fowler JF (1985) A review of alpha/beta ratios for experimental tumors: implications for clinical studies of altered fractionation. Int J Radiat Oncol Biol Phys 11:87–96

Withers HR, Thames HD Jr, Peters LJ (1983) A new isoeffect curve for change in dose per fraction. Radiother Oncol 1:187–191

Yarnold J, Bentzen SM, Coles C, Haviland J (2011) Hypofractionated whole-breast radiotherapy for women with early breast cancer: myths and realities. Int J Radiat Oncol Biol Phys 79:1–9

Technological Advance Enabling Alternate Fractionation

Olivier Gayou

Contents

O. Gayou
John D Cronin Cancer Center,
1401 Harrodsburg Rd, Lexington, KY, USA
e-mail: ogayou@lexclin.com

Abstract

Alternate fractionation can only be safely implemented when the target to normal tissue ratio is high. Recent advances in technology, such as improved localization using imaging, with or without fiducial placement, are combined with improved computer algorithms to allow safe delivery of high dose per fraction radiotherapy.

1 Introduction

It is inevitable that, in the process of killing tumor cells, many surrounding normal cells are also damaged. The radiobiological rationale underlying fractionation of radiation therapy is the fact that normal cells can repair sublethal damage faster than tumor cells, and therefore normal tissue has time to somewhat regenerate between fractions. The rate of fractionation is therefore directed primarily by the number of normal cells that are impacted by irradiation. A treatment course in which fewer normal cells are irradiated can benefit from "hypofractionated" treatment in a smaller number of higher dose irradiation sessions. A fractionation schedule around 2 Gy per fraction has historically been used as a clinically established compromise for most diseases as an intermediary optimal dose between tumor cell killing and normal cell regeneration, given the amount of dosimetric and geometrical uncertainties that surround radiation therapy.

Med Radiol Radiat Oncol (2017)
DOI 10.1007/174_2017_29, © Springer International Publishing AG
Published Online: 20 April 2017

To account for these uncertainties, different definitions of the treatment volume are commonly used (ICRU 1999). The gross tumor volume (GTV) is the primary disease that is visible directly on imaging; the clinical target volume (CTV) is an expansion of the GTV based on the physician's clinical intuition and knowledge to account for microscopic disease; the internal target volume (ITV) is an expansion of the CTV to account for internal tumor motion during treatment; the planning target volume (PTV) is an expansion of the ITV or CTV to account for uncertainties in day-to-day patient positioning and tumor localization. The PTV is the area to which the dose is prescribed and in which the treatment planner is confident that all tumor cells will receive the prescribed dose. By definition and design, the PTV also contains a large number of normal cells that will be damaged by receiving high dose.

Technological developments in treatment dose calculation and delivery, and in particular image guidance for tumor localization, have allowed for a significant reduction of these uncertainties for certain types of well-localized tumors, leading to small PTV expansions and smaller irradiated normal tissue volumes. Such a reduction allows for a clinically more efficient fractionation, which forms the basis of Stereotactic Body Radiation Therapy (SBRT).

This chapter presents a review of these technological improvements. It reprises a great deal of information and recommendations formulated by the American Association for Physicists in Medicine Task Group 101 titled "Stereotactic Body Radiation Therapy" (Benedict et al. 2000). This document is a must read for anyone contemplating the implementation of an SBRT program in their clinic. The members of this Task Group are hereby acknowledged and thanked for their contribution.

The general workflow for planning and delivering SBRT follows the same steps as conventional treatments: simulation imaging, planning, image guidance, and treatment delivery. What differentiates SBRT from conventional fractionation is the level of confidence in the accuracy in each of these steps, as well as confidence in the accuracy of the treatment process as a whole. Targets must be well defined, the planned dose to the target must be calculated accurately, the location of the target on the treatment couch must be known precisely throughout the treatment, and the dose must be delivered as intended.

2 Simulation and Contouring

2.1 Setting Up the Basis: CT Imaging

Similarly to for conventional treatments, there are two main reasons for which computed tomography (CT) imaging forms the basis of simulation imaging. First, in the energy range used for typical radiation treatments, Compton scattering is the dominant interaction of photons with tissue, which is mainly dependent on local tissue electron density. Since computed tomography measures X-ray photon attenuation, the image output signal is also essentially proportional to electron density and therefore is an ideal support for accurate dose calculation. Second, as will be developed later in this chapter, most image guidance systems are X-ray based. A planning image giving similar anatomical information is therefore ideal as a reference for the image guidance process.

In CT imaging, a rotating fan beam of low energy photons is directed at the patient, and attenuation of that beam is measured in an array of detectors located on the other side of the patient. In a single rotation, attenuation through multiple angles is mathematically combined to give a two-dimensional map of the attenuation properties of the anatomy inside the patient in a single transverse "slice." As the X-ray/detector system rotates around the patient, the couch moves along the axis of rotation. Multiple axial slices are thus acquired and put together to provide a three-dimensional "spiral" map. The image resolution of a CT image in the transverse direction (inside a given slice) is given by the size of the detectors and is typically on the order of 0.5–1 mm. The resolution in the cranio-caudal direction is given directly by the slice thickness and distance between two slices. In order to accurately identify targets, which are typically small in SBRT treatments, slice thickness of 1–3 mm are used in most cases.

Patient or tumor motion during imaging usually introduces artifacts and is detrimental to image quality. In particular respiratory motion, with amplitude reaching up to 5 cm, can lead to some significant misidentification of the tumor if not properly taken into account, which could potentially result in under-dosing and compromise of tumor control. Respiratory-correlated (RC) CT, also commonly known as four-dimensional (4D) CT, registers breathing motion using a surrogate device. During image acquisition, the couch motion along the scanner axis is slowed down, significantly increasing the number of acquired slices. The time stamps associated with each slice are then correlated with the breathing signal, which is divided in typically eight or ten inhalation and exhalation phases. Sorting the acquired slices into these phases allows reconstructing eight or ten separate CT sets, each corresponding to a breathing phase. The tumor and organs can then be delineated in each phase, and the contours can be combined into an internal target volume (ITV) which takes respiratory motion into account.

2.2 Gathering Additional Information: Multimodality Imaging

As mentioned before, tumors will respond well to SBRT treatment if they are well defined. In some instances, CT alone does not allow for correct identification of a tumor border and other imaging modalities may be necessary. X-ray-based imaging like CT offers great geometric representation of anatomy with differentiation of soft tissue, bony anatomy, and low density tissue such as lung and oral or nasal cavities. However, magnetic resonance imaging (MRI) allows for superior soft tissue differentiation. In MRI imaging, the patient is placed in a high intensity magnetic field, typically

1.5–3 Tesla units (T), which align the spin of hydrogen-rich tissue molecules in the same direction. In the imaging process a brief magnetic signal transverse to the original field is applied, disturbing the spin of the tissue molecules. The magnetic signal emitted by the molecule during relaxation while their spin is realigned is collected. Since different tissues will have different relaxation characteristics based on their compositions, they can be differentiated on the resulting image. These properties are particularly useful for tumor visualization inside the brain, prostate, abdomen, and around the spine.

Positron-emission tomography (PET) allows for visualization of metabolic activity, which is abnormally high for tumors even when the patient is resting. It is based on the uptake of the glucose-analog 5-fluorodeoxyglucose (5-FDG), tagged with positron-emitting fluorine-18 (^{18}F). Approximately 1 h following the 5-FDG injection, the patient is placed in the scanner which consists of a ring of photon detectors. These detect the two 0.511 MeV photons emitted in coincidence and in opposite directions following the recombination of the ^{18}F positron with an electron. Time of flight analysis combined with attenuation correction based on a CT acquired at the same time allows for accurate spatial representation of the site of emission of the positron, i.e., of high metabolic activity. While this technique is widely used for staging and restaging of cancer as well as evaluation of recurrence and response to treatment, it is also routinely used in the planning of radiation therapy as a secondary image to help delineate the target, particularly in head and neck, colorectal, and lung cancer.

Single photon emission computed tomography (SPECT) is a technique similar to PET in the sense that it uses gamma cameras at multiple angles to detect the gamma rays emitted by specific radionuclides. This technique is employed in SBRT treatment of metastatic liver cancer, with ^{99m}Tc-marked sulfur colloid, showing region of functional liver parenchyma. This information is used to direct radiation away from and thus spare healthy liver (Kirichenko et al. 2016).

3   Planning

3.1   Treatment Planning System, Beam Modeling, and Calculation Algorithm

Before any SBRT treatment plan can be calculated, special aspects of the planning system must be considered. Common to most modern techniques and systems, the issue of tissue heterogeneity and calculation algorithm has a particular importance in SBRT planning. As was recognized by the American Association of Physicists in Medicine (AAPM) Task Group 65 (Papanikolaou et al. 2004), any form of tissue heterogeneity correction is usually an improvement over an algorithm that ignores it, especially for tumors located in low density organs, such as the lung. However, simple corrections that ignore lateral electron transport are not appropriate, especially for small field calculations. Therefore calculation algorithms that use precalculated dose spread kernels, such as a superposition/convolution algorithm, algorithms that calculate transport by solving the Boltzmann equation, or Monte-Carlo algorithms should be used.

The second issue that is specific to SBRT is the measurement of small fields for beam modeling. As the field sizes used to treat small targets become smaller, special considerations must be taken into account both in the detector used and the measurement method. First the detector size is of primary importance to avoid volume averaging effects that tend to underestimate output factors and could potentially lead to systematic overdosing by more than 10%. In general the smallest possible detector should be used to measure small field dosimetry, and stereotactic diodes or diamond detectors are instruments of choice. Second, when the field size becomes very small (<2 cm), basic assumptions of standard broad beam geometry are violated. Lateral electron equilibrium is no longer present, and effects specific to linac and detector geometry related to collimator leaf edge and source size become important. The major impact these effects have is that the ratio of dose that defines scatter factors between two different field sizes is no longer equal to the ratio of detector readings. The AAPM Task Group dedicated to small field dosimetry developed a specific formalism introducing a correction factor that is detector and linac specific, and must be calculated by Monte Carlo (Francescon et al. 2011). These factors should be used to correct input data to the beam model.

3.2   Treatment Plan

Three dimensional conformal radiation therapy (3D-CRT), intensity modulated radiation therapy (IMRT), and volumetric modulated arc therapy (VMAT) are all techniques routinely used in SBRT. The emphasis in SBRT planning is the sharp dose gradient just outside the target, which requires creating a dose distribution that is as isotropic around the target as possible. This is usually achievable by using a higher number of beams than in conventional fractionation, with roughly equal weighting. The use of non-coplanar beams or arcs is fairly routine, which requires high confidence in the isocentricity of the treatment couch. A beam energy of 6 MV, which is widely available on most treatment units, offers a good compromise between beam penetration and penumbra characteristics, which is affected by lateral electron transport at high energies. The width of the multileaf collimator (MLC) leaf plays an important role in the conformity of the dose distribution, the smaller leaf being the most desirable, especially for the smallest targets. No MLC with leaves larger than 5 mm should be used for SBRT.

The cost of sharp falloff is high dose heterogeneity inside the target. In order to obtain a high dose gradient, a low isodose line is usually selected for normalization, typically 80%. This naturally results in hot spots on the order of 25%. However it is generally considered that hot spots may be a desirable feature of a plan as long as they are located inside the target, especially if it can help eradicate radioresistant hypoxic regions of the tumor (Fowler et al. 2004).

4 Treatment Delivery Systems

4.1 Dedicated Units

4.1.1 Gammaknife®

There are several dedicated systems that were designed specifically for hypofractionated treatment of small lesions. Historically the very first such dedicated unit is the Leksell Gammaknife® (Elekta AB, Stockholm, Sweden). Over the last half century the Gammaknife® has successfully treated thousands of primary or metastatic brain tumors as well as nonmalignant lesions all over the world. Precision in the brain has been technically achievable early with a stereotactic frame pressure-mounted directly to the patient skull, allowing for exact reproducibility of tumor position with respect to that frame between planning and treatment, with perfect intrafraction immobilization.

During treatment, the patient lies on the treatment couch in the supine position and the stereotactic frame attached to the skull is fixated inside the treatment unit. The treatment head consists of up to 201 ^{60}Co beams located in a hemisphere superior to the patient's head and converging onto the isocenter. The beams can be turned on and off and the beam size can be adjusted through the use of collimators, according to the treatment plan. When one area of the target has been irradiated to its prescribed level, the patient is moved slightly so that a different area of the target is located at isocenter, until the whole target is covered by the prescribed dose ("sphere packing" technique).

4.1.2 Cyberknife®

The Cyberknife® (Accuray, Sunnyvale, CA, USA) was developed as a robotic stereotactic radiosurgery device. It consists of a small X-band 6 MV linac mounted on an industrial robotic arm (Dieterich et al. 2011). Originally mounted with a fixed-size circular collimator, then a dynamically adjustable size collimator (IRIS) and now a 2.5 mm-leaf MLC, the Cyberknife® has evolved from specific device for brain and spinal tumors to a more versatile radiotherapy delivery unit. The robotic arm driven by the computer to follow the treatment plan travels along a definite path from node to node where the motion stops, the linac points toward the target area, and a given number of monitor units is delivered. The six degrees of freedom of motion of the arm allows for treatment to not only be non-coplanar, which helps building isotropic dose distribution with sharp falloff, but also nonisocentric, which allows for coverage of extended and oddly shaped targets.

4.1.3 Vero™

The Vero™ system was developed jointly by Mitsubishi (Mitsubishi Heavy Industry, Tokyo, Japan) and Brainlab (Brainlab AG, Feldkirche, Germany) as a dedicated SBRT device. It consists of a compact 6 MV linear accelerator mounted on an O-ring gantry (Kamino et al. 2006). The beam is able to rotate around the full gantry, which itself can rotate around the patient by ±60°, effectively giving access to a wide range of non-coplanar fields without moving the patient. The beam is shaped by a multileaf collimator (MLC) with variable leaf size, down to 3 mm at the center. The linac and MLC are mounted on the ring gantry using a gimbals-based mechanism, allowing pan-and-tilt motion of the beam. Coupled with a motion tracking system, this mechanism allows for the beam to follow tumor motion and deliver dynamic treatment more efficiently. Although this commercialization in the USA was abandoned by Brainlab, a few centers around the world use the device.

4.1.4 Gammapod™

Similar in concept to the Gammaknife®, the Gammapod™ is a new device under development by XCision LLC (Baltimore, MD, USA) dedicated for breast SBRT (Yu et al. 2013). It consists of 36 ^{60}Co sources converging toward and rotating around an isocenter. The patient is placed in prone position on the treatment couch, which continuously moves according to a path predetermined by the treatment planning system to create uniform and sharp dose distributions. The breast is immobilized using a tightly fit vacuum-assisted cup which remains in place between simulation and treatment. While the topic of breast SBRT is controversial, a consortium of five North American institutions is preparing to run clinical trials investigating the feasibility of surgery-free ablative radiation using the Gammapod™.

4.2 Gantry-Mounted Linac-Based SBRT

The most common way to deliver SBRT in many sites of the body is to use a gantry-mounted linac. The treatment delivery concept is the same as for conventional radiotherapy, with a gantry rotating around the isocenter, a multileaf collimator (MLC) shaping the beam, and a treatment couch able to rotate around the isocenter to achieve non-coplanar coverage. As was mentioned earlier, what differentiates an SBRT-capable linac from a conventional linac is the degree of confidence with which the dose can be delivered to the intended target. The prerequisites are the ability to deliver conformal dose distribution, a stable mechanical and radiation isocenter, and a way to ensure the intended target is located exactly where the dose is delivered. All current linac vendors (Varian, Palo Alto, CA; Elekta AB, Stockholm, Sweden; and Siemens Medical Solutions, Malvern, PA) have treatment machines that are capable of delivering SBRT or SRS plans. It should be noted that while Siemens linacs are still currently used for conventional and SBRT treatments, they are no longer commercialized.

Conformal distributions, especially for small tumors that are usually candidates for SBRT, require small MLC leaves. Elekta machines include the 5 mm-leaf Agility™ MLC. Its very low transmission (<0.3%) allows for better control of the dose outside the target. Siemens' Artiste™ also has an MLC with similar design. Varian's TrueBeam™, and more specifically its stereotactic version the Edge™, comes equipped with a high definition MLC with a leaf size of 2.5 mm around the central axis, for increased conformality of dose to very small targets, including small brain metastases.

Modern SBRT and SRS-capable linacs are installed using a specific stereotactic procedure ensuring the intersection of the three axes of rotation (gantry, collimator, and couch) is contained within a sphere of a 0.5 mm radius. This specification, which is tighter than that of conventional linacs, is reflected in the latest AAPM Task Group report on linac quality assurance, which proposes different tolerance values depending on whether the linac is meant to use modern techniques like IMRT and SRS/SBRT (Klein et al. 2009).

Ensuring that the target is located and remains where the dose is delivered requires the ability to visualize the target or a reliable surrogate immediately prior and possibly throughout the delivery. The topic of image guidance will be developed in detail in the next section. However, it should be added here that in the last few years, both Varian and Elekta have developed robotic couch tops that allow for patient position correction using six degrees of freedom: three translations and three rotations, thereby contributing to the high level of confidence in dose delivery according to intent.

5 Image Guidance Systems (Interfraction Motion)

Accurate image guidance is at the heart of the ability of modern units to deliver radiation with the precision required for stereotactic treatment. In order to be able to deliver a high dose of radiation to the target while sparing the surrounding tissue, treatment margins around the tumor are small and by design, dose gradients are high. Therefore, it is essential that the location of the tumor be known precisely at the time of treatment, to avoid underdosing the target, which would lower the chance of control and cure, or overdosing normal tissue, which would increase toxicity. The accuracy of target localization for SBRT treatment is of the order of 1 mm. Several solutions are offered on modern linacs to offer this type of accuracy.

5.1 2D Systems

There exist two planar image systems available on the market. One is from Accuray and comes with the Cyberknife®. The other one, called ExacTrac®, is available from Brainlab and is designed to be used in conjunction with a linac delivery system. The former system uses two ceiling-mounted X-ray tubes and two floor-mounted imagers, while the latter uses the opposite design. Either system allows for taking a pair of orthogonal X-ray images, which can be registered to digitally reconstructed radiographs (DRR) from the planning CT image. The computer computes the offsets and rotations required to align the two sets of images. The corrections are then applied either by a repositioning of the robotic arm in the case of the Cyberknife® or translation and rotation of the treatment couch in the case of the ExacTrac®. The reliable design of the floor/ceiling mounted systems is ideal for precise and reproducible localization, with sub-millimeter accuracy.

The image quality of early versions of the systems only allowed for visualization of bony structures, which was ideal for central nervous system tumors located in the brain or spine. Other sites required the implantation of high atomic number fiducial markers. Increased detection efficiency of the imager now allows for visualization of high contrast tumors, such as those located in the lung.

5.2 3D Systems

Cone beam computed tomography (CBCT) imaging systems are now commonly installed on most modern linacs. An X-ray/imager system is mounted on the gantry and rotates around the patient. The imager is a flat panel detector and thus acquires large field images. At regular intervals, typically every degree of rotation, an X-ray image is acquired. After completion of the rotation, all the images are filtered, back projected, and combined to reconstruct a volumetric image representative of photon attenuation in tissue inside the patient, similar to the planning CT process. The CBCT and planning CT are then co-registered and offsets and rotational corrections to be applied to the treatment couch are calculated.

Varian and Elekta offer kilo-voltage (kV) CBCT solutions (Jaffray 2005). The X-ray tube/imager system is mounted in the gantry 90° from the treatment beam. This configuration requires a quality control procedure to ensure that the treatment and imaging isocenter coincide within 1 mm or less. The image quality of the kV-CBCT system is not as high as that of conventional fan-beam CT, because of inherent scatter in the large field image. Image post-processing techniques are available and usually necessary to see soft tissue differentiation at the center of the image. Siemens offers a different solution with mega-voltage (MV) CBCT, where the X-ray generator is the treatment head itself (Pouliot et al. 2005), either with the clinical 6 MV beam in the early version or a modified 4.2 MV beam enhancing the low end of the energy spectrum. A MV-optimized amorphous Silicon portal imager detects beam attenuation through the patient. Image quality is lower than kV-CBCT because MV photons are less conducive to high contrast, and imaging dose has to be taken into account carefully. However MV-CBCT usually provides image quality sufficient for localization and is routinely used in SBRT applications.

The main advantage of CBCT over planar systems is the direct visualization of soft tissue, allowing for direct localization of the tumor for virtually all sites, rather than a surrogate or surrounding anatomy. Volumetric imaging also provides a way to monitor anatomical changes and possibly tumor response throughout the course of treatment, but this impact is lower in the typical short courses used in SBRT.

Submillimeter accuracy is difficult to obtain with gantry-mounted systems, because of the number of components subject to motion. The X-ray tube and imager have to be deployed prior to each image acquisition and the whole gantry is in motion during acquisition. Typical localization accuracy for CBCT systems is of the order of 1 mm.

Efforts to develop MRI-based image guidance solutions are underway. One commercially available solution is the MRIdian® system from ViewRay (Oakwood Village, OH), which combines a low field MRI (0.2 T) with a 3-head, MLC-shaped, ^{60}Co beam. Different projects combining high-field MRIs with 6 MV linacs are under development (Lagendijk et al. 2014). MRI is the modality of choice for imaging soft tissue and could eventually represent a gold standard for localization accuracy, using techniques to compensate for geometric distortions inherent to MRI imaging (Crijns et al. 2011).

6 Motion Management During Treatment (Intrafraction Motion)

For the same reasons that it is of vital importance that the patient is set up in the same location and position as at time of simulation, greatest care must be applied to ensure that they remain in that location and position throughout the delivery process. Yet patient and tumor are subject to different types of motion over a period of several minutes. The whole body may shift or move in undetectable yet clinically significant ways, or be subject to a more violent and difficult-to-control event such as a cough. Alternately the patient can remain still on the patient table but the tumor may be subject to internal motion. This internal motion may be periodic and predictable, like respiratory motion, or of a more random nature, such as swallowing or other digestive processes. A lot of these sources of motion do not matter very much in conventional therapy, where treatment margins are larger, and resulting dose deviations represent a small fraction of the total dose. However in accelerated SBRT treatment, it is necessary to minimize or otherwise manage random and periodic motion.

6.1 Minimizing Motion: Patient Immobilization

As was mentioned before, minimizing motion for intracranial SRS using a Gammaknife® or a linac

has historically been achieved using a stereotactic frame physically attached to the patient skull. This was necessary because no reliable way of visualizing the target in treatment position was available. With the development of image guidance techniques described earlier, noninvasive methods of patient setup are sufficient to reproduce the treatment position as it was defined during simulation, such as thermoplastic masks and body bags.

Thermoplastic masks become malleable when placed in a warm water bath and are placed over the head, neck, and shoulders at simulation time to espouse the external contour of the patient. The plastic then hardens upon cooling, and the head, neck, and shoulder positioning is captured and can be reproduced for each treatment session. Vacuum formed bags are typically used for positioning and immobilization of patients treated for thoracic, abdominal, and pelvic tumors. They consist of a polyurethane bag filled with polystyrene beads that form a tight-fit cradle when evacuated through a valve with the aid of an air pump.

In addition to minimizing whole body motion, it is possible to minimize and otherwise control respiratory motion through the use of an abdominal compression plate or a tight plastic sheet wrapped around the patient's body. These devices obviously do not eliminate breathing motion, but they can avoid wide excursions from the predictable baseline.

Overall patient motion can also be minimized simply by delivering more efficient treatment and decreasing the time the patient has to remain in the treatment position. The past few years have seen the development and increased use of flattening filter free beams. Flattening filters have historically been an important component of a linac's treatment head, whose purpose was to ensure the beam profile was "flat" when reaching the patient. They compensate for the forward-peaked photon distribution emerging from the target by preferentially absorbing photons at the center of the beam. Flattening of the beam made it possible to perform dose calculations intuitively and allowed to achieve familiar dose distributions from commonly used beam arrangements. However the advent of computer-based dose calculations, even more in the realm of inverse planning for intensity-modulated radiation therapy, rendered the initial purpose of the flattening filter irrelevant. Since it was a major source of photon absorption, removing the flattening filter allows for a more intense beam to reach the patient with the same amount of accelerator power, and therefore deposit a dose 3–6 times higher than flat beams in the same amount of time, leading to more efficient treatments less prone to intrafraction motion.

Random internal tumor motion, primarily seen in intra-abdominal or intrapelvic treatment, is more difficult to manage, especially in the prostate affected by rectal activity or the pancreas affected by stomach or bowel content. It is advisable to recommend patients to come to treatment with an empty digestive system, several hours after a meal and post bowel movement.

6.2   Managing Motion

Respiratory motion is not avoidable, but it may be predictable and therefore can be managed appropriately. As mentioned earlier, it is not recommended to treat a tumor affected by respiratory motion without a 4D-CT planning image that encompasses the entire motion through the ITV. However it should be recognized that by definition, while the ITV ensures that all tumor cells receive the prescribed lethal dose, a larger volume of normal tissue is contained in the ITV and therefore also receives high dose.

Gated treatment is the most common way to minimize the amount of normal tissue inside the ITV. The principle of gated treatment is to synchronize the beam with an external signal that is indicative of the respiratory phase. Based on that signal, the beam is turned off every time the tumor exits the treatment area, and back on when the tumor enters the treatment area. In this scenario, the ITV does not encompass the entire respiratory motion of the tumor but only a portion of it, typically around the more reliable full exhale phase.

Several devices to produce a respiratory signal are available on the market, both for gated treat-

ment and 4D-CT. The Real time Positioning Management™ (RPM) system from Varian consists of a reflective block placed on the patient's abdomen and whose position is read by an infrared camera mounted in the simulation or treatment room. The Anzai™ system (Anzai Medical, Tokyo, Japan) consists of a belt tightly fit around the patient's abdomen, containing a pressure sensor. The pressure increases during inhalation and decreases during exhalation, therefore indicating respiratory phases. A spirometer can also be used, measuring gas flow through the patient's mouth.

A different approach to decreasing the ITV size and reducing the amount of normal tissue irradiated consists of tracking the tumor, i.e., dynamically moving the beam to follow the predictable path of the tumor along the respiratory track. This is, in theory, a more efficient approach than gated treatment since the beam is on all the time. However it is technically more challenging and most solutions are currently in the development and trial phase. The most mature solution for tumor tracking is the Cyberknife® Synchrony Respiratory System. The patient wears a vest equipped with fiber optic markers whose position is recorded by a ceiling-mounted camera array, hereby capturing external breathing motion in real time. Immediately prior to treatment, a series of orthogonal kV image pairs of the treatment site are acquired and internal tumor motion is correlated with the external vest position. During treatment, the real time vest position is used as a surrogate signal for internal tumor position and the position and direction of the beam is adjusted accordingly using the robotic arm. Note that regular X-ray imaging is used throughout treatment delivery to correct and update the correlation between vest and tumor motion. Similar in principle, tumor tracking in the Vero™ system uses a combination and infrared and fluoroscopic cameras to reconstruct tumor position in real time, relaying the information to the gimbaled treatment head for tracking.

One of the advantages of a possible MR image guidance solution is the ability to capture real time 3D direct images of the anatomy during treatment. It could be envisioned in the future that these images could potentially be used for real time adaptation of the treatment beam, hereby further reducing the treatment margin and increasing the therapeutic ratio.

Conclusion

The field of radiation oncology has seen tremendous technological developments in the last 20 years. Tumor identification and delineation was enhanced through better integration of multimodality imaging, and treatment delivery capabilities focused on sharp dose gradient and delivery efficiency were developed. Most importantly the evolution of motion management from weekly portal imaging to accurate daily imaging with intrafraction monitoring has profoundly impacted the way we consider and apply treatment margins, opening the way for a radiobiological paradigm shift towards hypofractionation, resulting in shorter, more comfortable and more convenient treatment courses with better outcomes.

References

Benedict S, Yenice K, Followill D et al (2000) Stereotactic body radiation therapy: the report of AAPM Task Group 101. Med Phys 37(8):4078–4101

Crijns SPM, Bakker CJG, Seevinck PR et al (2011) Towards inherently distortion-free MR images for image-guided radiotherapy on an MRI accelerator. Phys Med Biol 57(5):1349–1358

Dieterich S, Cavedon C, Chuang C et al (2011) Report of AAPM TG 135: quality assurance for robotic radiosurgery. Med Phys 38(6):2914–2936

Fowler JF, Tome WA, Fenwick JD et al (2004) A challenge to traditional radiation oncology. Int J Radiat Oncol Biol Phys 60:1241–1256

Francescon P, Cora S, Satariano N (2011) Calculation of k (fclin,fmsr)(Qclin,Qmsr) for several small detectors and for two linear accelerators using Monte Carlo simulations. Med Phys 38:6513

International Commission on Radiation Units and Measurements (1999) ICRU report 62: prescribing, recording and reporting photon beam therapy (supplement to ICRU report 50). ICRU, Bethesda, MD, USA

Jaffray D (2005) Emergent technology for 3-dimensional image-guided radiation therapy. Semin Radiat Oncol 15:208–216

Kamino Y, Takayama K, Kokubo M et al (2006) Development of a four-dimensional image-guided radiotherapy system with a gimbaled X-ray head. Int J Radiat Oncol Biol Phys 66(1):271–278

Kirichenko A, Gayou O, Parda D et al (2016) Stereotactic body radiotherapy (SBRT) with or without surgery for primary and metastatic liver tumors. HPB 18(1):88–97

Klein E, Hanley J, Bayouth J et al (2009) Talk Group 142 report: quality assurance of medical accelerators. Med Phys 36(9):4197–4212

Lagendijk JJ, Raaymakers BW, van Vulpen M (2014) The magnetic resonance imaging-linac system. Semin Radiat Oncol 24(3):207–209

Papanikolaou N, Battista J, Boyer C et al (2004) AAPM Report No 85: tissue inhomogeneity corrections for megavoltage photon beams. American Association of Physicists in Medicine, Madison, WI. https://www.aapm.org/pubs/reports/RPT_85.pdf

Pouliot J, Bani-Hashemi A, Chen J et al (2005) Low-dose megavoltage cone-beam CT for radiation therapy. Int J Radiat Oncol Biol Phys 61:552–560

Yu C, Shao X, Zhang K et al (2013) Gammapod—a new device dedicated for stereotactic radiotherapy of breast cancer. Med Phys 40:051703

Workflow and Quality Assurance in Altered Fractionation

Geoffrey S. Ibbott

Contents

1   Introduction

There are significant differences between courses of "altered fractionation" and those using conventional fractionation, and some of these differences can affect the type of quality assurance (QA) performed and the schedule on which it is performed. Altered fractionation has been defined elsewhere in this book and won't be redefined here; suffice it to say that from a quality assurance perspective, changes in fractionation scheme should have no effect on the importance of quality assurance, or on the timeliness.

The term "quality assurance" is not universally defined, and is frequently mingled with the terms "quality control," "quality improvement," and "quality management," all of which have been defined by a number of authors, but which have somewhat overlapping definitions. For this chapter, the term "quality assurance" is being used to describe the actions taken to assure that treatment, simulation, and treatment planning equipment are performing to their specifications and consistent with their commissioning data, and that the instructions for treatment (whether transferred digitally or otherwise) are transmitted accurately. The role of quality assurance is to assure that the prescribed treatment is delivered safely and accurately, regardless of the fractionation scheme used or the time elapsed between the preparation of a written directive (a prescription for treatment) and the actual delivery of treatment.

A quality assurance program has many interacting parts but for this chapter; two components of a physical QA program will be considered: the routine QA of planning, simulation, and treatment equipment, and "patient-specific" QA procedures, intended to evaluate the quality of a specific treatment plan.

G.S. Ibbott, Ph.D.
Department of Radiation Physics, UT MD Anderson Cancer Center, 1400 Pressler St., Unit 1420, Houston, TX 77030, USA
e-mail: gibbott@mdanderson.org

Med Radiol Radiat Oncol (2017)
DOI 10.1007/174_2017_94, © Springer International Publishing AG
Published Online: 27 July 2017

2   Routine QA of Planning, Simulation, and Treatment Equipment

This topic has been addressed extensively elsewhere. Numerous recommendations exist for developing, conducting, and maintaining a program of routine quality assurance tests for radiation therapy equipment. The reader is referred to AAPM guidelines including the reports of its Task Groups 40 and 142 (Kutcher et al. 1994; Klein et al. 2009) as well as more specific recommendations for commissioning specific capabilities such as intensity-modulated radiation therapy (IMRT) that are contained in a report from AAPM Task Group 119 (Ezzell et al. 2009). Advice also appears in IAEA publications (IAEA 2008) and numerous texts (Pawlicki et al. 2016).

A rigorous, systematic, comprehensive equipment QA program is essential for any radiation therapy department, and is the foundation upon which the other recommendations made here are based. Such a program must address the fundamental aspects of operation of the equipment, as well as all components whose performance can affect the spatial or dosimetric accuracy of treatment. One example of such a component is a multileaf collimator (MLC). The performance of an MLC not only affects the spatial accuracy of delivery, but when used for intensity-modulated radiation therapy (IMRT), even small errors in calibration of the MLC can also lead to significant errors in dose delivery (Ling et al. 2008; Liu et al. 2008; Losasso 2008; Bayouth 2008; Nelms et al. 2011). For some IMRT techniques, a calibration error of 1 mm can lead to a dose delivery error of 10% or more (Liu et al. 2008). Consequently, for some treatment techniques, calibration of the MLC can have a large effect on patient dose distribution.

An equipment QA program must include procedures that effectively and efficiently address the requirements of the equipment and the department. While publications such as AAPM reports are excellent guidelines, they should be viewed as recommendations, not as a complete and adequate program for every department and piece of equipment. Instead, a department's QA program should be tailored to the needs of that department. This can be done by conducting a failure modes and effects analysis, as is described in and recommended by the report from AAPM Task Group 100 (Huq et al. 2016). The TG-100 report describes a framework and instructions for analyzing the processes and workflow in a department and determining the most likely and most impactful sources of error or failure. The QA program can then be designed to focus where it can provide the most benefit.

3   Independent Verification of the Treatment Delivery Process

An essential component of a quality assurance program is an independent evaluation of the treatment delivery process. It is important to stress that this verification should be much more than a check of treatment machine dosimetry calibration, although the basic output check is an important part of this evaluation. A good independent evaluation should comprise an end-to-end test of the entire simulation, planning, and delivery process. This can be accomplished by several methods, but the procedures developed by the Imaging and Radiation Oncology Core-Houston (IROC-Houston, formerly known as the Radiological Physics Center, or RPC) serve as an excellent model (Ibbott et al. 2008).

The approach of IROC-H when conducting an independent evaluation is to investigate the result rather than individual steps in the process of treatment delivery. To assist with credentialing for clinical trials, IROC-H has developed a family of anthropomorphic phantoms that are used to evaluate treatment delivery. These phantoms include a stereotactic brain phantom that has been used to evaluate the quality of stereotactic radiosurgery at more than 200 institutions (Balter et al. 1999), a head and neck phantom for IMRT (Molineu et al. 2005), a thorax phantom, and a pelvis phantom (Followill et al. 2007). The head and neck phantom has been irradiated more than 2000 times (Molineu 2017, Personal Communication), in most cases for credentialing purposes, but many times as part of an institution's own QA process (Molineu et al. 2013). The pelvis phantom and thorax phantom have been used to evaluate the ability of institutions to deliver SBRT to pelvic and lung lesions, respectively. Whether a service such as that offered by IROC-H is used, or an institution contracts with another group, such an independent end-to-end test can detect flaws or inconsistencies in a department's procedures that could lead to treatment errors. The time and resources required are a small investment to assure accurate treatment delivery (Ibbott et al. 2006).

4   Patient-Specific Quality Assurance

From the early days of radiation therapy, up through the implementation of 3D conformal therapy, most radiation therapy departments have performed "double-checks" of the treatment settings used to deliver treatments. In those early days, when electronic calculators were used to determine treatment times or monitor unit settings, it was common to repeat the calculation by hand to assure accuracy. Once computerized treatment planning systems became available, electronic calculators were used for redundant calculations of the monitor unit settings, to confirm accuracy. Shortly afterwards, it became common to use a second computer program, often a computerized version of the electronic calculator procedure, to check treatment plans for accuracy (Haslam et al. 2003).

The concept of patient-specific quality assurance emerged when IMRT was developed, and for the first time, it became clear that simple calculation techniques were no longer practical methods for checking the complex modulated, multi-field, inverse-planned treatments that were being generated. Instead, it became necessary to develop measurement-based techniques because confidence in calculation procedures was not sufficient. A variety of measurement-based techniques were conceived and implemented, ranging from simple point-dose measurements in a slab phantom to the use of radiochromic film or detector arrays in anthropomorphic phantoms.

Even after the widespread introduction of measurement-based IMRT QA, a considerable body of evidence emerged demonstrating that the QA procedures used at many institutions were inadequate (Nelms et al. 2011; Molineu et al. 2013; Chung et al. 2008). Data from IROC-H showed that of 1139 phantom irradiations, only 929 (81.6%) met IROC's acceptance criteria of ±7% dose agreement in a structure representing a PTV and 4 mm distance-to-agreement in regions of steep dose gradient (Molineu et al. 2013). Eighty-five percent of points at which the gamma index (Low and Dempsey 2003) was calculated were expected to meet these criteria. Two hundred and ten irradiations did not meet the criteria. Upon failure, some institutions repeated the irradiation and subsequently passed. Those repeat irradiations were included in the IROC analysis, increasing the apparent passing rate. Since the introduction of the head and neck IMRT phantom in 2001, the annual pass rate increased from an initial low of 66% to a high of 93% for a recent complete calendar year. The rate for the most recent year reported was somewhat lower, at 88.5%. Of the irradiations that did not meet the acceptance criteria, the majority (156 of 210) failed solely because the irradiations did not meet the dose criterion of ±7% of the planned dose. Three hundred and ninety-two repeat phantom irradiations were done. Several institutions reirradiated the phantom either because they wanted to improve their irradiation results after a failure, test different treatment planning system (TPS) algorithms, or test different treatment delivery systems. The pass rate for subsequent irradiations was still only 80.9% (Molineu et al. 2013).

Because of the risk, even today, that patient dose delivery can deviate from the treatment plan, a number of organizations and publications recommend measurement-based patient-specific quality assurance prior to the first treatment of any patient who will receive IMRT or volumetric arc therapy (VMAT). The American College of Radiology (ACR) recommends in a practice guideline that measurement-based QA be performed (Hartford et al. 2012). The American Society for Radiation Oncology (ASTRO) has published a guidance document (Ezzell et al.

2003) and also has published a guideline that advises "Before the first treatment or for any change in treatment, perform patient-specific QA to guarantee that data transfer between systems is correct before patient treatment begins." The ASTRO guideline suggests, but does not state, that the QA procedures must be measurement based (Moran et al. 2011). Together with the American Association of Physicists in Medicine (AAPM), ASTRO has published a guide that also strongly suggests measurement-based IMRT (Galvin et al. 2004).

Indeed, whether or not these patient-specific QA procedures should include a measurement of absolute or relative dose is a subject of intense debate (Childress et al. 2015; Siochi et al. 2013). The primary argument for substituting a calculation for a measurement is the time that can be saved this way. Not only does a redundant calculation generally require minimal staff time (regardless of the computer time needed) it avoids taking the treatment equipment to perform a measurement. In some departments, IMRT QA can be performed during gaps between patient treatments. Even when the patient load permits this, there is always the possibility that the schedule could change without notice, or that the QA could take longer than expected, resulting in the likelihood that the QA measurements are rushed, increasing the risk of errors or shortcuts. In busier departments, QA procedures must be performed after hours. This is expensive as it might require the payment of an overtime rate or shift differential. Alternatively, it might require salaried individuals to work extended hours, and this can contribute to stress, burnout, or an increased error rate.

Those who argue in favor of a measurement point out that a physical measurement of the dose distribution is the only way to confirm that the treatment equipment actually performed as intended for a particular treatment plan. Most calculation-based methods rely on "log files" (data collected while the treatment machine executes the treatment plan) (McDonald et al. 2017; Stell et al. 2004; Rangaraj et al. 2013). These log files contain data such as the number of monitor units (MU) delivered between "control points,"

or changes to machine settings such as gantry angle and multileaf collimator position. The log files must assume that the machine settings captured are properly calibrated. Certain important parameters are not captured, however, such as the actual radiation output of the treatment unit. Even if the relationship between monitor units and dose is correct, and the number of MU delivered between control points is correct, there is the possibility for the dose rate to fluctuate between control points in ways that make the delivered dose distribution incorrect. Such changes can only be detected through measurement.

Incorrect dose delivery due to discrepancies such as these can be minimized through a comprehensive QA program that detects errors in the calibration of MLC leaves and radiation output, as well as other parameters that can cause discrepancies between data saved in log files and actual delivery. Dose delivery errors can also be minimized by careful attention to the design of treatment plans, to increase the likelihood that the treatment equipment can reproduce the plan accurately. Discrepancies in dose delivery have been linked to the number of control points for IMRT plans; as the modulation of a plan increases, the number of segments and control points increases, and each dose delivery segment decreases in size (Nelms et al. 2011). Even small uncertainties in dose can accumulate, leading to large errors in the delivery of treatment.

5   When Patient-Specific Measurement-Based IMRT QA Is Not Practical

There are at least two situations in which measurement-based QA is unrealistic. The first occurs when a patient is being planned for a treatment that must be delivered urgently. In many departments, such urgent treatments are by definition simple treatments, and no unusual QA is required (Dennis et al. 2015). In other departments, CT-based simulation and planning have been implemented to allow 3D imaging to be used to define targets and structures of interest volumetrically and to deliver completed and conformal plans involving multiple beams (Driver et al. 2004; Haddad et al. 2006). An investigation of the use of onboard imaging was conducted at the Princess Margaret Hospital to evaluate the adequacy of cone beam CT for planning of 3D conformal palliative treatment of bone metastases (Létourneau et al. 2007; Wong et al. 2012). Similar studies have been conducted elsewhere (Ford et al. 2011). The treatments planned using these techniques were generally still very simple and did not require a QA procedure before delivery.

In yet other departments it was recognized that some patients requiring rapid palliative treatment for bone pain and similar concerns presented with challenging geometric configurations requiring highly conformal delivery. These challenges could be the result of a complex-shaped target volume, an adjacent sensitive structure or previously irradiated volume of tissue, or the desire to escalate beyond conventional doses. For these patients, an effort has been made to develop procedures that allow the preparation of a complex IMRT or VMAT treatment plan and delivery of the plan within a few hours. The rationale is apparent; even for an urgent treatment, or a palliative treatment to relieve symptoms such as pain, patients deserve the highest quality treatment we can provide, and sometimes that requires a plan that involves advanced treatment techniques.

A team at the Ottawa Hospital Cancer Center recognized this need and developed a workflow for developing and delivering image-guided highly conformal treatments over a short time span (Samant et al. 2008, 2009). A brief mention of delivery quality assurance was made, but no specifics were given, and the description of the procedure and workflow suggested that the measurements of dose delivery were made after the treatment was completed.

A team at the University of Virginia has developed a procedure for the use of advanced techniques to treat urgent patients (Jones et al. 2015). Their procedure allows for assessment, simulation, planning, QA, and treatment delivery in a single day, and generally much less. The method relies on assembling a team that is able to prioritize the procedures for these urgent cases, so that treatment planning can be performed and a plan approved within an hour after the simulation procedure is completed. A QA procedure is performed which relies entirely on an independent calculation of the treatment plan; in this case, an in-house-developed Monte Carlo planning system is used (Handsfield et al. 2014). Agreement between the two treatment plans to within a small error is considered confirmation of the original plan. This redundant plan can also be completed within a few minutes so that the patient can receive treatment within as little as 2 h after first being seen in the department.

The second set of conditions that make measurement-based QA impractical is that in which the patient remains on a single treatment table for the simulation, planning, and treatment delivery process. Such a procedure can arise in several different circumstances.

The first is again in the case of urgent treatment, such as required for painful bone metastases. Researchers at the University of Ottawa describe the experiences at a number of facilities, including their own, to improve the access to and rapid delivery of radiation therapy for treatment of painful metastases (Dennis et al. 2015).

A second case is that in which the patient again remains on the treatment table for the entire simulation, planning, and delivery process. But in this case, the purpose is adaptive treatment, rather than urgent radiotherapy. The development of adaptive radiotherapy has taken place over the past several decades, and the benefits have been proven (van de Schoot et al. 2017; Acharya et al. 2016). Modifying the treatment in response to changes in size, shape, or position of the tumor volume, or of nearby normal tissues, has been shown to improve treatment results (de Crevoisier et al. 2005). Many patients experience interfractional changes due to bowel or bladder filling, weight loss or gain, or tumor growth or shrinkage. Such changes can cause movement or distortion of target volumes as well as other organs at risk. Adaptive radiotherapy techniques employ state-of-the-art imaging that can detect such changes and enable reoptimization of the treatment plan.

Such image-guided adaptive radiotherapy can employ cone beam CT or CT-on-rails, for cases in which X-ray imaging can demonstrate the critical changes in anatomy. A recent development has been the marrying of a magnetic resonance (MR) imager with a treatment unit, to enable the superior quality of MR imaging to indicate anatomical and even physiological changes. As of this writing, two MR-guided treatment units are available: the MRIdian system (ViewRay, Oakwood Village, Ohio, USA) and the Unity system from Elekta (Elekta Inc., Stockholm, Sweden). Both devices combine a diagnostic MR imaging system with a treatment unit. Patients undergo conventional CT or MR simulation, and a "reference" treatment plan is created. When the patient returns for daily treatment, a new MR image study is performed, and is registered with the reference image-based treatment plan. The plan is modified (adapted) to the daily images, and the adapted plan is delivered to the patient. This implies that the patient could potentially be treated with a slightly different plan every day of treatment. The benefits of such daily MR-guided treatment appear to be substantial. Lagendijk and others have suggested that the confidence afforded by MR guidance might permit the target dose prescription to be tailored daily, based on the dose received by organs at risk (Lagendijk et al. 2014; van der Heide 2016).

The implications for QA are apparent when daily MR guidance is used in this fashion; the patient cannot be removed from the table between imaging and treatment, so measurement-based QA is not possible. The developers and early clinical users of these systems have implemented calculation-based methods of redundant planning to offer confidence in the daily adapted plan in a very short time, so that treatment is not delayed. The redundant calculation must be based on control point data as an opportunity to retrieve log files isn't available until after daily treatment is completed. Li et al. have described a system for QA of an MR-guided cobalt unit used for daily adaptive treatment (Li et al. 2015), and Bol et al. have described a similar calculation-based QA system for the MR-linac (Bol et al. 2012).

These QA programs include multiple components, as discussed above, including measurement-based systems for evaluating "class solutions" or representative treatment plans, as well as for confirming an initial or a reference plan for individual patients. Measurement in a magnetic field environment requires precautions that have not previously been encountered in radiation therapy physics practices, due to the influence of the magnetic field on secondary electrons resulting from photon interactions in the patient and other materials. Several authors have published on the effects of small air gaps around ionization chambers, such as are unavoidable when water-equivalent plastic phantoms are used (O'Brien et al. 2015; O'Brien and Sawakuchi 2017). At least one commercial QA device has been modified for use in magnetic fields, and has been demonstrated to provide acceptable results (Houweling et al. 2016). Finally, the use of gel dosimetry has been explored in MR-guided radiation therapy equipment (Maryanski et al. 1996; Baldock et al. 2010; Ibbott et al. 1997; Lee et al. 2016; Rankine et al. 2017). One large benefit of using gel dosimetry to evaluate dose distributions from an MR-Linac is that the gel is not affected by the magnetic field, but accurately reports the influence of the magnetic field on the dose distribution (Lee et al. 2016). The MR imager component of the device can be used to evaluate the dosimeter, which avoids having to move the dosimeter to another imaging system for readout (Roed et al. 2016).

For QA of daily adapted plans, both Li and Bol describe the use of a Monte Carlo-based calculation that uses, as input, the plan parameters and control point data from the original treatment plan (Li et al. 2015; Bol et al. 2012). This enables a rapid validation of the plan, while the patient is on the table and before the treatment is delivered. Rapid Monte Carlo codes exist that can provide calculations with sufficient spatial resolution and adequate accuracy for a comparison with the original treatment plan to be made in 1 or 2 min (Handsfield et al. 2014; Bol et al. 2012).

6 Summary

A QA program that provides sufficient confidence that treatment delivery will faithfully reproduce the approved treatment plan must consist of a number of components. These must include the recommended routine equipment QA called for by a number of existing publications (Kutcher et al. 1994; Klein et al. 2009; Huq et al. 2016) as well as patient-specific QA procedures that are tailored to the treatment technique to be used. It is therefore recommended that measurement-based QA be used when practical, and at a minimum to evaluate representative treatment plans. In situations in which measurements are not practical, the calculation of a redundant plan is an acceptable method to assure the veracity of the original. Such situations can occur when treatment must be delivered immediately after development of the plan, or when staff resources do not permit a measurement.

References

Acharya S, Fischer-Valuck BW, Kashani R et al (2016) Online magnetic resonance image guided adaptive radiation therapy: first clinical applications. Int J Radiat Oncol Biol Phys 94:394–403

Baldock C, De Deene Y, Doran S et al (2010) Polymer gel dosimetry. Phys Med Biol 55:R1–R63

Balter P, Stovall M, Hanson WF (1999) An anthropomorphic head phantom for remote monitoring of stereotactic radiosurgery at multiple institutions. Med Phys 26:1164

Bayouth JE (2008) Siemens multileaf collimator characterization and quality assurance approaches for intensity-modulated radiotherapy. Int J Radiat Oncol Biol Phys 71:S93–S97

Bol GH, Hissoiny S, Lagendijk JJ et al (2012) Fast online Monte Carlo-based IMRT planning for the MRI linear accelerator. Phys Med Biol 57:1375–1385

Childress N, Chen Q, Rong Y (2015) Parallel/opposed: IMRT QA using treatment log files is superior to conventional measurement-based method. J Appl Clin Med Phys 16:5385

Chung HT, Lee B, Park E et al (2008) Can all centers plan intensity-modulated radiotherapy (IMRT) effectively? An external audit of dosimetric comparisons between three-dimensional conformal radiotherapy and IMRT for adjuvant chemoradiation for gastric cancer. Int J Radiat Oncol Biol Phys 71:1167–1174

de Crevoisier R, Tucker SL, Dong L et al (2005) Increased risk of biochemical and local failure in patients with distended rectum on the planning CT for prostate cancer radiotherapy. Int J Radiat Oncol Biol Phys 62:965–973

Dennis K, Linden K, Balboni T et al (2015) Rapid access palliative radiation therapy programs: an efficient model of care. Future Oncol 11(17):2417–2426

Driver DM, Drzymala M, Dobbs HJ et al (2004) Virtual simulation in palliative lung radiotherapy. Clin Oncol 16(7):461–466

Ezzell GA, Galvin JM, Low D et al (2003) Guidance document on delivery, treatment planning, and clinical implementation of IMRT: report of the IMRT Subcommittee of the AAPM Radiation Therapy Committee. Med Phys 30:2089–2115

Ezzell GA, Burmeister JW, Dogan N et al (2009) IMRT commissioning: multiple institution planning and dosimetry comparisons, a report from AAPM Task Group 119. Med Phys 36(11):5359–5373

Followill D, Evans DR, Cherry C et al (2007) Design, development, and implementation of the Radiological Physics Center's pelvis and thorax anthropomorphic quality assurance phantoms. Med Phys 34:2070–2076

Ford A, Bydder S, Ebert MA (2011) The use of On-Board Imaging to plan and deliver palliative radiotherapy in a single cohesive patient appointment. J Med Imaging Radiat Oncol 55(6):633–638

Galvin JM, Ezzell G, Eisbrauch A et al (2004) Implementing IMRT in clinical practice: a joint document of the American Society for Therapeutic Radiology and Oncology and the American Association of Physicists in Medicine. Int J Radiat Oncol Biol Phys 58:1616–1634

Haddad P, Cheung F, Pond G et al (2006) Computerized tomographic simulation compared with clinical mark-up in palliative radiotherapy: a prospective study. Radiat Oncol Biol Phys 65(3):824–829

Handsfield LL, Jones R, Wilson DD et al (2014) Phantomless patient-specific TomoTherapy QA via delivery performance monitoring and a secondary Monte Carlo dose calculation. Med Phys 41:101703

Hartford AC, Galvin JM, Beyer DC, et al; American College of Radiology; American Society for Radiation Oncology. (2012) American College of Radiology (ACR) and American Society for Radiation Oncology (ASTRO) practice guideline for intensity-modulated radiation therapy (IMRT). Am J Clin Oncol 35:612–617

Haslam JJ, Bonta DV, Lujan AE et al (2003) Comparison of dose calculated by an intensity modulated radiotherapy treatment planning system and an independent monitor unit verification program. J Appl Clin Med Phys 4:224–230

U.A. van der Heide (2016) MR-guided radiation therapy. Phys Med Eur J Med Phys 32:175.

Houweling AC, de Vries JH, Wolthaus J et al (2016) Performance of a cylindrical diode array for use in a 1.5 T MR-linac. Phys Med Biol 61:N80–N89

Huq MS, Fraass BA, Dunscombe PB et al (2016) The report of Task Group 100 of the AAPM: application of risk analysis methods to radiation therapy quality management. Med Phys 43:4209

IAEA (2008) Setting up a radiotherapy programme. International Atomic Energy Agency, Vienna

Ibbott GS, Maryanski MJ, Eastman P et al (1997) Three-dimensional visualization and measurement of conformal dose distributions using magnetic resonance imaging of BANG polymer gel dosimeters. Int J Radiat Oncol Biol Phys 38:1097–1103

Ibbott GS, Molineu A, Followill DS (2006) Independent evaluations of IMRT through the use of an anthropomorphic phantom. Technol Cancer Res Treat 5:481–487

Ibbott GS, Followill DS, Molineu HA et al (2008) Challenges in credentialing institutions and participants in advanced technology multi-institutional clinical trials. Int J Radiat Oncol Biol Phys 71:S71–S75

Jones RT, Handsfield L, Read PW, Wilson DD et al (2015) Safety and feasibility of STAT RAD: improvement of a novel rapid tomotherapy-based radiation therapy workflow by failure mode and effects analysis. Pract Radiat Oncol 5:106–112

Klein EE, Hanley J, Bayouth J, Yin FF et al (2009) Task Group 142 report: quality assurance of medical accelerators. Med Phys 36:4197–4212

Kutcher GJ, Coia L, Gillin M et al (1994) Comprehensive QA for radiation oncology: report of AAPM Radiation Therapy Committee Task Group 40. Med Phys 21:581–618

Lagendijk JJ, Raaymakers BW, Van den Berg CA et al (2014) MR guidance in radiotherapy. Phys Med Biol 59:R349–R369

Lee HJ, Alqathami M, Kadbi M et al (2016) Novel iron-based radiation reporting systems as 4D dosimeters for MR-guided radiation therapy. Med Phys 43:3874

Létourneau D, Wong R, Moseley D et al (2007) Online planning and delivery technique for radiotherapy of spinal metastases using cone-beam CT: image quality and system performance. Int J Radiat Oncol Biol Phys 67(4):1229–1237

Li HH, Rodriguez VL, Green OL et al (2015) Patient-specific quality assurance for the delivery of (60)Co intensity modulated radiation therapy subject to a 0.35-T lateral magnetic field. Int J Radiat Oncol Biol Phys 91:65–72

Ling CC, Zhang P, Archambault Y et al (2008) Commissioning and quality assurance of RapidArc radiotherapy delivery system. Int J Radiat Oncol Biol Phys 72:575–581

Liu C, Simon TA, Fox C et al (2008) Multileaf collimator characteristics and reliability requirements for IMRT Elekta system. Int J Radiat Oncol Biol Phys 71:S89–S92

Losasso T (2008) IMRT delivery performance with a varian multileaf collimator. Int J Radiat Oncol Biol Phys 71:S85–S88

Low DA, Dempsey JF (2003) Evaluation of the gamma dose distribution comparison method. Med Phys 30:2455–2464

Maryanski MJ, Ibbott GS, Eastman P et al (1996) Radiation therapy dosimetry using magnetic resonance imaging of polymer gels. Med Phys 23:699–705

McDonald DG, Jacqmin DJ, Mart CJ et al (2017) Validation of a modern second-check dosimetry system using a novel verification phantom. J Appl Clin Med Phys 18:170–177

Molineu A, Followill DS, Balter PA et al (2005) Design and implementation of an anthropomorphic quality assurance phantom for intensity-modulated radiation therapy for the Radiation Therapy Oncology Group. Int J Radiat Oncol Biol Phys 63:577–583

Molineu A, Hernandez N, Nguyen T et al (2013) Credentialing results from IMRT irradiations of an anthropomorphic head and neck phantom. Med Phys 40:022101

Moran JM, Dempsey M, Eisbruch A, Fraass BA et al (2011) Safety considerations for IMRT: executive summary. Pract Radiat Oncol 1:190–195

Nelms BE, Zhen H, Tome WA (2011) Per-beam, planar IMRT QA passing rates do not predict clinically relevant patient dose errors. Med Phys 38:1037–1044

O'Brien DJ, Sawakuchi G (2017) Monte Carlo study of the chamber-phantom air gap effect in a magnetic field. Med Phys 44:3830–3838

O'Brien DJ, Hackett SL, van Asselen B et al (2015) Small air-gaps affect the response of ionization chambers in the presence of a 1.5 T magnetic field. Med Phys 42:3724–3724

Pawlicki T, Scanderbeg DJ, Starkschall G (2016) Hendee's radiation therapy physics, 4th edn. Wiley, New York

Rangaraj D, Zhu M, Yang D et al (2013) Catching errors with patient-specific pretreatment machine log file analysis. Pract Radiat Oncol 3:80–90

Rankine LJ, Mein S, Cai B et al (2017) Three-dimensional dosimetric validation of a magnetic resonance guided intensity modulated radiation therapy system. Int J Radiat Oncol Biol Phys 97(5):1095–1104

Roed Y, Kadbi M, Wang J et al (2016) Real-time imaging of 3-dimensional dose distributions with polymer gels using a magnetic resonance-guided linear accelerator. Radiat Oncol Biol 96(2):E633

Samant R, Gerig L, Montgomery L et al (2008) High-technology palliative radiotherapy using image-guided intensity-modulated radiotherapy. Clin Oncol 20(9):718–720

Samant R, Gerig L, Montgomery L et al (2009) The emerging role of IG-IMRT for palliative radiotherapy: a single-institution experience. Curr Oncol 16(3):40–45

van de Schoot A, de Boer P, Visser J et al (2017) Dosimetric advantages of a clinical daily adaptive plan selection strategy compared with a non-adaptive strategy in cervical cancer radiation therapy. Acta Oncol 56:667–674

Siochi RA, Molineu A, Orton CG (2013) Point/counterpoint: patient-specific QA for IMRT should be performed using software rather than hardware methods. Med Phys 40:070601

Stell AM, Li JG, Zeidan OA et al (2004) An extensive log-file analysis of step-and-shoot intensity modulated radiation therapy segment delivery errors. Med Phys 31:1593–1602

Wong RKS, Létourneau D, Varma A et al (2012) A one-step cone-beam CT-enabled planning-to-treatment model for palliative radiotherapy-from development to implementation. Int J Radiat Oncol Biol Phys 84(3):834–840

The Future of Altered Fractionation

Brian J. Gebhardt, Zachary D. Horne,
and Sushil Beriwal

Contents

Abstract

Radiotherapy remains at the core of treatment for a number of disease sites, especially breast, prostate, and lung cancers, the three most commonly diagnosed cancers in 2015 (Siegel et al. 2016). Radiotherapy (RT) has typically been delivered in multifraction regimens dating back to radiobiology experiments in the 1920s and 1930s which demonstrated that dividing the radiation dose into multiple treatments provides a balance between tumor control and normal tissue toxicity. Subsequent experimentation demonstrated that 1.8–2.0 Gy fractions of radiation delivered daily five times per week allows for repair of sublethal damage within normal tissues thereby reducing radiation toxicity while maximizing cell kill in most tumor types due to reassortment within radiosensitive phases of the cell cycle and reoxygenation of tissues (Hall and Giaccia 2012).

1   Introduction

Radiotherapy remains at the core of treatment for a number of disease sites, especially breast, prostate, and lung cancers, the three most commonly diagnosed cancers in 2015 (Siegel et al. 2016). Radiotherapy (RT) has typically been delivered in multifraction regimens dating back to radiobiology experiments in the 1920s and 1930s which demonstrated that dividing the radiation dose

B.J. Gebhardt, M.D. • Z.D. Horne, M.D.
S. Beriwal, M.D. (✉)
University of Pittsburgh Cancer Institute, Department
of Radiation Oncology, Pittsburgh, PA, USA
e-mail: beriwals@upmc.edu

Med Radiol Radiat Oncol (2017)
DOI 10.1007/174_2017_30, © Springer International Publishing AG
Published Online: 26 April 2017

into multiple treatments provides a balance between tumor control and normal tissue toxicity. Subsequent experimentation demonstrated that 1.8–2.0 Gy fractions of radiation delivered daily five times per week allows for repair of sublethal damage within normal tissues thereby reducing radiation toxicity while maximizing cell kill in most tumor types due to reassortment within radiosensitive phases of the cell cycle and reoxygenation of tissues (Hall and Giaccia 2012).

Various alternate fractionation schedules have been devised to increase the efficacy of radiation against particularly aggressive tumor types. Hyperfractionation is a method of altered fractionation in which smaller fractions of radiation are given twice daily to a higher absolute dose. This scheme is designed to increase the total dose to tumor cells while reducing late toxicity to normal tissues that are less sensitive to smaller fraction sizes. The Radiation Therapy Oncology Group (RTOG) 9003 trial compared several altered fractionation models and demonstrated that hyperfractionation can increase locoregional control at the cost of increased acute toxicity (Beitler et al. 2014).

Accelerated fractionation is a second alternate fractionation strategy that seeks to overcome tumor repopulation by delivering the same total dose of radiation over a shortened time period. Delivering radiation treatments six times per week has been shown to improve locoregional control of head and neck tumors while increasing acute but not late toxicity (Overgaard et al. 2003). Though associated with improved locoregional control of head and neck tumors, both fractionation schedules have been decreasingly utilized due to the growing use of concurrent chemotherapy regimens and a demonstrated lack of benefit when combining the two strategies (Adelstein et al. 2003; Bonner et al. 2010; Nguyen-Tan et al. 2014). Accelerated radiotherapy alone, however, is again being investigated as a method of treatment de-escalation for p16 positive oropharyngeal cancers compared with concurrent chemoradiotherapy (NRG Oncology 2000).

Conventional fractionation provides a balance between efficacy and toxicity in many tumor types. These regimens, however, are associated with protracted radiation courses of 6–9 weeks that are both inconvenient to patients and costly to the healthcare system. With an increasing population and improving survivorship, cancer care costs are estimated to rise between 27% and 39% between 2010 and 2020 (Mariotto et al. 2011). The financial burden of cancer care has an impact not only at a national level but also on a personal level in terms of quality of life. Rising costs coupled with bundled payments and accountable care organizations (ACOs) in the United States, as well as increasing evidence that shorter courses of radiotherapy are equally efficacious and sometimes superior in terms of disease control, have resulted in hypofractionated radiotherapy being investigated for a number of disease sites.

External beam radiotherapy (EBRT) has historically been delivered using 2-dimensional (2-D) treatment planning techniques with 2- to 4-field beam arrangements. As a result, a large volume of normal tissue receives the prescription radiation dose in addition to the target. Concerns for normal tissue toxicity have thus limited the ability to escalate the dose per fraction and total radiation dose, which could potentially enhance tumor control. One strategy to reduce treatment toxicity while escalating the dose to the tumor has been brachytherapy. This technique is characterized by intracavitary, intraluminal, or interstitial implantation of a radioactive source with low energy and rapid dose fall-off minimizing the dose to surrounding normal tissue.

Computed tomography (CT) based radiation planning techniques have been devised that utilize 3-dimensional (3-D) anatomic information as opposed to relying on traditional bony landmarks from 2-D imaging. These techniques allow the generation of complex dose distributions that conform to the planning target volume (PTV) while limiting the dose to surrounding critical structures. The development of intensity-modulated radiotherapy (IMRT) is a more sophisticated extension of 3-D planning techniques. The term IMRT refers to a method of inverse 3-D planning using computer algorithms to optimize the dose to the PTV while minimizing dose to critical structures. The integration of image guidance with orthogonal kilo-voltage and cone beam CT imaging with modern linear accelerators is another significant development in EBRT. Image guidance can decrease daily setup uncertainty and allow for further reductions in PTV margins and resultant exposure to normal tissue. This combination of technologies has enabled target dose escalation beyond what could be achieved with traditional planning methods while maintaining or potentially reducing treatment toxicity. CT-based planning and image guidance technologies have also been adapted to high-dose rate brachytherapy and have been shown to improve local control of cervical cancer, for example, while allowing reductions in the rectal dose and ultimately decreases in late toxicity (Potter et al. 2011).

Modern planning methods have thus obviated many of the concerns with hypofractionated RT that utilize fraction sizes greater than 2.0 Gy. For example, a concern with hypofractionated prostate cancer regimens has been late toxicity to the adjacent rectum. Use of IMRT has been shown to significantly reduce the volume of rectum receiving 45 Gy and has been associated with reduced late rectal toxicity (Ashman et al. 2005; Zelefsky et al. 2002). Recently, published randomized evidence suggests that shorter courses utilizing 2.5–3.0 Gy fractions are associated with similar levels of late toxicity and equivalent rates of tumor control (Lee et al. 2016; Dearnaley et al. 2016). Similar concerns have existed with hypofractionated whole-breast irradiation (WBI) and long-term cosmetic outcomes. The use of 3-D field-in-field and IMRT techniques has improved dose homogeneity of WBI compared with 2-D planning using wedges as compensators. Randomized evidence has shown equivalent or improved acute toxicity and late cosmetic outcomes with hypofractionated WBI (Bentzen et al. 2008; Whelan et al. 2010). This evidence has caused reexamination of radiobiological models that assume high alpha-beta ratios for prostate and breast cancer. These slowly proliferating tumors may have alpha-beta ratios that are similar to that of surrounding normal tissue, and thus hypofractionated treatment in conjunction with modern planning techniques may result in a higher therapeutic index from RT (Ray et al. 2015).

Stereotactic radiosurgery (SRS) is an advanced form of inverse planning that is characterized by highly conformal radiation fields and high doses per fraction. SRS is delivered over a course of 1–5 fractions and can be considered an extreme form of hypofractionated radiation. SRS was first developed for treatment of lesions within the brain and has been associated with improved local control of brain metastases (Andrews et al. 2004). Radiosurgical techniques have been adapted to extracranial sites including the lung, liver, spine, prostate, and pancreas. Improved local control has been demonstrated with lung radiosurgery to a dose of 54 Gy in three fractions in comparison to historical data with CF radiation, which is likely related to the relatively high biologically equivalent dose delivered to the tumor (Timmerman et al. 2014). Overall, hypofractionated RT regimens are associated with shorter treatment courses, increased patient convenience, and reduced healthcare expenditures in comparison with conventionally fractionated schedules. This is a significant area of ongoing clinical research in many disease sites including breast, prostate, lung, and high-grade glioma. A more detailed discussion of the future of altered fractionation and ongoing protocols investigating these disease sites will comprise the remainder of the present chapter.

2 Breast Cancer

As the most commonly diagnosed cancer among women in 2015 (Siegel et al. 2016b), breast cancer has been the subject of an increasing amount of research with regard to shortening radiotherapy treatment courses. The first randomized evidence emerged from France in the 1990s, comparing a course of conventional whole breast external beam radiotherapy—45 Gy in 25 fractions—to 23 Gy in 4 fractions (5.75 Gy/fraction) over 2 weeks in patients with varied stages of disease. The trial shows equivalent outcomes in terms of locoregional control and complication rates; however fibrosis rates were doubled in the hypofractionation arm, at 18% versus 9% for conventional fractionation (Baillet et al. 1990). Because of late effects, conventional fractionation remained the standard of care.

The Royal Marsden group initiated a trial in 1986 comparing two hypofractionated regimens against conventional fractionation, using 3.0 and 3.3 Gy fractions to total doses of 39 and 42.9 Gy, respectively. Important findings from this trial included a lack of significant difference in ipsilateral breast tumor recurrence between the two experimental arms and conventional fractionation (Owen et al. 2006). What was also uncovered with prolonged follow-up was that regular breast tissue likely has an α/β ratio of approximately 4.0 Gy for late cosmetic changes and an α/β ratio of 3.1 Gy for palpable induration (Owen et al. 2006; Yarnold et al. 2005). These results suggested that doses of higher than 2.0 Gy/fraction could be utilized with little impact on breast cosmesis compared to conventional fractionation. This trial was terminated early in favor of accruing to the START A/B trials which evaluated three hypofractionation schedules administered over the same time course as conventionally fractionated therapy: START A (41.6 Gy/13 fractions or 39 Gy/13 fractions) or START B (40 Gy/15 fractions). The results of these trials demonstrated excellent disease outcomes, improved late effects with the 39 Gy (hazard ratio 0.63) and 40 Gy (hazard ratio 0.76) regimens and equivalence of the 41.6 Gy regimen against conventional fractionation (START Trialists' Group et al. 2008a, b; Hopwood et al. 2010).

Most recently, the Canadian hypofractionation trial randomized women with T1-2N0 invasive breast cancer to a course of 50 Gy/25 fractions versus 42.56 Gy/16 fractions and again found equivalent disease outcomes and no differences in late effects from radiotherapy; ultimately concluding that a course of hypofractionated whole breast radiotherapy is not inferior to conventionally fractionated RT (Whelan et al. 2010, 2002).

The results of these trials has led to the adoption of hypofractionated radiotherapy as the preferred standard for women over 50 with T1-2N0 disease in the United States according to the NCCN (Gradishar et al. 2016) and supported by the ASTRO consensus statement (Smith et al. 2011). Despite these recommendations, utilization in the United States has increased slowly, from 5.4% in 2004 to only 22.8% in 2011 (Wang et al. 2014) compared to over 70% in Canada (Ashworth et al. 2013) possibly in part to results from the UK RAPID trial, which compared accelerated partial breast irradiation to 38.5 Gy in ten fractions BID with either conventionally fractionated or hypofractionated whole breast RT. The trial showed increased toxicity and worse fibrosis when compared to the other two schedules (Peterson et al. 2015; Olivotto et al.

2013). Despite reluctance to adopt hypofractionation more widely, some institutions have successfully implemented clinical pathways which help guide physician decision making with evidence summaries and decision trees, and have been found to increase utilization greatly (Rajagopalan et al. 2011; Chapman et al. 2015).

There are a number of ongoing clinical trials evaluating the role of hypofractionated regional nodal irradiation (RNI) and different dose fractionation schedules which would even further decrease the burden of adjuvant radiotherapy for women undergoing breast-conserving surgery with the potential to maintain excellent long-term cosmesis. In the United Kingdom, the Medical Research Council (MRC) FAST trial is comparing conventionally fractionated 50 Gy in 25 fractions to ultra-short courses of 28.5 or 30 Gy in 5 once-weekly fractions for women with completely resected, node-negative invasive tumors. At 3 year median follow-up, there was noted to be a significant increase in physician-scored moderate/marked fibrotic effect noted in photographic cosmetic assessments with the 30 Gy regimen compared to standard fractionation, but no difference with the 28.5 Gy regimen (FAST Trialists Group HD et al. 2011). An assessment of tumor control rates has not been published. A similar phase II study is being conducted by the University of Louisville for patients who meet criteria for financial hardship in an attempt to reduce the cost burden of adjuvant radiotherapy (James Graham Brown Cancer Center U of L 2011). They are enrolling women with DCIS and invasive stage I–II breast cancers who have undergone breast-conserving surgery with negative axillary nodes and administering radiotherapy once per week at 6 Gy per fraction over a 5-week period. The primary endpoint is ipsilateral breast tumor recurrence with cosmesis, toxicities, and survival as secondary endpoints.

To evaluate the role that treatment time course has on hypofractionated whole breast radiotherapy, the United Kingdom also conducted the FAST-Forward trial, which is accrued 4100 women in a trial of a hypofractionation consisting of 40 Gy in 15 fractions compared with two time-condensed courses of 27 or 26 Gy in 5 fractions over 1 week (5.4 and 5.2 Gy/fraction, respectively). They recently reported on toxicity in patients who did not require tumor bed boost and found that acute grade 2 toxicity rates were 50% for conventional hypofractionation, with 27% and 36% for the two condensed schedules (Brunt et al. 2016). Tumor recurrence outcomes are awaited.

Utilizing a different planning tactic, the MRC has also completed accrual to two separate trials which investigate differential dosing to the breast and tumor bed for patients with low- and high-risk tumors, the IMPORT LOW and HIGH trials, respectively (Institute of Cancer Research UK 2008, 2009). IMPORT LOW is evaluating women with low risk, completely excised breast cancer defined as: tumor size smaller than 3.0 cm without LVSI, negative axillary lymph nodes or isolated tumor cells up to 0.2 mm and a minimum margin of 2 mm. They are being randomized to hypofractionated whole breast RT (40 Gy/15 fractions) versus two experimental arms: (1) Reduced-dose whole breast RT (36 Gy/15 fractions) with standard dosing (40 Gy/15 fractions) via simultaneously integrated boost technique to the tumor bed and (2) Partial breast RT (40 Gy/15 fractions). The endpoints of this trial are ipsilateral breast tumor recurrence rates and cosmesis (Institute of Cancer Research UK 2008). IMPORT HIGH is examining women with T1-3 N0-1 disease at higher risk of recurrence who due to at least one of the following risk factors: Age <50, tumor >2.0 cm, any residual tumor after neoadjuvant chemotherapy, grade III disease, margins <5 mm, LVSI, or positive axillary lymph nodes. These patients are being randomized to: (1) Whole breast RT with a sequential tumor bed boost (56 Gy in 23 fractions; 2.43 Gy/fraction), (2) Whole breast RT with a concurrent boost (48 Gy/15 fractions; 3.2 Gy/fraction), and (3) Whole breast RT with a concurrent boost (53 Gy/15 fractions; 3.53 Gy/fraction) (Institute of Cancer Research UK 2009). The primary endpoint of IMPORT HIGH is the development of palpable induration within the boost volume, with secondary endpoints including IBTR, other late changes, and survival.

Similarly, the NRG/RTOG 1005 trial is evaluating women with stage 0–II breast cancer with or without neoadjuvant chemotherapy and breast-conserving surgery and the role of a simultaneously integrated boost to the lumpectomy cavity. The study is aimed at patients with higher than typical risk of local recurrence, i.e., age <50, node positive, presence of LVSI, EIC with <2 mm

margins, positive margins, or non-luminal-type histology. The control arm is conventionally (50 Gy/25 fractions) or hypofractionated (42.7 Gy/16 fractions) whole breast radiotherapy followed by a tumor bed boost versus a hypofractionated whole breast dose of 40 Gy/15 fractions with an integrated 3.2 Gy/fraction tumor bed dose to a total of 48.0 Gy (RTOG 2014). The primary endpoint of this study is non-inferior local control with secondary endpoints consisting of treatment toxicity, cosmesis, superior local control, and the development of dose-volume histogram guidelines for future patients.

Despite the increased toxicities and inferior fibrosis of the RAPID trial evaluating accelerated partial breast irradiation, there is continued interest in pursuing this technique. The currently accruing RTOG 0413/NSABP B-39 trial is comparing standardly fractionated whole-breast RT with three accelerated partial breast irradiation techniques: (1) 34 Gy/10 fractions BID via multicatheter interstitial brachytherapy, (2) 34 Gy/10 fractions BID via MammoSite balloon catheter, or (3) 38.5 Gy/10 fractions BID via external beam RT (RTOG 2013). The main endpoint of this trial is local control, with secondary endpoints including toxicity, cosmesis, and survival. Similar studies are being conducted in Canada (Group OCO 2006), Florence (Livi et al. 2010), and the UK (Institute of Cancer Research UK 2008). The Florence group published preliminary toxicity data which showed a reduction in grade 1–2 acute skin toxicity from 41% with whole breast irradiation to 5.8% with APBI (p value not given) (Livi et al. 2010).

3 Prostate Cancer

The most common EBRT treatment regimen for prostate cancer has utilized 1.8–2.0 Gy fractions delivered 5 days per week over a 7–8-week period (Zietman et al. 2001). This CF scheme has been favored due to the close proximity of the prostate to the rectum and bladder and concerns with acute and late treatment toxicity with larger fraction sizes, particularly when pelvic nodes are included within the RT fields. In recent years, multiple randomized trials have demonstrated the superiority of dose-escalated EBRT to 75 Gy or higher in terms of biochemical control (Dearnaley et al. 2014;

Peeters et al. 2006; Zietman et al. 2010; Pollack et al. 2002; Kuban et al. 2008; Michalski et al. 2014). While dose escalation improves cancer outcomes, it causes EBRT courses to become even more protracted to a total duration of 8–9 weeks. Hypofractionated treatment courses, by contrast, reduce the overall treatment course to 4–6 weeks or less and have been theorized to potentially improve treatment outcomes.

Radiobiology research in recent decades has suggested that the alpha-beta ratio of prostate cancer is much lower than that of other tumors and even surrounding normal tissue (Barendsen 1982; Brenner and Hall 1999; Duchesne and Peters 1999). Utilizing a HF approach has been hypothesized to produce improved tumor control and reduce treatment time without increasing late treatment toxicity (Brenner et al. 2002). An Australian trial compared the late morbidity of CF treatment with 64 Gy in 32 fractions to a HF course of 50 Gy in 20 fractions in patients with low-risk disease (Yeoh et al. 2003). This trial found no difference in biochemical failure, but the rate of rectal bleeding at 2 years was 27% among CF patients compared with 42% in the HF patients. This high rate may be attributed to the 2-dimensional planning techniques used in the study. A Canadian trial compared similar fractionation schedules in men with low- and intermediate-risk disease and found that the 5-year clinical and biochemical failure rate was higher in the HF arm (Lukka et al. 2005). The authors speculated the decreased tumor control rates may be due to prostate cancer having a lower alpha-beta ratio than initially suspected, which may have led to a discrepancy in the biological effective doses between the two arms. A limitation of both trials is that they were initiated prior to the publication of dose escalation data, and patients treated in both the CF and HF arms received lower doses than is currently standard.

An Italian trial of men with high-risk disease compared dose-escalated CF EBRT to 80 Gy with a HF regimen of 62 Gy at 3.1 Gy per fraction, which were estimated to be isoeffective based on an alpha-beta ratio of 1.5–1.8 (Arcangeli et al. 2012). The researchers found no difference in acute or late toxicity between the two arms. The

Fox Chase Cancer Center conducted a randomized trial of dose-escalated CF RT to 76 at 2 Gy per fraction with 70.2 Gy at 2.7 Gy per fraction (Pollack et al. 2013). The HF arm was hypothesized to deliver an additional 8.4 Gy biologically effective dose utilizing an alpha-beta ratio of 1.5. The trial was powered to show a 15% improvement in 5-year biochemical control but found no significant difference in tumor control or late toxicity between the arms. While the two approaches were found to be statistically equivalent, the results have been interpreted as a negative finding due to the superiority design of the trial.

RTOG 0415 was subsequently initiated to compare CF RT to 73.8 Gy in 41 fractions with a HF course of 70 Gy in 28 fractions. In contrast to prior studies, this trial was designed to test the non-inferiority of the HF arm in terms of biochemical control. The non-inferiority design was justified in light of the potential benefits in patient convenience and cost savings to the healthcare system with shorter treatment courses. Early results have demonstrated no difference in 7-year disease-free survival, but a small, nonsignificant increase in grade 3 or higher genitourinary and gastrointestinal toxicity was seen in the HF arm (Lee et al. 2016b).

The 5-year results of the CHHiP non-inferiority trial from the UK, randomizing patients to a CF schedule of 74 Gy in 2 Gy fractions with two HF arms of either 60 or 57 Gy in 3 Gy fractions, have now been reported (Dearnaley et al. 2016b). The 60 Gy HF arm was found to be non-inferior in terms of biochemical and clinical failure, though the 57 Gy arm exceeded the non-inferiority margin relative to 74 Gy. The HF schedules were associated with increased acute grade 2 or higher gastrointestinal toxicity with no difference in bowel, bladder, or sexual toxicities between the groups at 5 years. There was also no difference in patient-reported quality of life outcomes at 2 and 5 years. The authors concluded that the 60 Gy HF schedule should become the new standard of care for EBRT based upon the demonstrated non-inferiority of this schedule combined with the logistical benefits of a shorter radiation course.

Stereotactic body radiotherapy (SBRT) is a technique of high-dose per fraction, highly conformal RT that is delivered in 1–5 fractions and can be considered an extreme form of hypofractionation. A retrospective series of 304 patients with organ-confined prostate cancer treated with 5-fraction SBRT to 35–36.25 Gy found that rates of late grade 2 urinary and rectal toxicity rates were 5.8% and 2.9%, respectively, and only one patient experienced late grade 3 toxicity (Katz et al. 2010). At a median 30-month follow-up, a total of four patients experienced biochemical failures. Several other retrospective reports have found acceptable rates of toxicity and biochemical control (Townsend et al. 2011; Friedland et al. 2009; Morgia and De Renzis 2009).

A prospective study from Stanford analyzed 41 patients with low-risk prostate cancer treated with SBRT to 36.25 Gy in five fractions (King et al. 2009). Severe late complications were low with only three of the studied patients experiencing grade 3 late toxicities, though late grade 1–2 urinary and rectal toxicities were reported in 65% and 48% of patients, respectively. At a median follow-up of 33 months, no patients had experienced biochemical failure. A Phase I/II trial from Virginia Mason found similar rates of grade 1–2 late toxicity and did not report any late grade 3 or higher toxicity. The 4-year actuarial rate of biochemical control was 90% (Madsden et al. 2007). These data suggest that this technique is a safe and feasible option for patients. An analysis of Medicare data also found that SBRT may result in significant cost savings in comparison with IMRT, though at a cost of higher GU toxicity (Yu et al. 2014).

Several ongoing studies are currently investigating HF EBRT courses. Early results from the Canadian Prostate Fractionated Irradiation (PROFIT) trial comparing CF RT of 78 Gy in 39 fractions with a HF course of 60 Gy in 20 fractions were recently reported (Catton et al. 2016). At a median follow-up of 6 years, the HF course was non-inferior in terms of biochemical-clinical failure, and late toxicity favored the HF arm. The Polish HYPOPROST study is assessing outcomes with a HF boost dose in high-risk patients receiving nodal irradiation. All patients undergo CF IMRT to the whole pelvis to 46 Gy and then are randomized to receive either a CF boost dose

to a total of 76 Gy versus a HF regimen of 15 Gy in two fractions (The Greater Poland Cancer Centre 2000). Trials are also underway investigating outcomes with CF versus HF proton therapy regimens (Slater 2000). The HYPO study from the Netherlands is comparing CF EBRT to 78 Gy with a hypofractionated regimen of 43.7 Gy delivered in only seven fractions (Incrocci 2016). Some ongoing SBRT protocols include comparisons of 5-fraction SBRT with HF IMRT to 70.2 Gy in 26 fractions (Abramowitz 2000) and with single-fraction SBRT to 24 Gy (Fundacao Champalimaud 2000). Due to the significant benefits of these approaches in terms of patient convenience and reduced healthcare costs, both HF IMRT and SBRT will surely continue to be active areas of prostate cancer research in the coming years.

4 Lung Cancer

The standard radiotherapy dose for patients with locally advanced or medically inoperable non-small cell lung cancer was set early on by RTOG 7310, which established 60 Gy at 2 Gy per fraction as the recommended dose (Perez et al. 1986). Multiple clinical trials have shown the benefit of concurrent systemic therapy to this radiotherapy regimen (Auperin et al. 2010). Because local failures continue to be an issue, multiple attempts have been undertaken to increase the total radiation dose delivered, most recently in the form of RTOG 0617, which compared conventionally fractionated 60 versus 74 Gy with concurrent chemotherapy (Bradley et al. 2015). The trial unfortunately did not show a survival advantage for dose escalation, and in fact showed 2-year overall survival of 57% in the 60 Gy arm versus 44% in the dose-escalated arm.

Because concurrent chemoradiotherapy has been shown to be more toxic than sequential therapy (Auperin et al. 2010; Curran et al. 2011), this approach is often not utilized in frailer patients. Patients with locally advanced non-small cell lung cancer frequently have a performance status which precludes the use of any systemic therapy, and precluded their participation in past clinical trials, such as significant weight loss (>5%), KPS <70, and multiple medical comorbidities. Because of the known poor outcomes of a traditional 60 Gy regimen alone in this setting, alternative fractionation schedules have been utilized in select groups of patients in an attempt to increase otherwise poor rates of local control.

The MD Anderson Cancer Center conducted a study evaluating a conventional course of 60 Gy against 45 Gy in 15 fractions in good and poor performance patients, respectively. Despite differences in baseline characteristics, they did not find differences in toxicity, response rates, locoregional control, or survival, and adopted the hypofractionated 45 Gy course as their standard for patients who were unable to tolerate systemic therapy concurrent with radiotherapy (Nguyen et al. 1999). They later updated their experience and showed no differences in locoregional and distant control, but lower grade 2+ radiation dermatitis/pneumonitis, nausea/vomiting, and weight loss with the hypofractionated regimen compared to standard fractionation despite worse baseline characteristics. Further, after multivariate adjustment, there was no difference in survival between standard and hypofractionated radiotherapy despite a significantly increased relapse rate in the hypofractionated cohort (Amini et al. 2012).

In the United Kingdom, two approaches are commonly employed in patients with medically inoperable disease who are ineligible for chemotherapy: continuous hyperfractionated accelerated radiation therapy (CHART) and hypofractionation. Utilizing the CHART technique in unselected patients, they reported a 2-year survival of 34% with 0.7% grade 4+ toxicity with a fractionation of 1.5 Gy TID over 12 continuous days for a total dose of 54 Gy (Din et al. 2008). In a prospective comparison to conventionally fractionated 60 Gy, there was a 22% relative reduction in risk of death (2-year overall survival increased from 20% to 29%) (Saunders et al. 1999). This fractionation schedule has not gained wide acceptance in many centers due to the difficulties of treating TID over a continuous 12-day period.

In other UK centers, hypofractionation is utilized to rapidly complete a course of radical radiotherapy for patients in whom chemotherapy is not feasible. In a large series of patients who received 55 Gy/20 fractions (2.75 Gy/fraction), 2-year overall survival was 50% with survival for stage IA being 72%, dropping to 40% for stage III (Din et al. 2013). In the subset of patients in whom toxicity data was available, there was no grade 3+ toxicity, with 25% of patients receiving sequential chemotherapy. Similarly, a Canadian phase II trial evaluating a fractionation of 60 Gy/15 fractions was undertaken in medically inoperable patients with T1-3, node-negative lung cancers (Cheung et al. 2014). They found a tumor control rate of 87.4% and a 2-year overall survival of 68.7%. Grade 4 dyspnea or pneumonitis was seen in 5.1% and grade 3 toxicity in 32.6%.

As is evident, there is no defined hypofractionated dose schedule, with survival and toxicities dependent on patient baseline characteristics, disease stage, and dose fractionation. The Cancer and Leukemia Group-B (CALGB) conducted a phase I dose-escalation study in patients with T1-2N0 disease, treating to a nominal dose of 70 Gy with a successively decreasing number of fractions from 29 to 17 (2.41–4.11 Gy/fraction) (Bogart et al. 2010). Median survival was 38.5 months with a local failure rate of 7% and a 7.7% rate of grade 3+ acute toxicity and no late grade 3+ toxicity.

With these encouraging results from hypofractionated radiotherapy, attention has recently shifted towards the incorporation of systemic therapy. The All-India Institute recently reported on a phase II trial of hypofractionated radiotherapy (48 Gy/20 fractions) with neoadjuvant and concurrent chemotherapy versus standardly fractionated radiotherapy to 60 Gy following neoadjuvant chemotherapy (Roy et al. 2016). In this small study of 36 patients with locally advanced lung cancers, the overall response rate was significantly higher with hypofractionated radiotherapy and concurrent chemotherapy, at 72.2% versus 44%, as was median overall survival at 24.7 versus 12.3 months, though a prior randomized trial comparing hypofractionated radiotherapy with or without concurrent chemotherapy did not reveal a survival advantage to the addition of systemic agents (Maguire et al. 2014). A Dutch study of hypofractionated RT concurrent with low-dose daily cisplatin with or without cetuximab in locally advanced lung cancers revealed a median survival of 31.5 months with just over one third of patients surviving at 5 years (Walraven et al. 2016). The study showed no advantage to the addition of cetuximab and a decreased survival in patients who had poor performance status, more comorbidities, and a higher esophageal V35, indicating that the combination hypofractionated chemo-RT approach requires careful patient selection to derive the benefit of intensified therapy.

Because the hypofractionated approach has not been extensively studied with concurrent systemic therapy, a number of prospective trials are underway. Washington University is conducting a Phase I dose-escalation study of hypofractionated (15 fractions) proton beam radiotherapy with concurrent carboplatin and paclitaxel (Medicine WUS 2014). The State University of New York, Upstate, is also evaluating a regimen which incorporates carboplatin and paclitaxel with a course of radiotherapy to 70 Gy/20 fractions in patients with T1b-T2bN0 disease, again with toxicity as the main endpoint (University SU of NY-UM 2015). A third dose-escalation trial is underway at UCLA, evaluating a 10-day course of hypofractionated RT followed by a 5-fraction stereotactic escalating "boost," which is to reach a maximum total dose of 75 Gy (15 fractions total) (Institute JCCI and NC 2011). A similar phase I/II trial is being conducted in Poland, evaluating 58.8 Gy/21 fractions with or without concurrent cisplatin/vinorelbine with overall survival as the primary endpoint (Centre IPCHF 2015). The RTOG is also leading a phase II trial evaluating dose escalation in conjunction with chemotherapy and the use of mid-treatment PET-CT imaging for adaptive therapy (Institute NC 2012). Patients with stage III non-small cell lung cancer are being randomized to an initial phase of 50 Gy/25 fractions versus 46.2 Gy/21 fractions (2.2 Gy/fraction) with concurrent carboplatin and paclitaxel. Between fractions 18 and 19, a PET-CT is performed which is then used in the experimental arm to create an adaptive plan for the final 9 fractions of therapy. The boost dose is set to achieve a mean lung dose of 20 Gy and can range from 19.8 to 34.2 Gy (2.2–3.8 Gy/fraction), for a total dose of up to 80.4 Gy in 30 fractions. The control arm does not utilize the interim PET-CT and receives 10 Gy/5 fractions to a total dose of 60 Gy/30 fractions. All patients then receive three cycles of consolidative carboplatin and paclitaxel.

5 High-Grade Glioma

Glioblastoma is the most common primary malignant brain tumor in adults with an estimated annual incidence of approximately 23,000 cases in the USA (SEER Stat Fact Sheets 2016). Despite recent therapeutic advances, overall survival rates have been dismal (Grossman et al. 2010; Wang and Shi 2010). The standard of care for patients with good performance status has included maximal safe resection and postoperative RT. Prior to the publication of the data by Stupp et al. (2009) demonstrating a significant survival benefit with the addition of concurrent temozolomide (TMZ) to RT, many attempts were made at improving patient outcomes through optimizing radiation dose and fractionation schedules. Even with dose escalation to 90 Gy, the predominant pattern of failure remains within the treatment field (Chan et al. 2002).

Multiple studies have investigated altered fractionation regimens for high-grade gliomas. The Brain Tumor Cooperative Group (BTCG) study 7702 randomized patients with glioblastoma between hyperfractionated RT with carmustine to CF RT with either carmustine/misonidazole followed by carmustine or streptozocin (Deutsch et al. 1989). Hyperfractionated RT consisted of twice-daily 1.1 Gy fractions to a total dose of 66 Gy. The overall median survival was 10 months, and there was no significant difference between the four treatment arms. The RTOG later conducted a series of trials investigating different altered fractionation schedules. RTOG 8302 was a Phase I/II trial that explored dose escalation of two different RT fractionation schedules delivered with concurrent carmustine (Werner-Wasik et al. 1996). Patients with high-grade glioma were randomized to undergo either hyperfractionated RT using twice-daily 1.2 Gy fractions to a maximum total dose of 81.6 Gy or to an accelerated fraction RT regimen using twice-daily 1.6 Gy fractions to a maximum of 54.4 Gy. They found the regimens tolerable, though higher doses of hyperfractionated RT were associated with increased late toxicity.

Two additional trials were conducted to further investigate the hyperfractionated and accelerated fractionation schedules. RTOG 8302 demonstrated that 70.2 Gy was associated with the best survival outcome with hyperfractionation and was chosen as the experimental arm of RTOG 9006. This trial randomized patients to receive carmustine concurrently with either CF RT to 60 Gy or hyperfractionated RT to 70.2 Gy (Scott et al. 1998). There was no significant difference between the study arms in the overall treatment population, although decreased survival was demonstrated in patients younger than age 50 with hyperfractionation. It was speculated that the late side effects of hyperfractionated RT may have had a more deleterious impact on this cohort of younger patients with a better baseline prognosis. The accelerated fractionation arms of 8302 were associated with lower toxicity, and thus dose escalation beyond 54.4 Gy using this schema was felt to be possible. The RTOG 9411 trial was an attempt at dose escalation using the accelerated fractionation schedule from 8302 to either 64 or 70.4 Gy depending on tumor volume and was delivered with concurrent carmustine (Coughlin et al. 2000). The results demonstrated that although the treatment was tolerable, outcomes were not improved in comparison with historical controls.

An alternative treatment approach has been dose escalation through a stereotactic radiosurgery (SRS) boost in an attempt to overcome hypoxia-related treatment resistance. RTOG 9305 examined 203 patients with supratentorial glioblastoma who were randomized to receive either an upfront 15–24 Gy SRS boost followed by 60 Gy EBRT with concurrent carmustine or

60 Gy EBRT and carmustine alone (Souhami et al. 2004). At a median follow-up time of 61 months, there was no difference in survival, failure patterns, or quality of life deterioration between the two groups. Despite multiple attempts at finding an optimal dose fractionation schedule, no randomized trial has demonstrated a significant benefit over conventional 1.8–2.0 Gy daily fractions to a total dose of 60 Gy in patients with good performance status.

The most significant treatment advancement in recent years has been the addition of the oral alkylating agent TMZ to CF RT. Stupp et al. found that concurrent and adjuvant TMZ increased median and 5-year overall survival, and this regimen defines the current standard of care in younger patients with good performance status (Stupp et al. 2009). The ongoing NRG protocol BN001 is again investigating focal intensification of RT but in the context of radiosensitizing TMZ (NRG Oncology 2000). While previous trials have not demonstrated a benefit to dose escalation beyond 60 Gy, they were performed prior to the introduction of temozolomide, which may improve response to dose escalation. Tsien et al. (2012) published a dose-escalation trial that demonstrated a maximum tolerated dose of 75 Gy in 2.5 Gy fractions delivered with concurrent TMZ. The median survival in this trial was 20.1 months, which suggests increased efficacy in comparison with historical controls. Based upon these data, BN001 is currently randomizing patients with glioblastoma to CF photon or proton radiation therapy to 60 Gy with concurrent TMZ versus 50 Gy in 30 fractions with a simultaneous integrated boost to 75 Gy in 30 fractions with concurrent TMZ with a primary outcome of overall survival (NRG Oncology 2000).

While research efforts for patients with good performance status have focused on treatment intensification, attempts at improving outcomes in elderly and poor-performing patients have been concentrated on improving the tolerability of treatment. The trial conducted by Stupp et al. (2009) was limited to patients age 70 or less and found that the benefits of TMZ were reduced with increasing age. A French trial challenged the benefit of RT in elderly patients 70 years of age or older compared with supportive care alone but was closed early due to a significant survival benefit from CF RT to 50 Gy (Keime-Guibert et al. 2007). Though elderly patients with limited performance status have been shown to benefit from RT, life expectancy in this population is particularly poor (Li et al. 2011). A Canadian trial employed a hypofractionated course for patients of age 60 years or older with the objective of decreasing RT treatment time from 6 to 3 weeks by delivering 40 Gy in 2.67 Gy fractions (Roa et al. 2004). The non-inferiority design showed no survival difference between the hypofractionated and CF arms.

The Nordic trial compared a 6-week course of CF RT to a hypofractionated schedule of 34 Gy in 10 fractions and also included an arm that received TMZ alone (Malmstrom et al. 2012). This trial not only showed that the experimental arms did not compromise outcomes, but overall survival was superior in both the TMZ and hypofractionated RT arms in patients 70 years of age or older. The authors concluded that both TMZ alone and hypofractionated RT should be considered standard treatment options in this patient population. Having established the benefits of hypofractionated RT for frail and elderly patients, a subsequent trial sought to compare the Canadian hypofractionation schedule of 40 Gy in 15 fractions with an even more abbreviated course of 25 Gy in 5 fractions (Roa et al. 2015). The 1-week course was found to be statistically non-inferior to the 3-week course with median overall survival times of 6.4 and 7.9 months, respectively. There was also no difference in progression-free survival or quality of life following treatment, and the authors concluded that this shorter schedule can safely improve the survival-to-treatment time ratio in this group of patients with limited survival potential while also reducing resource utilization.

One limitation of the aforementioned trials is that none have addressed the potential benefit of concurrent TMZ with hypofractionation. Early results of a Phase III trial randomizing elderly patients to hypofractionated RT to 40 Gy in 15 fractions with or without concurrent TMZ have been presented (Perry et al. 2016). At this early stage, the addition of TMZ significantly improved overall survival compared with RT alone with no impact on functional quality of life domains. Overall, this series of trials has shown that hypofractionated RT is safe and feasible and should be considered the preferred management option for elderly or frail patients. Hypofractionated approaches are now being explored in patients with good performance status as well. One trial is comparing standard RT to 60 Gy in 30 fractions and concurrent TMZ with 60 Gy in 20 fractions and concurrent TMZ (AHS Cancer Control Alberta 2000). Another ongoing protocol is exploring the addition of metformin to this same hypofractionated RT regimen and TMZ, as this combination has been shown to stimulate 5-adenosine monophosphate-activated protein kinase (AMPK) leading to inhibition of cellular proliferation (McGill University Health Center 2000). Hypofractionation is likely to continue to be an important avenue of future research due to substantial benefits in patient comfort and convenience in a population with limited life expectancy.

6 High-Dose-Rate Brachytherapy

6.1 Prostate

Brachytherapy techniques involve the intracavitary or interstitial implantation of radioactive sources in order to deliver high doses of radiation to tumors while reducing the dose to normal tissue. Low-dose-rate (LDR) brachytherapy has been used as a treatment strategy for prostate cancer for many years. One benefit of this technique is that it reduces the number of treatment-related visits. Patients undergo a single procedure for implantation of radioactive seeds, which deliver a therapeutic radiation dose over several months. High rates of biochemical control have been demonstrated with LDR brachytherapy as monotherapy for low-risk disease (Blasko et al. 2000; Wallner et al. 1996; Sylvester et al. 2006). Recent data have also shown that the addition of LDR brachytherapy to EBRT improves relapse-free survival among intermediate- and high-risk patients, likely due to the ability to escalate the radiation dose to the prostate beyond what can be delivered with EBRT alone while respecting normal tissue tolerance (Morris et al. 2015). A downside to this approach is an extended period of urinary symptoms due to the long overall treatment duration as well as the need for patients to maintain radiation precautions for several months following implantation (Sanda et al. 2008).

High-dose-rate (HDR) brachytherapy is a form of hypofractionated (HF) RT that achieves similar levels of dose escalation while potentially ameliorating the long duration of side effects seen with LDR brachytherapy (Galalae et al. 2006). HDR prostate treatments deliver radiation in 1–3 fractions over the course of 1–2 days. Implantation is performed using an interstitial template and after-loading technique, and so patients are no longer radioactive following treatment. The ability to optimize the dose distribution by manipulating the source dwell times allows the planner to better account for the patient's anatomy and needle placement in the operating room (Martinez et al. 2002). Another potential advantage of HDR treatment is that the alpha-beta ratio of prostate cancer may be lower than most tumors and possibly lower than that of surrounding normal tissue (Barendsen 1982; Brenner and Hall 1999; Duchesne and Peters 1999b). Courses utilizing higher doses per fraction thus may improve the therapeutic ratio for prostate cancer radiation treatments.

Initial HDR brachytherapy publications described techniques using 2–3 fraction boosts following EBRT (Galalae et al. 2006; Martinez et al. 2002; Ares et al. 2009). The William Beaumont Hospital prospectively treated 207 patients with unfavorable risk prostate cancer with pelvic RT to 46 Gy followed by escalating doses of HDR brachytherapy delivered as 16.5–19.5 Gy in three fractions or 16.5–23.0 Gy in two fractions (Martinez et al. 2002). Comparing the 2- and 3-fraction cohorts, they found the 5-year biochemical control rates improved from 52% with the 3-fraction regimens to 87% with 2-fractions with no difference in toxicity. Early results of the RTOG 0321 prospective phase II

trial analyzing the addition of an HDR boost of 19 Gy in two fractions to 45 Gy EBRT demonstrated rates of severe acute and late adverse events of 2.4% and 2.6%, respectively (Hsu et al. 2010). Comparison of two prospective phase II clinical trials utilizing single- and 2-fraction boosts found no difference in biochemical control or late toxicity between the two regimens, and many centers are now adopting the single-fraction approach for HDR prostate boosts (Morton et al. 2011; Morton 2014). There is also recent evidence demonstrating the safety and feasibility of single-fraction brachytherapy as monotherapy for some prostate cancer patients (Hoskin et al. 2014).

6.2 Cervix

While there is growing evidence for the use of combination therapy for prostate cancer, the brachytherapy boost has been established as an integral component of concurrent chemoradiotherapy for treatment of locally advanced cervical cancer (Nag et al. 2000). This had traditionally involved the use of LDR planning techniques as defined by the Manchester system based upon 2-D imaging (Nag et al. 2002). The introduction of HDR techniques has had several benefits including reducing radiation exposure to healthcare workers through the use of an automated afterloader and avoiding lengthy hospitalizations during treatment delivery with resultant risk of venous thromboembolism. A randomized comparison of HDR and LDR techniques in cervical cancer patients demonstrated similar rates of local control, overall survival, and late toxicity (Patel et al. 1994). HDR brachytherapy also allows for 3-D image-based planning and functional image fusion. Accurate and individualized tumor and organ-at-risk delineation can enhance target coverage and sparing of critical organs and has been shown to improve local control and normal tissue toxicity in comparison with 2-D dosimetry (Charra-Brunaud et al. 2012).

A significant downside to the use of HDR techniques for cervical cancer is that they have traditionally required delivery over five to six treatments in order to maintain acceptable toxicity (Orton et al. 1991). Multifraction courses are naturally accompanied by increased discomfort and inconvenience to patients due to multiple intracavitary implantations as well as higher healthcare costs. In the developing world where cervical cancer screening is not widespread, physicians are faced with treating a large number of patients despite limited numbers of available radiation afterloader units and other necessary equipment. Hypofractionated courses that deliver treatment in fewer fractions could potentially help to offset this disadvantage and conserve scarce resources.

Prospective evidence for hypofractionated HDR brachytherapy is currently limited. A retrospective study of 49 patients treated with EBRT and chemotherapy followed by two fractions of 7–11 Gy HDR demonstrated comparable rates of local control, but was associated with grade 3–4 acute toxicity in 44% of patients (Sood et al. 2002). Modern image-based planning can achieve lower doses to critical organs, and the availability of necessary infrastructure is growing in countries such as India (Banerjee et al. 2014; Deshpande 2012). This can potentially improve the tolerability of hypofractionated HDR courses, which is an active area of ongoing research. A trial sponsored by the International Atomic Energy Agency randomized patients with FIGO Stage IIB-IIIB cervical cancer to EBRT followed by HDR brachytherapy to either 28 Gy in four fractions or 18 Gy in two fractions (International Atomic Energy Agency 2000). This study is now closed and the results are awaited. An ongoing protocol from Bangladesh is comparing two different HDR boost schedules. Patients with stage IIB to IVA cervical cancer undergo 50 Gy EBRT and then are randomized to receive either 21 Gy in three fractions or 18 Gy in two fractions (Bangabandhu Sheikh Mujib Medical University 2000).

Conclusions

Conventionally fractionated radiotherapy utilizing 1.8–2.0 Gy fractions has been the standard treatment paradigm for most cancer types for many years. Early research demonstrated that this scheme provided an optimal balance between treatment efficacy and normal tissue toxicity and thus maximized the therapeutic

ratio from radiotherapy. This research was predicated on the use of traditional radiotherapy planning techniques with 2-D imaging based on bony landmarks and 2- to 4-field treatment plans that included a large volume of normal tissue receiving the prescription dose. A significant downside of conventionally fractionated regimens is that they lead to protracted 7–9-week treatment courses that impose a significant burden on individual patients and an increased financial cost to the healthcare system. Investigations into altered fractionation schemes have historically focused on schemes that seek to enhance treatment efficacy by increasing the total radiation dose or decrease the overall treatment time while limiting late toxicity by using smaller fraction sizes. Some success has been demonstrated with these approaches, though acute treatment toxicity has often been a limiting factor and constrains the ability to combine these schemes with concurrent chemotherapy.

In recent years, the focus of altered fractionation research has shifted to hypofractionated courses, which utilize larger fraction sizes to deliver a biologically equivalent radiation dose over a shorter period of time. The advent of modern treatment techniques including IMRT, IGRT, and SRS has obviated many of the traditional concerns with toxicity and larger fraction sizes. Studies of hypofractionated radiotherapy for breast cancer have demonstrated equivalent cancer outcomes and comparable, or potentially improved, cosmetic outcomes compared with CF. Hypofractionation has also been shown to provide equivalent levels of biochemical control of prostate cancer at a potential cost of increased grade 2 bowel toxicity. In the areas of lung cancer and high-grade glioma, there is some evidence that hypofractionated courses may actually improve outcomes. Considering the growing concerns with healthcare expenditures and the increasing costs associated with cancer treatment, hypofractionated radiotherapy is likely to continue to be a very active avenue of research due to projected benefits in patient convenience and reduced economic burden on the healthcare system.

Prostate

Trial title	Organization/ Institution	Standard arm	Experimental arm	Endpoint	Anticipated accrual complete	Anticipated enrollment
Hypoprost: randomized, multicenter clinical trial comparing hypofractionated radiotherapy boost to conventionally fractionated in a high-risk group of prostate cancer patients	The Greater Poland Cancer Centre	46 Gy @ 2 Gy/fx to whole pelvis followed by 30 Gy @ 2 Gy/fx to prostate and proximal SV with neoadjuvant and concurrent ADT for up to 24 months	46 Gy @ 2 Gy/fx to whole pelvis followed by 15 Gy @ 7.5 Gy/fx to the prostate and proximal SV with neoadjuvant and concurrent ADT for up to 24 months	Phoenix PSA Failure	December 2016	465
Profit: prostate fractionated irradiation trial	Ontario Clinical Oncology Group	78 Gy @ 2 Gy/fx	60 Gy @ 2 Gy/fx	ASTRO PSA failure	March 2016	1204
Study of hypofractionated proton beam radiation therapy for prostate cancer	Loma Linda University	n/a	60 Cobalt gray equivalents (3CGE) @ 3CGE/fx	Late RTOG Grade 3+ toxicity	June 2018	200
Heat: a randomized study of radiation hypofractionation via extended vs. accelerated therapy for prostate cancer	University of Miami	36.25 Gy @ 7.25 Gy/fx to prostate and proximal SV	70.2 Gy @ 2.7 Gy/fx to prostate and proximal SV	2-year failure rates (biochemical, clinical, or biopsy)	February 2018	75
Prosint: phase II randomized study comparing ultra-high-dose hypofractionated vs. single-dose image-guided radiotherapy (IGRT) with urethral sparing for intermediate-risk prostate cancer	Fundacao Champalimaud	45 Gy @ 9 Gy/fx	24 Gy @ 24 Gy/fx	Late CTCAE v4.0Toxicity	September 2016	30

Lung

Trial title	Organization/Institution	Standard arm	Experimental arm	Endpoint	Anticipated accrual complete	Anticipated enrollment
A phase I study of radiation dose intensification with accelerated hypofractionated proton therapy and chemotherapy for non-small cell lung cancer (NSCLC)	Washington University School of Medicine (St. Louis, MO)	n/a	Hypofractionated proton beam RT (15 fraction course) with concurrent weekly carboplatin and paclitaxel followed by consolidation carboplatin and paclitaxel every 3 weeks ×2 cycles	Maximum tolerated dose	July 2016	20
Pilot study of the safety and feasibility of administering concurrent systemic chemotherapy with accelerated hypofractionated radiation therapy in the treatment of medically inoperable T1b and T2 NSCLC	State University of New York—Upstate Medical University	n/a	70 Gy/20 fractions with concurrent carboplatin AUC 2 and paclitaxel 45 mg/m^2 ×4 cycles	Late CTCAE grade 3+ toxicity	December 2017	12
Image-guided hypofractionated radiotherapy with stereotactic boost and chemotherapy for inoperable stage II–III NSCLC	Jonsson Comprehensive Cancer Center (University of California Los Angeles)	n/a	10 fractions hypofractionated RT over 2 weeks followed by 5 fractions of dose-escalated hypofractionated boost with concurrent weekly carboplatin AUC 2 and paclitaxel 45 mg/m^2	Maximum tolerated dose up to 75 Gy	May 2017	45
Hypofractionated accelerated radiotherapy with concomitant full dose chemotherapy for locally advanced NSCLC: phase I/II study	Independent Public Care Health Facility of the Ministry of the Interior and Warmian & Mazurian Oncology Centre (Poland)	n/a	58.8 Gy @ 2.8 Gy/fx with concurrent q3 weekly cisplatin and vinorelbine	Grade 3+ toxicity	December 2016	100
Randomized phase II trial of individualized adaptive radiotherapy using during-treatment FDG-PET/CT and modern technology in locally advanced NSCLC	RTOG/NRG/ECOG-ACRIN	60 Gy @ 2 Gy/fx with concurrent carboplatin AUC 2 and paclitaxel 45 mg/m^2 followed by three cycles of consolidation	46.2 Gy @ 2.2 Gy/fx followed by 9 fraction boost @ 2.2–3.8 Gy/fx to a total of up to 80.4 Gy with concurrent carboplatin AUC 2 and paclitaxel 45 mg/m^2 followed by 3 cycles of consolidation	Locoregional progression-free survival and relative change in SUV_{max} at mid-treatment PET-CT	November 2016	138

Breast

Trial title	Organization/ Institution	Standard arm	Experimental arm	Endpoint	Anticipated accrual complete	Anticipated enrollment
A phase II study of accelerated hypofractionated radiotherapy (AHF-RT) after breast conserving surgery (BCS) in medically underserved patients	James Graham Brown Cancer Center (University of Louisville)	n/a	30 Gy @ 6 Gy/ fx once per week	Ipsilateral breast tumor recurrence	December 2016	250
Import low: randomized trial testing intensity-modulated and partial organ radiotherapy after breast conservation surgery for early breast cancer	Institute of Cancer Research (United Kingdom)	Standard whole breast hypofractionated RT	1. Reduced-dose whole breast hypofractionated RT with standard dosing to tumor cavity (partial breast) 2. Partial breast hypofractionated RT	Ipsilateral breast tumor recurrence	June 2010	1935
Import high: randomized trial testing dose-escalated intensity-modulated radiotherapy for women treated by breast conservation surgery and appropriate systemic therapy for early breast cancer	Institute of Cancer Research (United Kingdom)	Whole breast RT to 56 Gy @ 2.43 Gy/ fx	1. Whole breast RT with SIB boost to tumor cavity to 48 Gy @ 3.2 Gy/fx 2. Whole breast RT with SIB boost to tumor cavity to 53 Gy @ 3.53 Gy/fx	Palpable induration at boost site	Unknown	840
RTOG/NRG 1005: a phase III trial of accelerated whole breast irradiation with hypofractionation plus concurrent boost vs. standard whole breast irradiation plus sequential boost for early-stage breast cancer	RTOG/NRG	Standard whole breast RT with conventional (50 Gy @ 2 Gy/fx) or hypofractionation (42.7 Gy @ 2.67 Gy/fx)	Accelerated hypofractionated whole breast RT to 40 Gy @ 2.67 Gy/fx with SIB to tumor cavity to 48.0 Gy @ 3.2 Gy/fx	Ipsilateral breast tumor recurrence	August 2020	2312
Rapid: a multicenter randomized trial to determine if accelerated partial breast irradiation, utilizing 3D CRT, is as effective as whole breast irradiation following breast-conserving surgery in women with ductal carcinoma in situ or invasive breast cancer with negative axillary lymph nodes	Ontario Clinical Oncology Group	Whole breast RT to 42.5 Gy/16 fx or 50 Gy/25 fx	Accelerated partial breast RT to 38.5 Gy/10 fx BID	Ipsilateral breast tumor recurrence	June 2020	2128
Randomized phase 3 trial of accelerated partial breast irradiation using intensity-modulated radiotherapy vs. whole breast irradiation	Azienda Ospedaliero-Universitaria Careggi (Florence, Italy)	Conventional whole breast RT to 50 Gy/25fx	Accelerated partial breast irradiation to 30 Gy/5fx	Ipsilateral breast tumor recurrence	February 2014	520

CNS

Trial title	Organization/ Institution	Standard arm	Experimental arm	Endpoint	Anticipated accrual complete	Anticipated enrollment
NRG-BN001: randomized phase II trial of hypofractionated dose-escalated photon IMRT or proton beam therapy vs. conventional photon irradiation with concomitant and adjuvant temozolomide in patients with newly diagnosed glioblastoma	NRG/RTOG	46 Gy @ 2 Gy/fx followed by 14 Gy boost @ 2 Gy/fx via photon or proton RT with concurrent/ adjuvant TMZ	50 Gy @ 1.67 Gy/fx with SIB to 75 Gy @ 2.5 Gy/fx via photon or proton RT with concurrent/ adjuvant TMZ	Overall survival	May 2019	576
A randomized controlled trial of conventional vs. hypofractionated radiation therapy with temozolomide for patients with newly diagnosed glioblastoma	AHS Cancer Control Alberta	60 Gy @ 2 Gy/fx with concurrent/ adjuvant TMZ	60 Gy @ 3 Gy/fx with concurrent/ adjuvant TMZ	Overall survival	August 2020	132
M-HARTT: Metformin and neo-adjuvant temozolomide and hypofractionated accelerated limited-margin radiotherapy followed by adjuvant temozolomide in patients with glioblastoma multiforme	McGill University Health Center	n/a	60 Gy @ 3 Gy/fx with concurrent/ adjuvant TMZ and metformin	Percent of patients completing therapy	December 2018	50

References

Abramowitz M (2000) Radiation hypofractionation via extended versus accelerated therapy (HEAT) for prostate cancer. In: ClinicalTrials.gov [Internet]. National Library of Medicine (US), Bethesda, MD [cited 1 Aug 2016]. https://clinicaltrials.gov/ct2/show/NCT01794403 NLM Identifier: NCT01794403

Adelstein DJ, Li Y, Adams GL et al (2003) An intergroup phase III comparison of standard radiation therapy and two schedules of concurrent chemoradiotherapy in patients with unresectable squamous cell head and neck cancer. J Clin Oncol 21(1):92–98

AHS Cancer Control Alberta (2000) Trial of hypofractionated radiation therapy for glioblastoma. In: ClinicalTrials.gov [Internet]. National Library of Medicine (US), Bethesda, MD [cited 3 Aug 2016]. http://clinicaltrials.gov/show/ NCT02206230. NLM Identifier: NCT02206230

Amini A, Lin SH, Wei C et al (2012) Accelerated hypofractionated radiation therapy compared to conventionally fractionated radiation therapy for the treatment of inoperable non-small cell lung cancer. Radiat Oncol 7(1):33. doi:10.1186/1748-717X-7-33

Andrews DW, Scott CB, Sperduto PW et al (2004) Whole brain radiation therapy with or without stereotactic radiosurgery boost for patients with one to three brain metastases: phase III results of the RTOG 9508 randomized trial. Lancet 363(9422):1665–1672

Arcangeli S, Strigari L, Gomellini S et al (2012) Updated results and patterns of failure in a randomized hypofractionation trial for high-risk prostate cancer. Int J Radiat Oncol Biol Phys 84(5):1172–1178

Ares C, Popowski Y, Pampallona S et al (2009) Hypofractionated boost with high-dose-rate brachytherapy and open magnetic resonance imaging-guided implants for locally aggressive prostate cancer: a sequential dose-escalation pilot study. Int J Radiat Oncol Biol Phys 75(3):656–663

Ashman JB, Zelefsky MJ, Hunt MS et al (2005) Whole pelvic radiotherapy for prostate cancer using 3D conformal and intensity-modulated radiotherapy. Int J Radiat Oncol Biol Phys 63(3):765–771

Ashworth A, Kong W, Whelan T et al (2013) A population-based study of the fractionation of postlumpectomy breast radiation therapy. Int J Radiat Oncol Biol Phys 86(1):51–57. doi:10.1016/j.ijrobp.2012.12.015

Auperin A, Le Pechoux C, Rolland E et al (2010) Meta-analysis of concomitant versus sequential radiochemotherapy in locally advanced non-small-cell lung cancer. J Clin Oncol 28(13):2181–2190. doi:10.1200/JCO.2009.26.2543

Baillet F, Housset M, Maylin C et al (1990) The use of a specific hypofractionated radiation therapy regimen versus classical fractionation in the treatment of breast cancer: a randomized study of 230 patients. Int J Radiat Oncol Biol Phys 19(5):1131–1133. doi:10.1016/0360-3016(90)90216-7

Banerjee S, Mahantshetty U, Shrivastava S (2014) Brachytherapy in India – A long road ahead. J Contemp Brachytherapy 6(3):331–335

Bangabandhu Sheikh Mujib Medical University (2000) A randomized controlled trial between two different HDR brachytherapy schedules in local advanced carcinoma of uterine cervix. In: ClinicalTrials.gov [Internet]. National Library of Medicine (US), Bethesda, MD [cited 15 Aug 2016]. http://clinicaltrials.gov/show/NCT02765919. NLM Identifier: NCT02765919

Barendsen GW (1982) Dose fractionation, dose rate and iso-effect relationships for normal tissue responses. Int J Radiat Oncol Biol Phys 8:1981–1997

Beitler JJ, Zhang Q, Fu KK et al (2014) Final results of local-regional control and late toxicity of RTOG 9003: a randomized trial of altered fractionation radiation for locally advanced head and neck cancer. Int J Radiat Oncol Biol Phys 89(1):13–20

Bentzen SM, Agrawal RK, Aird EG et al (2008) The UK Standardization of Breast Radiotherapy (START) Trial B of radiotherapy hypofractionation for treatment of early breast cancer: a randomized trial. Lancet 371(9618):1098–1107

Blasko JC, Grimm PD, Sylvester JE et al (2000) Palladium-103 brachytherapy for prostate carcinoma. Int J Radiat Oncol Biol Phys 46:839–850

Bogart JA, Hodgson L, Seagren SL et al (2010) Phase I study of accelerated conformal radiotherapy for stage I non-small-cell lung cancer in patients with pulmo-nary dysfunction: CALGB 39904. J Clin Oncol 28(2):202–206. doi:10.1200/JCO.2009.25.0753

Bonner JA, Harari PM, Giralt J et al (2010) Radiotherapy plus cetuximab for locoregionally advanced head and neck cancer: 5-year survival data from a phase 3 randomized trial, and relation between cetuximab-induced rash and survival. Lancet Oncol 11(1):21–28

Bradley J, Paulus R, Komaki R et al (2015) Standard-dose versus high-dose conformal radiotherapy with concurrent and consolidation carboplatin plus paclitaxel with or without cetuximab for patients with stage IIIA or IIIB non-small-cell lung cancer (RTOG 0617): a randomised, two-by-two factorial phase 3 study. Lancet Oncol 16(2):187–199

Brenner DJ, Hall EJ (1999) Fractionation and protraction for radiotherapy of prostate carcinoma. Int J Radiat Oncol Biol Phys 43:1095–1101

Brenner DJ, Martinez AA, Edmundson GK et al (2002) Direct evidence that prostate tumors show high sensitivity to fractionation (low alpha/beta ratio), similar to late-responding normal tissue. Int J Radiat Oncol Biol Phys 52:6–13

Brunt A, Yarnold J, Wheatly D, et al (2016) Acute skin toxicity reported in the FAST-Forward trial (HTA 09/01/47): a phase III randomised trial of 1-week whole breast radiotherapy compared to standard 3 weeks in patients with early breast cancer. Proceedings of the 10th National Cancer Research Conference. http://conference.ncri.org.uk/abstracts/2014/abstracts/LB116.html. Accessed 26 Aug 2016

Catton CN, Lukka H, Julian JA et al (2016) A randomized trial of a shorter radiation fractionation schedule for the treatment of localized prostate cancer. J Clin Oncol 34. (Suppl; abstr 5003)

Centre IPCHF of the M of the I and W& MO (2015) Hypofractionated accelerated radiotherapy with concomitant full dose chemotherapy for locally advanced non-small cell lung cancer: phase I/II study. ClinicalTrials.gov [Internet]. National Library of Medicine (US), Bethesda, MD. https://clinicaltrials.gov/ct2/show/NCT02367443. Accessed 8 Oct 2016

Chan JL, Lee SW, Fraass BA et al (2002) Survival and failure patterns of high-grade gliomas after three-dimensional conformal radiotherapy. J Clin Oncol 90(6):1635–1642

Chapman BV, Rajagopalan MS, Heron DE et al (2015) Clinical pathways: a catalyst for the adoption of hypofractionation for early-stage breast cancer. Int J Radiat Oncol Biol Phys 93(4):854–861. doi:10.1016/j.ijrobp.2015.08.013

Charra-Brunaud C, Harver V, Delannes M et al (2012) Impact of 3D image-based PDR brachytherapy on outcome of patients treated for cervix carcinoma in France: results of the French STIC prospective study. Radiother Oncol 103(3):305–313

Cheung P, Faria S, Ahmed S et al (2014) Phase II study of accelerated hypofractionated three-dimensional conformal radiotherapy for stage T1-3 N0 M0 non-small cell lung cancer: NCIC CTG BR.25. J Natl Cancer Inst 106(8):dju164. doi:10.1093/jnci/dju164

Coughlin C, Scott C, Langer C et al (2000) Phase II, two-arm RTOG trial (94-11) of bischloroethyl-nitrosourea plus accelerated hyperfractionated radiotherapy (64.0 or 70.4 Gy) based on tumor volume (> 20 or < or = 20 cm(2), respectively) in the treatment of newly-diagnosed radiosurgery-ineligible glioblastoma multiforme patients. Int J Radiat Oncol Biol Phys 48(5):1351–1358

Curran WJ, Paulus R, Langer CJ et al (2011) Sequential vs. concurrent chemoradiation for stage III non-small cell lung cancer: randomized phase III trial RTOG 9410. J Natl Cancer Inst 103(19):1452–1460. doi:10.1093/jnci/djr325

Dearnaley DP, Jovic G, Syndikus I et al (2014) Escalated-dose versus control-dose conformal radiotherapy for prostate cancer: long-term results from the MRC RT01 randomized controlled trial. Lancet Oncol 15(4):464–473

Dearnaley D, Syndikus I, Mossop H et al (2016) Conventional versus hypofractionated high-dose intensity-modulated radiotherapy for prostate cancer: 5-year outcomes of the randomized, non-inferiority, phase 3 CHHiP trial. Lancet Oncol 17(8):1047–1060

Deshpande D (2012) Will MR image-guided brachytherapy be a standard of care for cervical cancer in future? An Indian perspective. J Med Phys 37(1):1–3

Deutsch M, Green SB, Strike TA et al (1989) Results of a randomized trial comparing BCNU plus radiotherapy, streptozotocin plus radiotherapy, BCNU plus hyperfractionated radiotherapy, and BCNU following misonidazole plus radiotherapy in the postoperative treatment of malignant glioma. Int J Radiat Oncol Biol Phys 16(6):1389–1396

Din OS, Lester J, Cameron A et al (2008) Routine use of continuous, hyperfractionated, accelerated radiotherapy for non-small-cell lung cancer: a five-center experience. Int J Radiat Oncol Biol Phys 72(3):716–722

Din OS, Harden SV, Hudson E et al (2013) Accelerated hypo-fractionated radiotherapy for non small cell lung cancer: results from 4 UK centres. Radiother Oncol 109(1):8–12. doi:10.1016/j.radonc.2013.07.014

Duchesne GM, Peters LJ (1999) What is the alpha/beta ratio for prostate cancer? Rationale for hypofractionated high dose rate brachytherapy. Int J Radiat Oncol Biol Phys 44:747–748

FAST Trialists Group HD, Agrawal RK, Alhasso A et al (2011) First results of the randomised UK FAST Trial of radiotherapy hypofractionation for treatment of early breast cancer (CRUKE/04/015). Radiother Oncol 100(1):93–100. doi:10.1016/j.radonc.2011.06.026

Friedland JL, Freeman DE, Masterson-McGary ME, Spellberg DM (2009) Stereotactic body radiotherapy: an emerging treatment approach for localized prostate cancer. Technol Cancer Res Treat 8(5):387–392

Fundacao Champalimaud (2000) Phase II study of ultra-high-dose hypofractionated vs. single-dose image-guided radiotherapy for prostate cancer (PROSINT). In: ClinicalTrials.gov [Internet]. National Library of Medicine (US), Bethesda, MD [cited 1 Aug 2016]. https://clinicaltrials.gov/ct2/show/NCT02570919

Galalae RM, Martinez A, Nuernberg N et al (2006) Hypofractionated conformal HDR brachytherapy in hormone naive men with localized prostate cancer. Is escalation to very high biologically equivalent dose beneficial in all prognostic risk groups? Strahlenther Onkol 182(3):135–141

Gradishar WJ, Robert CH, Anderson BO, et al (2016) NCCN guidelines version 2.2016 Breast cancer panel members. http:NCCN.org

Grossman SA, Ye X, Piantadosi S et al (2010) Survival of patients with newly diagnosed glioblastoma treated with radiation and temozolomide in research studies in the United States. Clin Cancer Res 16(8):2443–2449

Group OCO (2006) RAPID: Randomized trial of accelerated partial breast irradiation. ClinicalTrials.gov [Internet]. National Library of Medicine (US), Bethesda, MD. https://clinicaltrials.gov/ct2/show/NCT00282035. Accessed 8 Aug 2016

Hall EJ, Giaccia AK (2012) Time, dose, and fractionation in radiotherapy. In: Radiobiology for the radiologist, 7th edn. Lippincott, Williams & Wilkins, Philadelphia, pp 391–418

Hopwood P, Haviland JS, Sumo G et al (2010) Comparison of patient-reported breast, arm, and shoulder symptoms and body image after radiotherapy for early breast cancer: 5-year follow-up in the randomised Standardisation of Breast Radiotherapy (START) trials. Lancet Oncol 11(3):231–240. doi:10.1016/S1470-2045(09)70382-1

Hoskin P, Rojas A, Ostler P et al (2014) High-dose-rate brachytherapy alone given as two or one fraction to patients for locally advanced prostate cancer: acute toxicity. Radiother Oncol 110(2):268–271

Hsu IC, Bae K, Shinohara K et al (2010) Phase II trial of high-dose-rate brachytherapy and external beam radiotherapy for adenocarcinoma of the prostate: preliminary results of RTOG 0321. Int J Radiat Oncol Biol Phys 78(3):751–758

Incrocci L (2016) Hypofractionated irradiation for prostate cancer: a randomized multicenter phase III study. In: ISRCTN Registry [Internet] [cited 1 Aug 2016]. http://www.isrctn.com/ISRCTN85138529. ISRCTN Identifier: N85138529

Institute JCCI and NC (2011) Image-guided hypofractionated radiotherapy with stereotactic boost and chemotherapy for inoperable stage II–III non-small cell lung cancer. ClinicalTrials.gov [Internet]. National Library of Medicine (US), Bethesda, MD. https://clinicaltrials.gov/ct2/show/NCT01345851. Accessed 8 Oct 2016

Institute NC (2012) Study of positron emission tomography and computed tomography in guiding radiation therapy in patients with stage III non-small cell lung cancer. ClinicalTrials.gov [Internet]. National Library of Medicine (US), Bethesda, MD. https://clinicaltrials.gov/ct2/show/NCT01507428. Accessed 26 Aug 2016

Institute of Cancer Research UK (2008) Radiation therapy in treating women with early-stage breast cancer who have undergone breast conservation surgery.

ClinicalTrials.gov [Internet]. National Library of Medicine (US), Bethesda, MD. https://clinicaltrials.gov/ct2/show/NCT00814567. Accessed 2 Aug 2016

Institute of Cancer Research UK (2009) Radiation therapy in treating women who have undergone breast conservation surgery and systemic therapy for early breast cancer. ClinicalTrials.gov [Internet]. National Library of Medicine (US), Bethesda, MD. https://clinicaltrials.gov/ct2/show/NCT00818051. Accessed 2 Aug 2016

International Atomic Energy Agency (2000) CRP on radiobiological and clinical studies on viral-induced cancer's response to radiotherapy. In: ClinicalTrials.gov [Internet]. National Library of Medicine (US), Bethesda, MD [cited 15 Aug 2016]. http://clinicaltrials.gov/show/NCT00122772. NLM Identifier: NCT00122772

James Graham Brown Cancer Center U of L (2011) Accelerated Hypofractionated Radiotherapy (AHF-RT) for the treatment of breast cancer. ClinicalTrials.gov [Internet]. National Library of Medicine (US), Bethesda, MD. https://clinicaltrials.gov/ct2/show/NCT01278212. Accessed 2 Aug 2016

Katz AJ, Santoro M, Ashley R et al (2010) Stereotactic body radiotherapy for organ-confined prostate cancer. BMC Urol 10(1):1–10

Keime-Guibert F, Chinot O, Taillandier L et al (2007) Radiotherapy for glioblastoma in the elderly. N Engl J Med 356(15):1527–1535

King CR, Brooks JD, Gill H et al (2009) Stereotactic body radiotherapy for localized prostate cancer: interim results of a prospective phase II clinical trial. Int J Radiat Oncol Biol Phys 73(4):1043–1048

Kuban DA, Tucker SL, Dong L et al (2008) Long-term results of the M.D. Anderson randomized dose-escalation trial for prostate cancer. Int J Radiat Oncol Biol Phys 70(1):67–74

Lee WR, Dignam JJ, Amin M et al (2016a) NRG Oncology ROTG 0415: a randomized phase 3 noninferiority study comparing 2 fractionation schedules in patients with low-risk prostate cancer. J Clin Oncol 34(20):2325–2332

Lee WR, Dignam JJ, Amin M et al (2016b) NRG Oncology ROTG 0415: a randomized phase III noninferiority study comparing 2 fractionation schedules in patients with low-risk prostate cancer. J Clin Oncol 34. (Suppl 2S; abstr 1)

Li J, Wang M, Won M et al (2011) Validation and simplification of the Radiation Therapy Oncology Group recursive partitioning analysis classification for glioblastoma. Int J Radiat Oncol Biol Phys 81(3):623–630

Livi L, Buonamici FB, Simontacchi G et al (2010) Accelerated partial breast irradiation with IMRT: new technical approach and interim analysis of acute toxicity in a phase III randomized clinical trial. Int J Radiat Oncol Biol Phys 77(2):509–515. doi:10.1016/j.ijrobp.2009.04.070

Lukka H, Hayter C, Julian JA et al (2005) Randomized trial comparing two fractionation schedules for patients with localized prostate cancer. J Clin Oncol 23:6132–6138

Madsden BL, His RA, Pham HT et al (2007) Stereotactic hypofractionated accurate radiotherapy of the prostate (SHARP), 33.5 Gy in five fractions for localized disease: first clinical trial results. Int J Radiat Oncol Biol Phys 67(4):1099–1105

Maguire J, Khan I, McMenemin R et al (2014) SOCCAR: A randomised phase II trial comparing sequential versus concurrent chemotherapy and radical hypofractionated radiotherapy in patients with inoperable stage III non-small cell lung cancer and good performance status. Eur J Cancer 50(17):2939–2949. doi:10.1016/j.ejca.2014.07.009

Malmstrom A, Gronberg BH, Marosi C et al (2012) Temozolomide versus standard 6-week radiotherapy versus hypofractionated radiotherapy in patients older than 60 years with glioblastoma: the Nordic randomized, phase 3 trial. Lancet Oncol 13(9):916–926

Mariotto AB, Yabroff KR, Shao Y et al (2011) Projections of the cost of cancer care in the United States: 2010–2020. J Natl Cancer Inst 103(2):117–128. doi:10.1093/jnci/djq495

Martinez AA, Gustafson G, Gonzalez J et al (2002) Dose escalation using conformal high-dose-rate brachytherapy improves outcome in unfavorable prostate cancer. Int J Radiat Oncol Biol Phys 53(2):316–327

McGill University Health Center (2000) Metformin, neoadjuvant temozolomide and hypo- accelerated radiotherapy followed by adjuvant TMZ in patients with GBM. In: ClinicalTrials.gov [Internet]. National Library of Medicine (US), Bethesda, MD [cited 3 Aug 2016]. http://clinicaltrials.gov/show/NCT02780024. NLM Identifier: NCT02780024

Medicine WUS (2014) A phase I study of radiation dose intensification with accelerated hypofractionated proton therapy and chemotherapy for non-small cell lung cancer. ClinicalTrials.gov [Internet]. National Library of Medicine (US), Bethesda, MD. https://clinicaltrials.gov/ct2/show/NCT02172846. Accessed 8 Oct 2016

Michalski JM, Moughan J, Purdy JA et al (2014) Initial results of a phase 3 randomized study of high dose 3DCRT/IMRT versus standard dose 3D-CRT/IMRT in patients treated for localized prostate cancer. Int J Radiat Oncol Biol Phys 90(5):1263

Morgia G, De Renzis C (2009) Cyberknife in the treatment of prostate cancer: a revolutionary system. Eur Urol 56(1):40–42

Morris JW, Tyldesley S, Pai HH et al (2015) ASCENDE-RT: a multicenter, randomized trial of dose-escalated external beam radiation therapy (EBRT-B) versus low-dose-rate brachytherapy (LDR-B) for men with unfavorable-risk localized prostate cancer. J Clin Oncol 33

Morton GC (2014) High-dose-rate brachytherapy boost for prostate cancer: rationale and technique. J Contemp Brachytherapy 6(3):323–330

Morton GC, Loblaw A, Cheung P et al (2011) Is single fraction 15 Gy the preferred high dose-rate brachytherapy boost dose for prostate cancer? Radiother Oncol 100(3):463–467

Nag S, Erickson B, Thomadsen B et al (2000) The American Brachytherapy Society recommendations for high-dose-rate brachytherapy for carcinoma of the cervix. Int J Radiat Oncol Biol Phys 48(1):201–211

Nag S, Chao C, Erickson B et al (2002) The American Brachytherapy Society recommendations for low-dose-rate brachytherapy for carcinoma of the cervix. Int J Radiat Oncol Biol Phys 52(1):33–48

Nguyen LN, Komaki R, Allen P et al (1999) Effectiveness of accelerated radiotherapy for patients with inoperable non-small cell lung cancer (NSCLC) and borderline prognostic factors without distant metastasis: a retrospective review. Int J Radiat Oncol Biol Phys 44(5):1053–1056. doi:10.1016/s0360-3016(99)00130-3

National Research Group/Radiation Therapy Oncology Group (2014) RTOG 1005 Protocol Information. https://www.rtog.org/clinicaltrials/protocoltable/studydetails.aspx?study=1005. Accessed 3 Aug 2016

Nguyen-Tan PH, Zhang Q, Ang KK et al (2014) Randomized phase III trial to test accelerated versus standard fractionation in combination with concurrent cisplatin for head and neck carcinomas in the Radiation Therapy Oncology Group 0129 trial: long-term report of efficacy and toxicity. J Clin Oncol 34(23):1–10

NRG Oncology (2000a) Reduced-dose intensity-modulated radiation therapy with or without cisplatin in treating patients with advanced oropharyngeal cancer. In: ClinicalTrials.gov [Internet]. National Library of Medicine (US), Bethesda, MD [cited 8 Aug 2016]. http://clinicaltrials.gov/show/NCT02254278. NLM Identifier: NCT02254278

NRG Oncology (2000b) Dose-escalated photon IMRT or proton beam radiation therapy versus standard-dose radiation therapy and temozolomide in treating patients with newly diagnosed glioblastoma. In: ClinicalTrials.gov [Internet]. National Library of Medicine (US), Bethesda, MD [cited 3 Aug 2016]. http://clinicaltrials.gov/show/NCT02179086. NLM Identifier: NCT02179086

Olivotto IA, Whelan TJ, Parpia S et al (2013) Interim cosmetic and toxicity results from RAPID: a randomized trial of accelerated partial breast irradiation using three-dimensional conformal external beam radiation therapy. J Clin Oncol 31(32):4038–4045. doi:10.1200/JCO.2013.50.5511

Orton CG, Seyedsadr M, Somnay A (1991) Comparison of high and low dose rate remote afterloading for cervix cancer and the importance of fractionation. Int J Radiat Oncol Biol Phys 21(6):1425–1434

Overgaard J, Hansen HS, Specht L et al (2003) Five compared with six fractions per week of conventional radiotherapy of squamous-cell carcinoma of head and neck: DAHANCA 6 and 7 randomized controlled trials. Lancet 362(9388):933–940

Owen JR, Ashton A, Bliss JM et al (2006) Effect of radiotherapy fraction size on tumour control in patients with early-stage breast cancer after local tumour excision: long-term results of a randomised trial. Lancet Oncol 7(6):467–471. doi:10.1016/S1470-2045(06)70699-4

Patel FD, Sharma SC, Negi PS et al (1994) Low dose rate vs. high dose rate brachytherapy in the treatment of carcinoma of the uterine cervix: a clinical trial. Int J Radiat Oncol Biol Phys 28(2):335–341

Peeters ST, Heemsbergen WD, Koper PC et al (2006) Dose-response in radiotherapy for localized prostate cancer: results of the Dutch multicenter randomized phase III trial comparing 68 Gy of radiotherapy with 78 Gy. J Clin Oncol 24(13):1990–1996

Perez CA, Bauer M, Edelstein S et al (1986) Impact of tumor control on survival in carcinoma of the lung treated with irradiation. Int J Radiat Oncol 12(4):539–547. doi:10.1016/0360-3016(86)90061-1

Perry JR, Laperriere N, O'Callaghan CJ et al (2016) A phase III randomized controlled trial of short-course radiotherapy with or without concomitant and adjuvant temozolomide in elderly patients with glioblastoma. J Clin Oncol 34. Suppl abstr LBA2

Peterson D, Truong PT, Parpia S et al (2015) Predictors of adverse cosmetic outcome in the RAPID trial: an exploratory analysis. Int J Radiat Oncol Biol Phys 91(5):968–976. doi:10.1016/j.ijrobp.2014.12.040

Pollack A, Zagars GK, Starkschall G et al (2002) Prostate cancer radiation dose response: results of the M. D. Anderson phase III randomized trial. Int J Radiat Oncol Biol Phys 53:1097–1105

Pollack A, Walker G, Horwitz EM et al (2013) Randomized trial of hypofractionated external-beam radiotherapy for prostate cancer. J Clin Oncol 31(31):3860–3868

Potter R, Georg P, Dimopoulos JC et al (2011) Clinical outcome of protocol based image (MRI) guided adaptive brachytherapy combined with 3D conformal radiotherapy with or without chemotherapy in patients with locally advanced cervical cancer. Radiother Oncol 100(1):116–123

Rajagopalan MS, Flickinger JC, Heron DE et al (2011) Changing practice patterns for breast cancer radiation therapy with clinical pathways: an analysis of hypofractionation in a large, integrated cancer center network. Pract Radiat Oncol 5(2):63–69. doi:10.1016/j.prro.2014.10.004

Ray KJ, Sibson NR, Kiltie AE (2015) Treatment of breast and prostate cancer by hypofractionated radiotherapy: potential risks and benefits. Clin Oncol 27(7):420–426

Roa W, Brasher PM, Bauman G et al (2004) Abbreviated course of radiation therapy in older patients with glioblastoma multiforme: a prospective randomized clinical trial. J Clin Oncol 22:1583–1588

Roa W, Kepka L, Kumar N et al (2015) International Atomic Energy Agency randomized phase III study of radiation therapy in elderly and/or frail patients with newly diagnosed glioblastoma multiforme. J Clin Oncol 33:1–6

Roy S, Pathy S, Mohanti BK et al (2016) Accelerated hypofractionated radiotherapy with concomitant chemotherapy in locally advanced squamous cell carcinoma of lung: evaluation of response, survival, toxicity and quality of life from a Phase II randomized study. Br J Radiol 89(1062):20150966. doi:10.1259/bjr.20150966

Radiation Therapy Oncology Group/National Surgical Adjuvant Breast and Bowel Project (2013) RTOG 0413/NSABP-39 Protocol. https://www.rtog.org/ClinicalTrials/ProtocolTable/StudyDetails.aspx?study=0413. Accessed 3 Aug 2016

Sanda MG, Dunn RL, Michalski J et al (2008) Quality of life and satisfaction with outcome among prostate-cancer survivors. N Engl J Med 358(12):1250–1261

Saunders M, Dische S, Barrett A et al (1999) Continuous, hyperfractionated, accelerated radiotherapy (CHART) versus conventional radiotherapy in non-small cell lung cancer: mature data from the randomised multi-centre trial. Radiother Oncol 52(2):137–148. doi:10.1016/S0167-8140(99)00087-0

Scott C, Curran W, Yung W et al (1998) Long term results of RTOG 90-06: a randomized trial of hyperfractionated radiotherapy (RT) to 72.0 Gy and carmustine versus standard RT and carmustine for malignant glioma patients with emphasis on anaplastic astrocytoma (AA) patients. J Clin Oncol 17:401a

SEER Stat Fact Sheets (2016) Brain and other nervous system cancer. National Cancer Institute. Surveillance, Epidemiology, and End Results Program. http://seer.cancer.gov/statfacts/html/brain.html#risk. Accessed 2 Aug 2016

Siegel RL, Miller KD, Jemal A (2016) Cancer statistics. CA Cancer J Clin 66(1):7–30. doi:10.3322/caac.21332

Slater D (2000) Study of hypofractionated proton beam radiation therapy for prostate cancer. In: ClinicalTrials.gov [Internet]. National Library of Medicine (US), Bethesda, MD [cited 1 Aug 2016]. https://clinicaltrials.gov/ct2/show/NCT00831623. NLM Identifier: NCT00831623

Smith BD, Bentzen SM, Correa CR et al (2011) Fractionation for whole breast irradiation: An American Society for Radiation Oncology (ASTRO) evidence-based guideline. Int J Radiat Oncol Biol Phys 81(1):59–68. doi:10.1016/j.ijrobp.2010.04.042

Sood BM, Gorla G, Gupta S et al (2002) Two fractions of high-dose-rate brachytherapy in the management of cervix cancer: clinical experience with and without chemotherapy. Int J Radiat Oncol Biol Phys 53(3):702–706

Souhami L, Seiferheld W, Brachman D et al (2004) Randomized comparison of stereotactic radiosurgery followed by conventional radiotherapy with carmustine to conventional radiotherapy with carmustine for patients with glioblastoma multiforme: report of Radiation Therapy Oncology Group 93-05 protocol. Int J Radiat Oncol Biol Phys 60(3):853–860

START Trialists' Group, Bentzen SM, Agrawal RK et al (2008a) The UK Standardisation of Breast Radiotherapy (START) Trial A of radiotherapy hypofractionation for treatment of early breast cancer: a randomised trial. Lancet Oncol 9(4):331–341. doi:10.1016/S1470-2045(08)70077-9

START Trialists' Group, Bentzen SM, Agrawal RK et al (2008b) The UK Standardisation of Breast Radiotherapy (START) Trial B of radiotherapy hypofractionation for treatment of early breast cancer: a randomised trial. Lancet 371(9618):1098–1107. doi:10.1016/S0140-6736(08)60348-7

Stupp R, Hegi ME, Mason WP et al (2009) Effects of radiotherapy with concomitant and adjuvant temozolomide versus radiotherapy alone on survival in glioblastoma in a randomized phase III study: 5-year analysis of the EORTC-NCIC trial. Lancet Oncol 10(5):459–466

Sylvester JE, Grimm PD, Blasko JC et al (2006) 15-year biochemical relapse free survival in clinical stage T1-T3 prostate cancer following combined external beam radiotherapy and brachytherapy; Seattle experience. Int J Radiat Oncol Biol Phys 67:57–64

The Greater Poland Cancer Centre (2000) Randomized, multi-center clinical trial comparing hypofractionated radiotherapy boost to conventionally fractionated combined with androgen deprivation therapy in a high risk group of prostate cancer patients (HYPOPROST). In: ClinicalTrials.gov [Internet]. National Library of Medicine (US), Bethesda, MD [cited 1 Aug 2016]. https://clinicaltrials.gov/ct2/show/NCT02300389. NLM Identifier: NCT02300389

Timmerman RD, Hu C, Michalski J et al (2014) Long-term results of RTOG 0236: a phase II trial of stereotactic body radiation therapy (SBRT) in the treatment of patients with medically inoperable stage I non-small cell lung cancer. Int J Radiat Oncol Biol Phys 90(Suppl 1):S30

Townsend NC, Huth BJ, Ding W et al (2011) Acute toxicity after cyberknife-delivered hypofractionated radiotherapy for treatment of prostate cancer. Am J Clin Oncol 34(1):6–10

Tsien CI, Brown D, Normolle D et al (2012) Concurrent temozolomide and dose-escalated intensity-modulated radiation therapy in newly diagnosed glioblastoma. Clin Cancer Res 18(1):273–279

University SU of NY-UM (2015) Pilot study of the safety and feasibility of administering concurrent systemic chemotherapy with accelerated hypofractionated radiation therapy in the treatment of medically inoperable T1b and T2 non-small cell lung cancer. ClinicalTrials.gov [Internet]. National Library of Medicine (US), Bethesda, MD. https://clinicaltrials.gov/ct2/show/NCT02619448. Accessed 8 Oct 2016

Wallner K, Roy J, Harrison L (1996) Tumor control and morbidity following transperineal I-125 implantation for Stage T1/T2 prostate carcinoma. J Clin Oncol 14:449–453

Walraven I, van den Heuvel M, van Diessen J et al (2016) Long-term follow-up of patients with locally advanced non-small cell lung cancer receiving concurrent hypofractionated chemoradiotherapy with or without cetuximab. Radiother Oncol 118(3):442–446. doi:10.1016/j.radonc.2016.02.011

Wang XS, Shi Q, Lu C et al (2010) Prognostic value of symptom burden for overall survival in patients receiving chemotherapy for advanced non-small cell lung cancer. Cancer 116(1):137–145

Wang EH, Mougalian SS, Soulos PR et al (2014) Adoption of hypofractionated whole-breast irradiation for early-stage breast cancer: a National Cancer Data Base analysis. Int J Radiat Oncol Biol Phys 90(5):993–1000. doi:10.1016/j.ijrobp.2014.06.038

Werner-Wasik M, Scott CB, Nelson DF (1996) Final report of a phase I/II trial of hyperfractionated and accelerated hyperfractionated radiation therapy with carmustine for adults with supratentorial malignant gliomas. Radiation Therapy Oncology Group Study 83-02. Cancer 77(8):1535–1543

Whelan T, MacKenzie R, Julian J et al (2002) Randomized trial of breast irradiation schedules after lumpectomy for women with lymph node-negative breast cancer. J Natl Cancer Inst 94(15):1143–1150. doi:10.1093/jnci/94.15.1143

Whelan TJ, Pignol JP, Levine MN et al (2010a) Long-term results of hypofractionated radiation therapy for breast cancer. N Engl J Med 362(6):513–520

Whelan TJ, Pignol JP, Levine MN, et al (2010b) Long-term results of hypofractionated radiation therapy for breast cancer. http://dx.doi.org/101056/NEJMoa0906260

Yarnold J, Ashton A, Bliss J et al (2005) Fractionation sensitivity and dose response of late adverse effects in the breast after radiotherapy for early breast can-cer: long-term results of a randomised trial. Radiother Oncol 75(1):9–17. doi:10.1016/j.radonc.2005.01.005

Yeoh EE, Fraser RJ, McGowan RE et al (2003) Evidence for efficacy without increased toxicity of hypofractionated radiotherapy for prostate carcinoma: early results of a phase III randomized trial. Int J Radiat Oncol Biol Phys 55:943–955

Yu JB, Cramer LD, Herrin J et al (2014) Stereotactic body radiation therapy versus intensity-modulated radiation therapy for prostate cancer: comparison of toxicity. J Clin Oncol 32(12):1195–1201

Zelefsky MJ, Fuks Z, Hunt M et al (2002) High-dose intensity modulated radiation therapy for prostate cancer: early toxicity and biochemical outcome in 772 patients. Int J Radiat Oncol Biol Phys 53(5):1111–1116

Zietman A, Moughan J, Owen J, Hanks G (2001) The Patterns of Care Survey of radiation therapy in localized prostate cancer: similarities between the practice nationally and in minority-rich areas. Int J Radiat Oncol Biol Phys 50:75–80

Zietman AL, Bae K, Slater JD et al (2010) Randomized trial comparing conventional-dose with high-dose conformal radiation therapy in early-stage adenocarcinoma of the prostate: long-term results from proton radiation oncology group/American college of radiology 95-09. J Clin Oncol 28(7):1106–1111

Brachytherapy: The Original Altered Fractionation

Mark Trombetta and Janusz Skowronek

Contents

M. Trombetta (✉)
Allegheny General Hospital,
Allegheny Health Network Cancer Institute,
Professor of Radiation Oncology, Drexel University
College of Medicine, Pittsburgh, Pennsylvania, USA
e-mail: mtrombet@wpahs.org

J. Skowronek
Professor, Head of Brachytherapy Department,
Greater Poland Cancer Centre, Associate Professor,
Electroradiology Department (secondary), Poznan
University of Medical Science, Poznań, Poland

1 The Evolution of Brachytherapy as a Discipline

Brachytherapy was first used for skin cancer in 1901 by Abbe (New York) and Strebel (Munich) reported the use of radium in the treatment of skin cancer and keloids (Curie and Curie 1898; Curie 1937; Mould 1997). In 1905, radium was used in interstitial brachytherapy, and radium was used for the first time in gynecology shortly afterward. The Institut du Radium was founded by the Polish scientist Marie Curie in Paris in 1909 and the Holt Radium Institute was created in Manchester in 1921. The first "cure" was identified in the United States by Robert Abbe in 1905 who reported on the treatment of cervix cancer. The excitement for such a "miracle" therapy was so great that no less than the inventor of the telephone, Alexander Graham Bell, postulated the use of tiny slivers of radium, sealed within a glass tube, to be placed interstitially and directly into a cancer. The rest is, as they say, history.

For nearly one-half of a century, brachytherapy enjoyed a parallel but superior role in the radiotherapeutic management of cancer until the post-World War II era which saw the development of teletherapy devices that could be manipulated to deliver photons precisely to tumors with less technical skill required by the operator. The emergence of megavoltage therapy, beginning with ^{60}Co devices, began the new era of radiotherapy by reducing skin reactions and increasing penetrance with improved precision. The dawn of the megavoltage betatron and

Med Radiol Radiat Oncol (2017)
DOI 10.1007/174_2017_95, © Springer International Publishing AG
Published Online: 08 August 2017

finally the linear accelerator seemed to signal the demise of brachytherapy … almost.

2 A Change in the Wind

With the advent of modern teletherapy devices, so began the change of focus from highly tactile and time-consuming brachytherapy approaches to more streamlined and high-throughput devices that incorporated the use of technicians and dosimetrists and adjunct personnel that allowed the radiotherapist (the term of the day) to become more efficient in the delivery of radiation to larger volumes of patients daily. As payors (whether governmental or private) developed reimbursements based on procedural metrics, a natural direction toward following convenience and increased revenue efficiency emerged. As computer algorithms and more accurate targeting of tumors due to superior imaging and localization improved the therapeutic ratio, brachytherapy was considered by some an almost "cult" therapy. With this newfound ability to safely deliver highly conformal, fractionated high-dose therapy, the total number of fractions increased significantly. While this technology allowed improved delivery and better local control, the impact on patients was significant in this modern day. Long courses of therapy, while improving local control and curability, are fraught with increased inconvenience and patient fatigue, especially for patients receiving multi-modality extended-course therapies.

3 The Era of Hypofractionation

Hypofractionation has appeared throughout the literature and in clinical practice in many forms over the years. The skin was a favorite site for early hypofractionated schedules due to its relative tolerance to irradiation (Zagrodnik et al. 2003; Kharofa et al. 2013; Avril et al. 1997). Additional roles in palliative radiotherapy have been well documented (Lutz et al. 2007; Jones 2013; Rades et al. 2011) and are considered the gold standard. In fact, traditionally fractionated regimens are felt by most radiation oncologists to be excessive and unnecessary. A seminal device in the application of hypofractionated (altered) fraction radiation was the Gamma Knife® (Elekta AB, Stockholm, Sweden). Introduced by Leksell in 1968 (Leksell 1983), this device has proven invaluable in the application of focused, altered fraction radiotherapy (Petrovich et al. 2003; Kruyt et al. 2017; Dong et al. 2016; McTyre et al. 2017). Increasingly and concurrent with improved skin dosing and targeting, "altered fraction" regimens have developed in the treatment of cancers of the lung (Fakiris et al. 2009; Timmerman et al. 2010), breast (Shah et al. 2013; Whelan et al. 2010; Smith et al. 2009, 2011; Skowronek et al. 2012), pancreas (De Baria et al. 2016; Crane 2016), liver (Kirichenko et al. 2016; Katz et al. 2007), prostate (Chadha et al. 2008; Hannoun-Levi et al. 2013), and nearly every disease site. The improvements in local control, decreases in morbidity, and patient satisfaction are well documented.

4 The Resurgence of the "Ultimate Conformal Therapy"

Brachytherapy has been termed by many as the "ultimate conformal therapy," and rightly so. Instead of delivering high energy through organs at risk that necessarily receive unwanted radiotherapy from without the body to within as is the case for teletherapy, the energy of brachytherapy emerges from the "inside-out" of the tumor. This "ultimate" form of delivery delivers better conformality and maximal effect from within the tumor while lessening such exposures to organs at risk. While gynecologic brachytherapy has enjoyed continual primary importance in the treatment role, other body site brachytherapy has decreased in usage. With the development of sophisticated computer algorithms and high-image-quality sonography, prostate brachytherapy enjoyed a strong resurgence in the 1980s which has continued to the present day. The emergence of breast brachytherapy as primary (Polgar et al. 2013; Strnad et al. 2016; Wenz et al. 2015; Cuttino et al. 2014; Shah et al. 2013; Polgar et al. 2016) therapy or in the event of ipsilateral breast tumor recurrences (Trombetta et al. 2011, 2016; Hannoun-Levi et al. 2011; Guix et al. 2010) has once again pushed brachytherapy to the forefront of clinical relevance.

5 Clinical Usage of Brachytherapy

5.1 Altered Fractionation in Clinical Brachytherapy

The efficacy of brachytherapy (BT) is attributed to the ability of radioactive sources to be placed close to or within the target to deliver higher radiation doses more precisely to the target than external beam radiotherapy (EBRT). As in EBRT, the biological effects depend on similar parameters such as total dose delivered, dose rate, fractionation schedule, overall treatment time, and volume parameters such as total volume treated to certain doses and the dose distribution within that treated volume. In BT, the dose is prescribed to an isodose encircling a small target volume, either D100 (100% of the minimum target dose, MTD), D98%, or D90 of the MTD. High doses delivered by BT are accepted only because the volumes treated are usually very small as compared to EBRT. Time-dose factors may also differ widely between EBRT and BT. In EBRT, the total dose is delivered in small daily exposure times of a few seconds or minutes, allowing for full repair between fractions. In the last few years, new machines such as Cyberknife® (Accuray Inc. Sunnyvale, California, USA) try to diminish this difference. In EBRT the overall treatment time is several weeks. In BT, by contrast, the dose is delivered either continuously (LDR, MDR) or discontinuously (PDR, HDR), and overall treatment times tend to be short (several hours to several days). This makes it possible to shorten patient's treatment time substantially (Skowronek et al. 2009a, 2010a, b). The following

are some disease site-based examples of altered treatment schedules.

5.2 Prostate Cancer

It's one of the best described examples of altered fractionation. First cases of BT in this location were performed with radium (1909 Zuckerkandl in Vienna, 1910 Paschkis, Titinger, Pasteau, Degais) (Skowronek 2009). The results were so bad for so many years that this technique was criticized. In 1952, for the first time Au-198 was used intraoperatively. An important step forward was made by Syed and Holm in 1983 when they incorporated perineal application of seeds (LDR-BT) under transrectal ultrasonography (TRUS) guidance (Skowronek 2013). In 1985, Bertelmann performed the first HDR Ir-192 application. For more than 30 years, both techniques (and later PDR-BT—pulsed-dose-rate brachytherapy) were used in hundreds of thousands of patients (King 2002). Additionally, LDR-BT is currently under research in breast, lung, pancreas, and head and neck cancers.

LDR-BT is one of the radiation methods known for almost 30 years in the treatment of localized prostate cancer. The main idea of this method is to implant small radioactive seeds as a source of radiation, directly into the prostate gland. LDR-BT can be applied as monotherapy and also used along with EBRT as a boost. It is used as a sole radical treatment modality, and however not as a palliative treatment. The application of permanent seed implants is a curative treatment alternative in patients with organ-confined cancer, without extracapsular extension of the tumor. Recommendations are based on risk groups which are confirmed by several societies (Nag et al. 1999; Ash et al. 2000; Grimm et al. 2012; Davis et al. 2012). This is an example of so-called continuous brachytherapy. LDR-BT has been a gold standard for prostate brachytherapy in low-risk patients for many years.

HDR-BT is a temporary type of brachytherapy where the high-dose-rate radioactive source (usually iridium 192 (^{192}Ir) or cobalt 60 (^{60}Co)) is put in the gland during the applicator implantation procedure. In Europe since at least 30 years, HDR-BT has been developed parallel to LDR-BT (Kovacs et al. 2005; Yamada et al. 2012; Burchardt et al. 2012); in the last few years it has also developed in the United States with growing interest. HDR equipment is commonly available and the radioactive source used for treatment is the same as in the case of other neoplasms. The dwell-time position of the source in the applicators may be freely programmed during the procedure, and the dwell time may be adapted to the requirements of treatment. In the course of treatment and real-time planning, the possibility of imprecise indication of the applicators position in relation to the treated gland is minimal, which ensures high precision of the treatment.

Initially HDR-BT was introduced as a high-dose-rate supplement for EBRT and proved to be an effective and safe method of treatment (Martinez et al. 2002; Demanes et al. 2000, 2005). Treatment of patients from the low- and intermediate-risk groups with HDR-BT monotherapy was initiated at the end of the previous decade (Demanes et al. 2011; Martinez et al. 2010; Rogers and Rogers 2010; Yoshioka et al. 2006; Zamboglou et al. 2013). Comparing discussed recommendations, we can clearly observe a tendency to shorten treatment time and number of fractions, typically in size of 7–11.5 Gy for monotherapy or 1–2 fractions of 10–15 Gy as a boost after EBRT. A recently published study found that a single, escalated dose of 19 Gray (Gy) may be a safe and effective alternative to longer courses of HDR treatment for men with localized prostate cancer (Krauss et al. 2017). Morton et al. compared two arms regarding early toxicity and quality-of-life results from a randomized phase II clinical trial of one fraction of 19 Gy or two fractions of 13.5 Gy. They concluded that both schedules—single 19 Gy and 13.5 Gy/2 fractions—are well tolerated. During the first 12 months, urinary symptoms and erectile dysfunction were more common in the two-fraction arm (Morton et al. 2017). Hoskin et al. also compared one single fraction of 19 Gy with two fractions of 13 Gy with the conclusion that single-dose HDR-BT is feasible with acceptable

levels of acute complications, and that tolerance may have been reached with the single 19 Gy schedule. Another single-HDR-fraction trial is ongoing (Hoskin et al. 2014).

5.3   Breast Cancer

With the prevalence of screening and increasing awareness of the disease, more and more women may be treated with breast-conserving surgery (BCS) with a complementary whole-breast EBRT and a boost to the tumor bed (Shaitelman et al. 2016). Results of conservative surgical treatment supplemented by radiation therapy are as good as the results obtained after mastectomy. Despite the evident equivalence of breast-conserving therapy with adjuvant whole-breast irradiation compared with mastectomy alone, up to 50% of patients in the United States who are clinically qualified for breast conservation still undergo mastectomy with the goal to omit radiation therapy. One of the most important reasons for the underuse of breast-conserving treatment is the length of adjuvant radiation therapy. "Boost" dose can be applied using different devices (interstitial flexible, reusable applicators) and HDR or PDR techniques. In HDR the advantages are as follows: one single high conformed fraction—dose ranged from 10 to 16 Gy and treatment on an outpatient basis. Further advances in radiotherapy techniques and knowledge of the biology of breast cancer increase the spectrum of application of accelerated partial breast irradiation (APBI) as a radical treatment in particular cases in addition to the standard methods of combination therapy (WBRT and "boost") (Strnad et al. 2016; Shah et al. 2013; Skowronek et al. 2012; Vicini et al. 2016; Ott et al. 2016). The first APBI treatments were done by Kuske and Vicini in 1992. This method of radiation therapy was used on a selected group of patients in the early stages of the disease. The advantage of APBI is also a shorter time of treatment from 5–7 weeks; (WBRT + boost) to 4–5 days of APBI. The number of fractions ranges from 8 to 10, at a fractional dose 3.4–4 Gy, twice daily. For many women such a short treatment is a favored treatment of choice.

5.4 Gynecological Cancer

Brachytherapy plays an essential role in the treatment of all gynecological tumors (Lee et al. 2016; Viswanathan and Thomadsen 2012; Viswanathan et al. 2012; Kirisits et al. 2014; Hellebust et al. 2010). In radical treatment, brachytherapy is usually combined with external beam radiation, but it can also be combined with surgery pre- and/or postoperatively. Brachytherapy is mainly applied as an intracavitary procedure, or in some cases done as interstitial implants. Radical brachytherapy for cervical and endometrial cancer is based on the use of intrauterine and intravaginal sources. There are several variations and choices available including a wide range of applicators (individualized molded applicators; different sized standard applicators with ovoids or with a ring Interstitial needles), different dose-prescribing and reporting systems related to historical traditions (depending also of country or technique preferred in specific region), different dose rates used (LDR, MDR (historical), PDR, HDR), and different schedules of dose (rate) and fractionation (Tanderup et al. 2016, 2017; Murakami et al. 2016). High-fraction doses are typical in HDR techniques, such as 3 fractions of 6 Gy in postoperative patients, 4 fractions of 7–7.5 Gy in radical sole treatment, and 5–6 fractions of 6 Gy frequently used in interstitial techniques.

5.5 Lung Cancer

Brachytherapy (BT) plays an important role in the palliative treatment of obstructive disease, sometimes in conjunction with endobronchial laser therapy or stent implantation (Stewart et al. 2016; Skowronek et al. 2009b, 2013; Skowronek 2015). Removal of an endobronchial obstruction often leads to quick improvement of clinical status and quality of life (QoL). Efforts to relieve this obstructive process are worthwhile, because patients may experience improved QoL in days or even hours after treatment. For patients with a bad performance status (Zubrod-ECOG-WHO score $\geq$ 2), single high doses ranging from 10 to 15 Gy may be applied. Brachytherapy plays a limited but specific role in definitive treatment with curative intent in selected cases of early endobronchial disease, in selected advanced inoperable tumors combined with EBRT, or in the postoperative treatment of small residual peribronchial disease. A less common indication is interstitial BT for peripheral tumors using permanent implants. In radical treatment combined with EBRT, 2–3 single "boost" doses are used in fraction sizes of 6–10 Gy. In radical sole treatment, radiologically occult cancer, such as T1-2N0, a total dose of 36–42 Gy in 6–7 fractions with an interval of 4–7 days between fractions is accepted but only in clinical studies (USA, Japan).

5.6 Esophageal Cancer

Endoesophageal brachytherapy allows the application of high doses of radiation to the tumor itself with concurrent protection of adjoining healthy tissues due to the rapid fall of dose by the inverse square of the distance from the center of the applicator. The above treatment is also associated with a relatively small proportion of late radiation complications. In the treatment of esophageal cancers, occasionally brachytherapy is used along with ERBT in doses of 10–40 Gy, which may extend the palliative effects of improved swallowing or decreased pain among patients. Brachytherapy used alone as an individual mode of treatment, in comparison to EBRT, gives a lower percentage of complications, out of which the most common problems are ulcerations and bleeding and bronchoesophageal fistulas. The aims of palliative brachytherapy are maintenance of oral intake, minimization of hospital stay, relief of pain, elimination of reflux and regurgitation, prevention of aspiration, and improvement of the patient's well-being. The HDR-BT doses proposed by the American Brachytherapy Society in 1997 and others are 1–3 fractions of 5–7.5 Gy (Kanikowski et al. 2009; Gaspar et al. 1997).

5.7 Head and Neck Cancer

The patients with locally recurrent head and neck cancers remain a challenge for oncologists. Treatment options are frequently limited for this group because of the extent of tumor precluding complete resection with clear surgical margins or the complicating factor of full-dose EBRT applied during first-line therapy. Brachytherapy (BT) alone or in combination with EBRT and chemotherapy may allow local dose escalation over the possibilities of EBRT alone. Major advantages of EBRT are the use of imaging targeting and organ at risk definition, the implementation of stepping source technology with the potential for intensity modulation, and the developments in medical and physics quality assurance (QA). Similarly, BT can provide specific intensive local interstitial irradiation allowing for the protection of surrounding structures, preserving organ function, and giving a good palliative effect. Both HDR and PDR techniques can be used depending on the location of the tumor. Seeds (LDR) are used only in clinical studies. Many different fractionation schemes can be used, sometimes shortening treatment time and using twice-daily fractions. Fractional doses are used extensively according to the studies recommended in the given center (Lukens et al. 2016; Mazeron et al. 2009; Kovács et al. 2017; Bartochowska et al. 2012).

Conclusion

Brachytherapy can be considered the original "altered fractionation" when considering current trends in modern radiotherapy. The role of brachytherapy is increasing in scope, but requires dedicated physicians committed to a "handcrafted" approach to personalized care and who are also committed to investing significant training and dedication to this original and resurgent art form.

References

Ash D, Flynn A, Battermann J, de Reijke T et al (2000) ESTRO/EAU/EORTC recommendations on permanent seed implantation for localized prostate cancer. Radiother Oncol 57:315–321

Avril M, Auperin A, Margulis A (1997) Basal cell carcinoma of the face: surgery or radiotherapy? Results of a randomized study. Br J Cancer 76(1):100–106

Bartochowska A, Wierzbicka M, Skowronek J et al (2012) High-dose-rate and pulsed-dose-rate brachytherapy in palliative treatment of head-and-neck cancers. Brachytherapy 11:137–143

Burchardt W, Skowronek J, Łyczek J (2012) Samodzielna brachyterapia HDR raka gruczołu krokowego—alternatywa we wczesnym stopniu zaawansowania. Przegl Urol 4:33–38. [in Polish]

Chadha M, Feldman S, Boolbol S et al (2008) The feasibility of a second lumpectomy and breast brachytherapy for localized cancer in a breast previously treated with lumpectomy and radiation therapy for breast cancer. Brachytherapy 7:22–28

Crane C (2016) Hypofractionated ablative radiotherapy for locally advanced pancreatic cancer. J Radiat Res 57(Suppl 1):i53–i57

Curie P, Curie M (1898) Proceedings of the academy of science

Curie, E (1937) Madame Curie: a biography by Eve Curie. Doubleday, Doran and Company, Inc., Country Life Press, Garden City, New York

Cuttino L, Arthur D, Vicini F et al (2014) Long term results from the Contura® multi-lumen balloon breast brachytherapy catheter phase 4 registry trial. Int J Radiat Oncol Biol Phys 90(5):1025–1029

Davis BJ, Horwitz EM, Lee WR et al (2012) American Brachytherapy Society consensus guidelines for transrectal ultrasound-guided permanent prostate brachytherapy. Brachytherapy 11:6–19

De Baria B, Portaa L, Mazzolab R et al (2016) Hypofractionated radiotherapy in pancreatic cancer: lessons from the past in the era of stereotactic body radiation therapy. Crit Rev Oncol Hematol 103:49–61

Demanes DJ, Rodriguez RR, Altieri GA (2000) High dose rate prostate brachytherapy: the California Endocurietherapy (CET) Method. Radiother Oncol 57:289–296

Demanes DJ, Rodriguez RR, Schour L et al (2005) High-dose-rate intensity-modulated brachytherapy with external beam radiotherapy for prostate cancer: California endocurietherapy's 10-year results. Int J Radiat Oncol Biol Phys 61(5):1306–1316

Demanes DJ, Martinez AA, Ghilezan M et al (2011) High-dose-rate monotherapy: safe and effective brachytherapy for patients with localized prostate cancer. Int J Radiat Oncol Biol Phys 81:1286–1292

Dong P, Pérez-Andújar A, Pinnaduwage D et al (2016) Dosimetric characterization of hypofractionated Gamma Knife radiosurgery of large or complex brain tumors versus linear accelerator-based treatments. J Neurosurg 125(Suppl 1):97–103

Fakiris A, McGarry RC, Yiannoutsos C et al (2009) Stereotactic body radiation therapy for early-stage non-small-cell lung carcinoma: four-year results of a prospective phase II trial. Int J Radiat Oncol Biol Phys 75(3):677–682

Gaspar LE, Nag S, Herskovic A et al (1997) American Brachytherapy Society (ABS) consensus guidelines for brachytherapy of esophageal cancer. Int J Radiat Oncol Biol Phys 38:127–132

Grimm P, Billiet I, Bostwick D et al (2012) Comparative analysis of prostate-specific antigen free survival outcomes for patients with low, intermediate and high risk prostate cancer treatment by radical therapy. Results from the Prostate Cancer Results Study Group. BJU Int 109(Suppl 1):22–29

Guix B, Lejarcegui JA, Tello JI et al (2010) Excision and brachytherapy as salvage treatment for local recurrence after conservative treatment for breast cancer: results of a ten-year pilot study. Int J Radiat Oncol Biol Phys 78:804–810

Hannoun-Levi JM, Castelli J, Plesu A et al (2011) Second conservative treatment for ipsilateral breast cancer recurrence using high-dose rate interstitial brachytherapy: preliminary clinical results and evaluation of patient satisfaction. Brachytherapy 10:171–177

Hannoun-Levi JM, Resch A, Gal J et al (2013) Accelerated partial breast irradiation with interstitial brachytherapy as second conservative treatment for ipsilateral breast tumor recurrence: multicentric study of the GEC-ESTRO Breast Cancer Working Group. Radiother Oncol 108(2):226–231

Hellebust TP, Kirisits C, Berger D et al (2010) Recommendations from Gynaecological (GYN) GEC-ESTRO Working Group: considerations and pitfalls in commissioning and applicator reconstruction in 3D image-based treatment planning of cervix cancer brachytherapy. Radiother Oncol 96(2):153–160

Hoskin P, Rojas A, Ostler P et al (2014) High-dose-rate brachytherapy alone given as two or one fraction to patients for locally advanced prostate cancer: acute toxicity. Radiother Oncol 110:268–271

Jones J (2013) A brief history of palliative radiation oncology. In: Lutz S, Chow E, Hoskin P (eds) Radiation oncology in palliative cancer care. Wiley-Blackwell, West Sussex

Kanikowski M, Skowronek J, Kubaszewska M, Chicheł A, Piotrowski T (2009) HDR brachytherapy (HDR-BT) combined with stent placement in palliative treatment of esophageal cancer. J Contemp Brachytheraphy 1(1):25–32

Katz A, Carey-Sampson M, Muhs AG et al (2007) Stereotactic body radiotherapy (SBRT) with or without surgery for primary and metastatic liver tumors. Int J Radiat Oncol Biol Phys 67(3):793–798

Kharofa J, Currey A, Wilson JF (2013) Patient-reported outcomes in patients with non-melanomatous skin cancers of the face treated with ortho-voltage radiation therapy: a cross-sectional study. Int J Radiat Oncol Biol Phys 87(4):636–637

King CR (2002) LDR vs HDR brachytherapy for localized prostate cancer—the view from radiobiological models. Brachytherapy 1:219–228

Kirichenko AV, Gayou O, Parda D et al (2016) Stereotactic body radiotherapy (SBRT) with or without surgery for primary and metastatic liver tumors. HPB 18(1):88–97

Kirisits C, Rivard MJ, Baltas D et al (2014) Review of clinical brachytherapy uncertainties: analysis guidelines of GEC-ESTRO and the AAPM. Radiother Oncol 110:199–212

Kovacs G, Potter R, Tillmann L et al (2005) GEC/ESTRO-EAU recommendations on temporary brachytherapy using stepping sources for localized prostate cancer. Radiother Oncol 74(2):137–148

Kovács G, Martinez-Monge R, Budrukkar A et al (2017) GEC-ESTRO ACROP recommendations for head & neck brachytherapy in squamous cell carcinomas: 1st update—improvement by cross sectional imaging based treatment planning and stepping source technology. Radiother Oncol 122:248–254

Krauss DJ, Ye H, Martinez AA et al (2017) Favorable preliminary outcomes for men with low- and intermediate-risk prostate cancer treated with 19-Gy single-fraction high-dose-rate brachytherapy. Int J Radiat Oncol Biol Phys 97:98–106

Kruyt IJ, Verheul JB, Hanssens PE et al (2017) Gamma Knife radiosurgery for treatment of growing vestibular Schwannomas in patients with neurofibromatosis Type 2: a matched cohort study with sporadic vestibular schwannomas. J Neurosurg 27:1–11

Lee LJ, Damato AL, Viswanathan AN (2016) Gynecologic brachytherapy. In: Devlin PM, Cormack RA, Holloway CL, Stewart AJ (eds) Brachytherapy. Applications and techniques, vol vol 2016, 2nd edn. Demos Medical Publishing, LLC, New York, pp 139–164

Leksell L (1983) Stereotactic radiosurgery. J Neurol Neurosurg Psychiatry 46(9):797–803

Lukens JN, Hu KS, Levendag PC, Teguh DN, Busse PM, Harrison LB (2016) Head and neck brachytherapy. In: Devlin PM, Cormack RA, Holloway CL, Stewart AJ (eds) Brachytherapy. Applications and techniques, vol vol 2016, 2nd edn. Demos Medical Publishing, LLC, New York, pp 235–292

Lutz ST, Chow EL, Hartsell WF et al (2007) A review of hypofractionated palliative radiotherapy. Cancer 109(8):1462–1470

Martinez AA, Gustafson G, Gonzalez J et al (2002) Dose escalation using conformal high-dose-rate brachytherapy improves outcome in unfavorable prostate cancer. Int J Radiat Oncol Biol Phys 53(2):316–327

Martinez AA, Demanes J, Vargas C et al (2010) High-dose-rate prostate brachytherapy: an excellent accelerated-hypofractionated treatment for favorable prostate cancer. Am J Clin Oncol 33(5):481–488

Mazeron J-J, Ardiet J-M, Haie-Méder C et al (2009) GEC-ESTRO recommendations for brachytherapy for head and neck squamous cell carcinomas. Radiother Oncol 91:150–156

McTyre E, Helis CA, Farris M et al (2017) Emerging indications for fractionated Gamma Knife radiosurgery. Neurosurgery 80(2):210–216

Morton G, Chung HT, McGuffin M et al (2017) Prostate high dose-rate brachytherapy as monotherapy for low and intermediate risk prostate cancer: early toxicity and quality-of life results from a randomized phase II clinical trial of one fraction of 19 Gy or two fractions of 13.5 Gy. Radiother Oncol 122:87–92

Mould RF (1997) In: Vahrson HW (ed) Radiation oncology of gynecological cancer. Springer, Berlin.

Murakami N, Kobayashi K, Kato T et al (2016) The role of interstitial brachytherapy in the management of primary radiation therapy for uterine cervical cancer. J Contemp Brachytherapy 8:391–398

Nag S, Beyer D, Friedland J et al (1999) American Brachytherapy Society (ABS) recommendations for transperineal permanent brachytherapy of prostate cancer. Int J Radiat Oncol Biol Phys 44(4):789–799

Ott OJ, Strnad V, Hildebrandt G et al (2016) GEC-ESTRO multicenter phase 3-trial: accelerated partial breast irradiation with interstitial multicatheter brachytherapy versus external beam whole breast irradiation: early toxicity and patient compliance. Radiother Oncol 120(1):119–123

Petrovich Z, Yu C, Giannotta SL et al (2003 Jul) Gamma knife radiosurgery for pituitary adenoma: early results. Neurosurgery 53(1):51–59

Polgar C, Fodor J, Major T et al (2013) Breast-conserving therapy with partial or whole breast irradiation: ten-year results of the Budapest randomized trial. Radiother Oncol 108:197–202

Polgar C, Hepel J, Pignol JP (2016) In: Montemaggi P, Trombetta M, Brady LW (eds) Brachytherapy: an international perspective. Springer, Berlin.

Rades D, Lange M, Veninga T et al (2011) Final results of a prospective study comparing the local control of short-course and long-course radiotherapy for metastatic spinal cord compression. Int J Radiat Oncol Biol Phys 79:524–530

Rogers L, Rogers LI (2010) Extended follow-up of high-dose-rate brachytherapy as monotherapy for intermediate-risk prostate cancer. Brachytherapy 9(Suppl. 1):S55–S56

Shah C, Vicini F, Wazer D et al (2013) The American Brachytherapy Society consensus statement for accelerated partial breast radiation. Brachytherapy 12:267–277

Shaitelman SF, Shah C, Kim LH, Vicini FA, Arthur DW, Khan AJ (2016) Breast brachytherapy. In: Devlin PM, Cormack RA, Holloway CL, Stewart AJ (eds) Brachytherapy. Applications and techniques, vol vol 2016, 2nd edn. Demos Medical Publishing, LLC, New York, pp 165–186

Skowronek J (2009) Brachytherapy in Greater Poland Cancer Centre and in Poznań—the past and the presence. J Contemp Brachytherapy 1(1):50–56

Skowronek J (2013) Low-dose-rate or high-dose-rate brachytherapy in treatment of prostate cancer—between options. J Contemp Brachytherapy 5(1):33–41

Skowronek J (2015) Brachytherapy in the treatment of lung cancer—a valuable solution. J Contemp Brachytherapy 4:297–311

Skowronek J, Zwierzchowski G, Piotrowski T (2009a) Hyperfractionation of HDR brachytherapy—influence on dose and biologically equivalent dose in clinical target volume and healthy tissues. J Contemp Brachytherapy 1(2):109–116

Skowronek J, Kubaszewska M, Kanikowski M, Chicheł A, Młynarczyk W (2009b) HDR endobronchial brachytherapy (HDRBT) in the management of advanced lung cancer—comparison of two different dose schedules. Radiother Oncol 93:436–440

Skowronek J, Zwierzchowski G, Piotrowski T, Milecki P (2010a) Optimization and it's influence on value of doses in HDR and PDR brachytherapy. Neoplasma 57(4):369–376

Skowronek J, Malicki J, Piotrowski T (2010b) Values of biologically equivalent doses in healthy tissues: comparison of PDR and HDR brachytherapy techniques. Brachytherapy 9:165–170

Skowronek J, Wawrzyniak-Hojczyk M, Ambrochowicz K (2012) Brachytherapy in accelerated partial breast irradiation (APBI): review of treatment methods. J Contemp Brachytherapy 4(3):152–164

Skowronek J, Piorunek T, Kanikowski M, Chicheł A, Bie|ęda G (2013) Definitive high-dose-rate endobronchial brachytherapy of bronchial stump for lung cancer after surgery. Brachytherapy 12:560–566

Smith B, Arthur D, Buchholz T et al (2009) Accelerated partial breast irradiation consensus statement from the American Society for Radiation Oncology (ASTRO). Int J Radiat Oncol Biol Phys 74(4):987–1001

Smith B, Bentzen SM, Correa C et al (2011) Fractionation for whole breast irradiation: an American Society for Radiation Oncology (ASTRO) evidence-based guideline. Int J Radiat Oncol Biol Phys 81(1):59–68

Stewart A, Parashar B, Patel M (2016) American Brachytherapy Society consensus guidelines for thoracic brachytherapy for lung cancer. Brachytherapy 15:1–11

Strnad V, Ott OJ, Hildebrandt G et al (2016) Five-year results of accelerated partial breast irradiation using sole interstitial multicatheter brachytherapy versus whole breast irradiation with boost after breast conserving surgery for low-risk invasive and in-situ carcinoma of the female breast: a randomized phase 3, non-inferiority trial. Lancet 387:229–238

Tanderup K, Lindegaard JC, Kirisits C et al (2016) Image Guided Adaptive Brachytherapy in cervix cancer: a new paradigm changing clinical practice and outcome. Radiother Oncol 120(3):365–369

Tanderup K, Ménard C, Polgar C et al (2017) Advancements in brachytherapy. Adv Drug Deliv Rev 109:15–25

Timmerman R, Paulus R, Galvin J et al (2010) Stereotactic body radiation therapy for inoperable early stage lung cancer. JAMA 303(11):1070–1076

Trombetta M, Julian TB, Werts ED et al (2011) Comparison of conservative management techniques in the retreatment of ipsilateral breast tumor recurrence. Brachytherapy 10:74–80

Trombetta M, Julian TB, Hannoun-Levi JM (2016) Breast brachytherapy: brachytherapy in the management of ipsilateral breast tumor recurrence. In: Montemaggi P, Trombetta M (eds) Brachytherapy: an international perspective. Springer, Brady LW

Vicini F, Shah C, Tendulkar R et al (2016) Accelerated partial breast irradiation: an update on published Level I evidence. Brachytherapy 15(5):607–615

Viswanathan AN, Thomadsen B (2012) American Brachytherapy Society consensus guidelines for locally advanced carcinoma of the cervix. Part I: General principles. Brachytherapy 11:33–46

Viswanathan AN, Beriwal S, De Los Santos JF et al (2012) American Brachytherapy Society consensus guidelines for locally advanced carcinoma of the cervix. Part II: High-dose-rate brachytherapy. Brachytherapy 11:47–52

Wenz F, Sedlmayer F, Herskind C et al (2015) Accelerated partial breast irradiation in clinical practice. Breast Care 10:247S2

Whelan T, Pignol JP, Levine M et al (2010) Long-term results of hypofractionated radiation therapy for breast cancer. N Engl J Med 362:513–520

Yamada Y, Rogers L, Demanes DJ et al (2012) American Brachytherapy Society consensus guidelines for high-dose-rate prostate brachytherapy. Brachytherapy 11:20–32

Yoshioka Y, Konishi K, Oh RJ et al (2006) High-dose-rate brachytherapy without external beam irradiation for locally advanced prostate cancer. Radiother Oncol 80(1):62–68

Zagrodnik B, Kempf W, Seifert E et al (2003) Superficial radiotherapy for patients with basal cell carcinoma. Cancer 98(12):2708–2714

Zamboglou N, Tselis N, Baltas D (2013) High-dose-rate interstitial brachytherapy as monotherapy for clinically localized prostate. Cancer: treatment evolution and mature results. Int J Radiat Oncol Biol Phys 85:672–678

Part I

Disease Site Specific Topics

Altered Fractionation in Radiotherapy of CNS Tumors

John C. Flickinger

Contents

Abstract

Hypofractionated radiotherapy approaches varying from single-fraction radiosurgery to 15-fraction short-course radiotherapy have been used with increasing frequency for managing a wide spectrum of benign and malignant primary tumors of the brain and skull base. Tumor control rates and complication rates appear comparable to those for fractionated conventional radiotherapy in most reports.

1 Introduction

There are a number of reasons why radiation oncologists have favored conventional fractionation with standard dose fractions of 1.8–2.0 Gy in the treatment of brain tumors. First and foremost is the fear of causing radiation necrosis in the brain. Worries about dose fractions greater than 2.0 Gy were firmly established in 1976 by Harris and Levene (Harris and Levene 1976) from an analysis of five cases of optic neuropathy that all received dose fractions of ≥ 2.5 Gy/fraction among 55 patients treated with different fractionation schedules. At that time, the existing radiobiological formulas to account for altered fractionation were based on skin reactions and none were fully developed for CNS tolerance. They, therefore, underestimated the effect of larger dose fractions on late-responding tissues like brain, and specifically optic nerve. This was interpreted as a clear danger signal for using any dose fraction >2 Gy in the

J.C. Flickinger
University of Pittsburgh, Pittsburgh, PA, USA
e-mail: flickingerjc@upmc.edu

Med Radiol Radiat Oncol (2017)
DOI 10.1007/174_2017_31, © Springer International Publishing AG
Published Online: 07 April 2017

treatment of brain tumors with the exception of whole-brain radiotherapy where the standard dose of 30 Gy in ten fractions was in wide use. Other reasons for favoring conventional fractionation are reluctance to change established practice and conformity with historical treatments. Presently treatment of glioblastoma patients with reasonably well-established hypofractionated schedules (5, 10, or 15 fractions which have similar efficacy as 60 Gy in 30 fractions in trials without temozolomide) is discouraged by the fact that most experimental protocols of drug treatments used after initial chemoradiotherapy require that standard fractionation be used.

Two developments have changed our rigidity with avoiding larger dose fractions. The first is the development of the linear quadratic formula (Douglas and Fowler 1976) around 1972 with delineation of parameters for predicting radiation injury in different organs including CNS. The second is the introduction of stereotactic radiosurgery. Radiosurgery was catalyzed by Leksell's seminal work in Sweden in the late 1950s, starting with orthovoltage radiation before moving to proton beam radiotherapy and then developing the Gamma Knife. Aside from the first use in treating trigeminal neuralgia, most of the early work in radiosurgery was with arteriovenous malformations and acoustic schwannomas, which were previously regarded as radioresistant, with very few patients treated by fractionated radiotherapy at the time. Pituitary adenomas, craniopharyingiomas, and meningiomas were also treated with early radiosurgery. The rapid integration of radiosurgery into widespread use in the United States and other countries accelerated in the late 1980s with frame-based Gamma Knife and linear accelerator single-fraction radiosurgery of brain tumors including brain metastases.

1.1 Linear Quadratic Formula

The linear quadratic formula is widely accepted as accounting for the effects of altered fractionation in radiotherapy. It allows equivalent doses for effects on different tumors and different normal tissues to be estimated for different dose fractions. The following formula is used to calculate the 2 Gy/fraction equivalent dose:

$$ED\left(2\ Gy\,/\,fr, \alpha\,/\,\beta\right)$$
$$= D_{\mathrm{d}}\left[1 + d\,/\left(\alpha\,/\,\beta\right) + RF\right]\,/\left[1 + 2\,/\left(\alpha\,/\,\beta\right) + RF\right]$$

where ED (2 Gy, α/β) is the equivalent total dose at 2 Gy/fraction for a specific effect on a specific tissue or tumor with a given alpha/beta ratio (α/β) value, d is the alternate dose/fraction, and D_{d} is the total dose at d-Gy per fraction. RF is a repopulation factor that can usually be omitted for treatment times shorter than 2–3 weeks when accelerated repopulation begins, at least for rapidly responding tissues like head-and-neck tumors where it has been demonstrated from analysis of radiotherapy series with varied treatment breaks.

Table 1 displays the 2 Gy/fraction equivalent doses for different tissues for several commonly used hypofractionated treatment schedules used for treatment of benign and malignant brain tumors. The dose schedules of 10 Gy in one fraction, 18 Gy in three fractions, and 25 Gy in five fractions are accepted dose limits for optic chiasm/optic nerve tolerance. Doses of 30–40 Gy in five fractions have been used with Cyberknife® (Accuray Inc, Sunnyvale, Ca. USA) treatment of skull base chordomas and chondrosarcomas. Doses of 25, 34, and 40 Gy in 5, 10, and 15 fractions have been used extensively in treating elderly and other risk patients with glioblastoma. To limit risks of radiation injury with hypofractionation to sensitive structures such as the optic chiasm, brainstem, or spinal cord, it is best to use the most conservative 2 Gy/fraction dose-equivalent estimates with alpha/beta = 1, even though $\alpha/\beta = 2$ is more commonly used for brain tissue.

There are several limitations of the linear quadratic formula for comparing radiation schedules with different fractionation. First of all the alpha/beta ratios for different tumors are not well characterized because they are difficult to calculate without widely varying the dose per fraction used. Most of the earliest tumor alpha/beta ratios came from cell culture studies with the limited numbers of tumors that could be grown in cell culture, which were all rapidly growing tumors. Benign tumors are very difficult to grow in cell culture. Although there is quite a bit of variation in alpha/beta ratios for different tumors, the average value for most cell cultures lines is around $\alpha/\beta = 10$ and that became the standard value used

Table 1 2-Gy/fraction equivalent dose calculations for several commonly used hypofractionated radiation treatment schedules that were calculated for different alpha/beta ratio values of 1, 2, 7.5, and 10 used to represent responses of spinal cord (1), brain (2), skin erythema/mucositis (7.5), or possible tumor control (10) respectively

Total dose	Fractions	Dose/fr	ED2Gy (1)	ED2Gy (2)	ED2Gy (7.5)	ED2Gy (10)
10	1	10	36.7	30.0	18.4	16.7
18	3	6	42.0	36.0	25.6	24.0
21	3	7	56.0	47.3	32.0	29.8
24	3	8	72.0	60.0	39.1	36.0
27	3	9	90.0	74.3	46.9	42.8
20	5	4	33.3	30.0	24.2	23.3
25	5	5	50.0	43.8	32.9	31.3
30	5	6	70.0	60.0	42.6	40.0
35	5	7	93.3	78.8	53.4	49.6
40	5	8	120.0	100.0	65.2	60.0
34	10	3.4	49.9	45.9	39.0	38.0
40	15	2.67	48.9	46.7	42.8	42.2
42	14	3	56.0	52.5	46.4	45.5
45	15	3	60.0	56.3	49.7	48.8

to represent tumors. Recent analyses of hypofractionated radiotherapy of prostate cancer and even of breast cancer have supported alpha/beta ratios around 1.5–3 Gy for prostate cancer and 3 Gy for breast cancer (Haviland et al. 2013). Using a model with apoptotic-resistant mice, Garcia-Barros et al. (2003) demonstrated that most of the response treatment of tumors to single high dose fractions of radiation is from supporting endothelial cells within tumors. This explains why brain metastases from tumors that are known to be relatively resistant to standard radiotherapy, like melanoma and sarcoma, have radiosurgery responses that are similar to more responsive tumors like breast cancer and small-cell lung cancer. Another limitation of the linear quadratic formula is that it overestimates the effect of large dose fractions, particularly above 8–10 Gy per fraction (Park et al. 2008).

1.2 Possible Advantages of Hypofractionated Radiotherapy

Table 2 lists possible advantages versus disadvantages of hypofractionated radiotherapy compared to conventional radiotherapy. Presently the only accepted clinical models for predicting tumor formation after exposure to radiation calculate risk based on total dose

Table 2 Advantages versus disadvantages of hypofractionated radiotherapy

Advantages
1. Fewer fractions
a. Lower cost and greater convenience
b. Five or less fractions allows for radiosurgery
2. Lower total dose
a. Lower risk of second tumor formation
b. Possibly less immune suppression
3. Possible reduced acute radiation effects
4. Shorter overall treatment time should limit tumor repopulation

Disadvantages
1. Less published experience with hypofractionated radiotherapy shedules than with standard fractionation.
2. Some dose schedules calculated to respect radiation tolerance dose-limits of normal structures may be less effective for rapidly growing malignant tumors
3. Ineligibility for many clinical trials in glioblastoma with hypofractionated chemo-radio-therapy
4. Lower reimbursement for physicians and hospitals

without respect for the dose per fraction used. Compared to conventionally fractionated radiotherapy, the lower total doses for hypofractionated radiotherapy and especially single-fraction radiosurgery mean lower risk of second tumor formation. This is a special concern for young patients with benign tumors. The paper by Yovino et al. (2013) correlating immunosuppression in glioblastoma patients with radiation treatment volume also suggests that the lower doses used with hypofractionated radiotherapy schedules and smaller treatment volumes used with radiosurgery techniques should result in less immunosuppression.

1.3 High-Grade Gliomas

Table 3 compares median survivals for elderly and poor-risk patients with glioblastoma or other high-grade glioma (anaplastic astrocytoma) in several randomized trials of hypofractionated radiotherapy (Roa et al. 2004, 2015; Phillips et al. 2003; Malmström et al. 2012; Perry et al. 2016). The 2 Gy/fraction dose equivalents for all these different schedules are listed in Table 1 and generally correspond to a dose of 50 Gy/25 fractions which is below the tolerance for radiation injury to the optic chiasm or brain stem. Curiously, the equivalent doses calculated for tumor control with an estimated $\alpha/\beta = 10$ predict tumor control effects comparable to 31, 38, and 42 Gy for the 25, 34, and 40 Gy schedules with 5, 10, and 15 fractions, respectively. Nevertheless the observed tumor control in these randomized trials was no different than that observed for 60 Gy in 30 fractions. One possible explanation is that tumor repopulation during the more protracted 6-week fractionation balances any potential gain in tumor cell killing from the higher dose of 60 Gy, and allows treatment with more economical 3D treatment techniques which usually can be planned and started more quickly than IMRT plans. Another alternative explanation is that the α/β ratio for tumor cell killing is lower and closer to that for normal brain. The study arm of the last trial receiving 3 weeks of temozolomide plus radiotherapy to 40 Gy in 15 fractions had a similar survival to most series of better-risk patients getting 6 weeks of temozolomide plus 60 Gy in 30 fractions. Thus, there is strong reason to believe that hypofractionated chemoradiotherapy with temozolomide should have similar effectiveness to standard chemoradiotherapy (60 Gy in 6 weeks with temozolomide) in both poor-risk patients and in younger better-risk patients.

Figure 1 shows a treatment plan for short-course radiotherapy with 25 Gy in five fractions and the 6-week follow-up scan response. Because of the lower costs, improved patient convenience, and lower risks of brain injury expected with the shorter course hypofractionated radiotherapy schedules, there are good reasons to compare one or more of these schedules with standard chemoradiotherapy in a large clinical trial and to offer younger and better-risk patients the option of short-course chemoradiotherapy for initial postoperative management of their glioblastoma.

Table 3 Summary of randomized trials of hypofractionated radiotherapy in elderly and poor-risk glioblastoma/high-grade glioma patients

Trial	Pts	Dose	Tmz	Med OS
Roa: Canada (Roa et al. 2004)	47	40 Gy/15 fr	No	5.6 mo
	48	60 Gy/30fr	No	5.1 mo
Phillips: Australia (Phillips et al. 2003)	32	35 Gy/10 fr	No	8.7 mo
	36	60 Gy/30 fr	No	10.3 mo
Nordic (Malmström et al. 2012)	93	34 Gy/10 fr	No	7.4 mo
	98	60 Gy/30 fr	No	6.0 mo
	100	No XRT	Yes	8.4 mo
IAEA (Roa et al. 2015)	49	25 Gy/5 fr	No	7.9 mo
	49	40 Gy/15	No	6.4 mo
Perry (abstract) (Perry et al. 2016)	281	40 Gy/15	Yes	13.5 mo
	281	40 Gy/ 15	No	7.7 mo

TMZ Temazolomide

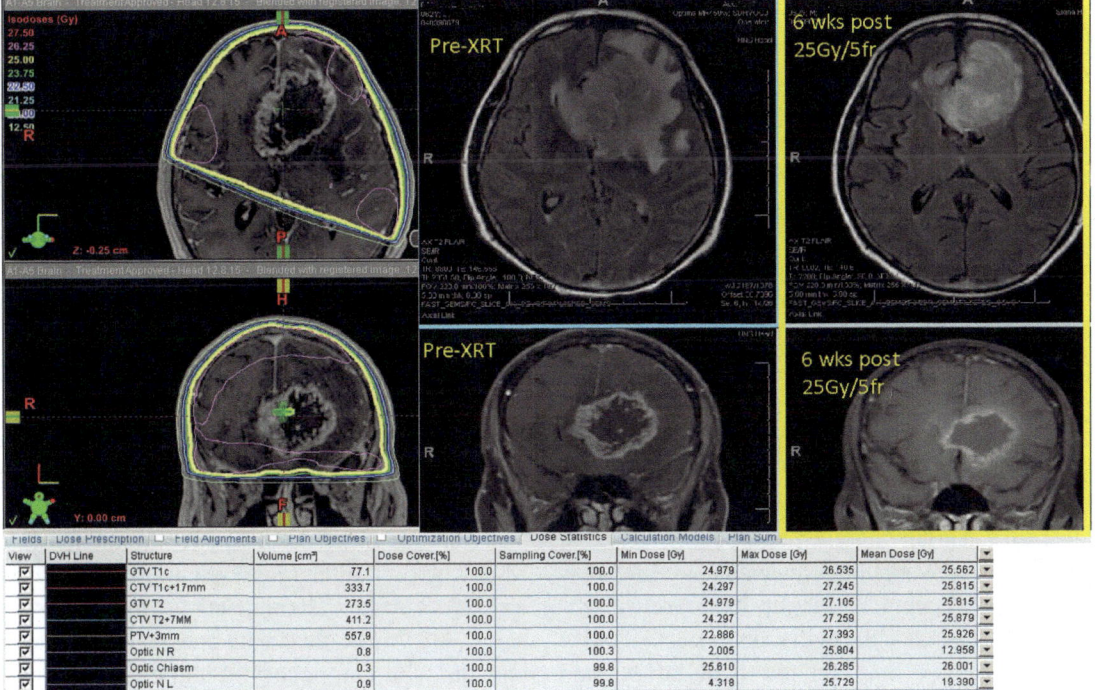

View	DVH Line	Structure	Volume [cm³]	Dose Cover.[%]	Sampling Cover.[%]	Min Dose [Gy]	Max Dose [Gy]	Mean Dose [Gy]	
☑		GTV T1c	77.1	100.0	100.0	24.979	26.535	25.562	▼
☑		CTV T1c+17mm	333.7	100.0	100.0	24.297	27.245	25.815	▼
☑		GTV T2	273.5	100.0	100.0	24.979	27.105	25.815	▼
☑		CTV T2+7MM	411.2	100.0	100.0	24.297	27.259	25.879	▼
☑		PTV+3mm	557.9	100.0	100.0	22.886	27.393	25.926	▼
☑		Optic N R	0.8	100.0	100.3	2.005	25.804	12.958	▼
☑		Optic Chiasm	0.3	100.0	99.8	25.610	26.285	26.001	▼
☑		Optic N L	0.9	100.0	99.8	4.318	25.729	19.390	▼

Fig. 1 Radiotherapy treatment plan (*left* axial and coronal images) for hypofractionated radiotherapy to a MGMT-positive glioblastoma with 25 Gy in five fractions. Patient was 62 years old and because of poor liver function from metastatic colon carcinoma and recurrent cholangitis, he was unable to be treated with temozolomide chemotherapy. *Right*-sided axial and coronal panels show the response 6 weeks after short-course radiotherapy alone with reduced T2-Flair signals, and reduced midline shift, while follow-up evaluation showed resolution of confusion and return of ambulation. Six months after treatment, he became confused again and was placed into hospice care after follow-up scans showed tumor progression

1.4 Pontine Glioma

Diffuse intrinsic pontine glioma (DIPG) has a poor prognosis in both children, where it comprises 10–15% of pediatric brain tumors and in adults where it is much more uncommon. Because of this, hypofractionated radiotherapy has been explored in pediatric DIPG. Zaghloul et al. (2014) randomized 71 newly diagnosed Egyptian cases of DIPG involving >50% of the pons in subjects <18 years old with ≤3-month history of symptoms between standard XRT to 54 Gy in 30 fractions and short-course hypofractionated XRT to 39 Gy in 13 fractions. The 2 Gy per fraction equivalent doses for the short course calculated with alpha/beta values of 1, 2, or 10 are 52, 48.75, and 42.25 Gy, respectively. The hypofractionated arm compared to the standard arm had slightly poorer median overall survival (6.6 vs. 7.3 months), but slightly better 1-year overall survival (22.5% vs. 17.9%) with the differences not reaching significance. They could not exclude 20% inferiority of the hypofractionated arm in this study with the number of patients enrolled.

1.5 Vestibular Schwannomas

Vestibular schwannomas, also known as acoustic neuromas, are benign tumors of the eighth cranial nerve composed of proliferating Schwann cells and are therefore not true neuromas. Left untreated, they can cause imbalance, hearing loss, tinnitus, facial weakness, numbness, and eventually brainstem compression with hydrocephalus. Unlike in meningiomas and glioblastomas, hypofractionated radiotherapy starting with single-fraction radiotherapy became more widely accepted for managing them before conventionally fractionated radiotherapy. Up until the 1980s, when radiosurgery started to move towards more widespread use, vestibular schwannomas were regarded by otoneurologists and neurosurgeons as radioresistant, which left surgery and observation as the only accepted options. Until the introduction of CT and later MR imaging, spontaneous cases of vestibular schwannomas (not related to type 2 neurofibromatosis) were difficult to diagnose until they were relatively large and compressing the brain stem. Most benign tumors like meningiomas or schwannomas shrink very slowly, if at all, after radiotherapy. If patients and surgeons expected clinical improvement, (relief of hydrocephalus, hearing improvement, etc.) as a result of treating large vestibular schwannomas with radiotherapy, they would normally have been disappointed. This made the high risks of postoperative facial weakness and limited hope of hearing preservation with most surgical resections seem acceptable at the time. After early single-fraction radiosurgery series started reporting better patient outcomes for small- and medium-sized vestibular schwannomas, surgical resection became less attractive to patients and the majority of vestibular schwannomas are now managed with some form of radiation treatment with either single-fraction radiosurgery, usually to 12–12.5 Gy, hypofractionated radiosurgery to 18–21 Gy in 3 fractions, 20–25 Gy in 5 fractions, or 45–50.4 Gy at 1.8 Gy/fraction. While some series report improved hearing control with fractionated radiation treatment versus single-fraction radiosurgery, no controlled randomized trials have been performed to settle the controversy. Moussavi et al. (2016) reported the highest rates of postradiosurgery hearing preservation in patients with the highest levels of hearing in the University of Pittsburgh series. Serviceable hearing preservation rates after radiosurgery were 98%, 73%, and 33% for patients with Class I-A, I-B1, and I-B2 hearing, respectively. No comparisons of hearing preservation following single-fraction versus hypofractionated radiosurgery that are matched for hearing levels to this degree have been performed.

1.6 Pituitary Adenomas

Conventional radiotherapy of pituitary adenomas was in widespread use even before the development of CT and MR imaging, since the pituitary fossa is easy to identify on plain AP and lateral X-ray films. Conventional external beam radiotherapy with doses of 45–50.4 Gy at 1.8 Gy/fraction is presently used for treatment of nonfunctional and hormone-secreting pituitary adenomas. The University of Pittsburgh series (Breen et al. 1998) analyzed 120 nonfunctional pituitary adenoma patients treated to 37.6–65.6 Gy, with 15 recurrences at 1–25 years and a median of 9 years of follow-up (range 0.1–32 years). Actuarial tumor control rates at 10, 20, and 30 years were 87.5%, 77.6%, and 64.7%, respectively. Tumor progression after radiotherapy occurred significantly more often ($p = 0.0397$) in patients with oncocytomas than in patients with non-oncocytic null-cell adenomas. No other factors correlated significantly with tumor control. One case of optic and oculomotor neuropathy developed 4.5 years after a maximum dose of 50 Gy in 25 fractions. Patients who received higher doses of radiation than the median 1.8 Gy/fraction dose equivalent of 48 Gy actually had slightly poorer tumor control than patients who received lower doses (many of whom received 40 Gy in 20 fractions). This was apparently by chance, as the difference was not statistically significant ($p = 0.225$). The rate of second tumor formation (meningioma and glioblastoma) was 2.7% by 20–30 years. Follow-up of all the pituitary adenoma patients irradiated at the University of Pittsburgh also identified a higher-than-expected rate of stroke which was later confirmed in the larger series of Brada et al. (1999) and Flickinger et al. (1989). Both of these problems in follow-up are reasons to consider stereotactic radiosurgery of hypofractionated radiotherapy with smaller treatment volumes and lower total radiation doses than those used with standard fractionated radiotherapy.

Sheehan et al. (2005) published an excellent review of pituitary adenoma radiosurgery in 2005. From 1998 to 2004, 17 nonfunctional pituitary adenoma radiosurgery series with 416 patients were published. Median follow-up varied from 16 to 49 months with a mean of 36.5 months. Median tumor margin doses varied from 14 to 25 Gy with a mean value of 16 Gy. Tumor control rates varied from 92 to 100% with a median of 96%. From 1991 to 2003, 22 radiosurgery radiosurgery series for ACTH producing pituitary adenomas with 310 patients were published. Median follow-up varied from 16 to 204 months with a median of 41.5 months. Median reported growth control was 95% (68–100%). Endocrine cure rates with varying criteria for cure varied widely from 10 to 100% with a median rate of 56%. Out of 25 reports of radiosurgery for acromegaly in 420 patients with median follow-up values of 12–55 months (34-month median), growth control rates varied from 66 to 100% with mean and median values of 96 and 100%. Endocrinological cure rates according to differing criteria varied as widely as possible from 0 to 100% with a median cure rate of 44%. With a median follow-up of 30 months (range 12–55 months) and doses of 13.3–33 Gy (median 21 Gy) in 22 series for prolactinoma radiosurgery (total of 393 patients), the growth control varied from 68 to 100% (median = 96%) and endocrine cure rates according to differing criteria varied from 0 to 84% (median = 19%).

In 2011, Park et al. (2011) reported a series of 125 patients with nonfunctional pituitary adenomas who underwent Gamma Knife radiosurgery to a median dose of 13 Gy (range: 10–25 Gy) at the University of Pittsburgh with median follow-up of 62 months and maximum of 22 years. The Kaplan-Meier-assessed tumor control rates at 5 and 10 years were 94%, and 76%, respectively. Decreased progression-free survival correlated with larger tumor volume ($\geq$4.5 cm^3) and $\geq$2 prior recurrences. Out of 88 patients with residual pituitary function, 21 (24%) developed new hormonal deficits at a median of 24 months (range: 3–114 months). The risk of developing decreased pituitary hormones was higher among 17 patients who had prior radiotherapy. One patient (0.8%) had a decline in visual function, and two (1.6%) developed new cranial neuropathies without tumor progression.

Lee et al. (2014a) reported the North American Gamma Knife Consortium analysis of 569 patients with nonfunctional pituitary adenomas irradiated to a median marginal dose of 16 Gy (range: 5–35 Gy) with a median follow-up of 36 months (range: 1–223 months). Treatment volumes varied from 0.08 to 35.2 cm^3 with a median of 3.3 cm^3. Maximum optic doses varied from 0 to 21 Gy with a median of 7.4 Gy. Tumor control rates (Kaplan-Meier) at 5 and 10 years were 85% and 85%, respectively. Tumor progression developed in 9/34 (26.5%) of patients treated with <12 Gy, 17/355 (4.5%) receiving 12–20 Gy, and 5/60 (8%) receiving >20 Gy.

Iwata et al. (2016) reported on long-term results with hypofractionated Cyberknife® radiosurgery for Cushing's disease. Marginal doses were 17.4–26.8 Gy in three fractions and 20.0–32.0 Gy in five fractions. Median follow-up was 60 months (range 27–137). The 5-year overall survival, local control, and disease-free survival rates (Kaplan-Meier) were 100%, 100%, and 96%, respectively. Only 9/52 (17%) patients met the Cortina consensus criteria for remission (random GH <1 ng/mL or <0.4 mg/mL after a glucose tolerance test and normal IGF-1). No post-SRT grade 2 or higher visual disorder developed.

Figure 2 shows an example of a four-fraction hypofractionated radiosurgery plan for recurrent/persistent invasive Cushing's disease after two transsphenoidal resections. The plan was designed to cover all possible occult diseases within the standard target volume that would have been used for fractionated conventional radiotherapy, as opposed to standard single-fraction radiosurgery plans which are designed to deliver the highest possible safe dose to only suspected gross tumor.

Haghighi et al. (2015) reported their experience in Australia treating 112 cavernous sinus region tumors (55 pituitary adenomas and 57 meningiomas) with short-course hypofractionated radiotherapy to mean dose of 38 Gy (range: 37.5–40 Gy) in 15 fractions (similar to one of the schedules used for poor-risk glioblastoma patients) (Haghighi et al. 2015). The 2 Gy/fr dose equivalents for 37.5–40 Gy in 15 fractions are

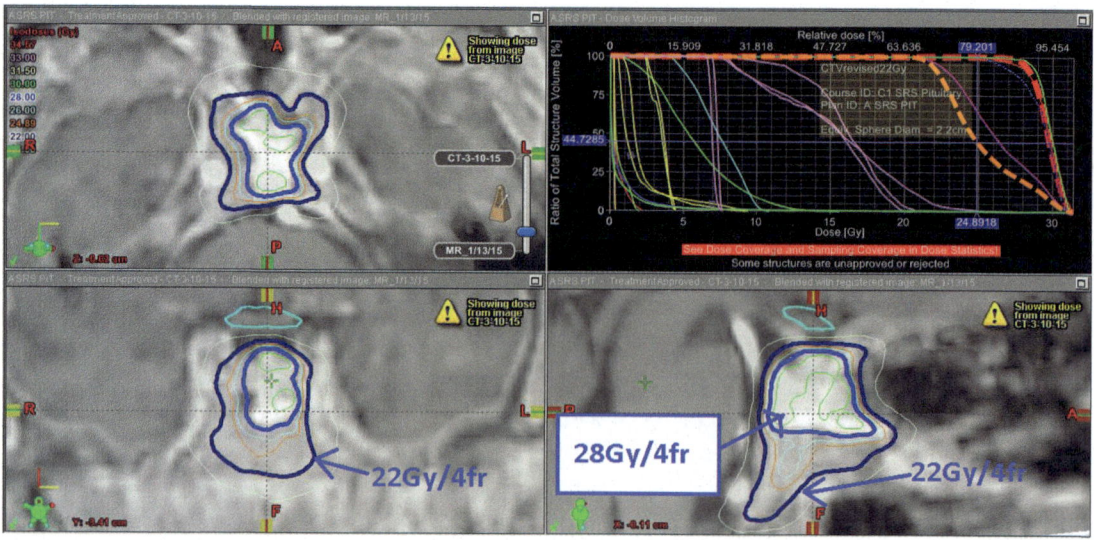

Fig. 2 Four-fraction radiosurgery plan for invasive Cushing's disease persisting after two transsphenoidal resections. The treatment plan was designed to cover the same treatment volume that would have been treated with conventionally fractionated radiotherapy to a marginal dose of 22 Gy and the suspected gross tumor to a marginal dose of 28 Gy. The 2 Gy/fraction dose equivalents were 47.7 and 35.8 Gy for 22 Gy/4 fr compared to 75.7 and 63 Gy for 28 Gy/4 fr using alpha/beta values of 1 and 2, respectively. The maximum doses to optic chiasm, and right and left optic nerves, were only 10.5, 9.3, and 9.5 Gy in four fractions, respectively

43.75–48.9 Gy and 42.1–46.7 Gy for alpha/beta values of 1 and 2, respectively. The median follow-up was 77 months (range: 2.3–177). After hypofractionated short-course radiotherapy, pre-existing cranial neuropathies resolved or improved in 57% and 38%, respectively; remained stable in 38%; and worsened in 5%. The diagnosis of meningioma was associated with potential recovery of cranial neuropathy ($p < 0.001$). Permanent cranial neuropathies associated with radiotherapy developed in three patients (3%). The 5- and 10-year tumor control rates (Kaplan-Meier) were 96% and 96%, respectively, for pituitary adenomas compared to 98% and 93%, respectively, for meningiomas.

1.7 Meningiomas

Because meningiomas commonly occur in elderly patients, some of whom may have transportation difficulties, hypofractionated radiotherapy schedules, including single-fraction radiosurgery, may be more attractive than conventional radiotherapy. The lowest possible expected risk of second tumor formation with single-fraction radiosurgery makes that especially attractive in patients with radiation-induced and multiple meningiomas.

Navarria et al. (2015) reported their experience in Milan treating 26 patients with skull-based meningiomas with volumetric modulated rapid-arc (VMAT) 30 Gy in five fractions. The 2 Gy/fr equivalent doses for that schedule would be 70 Gy or 60 Gy for alpha/beta ratios of 1 or 2, respectively. Nine patients were treated after prior resection and 17 received primary radiotherapy with no resection. After a median follow-up of 24.5 months (range 5–57 months) complete symptom remission developed in 9/18 (50%) symptomatic patients and partial improvement in the remaining 9 (50%). The eight asymptomatic patients remained so after treatment. No grade 3–4 neurological toxicity developed.

Maranzano et al. (2015) from Terni, Italy, reported their experience with hypofractionated short-course radiotherapy using 3 Gy fractions to either 42 Gy ($n = 49$) or 45 Gy ($n = 31$) in 77 meningioma patients (37 WHO-Grade 1, 12 WHO Gr 2, and 28 unbiopsied) with a median follow-up of 56 months. The 2 Gy/fr dose equivalents for 42 and 45 Gy at 3 Gy/fraction are 56 and 60 Gy versus 52.5 and 56.3 Gy with alpha/beta values of 1 versus 2, respectively. Local control was 84% at both 5 and 10 years.

Han et al. at UCLA (Han et al. 2014) reviewed 220 basal meningiomas in 213 patients treated by stereotactic radiosurgery and hypofractionated and fractionated radiotherapy in 55, 22, and 143 cases, respectively, with median volumes of 2.8, 4.8, and 11.1 cm^3 to median doses of 12.5 Gy, 25 Gy, and 50.4 Gy in 1, 5, and 28 fractions. With a median follow-up of 32 months (range 7–97 months), they reported tumor control in 91%, 94%, and 94%, respectively, for the SRS, hypofractionated, and conventional radiotherapy groups with no significant differences.

Concern about postradiosurgery edema is often the reason for choosing conventional or hypofractionated radiotherapy over single-fraction radiosurgery in the treatment of meningiomas particularly with parafalcine or parasagittal locations, Schulz-Ertner et al. (2007) analyzed postradiosurgery edema in 212 patients from multiple centers in the International Gamma Knife Research Foundation with a median of 20 (range: 6–158) months of follow-up. Median dose was 14 Gy (8–20 Gy) and median volume was 5.2 mL. Tumor edema was stable or regressed in 53%, temporarily increased and then regressed in 33%, and worsened without regressing in 5%. Worsening of edema correlated with venous sinus invasion or compression, as well as with increasing volume, and marginal and maximum doses.

1.8 Chordomas

Early attempts at controlling chordoma with conventional radiotherapy were limited to maximum doses of 54–60 Gy to avoid brainstem injury and produced poor tumor control. The development of 3D conformal radiotherapy treatment planning and delivery techniques for proton beam radiotherapy during the 1970s allowed for dose escalation to cobalt dose equivalents of 72–78 Gy at 1.8–2 Gy per fraction of skull base chordomas

and chondrosarcomas. As a result, proton beam radiotherapy became the standard of care for postoperative management of these tumors. Sheehan et al. (2015) performed a dose-response analysis from published literature and recommended a 2 Gy/fraction Co^{60} dose equivalent of 75 Gy for chordoma.

Stereotactic radiotherapy has also been used to manage these tumors when they are sufficiently small either in place of proton beam radiotherapy or for tumor recurrence after initial postoperative radiotherapy. Kano et al. (2011) analyzed data for 71 skull base chordoma patients from 6 centers in the North American Gamma Knife® Consortium managed by single-fraction radiosurgery. The median target volume was 7.1 cm^3 (range 0.9–109 cm^3) and median marginal dose was 15.0 Gy (range 9–25 Gy). Five-year local control (LC) and overall survival (OS) rates were 69 and 93% for 50 patients with no prior fractionated radiotherapy. For 21 patients treated for salvage after prior radiotherapy, the 5-year rates of LC and OS were 62% and 43%, respectively.

Henderson et al. (2009) reported the Georgetown University experience with Cyberknife® treatment of 18 patients with chordoma in the clivus (39%), sacrum (17%), or mobile spine (44%). Mean tumor volume was 128 cm^3 (range: 12–457 cm^3) and median marginal dose was 35 Gy (range: 24–40 Gy). One patient with a C3–C4 tumor was treated primarily without resection and was reported as free of recurrence at 65 months. The other 17 patients had surgical resections. In general, patients who received prior radiotherapy were treated with 7 Gy × 4 fractions. Patients with no prior radiotherapy received 5 fractions of 7 or 7.5 Gy before 2007 and 8 Gy × 5 fractions after 2007. The authors recommend treatment with 8 Gy × 5 fractions to gross tumor with at least a 1 cm margin. From their data, the author's estimated that for chordomas $\alpha/\beta = 2.45$, not much different than values of 2.0–2.5 that have been used for normal brain, As shown in Table 1 the 2 Gy/fraction equivalent doses for 35 and 40 Gy in five fractions for $\alpha/\beta = 2$ are 78.8 and 100 Gy, respectively. Three previously irradiated patients developed decreased vision with additional diplopia in two of those three. One patient developed C3–C4 hypoesthesia after radiosurgery. Odynophagia and/or esophagitis were reported in three patients, undoubtedly from the radiosurgery. Pain was listed as a complication from surgery and radiation in two patients with spine tumors.

Because there is a greater published experience with proton beam irradiation of skull base chordomas with standard fractionation than with 1–5 fractions of radiosurgery or other hypofractionated schedules, it is widely regarded as the adjuvant treatment of choice following maximal resection. Radiosurgery with one or five fractions, depending on volume, appears reasonable for recurrent tumors or for initial treatment of patients who are unwilling or unable to travel to a proton center, if the treatment volume is reasonable for radiosurgery. IMRT with standard fractionation could be considered for larger tumors if proton beam irradiation can't be given.

1.9 Chondrosarcomas

Chondrosarcomas behave somewhat similar to chordomas except that it appears from the proton beam literature that they can be more easily controlled with radiotherapy (particularly if a complete resection has not been achieved) and with slightly lower doses of radiation. Radiosurgery has been used for treating skull base chondrosarcomas that are small at diagnosis or small recurrences after conventional proton beam radiotherapy. Kano et al. (2015) analyzed the outcome in 46 patients for the North American Gamma Knife® Consortium with a median follow-up of 75 months. Prior resections were performed in 36 and prior fractionated radiotherapy in 5 patients. Median marginal dose was 15 Gy (range: 10.5–20 Gy) and median tumor volume was 8.0 cm³ (range: 0.9–28.2 cm³). Five- and ten-year overall survivals calculated by Kaplan-Meier were 86% and 76%, respectively, with progression-free survivals of 85% and 70%. Prior radiotherapy was associated with poorer local control. Among the 41 patients with no prior radiotherapy, tumor control was higher in patients treated with ≥15 Gy and with tumors <8 cm³ (where it was 100% at 10 years in both groups but with two later recurrences). Only three patients (7%) developed adverse postradiosurgery injury. Pre-SRS cranial nerve deficits improved in 22 (56%) of the 39 patients after SRS.

The published experience with hypofractionated radiation in chondrosarcoma is somewhat more limited. Jiang et al. (2013) reported Stanford's Cyberknife® experience from 1996 to 2011 with treating 20 chondrosarcomas (12 cranial and 8 spinal), with a median follow-up of 33 months. Median tumor volume was 11 cm³ and median marginal doses were 22, 24, 26, 27, and 30 Gy for 1, 2, 3, 4, and 5 fractions, respectively. The corresponding 2 Gy/fraction equivalent doses would be 169, 104, 84, 70, and 70 Gy for $\alpha/\beta = 1$ (cord injury) and 132, 84, 69, 59, and 60 Gy for $\alpha/\beta = 2$ (brain injury). Five- and ten-year survivals were 80% and 60%, respectively. Five-year tumor control (Kaplan-Meier) was only 41%. They reported better tumor control for cranial versus spinal tumors (58% vs. 38%). Radiation injury developed in one patient.

1.10 Paragangliomas/Glomus Tumor

Although paragangliomas have relatively high control rates with standard fractionated radiotherapy doses of 45–50 Gy in 25–28 fractions, both radiosurgery and short-course hypofractionated radiotherapy offer tumor control with greater convenience, lower risk of secondary tumor formation, and possibly less mucositis for the largest tumors extending down into the neck. Sheehan et al. (2012) reported the North American Gamma Knife® Consortium experience in 132 patients with a median follow-up of 50.5 months (range 5–220 months). Six patients had prior fractionated radiotherapy and 51 had prior resection. Median tumor dose was 15 Gy. Five-year tumor control (Kaplan-Meier) was 88% and was associated with the absence of trigeminal nerve dysfunction. Pulsatile tinnitus (present in 40% of patients at the time of radiosurgery) improved in

49% post-SRS. New or progressing cranial nerve deficits developed in 11% of patients, usually associated with recurrence. No patients died from tumor progression.

Chun et al. (2014) reported the UT-Southwestern experience in 31 skull base paragangliomas treated by Cyberknife® with 25 Gy in five fractions (2 Gy fraction equivalents of 50, 44, and 32.5 Gy for alpha/beta values of 1, 2, and 8, respectively, corresponding to cord, brain, and mucosa). Local control was 100% with a median follow-up of 24 months (range 4–78 months). Out of 20 patients with tinnitus, 30% developed partial resolution and another 30% developed complete resolution. Tumor volume shrunk by 37% in patients with >2 years of follow-up.

1.11 Craniopharyngiomas

Radiosurgery and hypofractionated stereotactic radiotherapy may be preferable to conventional radiotherapy in managing craniopharyingiomas as a strategy to limit radiation dose to optic and memory pathways, adjacent vasculature, pituitary gland, and all normal tissue at risk for development of secondary neoplasms. Niranjan et al. (2010) reported the University of Pittsburgh Gamma Knife® (Elekta AB, Stockholm, Sweden) experience with 51 craniopharyngiomas with a median follow-up of 62 months (range 12–232 months). Median marginal dose was 13 Gy (range 9–20 Gy) and median treatment volume was 1.0 cm^3 (range 0.07–8.0 cm^3). Local control (Kaplan-Meier) at 5 years was 91.6% for solid tumor but was 68% when cyst control was included. Not all cysts were covered by the radiosurgery treatment volumes used. Post-SRS visual deterioration occurred in two patients who developed homonymous hemianopsia from tumor progression. No patients developed any new hypopituitarism. Kobayashi et al. (2015) reported 30 craniopharyngioma patients treated to a mean marginal dose of 11.7 Gy with a mean follow-up of 80 months. Progression-free survival at both 5 and 10 years was 76%. Lee's et al. (2014b) series of 137 craniopharyngioma patients treated with a

median dose of 12 Gy (range: 9.5–16 Gy) was less favorable with 5- and 10-year local control rates of 70% and 40%, respectively.

Iwata et al. (2012) reported the Cyberknife® experience with 43 cases at a median follow-up of 40 months (range 12–92 months). Median tumor volume was 2.0 cm^3 (range 0.09–11 cm^3). Three cases underwent single-fraction SRS to 13–16 Gy. Hypofractionated SRS was delivered to doses of 16, 21, and 25 Gy in 2, 3, and 5 fractions in 2, 33, and 5 cases corresponding to 2 Gy fraction equivalent doses of 48, 56, and 50 Gy for $\alpha/\beta = 1$ and 40, 47, and 44 Gy for $\alpha/\beta = 2$, respectively.

Hashizume et al. (2010) reported the Nagoya experience with short-course hypofractionated radiotherapy using a Novalis® stereotactic system (Brainlab, Munich, Germany) in ten craniopharyngioma patients with median tumor volumes of 8 cm^3 (range: 1.1–21 cm^3) and median follow-up of 25.5 months (range 9–36 months). Doses of 30–39 Gy in 10–15 fractions (median 33 Gy) were delivered with 2 Gy/fraction equivalents of 46–68 Gy (median 60.2) for $\alpha/\beta = 4$ and relatively high maximum optic system 2 Gy fraction dose equivalents of 45–89 Gy (median 79 Gy) for $\alpha/\beta = 2$. All tumors were controlled, 8/10 showed response, and no complications had yet developed at the time of publication.

Conclusions

Alternate fractionation radiotherapy has changed the paradigm for site-specific CNS more than any other anatomic region of the body. It should be a prime consideration for intracranial and spinal tumors, benign and malignant.

References

Brada M, Burchell L, Ashley S et al (1999) The incidence of cerebrovascular accidents in patients with pituitary adenoma. Int J Radiat Oncol Biol Phys 45(3):693–698

Breen P, Flickinger JC, Kondziolka D et al (1998) Radiotherapy for nonfunctional pituitary adenoma: analysis of long-term tumor control. J Neurosurg 89(6):933–938

Chun SG, Nedzi LA, Choe KS et al (2014) A retrospective analysis of tumor volumetric responses to five-fraction stereotactic radiotherapy for paragangliomas of the head and neck (glomus tumors). Stereotact Funct Neurosurg 92(3):153–159

Douglas BG, Fowler JF (1976) The effect of multiple small doses of X-rays on skin reactions in the mouse and a basic interpretation. Radiat Res 66:401–426

Flickinger JC, Nelson PB, Taylor FH et al (1989) Incidence of cerebral infarction after radiotherapy for pituitary adenoma. Cancer 63(12):2404–2408

Garcia-Barros M, Paris F, Cordon-Cardo C, Lyden D et al (2003) Tumor response to radiotherapy regulated by endothelial cell apoptosis. Science 300(5622):1155–1159

Haghighi N, Seely A, Paul E et al (2015) Hypofractionated stereotactic radiotherapy for benign intracranial tumours of the cavernous sinus. J Clin Neurosci 22(9):1450–1455

Han J, Girvigian MR, Chen JC et al (2014) A comparative study of stereotactic radiosurgery, hypofractionated, and fractionated stereotactic radiotherapy in the treatment of skull base meningioma. Am J Clin Oncol 37(3):255–260

Harris JR, Levene MB (1976) Visual complications following irradiation for pituitary adenomas and craniopharyngiomas. Radiology 120(1):167–171

Hashizume C, Mori Y, Kobayashi T et al (2010) Stereotactic radiotherapy using Novalis for craniopharyngioma adjacent to optic pathways. J Neuro-Oncol 98(2):239–247

Haviland JS, Owen JR, Dewar JA et al (2013) The UK Standardization of Breast Radiotherapy (START) trials of radiotherapy hypofractionation for treatment of early breast cancer: 10-year follow-up results of two randomized controlled trials. Lancet Oncol 14(11):1086–1094

Henderson FC, McCool K, Seigle J et al (2009) Treatment of chordomas with CyberKnife: Georgetown university experience and treatment recommendations. Neurosurgery 64(2 Suppl):A44–A53

Iwata H, Tatewaki K, Inoue M et al (2012) Single and hypofractionated stereotactic radiotherapy with CyberKnife for craniopharyngioma. J Neuro-Oncol 106(3):571–577

Iwata H, Sato K, Nomura R et al (2016) Long-term results of hypofractionated stereotactic radiotherapy with CyberKnife for growth hormone-secreting pituitary adenoma: evaluation by the Cortina consensus. J Neuro-Oncol 128(2):267–275

Jiang B, Veeravagu A, Feroze AH et al (2013) CyberKnife radiosurgery for the management of skull base and spinal chondrosarcomas. J Neuro-Oncol 114(2):209–218

Kano H, Iqbal FO, Sheehan J et al (2011) Stereotactic radiosurgery for chordoma: a report from the North American Gamma Knife Consortium. Neurosurgery 68(2):379–389

Kano H, Sheehan J, Sneed PK et al (2015) Skull base chondrosarcoma radiosurgery: report of the North

American Gamma Knife Consortium. J Neurosurg 123(5):1268–1275

Kobayashi T, Tsugawa T, Hatano M et al (2015) Gamma knife radiosurgery of craniopharyngioma: results of 30 cases treated at Nagoya Radiosurgery Center. Nagoya J Med Sci 77(3):447–454

Lee CC, Kano H, Yang HC et al (2014a) Initial Gamma Knife radiosurgery for nonfunctioning pituitary adenomas. J Neurosurg 120(3):647–654

Lee CC, Yang HC, Chen CJ et al (2014b) Gamma knife surgery for craniopharyngioma: report on a 20-year experience. J Neurosurg 121(Suppl):167–178

Malmström A, Grønberg BH, Marosi C et al (2012 Sep) Nordic Clinical Brain Tumour Study Group (NCBTSG). Temozolomide versus standard 6-week radiotherapy versus hypofractionated radiotherapy in patients older than 60 years with glioblastoma: the Nordic randomized, phase 3 trial. Lancet Oncol 13(9):916–926

Maranzano E, Draghini L, Casale M et al (2015 Dec) Long-term outcome of moderate hypofractionated stereotactic radiotherapy for meningiomas. Strahlenther Onkol 191(12):953–960

Mousavi SH, Niranjan A, Akpinar B et al (2016) Hearing sub-classification may predict long-term auditory outcomes after radiosurgery for vestibular schwannoma patients with good hearing. J Neurosurg 125(4):845–852

Navarria P, Pessina F, Cozzi L et al (2015) Hypofractionated stereotactic radiation therapy in skull base meningiomas. J Neuro-Oncol 124(2):283–289

Niranjan A, Kano H, Mathieu D et al (2010) Radiosurgery for craniopharyngioma. Int J Radiat Oncol Biol Phys 78(1):64–71

Park C, Papiez L, Zhang S et al (2008) Universal survival curve and single fraction equivalent dose: useful tools in understanding potency of ablative radiotherapy. Int J Radiat Oncol Biol Phys 70(3):847–852

Park KJ, Kano H, Parry PV et al (2011) Long-term outcomes after gamma knife stereotactic radiosurgery for nonfunctional pituitary adenomas. Neurosurgery 69(6):1188–1199

Perry JR, Laperriere N, O'Callaghan CJ et al (2016) A phase III randomized controlled trial of short-course radiotherapy with or without concomitant and adjuvant temozolomide in elderly patients with glioblastoma (CCTG CE.6, EORTC 26062-22061, TROG 08.02, NCT00482677). J Clin Oncol 34 (suppl; abstr LBA2)

Phillips C, Guiney M, Smith J et al (2003) A randomized trial comparing 35Gy in ten fractions with 60Gy in 30 fractions of cerebral irradiation for glioblastoma multiforme and older patients with anaplastic astrocytoma. Radiother Oncol 68(1):23–26

Roa W, Brasher PM, Bauman G et al (2004) Abbreviated course of radiation therapy in older patients with glioblastoma multiforme: a prospective randomized clinical trial. J Clin Oncol 22(9):1583–1588

Roa W, Kepka L, Kumar N et al (2015) International Atomic Energy Agency randomized phase III study of radiation therapy in elderly and/or frail patients with newly diagnosed glioblastoma multiforme. J Clin Oncol 33(35):4145–4150

Schulz-Ertner D, Karger CP, Feuerhake A et al (2007) Effectiveness of carbon ion radiotherapy in the treatment of skull-base chordomas. Int J Radiat Oncol Biol Phys 68(2):449–457

Sheehan JP, Niranjan A, Sheehan JM et al (2005) Stereotactic radiosurgery for pituitary adenomas: an intermediate review of its safety, efficacy, and role in the neurosurgical treatment armamentarium. J Neurosurg 102(4):678–691

Sheehan JP, Tanaka S, Link MJ et al (2012) Gamma Knife surgery for the management of glomus tumors: a multicenter study. J Neurosurg 117(2):246–254

Sheehan JP, Cohen-Inbar O, Ruangkanchanasetr R et al (2015) Post-radiosurgical edema associated with parasagittal and parafalcine meningiomas: a multicenter study. J Neuro-Oncol 125(2):317–324

Yovino S, Kleinberg L, Grossman SA et al (2013) The etiology of treatment-related lymphopenia in patients with malignant gliomas: modeling radiation dose to circulating lymphocytes explains clinical observations and suggests methods of modifying the impact of radiation on immune cells. Cancer Investig 31(2):140–144

Zaghloul MS, Eldebawy E, Ahmed S et al (2014) Hypofractionated conformal radiotherapy for pediatric diffuse intrinsic pontine glioma (DIPG): a randomized controlled trial. Radiother Oncol 111(1):35–40

Head and Neck Cancer

Olgun Elicin and E. Mahmut Ozsahin

Contents

O. Elicin (✉)
Department of Radiation Oncology, Inselspital,
University Hospital of Bern, University of Bern,
Bern, Switzerland
e-mail: Olgun.Elicin@insel.ch

E. Mahmut Ozsahin
Department of Radiation Oncology, Lausanne
University Hospital, University of Lausanne,
Lausanne, Switzerland
e-mail: mahmut.ozsahin@chuv.ch

Abstract

In this chapter, various altered fractionation schedules are categorized and discussed within the landscape of clinical trials. Today, modern radiotherapy (RT) techniques are offering new avenues to exploit the advantages of altered fractionation not only for the primary treatment of treatment-naïve patients, but also in reirradiation and palliative situations. Novel agents, which are at least as effective but less toxic than platinum compounds, can be combined with contemporary RT techniques to widen the therapeutic window. Radiotherapy

Med Radiol Radiat Oncol (2017)
DOI 10.1007/174_2017_32, © Springer International Publishing AG
Published Online: 11 May 2017

with altered fractionation, both alone or as part of combined modalities with systemic therapy (ST), offers many opportunities to the head and neck oncologists.

1 Introduction

Head and neck cancer is the sixth most common cancer with an annual global incidence of about 600,000 cases (Siegel et al. 2015) and an age-standardized incidence of 15–20 per 100,000 (Ferlay et al. 2010). Squamous cell carcinoma is the dominant histology, for which alcohol and tobacco consumption are the main factors followed by the oncogenic human papillomavirus. About 80% of the new cases present in locoregionally advanced stages (Mohanti et al. 2007). Surgery, RT, or both remain as the main treatment modalities for locoregional disease. Despite aggressive curative treatments, over 80% of head and neck squamous cell carcinoma (HNSCC) recurrences occur above the clavicles (Carvalho et al. 2005). Another problem with similar therapeutic challenges is the development of second primary HNSCC (Cooper et al. 1989; Yamamoto et al. 2002), mainly because of "field cancerization" (Dakubo et al. 2007). There has been a continuous search for better local treatment alternatives with single or combined modalities involving surgery and RT with or without the combination of ST. Because it is deemed as a radiocurable disease, HNSCC has been considered as an ideal target for both preclinical and clinical research.

In addition to tumor stage and etiology, tumor volume, repopulation, and intrinsic and hypoxia-driven radioresistance are the main causes of RT failure (Good and Harrington 2013; Rischin et al. 2015). Traditionally, delivery of daily doses within the range of 1.8–2.2 Gy is considered as "normofractionation" (N). Based on clinical data and cell survival models (Thames et al. 1989), the most common regimens used to treat HNSCC were delivered using 1.8–2 Gy daily doses administered five times a week up to a total dose of around 60 to 70 Gy to the high-risk treatment volume in 6–7 weeks. With the emergence of dose painting techniques by intensity-modulated

radiotherapy (IMRT), slightly increased daily doses around 2.1 Gy were more frequently used in routine clinical practice.

Numerous randomized studies demonstrated the benefit of chemotherapy added to RT, which was confirmed with several meta-analyses (Budach et al. 2006; Blanchard et al. 2015), the most extensive and up to date being the MACH-NC meta-analysis ($n = 16,485$ patients) (Pignon et al. 2009). Without any significant beneficial effect of induction or adjuvant chemotherapy, only concomitant chemotherapy showed a significant increase in overall survival at 5 years: 6.5% absolute increase (hazard ratio [HR] 0.81; 95% confidence interval [CI] 0.78–0.86, $p < 0.0001$). No significant difference between mono- versus poly-chemotherapy regimens was observed. However, concomitant chemotherapy comes with the price of increased toxicity (Trotti et al. 2007). Therefore, RT with altered fractionation (AFRT) may be a feasible and safer alternative to chemo-RT, especially for "fragile" patients (Bentzen and Trotti 2007). Parallel to the MACH-NC, the large MARCH meta-analysis ($n = 6515$) showed the superiority of AFRT over N with an absolute overall survival benefit of 3.4% in 5 years (Baujat et al. 2010). Maximal effect was shown by hyperfractionation (HE) with an 8% increase in overall survival at 5 years (Baujat et al. 2010; Bourhis et al. 2006a). The most extensively investigated alternative schedules for HNSCC were HE and accelerated fractionation (AC). Generally, the main argument against the use of HE is logistical, for both the RT departments and patients (Rosenthal et al. 2015).

1.1 Radiobiologic Consequences of Altered Fractionation

Today, the use of hypofractionation (HO) schedules to treat HNSCC is rather uncommon and restricted to some special treatment settings. Most of the time, the reason to use HO is either logistical or to accelerate the treatment especially when the α/β of the tumor is low and the α/β of the surrounding healthy tissue is around the same level or ideally higher than that of the tumor.

Another reasonable goal of HO would be palliation, where long-term toxicity is not a concern, but may lead to a shorter hospital stay for some patients.

The biological rationale of fractionation was discussed in Chap. 2 in detail. According to the linear-quadratic model, each tissue is characterized by two parameters: α and β, where α represents the cell kill per dose resulting from nonreparable damage and based on the linear component of the survival curve, and β the cell kill per dose representing cumulative reparable damage and based on the quadratic component. The α/β ratio is inversely proportional to biological sensitivity to different fractionation regimens. Compared to the early-responding tissues, the dose-response relationship for late-responding tissues is influenced more from the curved β component. The main advantages of fractionation are reduced normal tissue reactions, allowance of tissue reoxygenation, and redistribution, whereas it may hamper the tumor control probability due to repair and repopulation occurring during an extended treatment time. Moreover, because of accelerated repopulation beginning after a 4-week lag phase, the effectiveness of later dose fractions will be compromised.

If an RT scheme is changed from many small doses to fewer large fractions, while the total dose is kept at an isoeffective level for tumor control probability and/or early effects, this new scheme will have more severe late effects. On the other hand, HE will result in reduced late effects, if the total dose is kept at a level to produce equal or slightly more severe early effects. Tumor control will be the same or slightly improved. Dose per fraction, total dose, and treatment volume are the most important factors for the late effects, on which the total treatment time has less impact. Similarly, total dose, treatment volume, but also the treatment time determine the severity of acute toxicities and the tumor control probability. One exception is the "consequential late toxicity" resulting from excess acute toxicity induced by over-acceleration (Peters et al. 1988). In summary, the difference in α/β ratios between HNSCC and late-responding tissues grants the opportunity to widen the therapeutic window.

1.2 Corresponding Therapeutic Implications of Altered Fractionation

There are countless combinations and confusing definitions of AC, HE, HO, and RT schedules. Roughly summarized, pure HE gives the same total dose in the same time, but with twice number of fractions, whereas impure HE increases the total dose with even more fractions in the same or longer time. Similarly, pure AC only shortens the treatment time without changing the fraction size (e.g., by continuously treating patients without pausing on the weekends), whereas hybrid AC may involve changes in other fractionation parameters throughout the whole or a part of the treatment course and can also fully (e.g., CHART) or partially incorporate HE (e.g., concomitant boost) with the aim of quickly completing the treatment. HO may be chosen with the intention of shortening the overall treatment time (i.e., AC), due to logistic reasons or patient comfort (e.g., HO for relatively small target volumes in reirradiation setting).

In the rest of this chapter, comparisons of different fractionation strategies in HNSCC are presented mainly within the context of prospective clinical trials published in the last three decades. Due to the bulk of unfavorable evidence collected in the past, "split-course" RT in the curative setting is not discussed in detail. Likewise, older studies using obsolete dose fractionation schedules are not included in the discussion. The meta-analyses will be discussed together toward the end of this chapter and not in the previous sections as scattered chunks of information. Throughout the chapter, all HRs and percentages with differences have p values under 0.05, if not otherwise stated.

2 Radiotherapy Alone, with or without Altered Fractionation

The majority of the clinical studies involving AFRT were designed to compare its effectiveness to N. Some of them directly compared N to a specific AFRT schedule, whereas others had multiple parallel arms trying to answer other questions about the possible benefits of ST and/or various AFRT schedules.

2.1 Pure Acceleration

The most straightforward approach to shorten the overall treatment time without changing any other fractionation parameter is omitting the weekend breaks. Investigators from Gliwice, Poland, conducted a randomized trial comparing N (5 days-a-week over 7 weeks) to "7-days-a-week fractionation continuous accelerated irradiation" (CAIR) with the same total and daily doses for locally advanced HNSCC (Skladowski et al. 2000, 2006). The primary endpoint was local control. This study demonstrated significant improvement in local control and progression-free and overall survival, but also increased acute mucositis with AC. Late toxicities remained similar to each other. Around the same period of time, another Polish group from Warsaw conducted a similar study, KBN PO 79 (Hliniak et al. 2002). The main differences were the selection of only laryngeal primaries in stages I–III and the AC methodology. Instead of treating seven daily fractions a week like CAIR, they performed bi-fractionation on Thursdays (i.e., 6 fractions a week). Interestingly, this study demonstrated increased rates of severe mucositis, odynophagia, and telangiectasia without any oncological benefit. Later, these two AC approaches were also compared head to head, which is discussed in the next section.

One of the landmark studies in this context is the DAHANCA 6 and 7 (Overgaard et al. 2003). This large study consisted of two parts: 6 and 7. Six hundred and ninety-four patients with glottic larynx primaries and 791 with various primary subsites were enrolled into DAHANCA 6 and 7, respectively. The treatment in the experimental arm was identical to the control arm except for overall treatment time (5.5 instead of 6.5 weeks by means of 6 instead of 5 weekly fractions). Patients in DAHANCA 7 also received oral nimorazole, a hypoxic cell radiosensitizer. With the primary endpoint of locoregional control, six compared with five fractions per week increased the 5-year locoregional control and progression-free survival. Accelerated fractionation also improved voice preservation among patients with laryngeal cancer (80 vs. 68%, $p < 0.01$). Acute grade ≥ 3 mucosal reactions were higher with AC,

all being reversible. Late toxicities were comparable (Mortensen et al. 2012). Post hoc analysis showed the lack of predictive value of p16 status concerning AC (Lassen et al. 2011). When the results of DAHANCA 6 were reported separately, the impact of AC on locoregional control and acute toxicities was significant too (Lyhne et al. 2015). The investigators showed a more prominent impact of AC on well-differentiated as well as early-stage (T1–2) tumors. Interestingly, no single isolated neck failure was reported in this large cohort. Recently, a similarly designed international trial (IAEA-ACC), led by the same group of investigators, confirmed the results of the Danish trial (Overgaard et al. 2010). Another landmark study, RTOG 9003, will be discussed exclusively in a dedicated section ahead.

The same question in the postoperative radiotherapy (PORT) setting was raised in two studies. The first study p-CAIR-1, conducted by the Polish team, compared the CAIR schedule with N in the high-risk postoperative oral cavity, oropharynx, and larynx cancer patients. With the primary endpoint of locoregional control, they could only show almost doubled acute grade ≥ 3 mucositis with CAIR (Suwiński et al. 2008). The second study, OCAT, was published only as a Congress abstract to date (Ghosh-Laskar et al. 2016a). Seven hundred patients diagnosed with stage III–IVB oropharynx cancer were randomized into three arms with the primary endpoint of locoregional control. Two arms compared N to AC PORT (5 vs. 6 fractions per week). No significant difference in outcome or toxicity was demonstrated.

Most of the head and neck trials involving mixed disease subsites exclude nasopharynx cancer, because it is considered as a distinct entity with different etiology and endemic incidence rates. NPC 9902 compared AC to N in two of its four arms (Lee et al. 2011). Unfortunately, the trial had to be closed prematurely due to slow accrual after recruiting 189 out of planned 464 patients. No difference could be shown in terms of outcome or late toxicity.

Despite the varying results, it is worthy to note that none of these trials comparing N versus pure AC showed any oncological/survival outcome favoring N (Table 1).

Table 1 Studies comparing normofractionation with pure acceleration

Authors (year)	Name or location	Sites	UICC stage[a]	n	Median follow-up (y)	Arm	Radiotherapy	Outcome in %[b] OS	PFS	LC	LRC	at y	Grade ≥3 toxicity[b]	Remarks
Skladowski et al. (2000)	CAIR-1	OC, OP, HP, L	II–IV	100	8	1	N: 66–72 Gy/33–36 f/7 w	20	18	33[c]		5	Increased acute mucositis in arm 2. LT comparable	
Skladowski et al. (2006)						2	AC: 66–72 Gy/33–36 f/5 w	62	60	75[c]				
Hliniak et al. (2002)	KBN PO 79	L	I–III	395	4.1	1	N: 66 Gy/33 f/6 w				NS[c]	2	Increased acute mucositis, odynophagia, and late telangiectasia in arm 2	
						2	AC: 66 Gy/33 f/5 w							
Overgaard et al. (2003) Mortensen et al. (2012)	DAHANCA 6&7	OC, OP, HP, L, NP	I–IV	1485	6.8	1	N: 66–68 Gy/33–34 f/6.5 w		66	64	60[c]	5	Increased acute mucositis in arm 2 LT comparable. Improved preservation of the voice in patients with L (80 vs. 68%) in arm 2	Patients in DAHANCA 7 also received nimorazole. p16 status not predictive (Lassen et al. 2011)
						2	AC: 66–68 Gy/33–34 f/5.5 w		73	76	70[c]			
Ezzat et al. (2005)	NCI Cairo	OC, OP, HP, L	III–IV	40	10.5	1	N: 68 Gy/34 f/6.5 w					2	Acute mucositis in arm 1 vs. 2 and 3. Hematological toxicities higher in arm 3. LT comparable	Not defined[c]
						2	AC: 68 Gy/34 f/5.5 w							
						3		Irrelevant						
Lee et al. (2006) Lee et al. (2011)	NPC 9902	NP	III–IV (T3–4, N0–1)	189	6.3	1	N: 70 Gy/35 f/7 w				NS[c]	5	Nonsignificant differences in AT and LT among arms 1 and 4	Terminated due to slow accrual (planned 464). The trial was designed to detect any difference in PFS compared to arm 1
						2		Irrelevant						
						3								
						4	AC: 70 Gy/35 f/6 w				NS[c]			

(continued)

Table 1 (continued)

Authors (year)	Name or location	Sites	UICC stage[a]	n	Median follow-up (y)	Arm	Radiotherapy	OS	PFS	LC	LRC	at y	Grade ≥3 toxicity[b]	Remarks
Suwiński et al. (2008)	p-CAIR-1	OC, OP, L	PORT, "high risk"	279	4	1	N: 63 Gy/35 f/7 w				NS[c]	3		
						2	AC: 63 Gy/35 f/5 w							
Overgaard et al. (2010)	IAEA-ACC	OC, OP, HP, L	I–IV	458	8.3	1	N: 66–70 Gy/33–35 f/7 w		40		30[c]	5	Increased AT and tube feeding in arm 2	Impact of AC on the primary site more prominent
						2	AC: 66–70 Gy/33–35 f/6 w		50		43[c]			
Lyhne et al. (2015)	DAHANCA 6	L (glottic)	I–IV	694	14.5	1	N: 66–68 Gy/33–34 f/6.5 w			78[d]	71[c]	10	Increased rate and duration of AT in arm 2 LT comparable	@: T1–2 primaries
						2	AC: 66–68 Gy/33–34 f/5.5 w			86[d]	78[c]			
Ghosh-Laskar et al. (2016a)	OCAT	OC	PORT III–IV	700	4.8	1	N: 56–60 Gy/28–30 f/6 w				NS[c]	5	All toxicities were comparable	
						2		Irrelevant						
						3	AC: 56–60 Gy/28–30 f/5 w				NS[c]			

[a]Nonmetastatic if not otherwise stated

[b]Only differences with $p \leq 0.05$ given, if not stated otherwise

[c]Primary endpoint

[d]See remarks

AC accelerated fractionation, *AT* acute toxicity, *f* fractions, *HP* hypopharynx, *L* larynx, *LT* late toxicity, *N* normofractionation, *NS* statistically not significant, *NP* nasopharynx, *O* other sites, *OC* oral cavity, *OP* oropharynx, *PORT* postoperative radiotherapy, *y* year, *w* weeks

2.2 Hybrid Acceleration

In the definitive RT setting, relatively fewer trials comparing AC to N yielded positive results. These trials often used concomitant boost (CB) technique, which can be described as a kind of partial HE. Others also used HE throughout the whole course of the treatment. But the main aim to use HE was not to (further) protect the normal tissue from late radiation damage or dose escalation, but to complete the treatment earlier than the planned time of the N schedule. One argument is finishing the treatment before accelerated repopulation starts; another argument is feasibility and optimization of financial resources. This concept is called accelerated-hyperfractionation (AC-HE). Therefore, the fraction doses were not as low as used in genuine HE schedules. Because of that, the acute toxicities sometimes reached an unbearable level. In order to overcome this problem, some investigators suggested incorporating a split-course concept, which is known to have a detrimental effect on tumor control due to accelerated repopulation. Like a vicious circle, to overcome the split and finish the treatment in 6–7 weeks, the dose fractionation had to be more aggressive. Consequently, this strategy brought more toxicity than benefit (Overgaard et al. 1988).

Two extreme examples to AC-HE are the CHART and V-CHART trials. In CHART, 918 patients with locally advanced HNSCC were randomized to receive 66 Gy in 33 fractions over 6.5 weeks or 54 Gy in 36 fractions, 3 days per week over 12 consecutive days (Dische et al. 1997). No significant difference was shown in local control, which was the primary endpoint. As expected, significantly more acute grade ≥3 toxicities were observed with CHART. However, late toxicities were significantly lower (Saunders et al. 2010). This may be explained with the lower total dose and strict compliance to the 6-hourly interfractional gaps. The latter trial, V-CHART, was conducted around the same time interval as CHART. It contained three randomized arms: N up to 70 Gy over 7 weeks and AC-HE, 55.3 Gy in 33 fractions over 17 consecutive days (Dobrowsky and Naudé 2000), and a third arm identical to the AC-HE plus mitomycin. In both AC-HE arms,

90% acute grade ≥3 mucositis was reported. The locoregional control or overall survival (primary endpoint) did not improve with AC-HE. Late toxicities were not reported.

It is important to note that the above-mentioned trials reduced the total dose in the AC arms. As a demonstrative example, the EORTC 22851 ($n = 512$) compared N using 70 Gy over 7 weeks against AC-HE up to 72 Gy in 45 fractions over 5 weeks (which included a 2-week split) (Horiot et al. 1997). The primary endpoint locoregional control at 5 years was significantly improved with AC-HE (59% vs. 46%). However, late grade ≥3 toxicity tripled (14% vs. 4%, respectively).

Similar results were reproduced in most of the other trials evaluating potential benefits of various AC strategies (i.e., AC with CB, AC-HE with or without split course) in definitive RT or PORT for locally advanced HNSCC. Regardless of the details of the AC method, if the total biologically equivalent dose was similar to the N schedule the oncological outcome improved at the cost of increased toxicity. If the total dose was reduced, the oncological outcome was similar or inferior to N, but the late toxicity profile improved (Table 2).

2.3 Hyperfractionation

Hyperfractionation (HE) is generally used in its "impure" form for dose escalation in order to increase tumor control probability without hampering late toxicity. Trials containing pure HE arms are rather rare and serve the purpose of decreasing toxicity (e.g., in reirradiation setting) or served as early phases of dose escalation projects with HE. When using multiple daily fractions, even though the fraction sizes are small, extreme care should be taken of intrafractional gap, as repeatedly demonstrated by two consecutive RTOG trials: 7913 and 8313 (Marcial et al. 1987; Fu et al. 2000).

A typical example for a trial comparing impure HE to N was EORTC 22791 (Horiot et al. 1992): In a homogenous cohort of 356 patients with stage II–III oropharynx cancer, 70 Gy (N)

Table 2 Studies comparing normofractionation with hybrid acceleration

Authors (year)	Name or location	Sites	UICC stage[a]	n	Median follow-up (y)	Arm	Radiotherapy	OS	PFS	LC	LRC	At y	Grade ≥3 toxicity and QoL[b]	Remarks
Awwad et al. (1992)	NCI Cairo PORT-1	OC, OP, HP, L, O	PORT III–IV	52	NR	1	N: 50 Gy/25 f/5 w					3	LT lower in arm 2	Not defined[c]
						2	AC.HE: 42 Gy/30 f/2.2 w							
Johnson et al. (1995)	Richmond	NR	III–IV	34	1.1	1	N: 70 Gy/35 f/7 w			31		1.3		Not defined[c]
						2	AC.CB: 74.8 Gy/5 w (details NR)			66				
Jackson et al. (1997)	Jackson	OC, OP, HP, L	III–IV	82	7.8	1	N: 66 Gy/33 f/6.5 w				NS[c]	NR	Early termination of the trial due to excessive toxicity	
						2	AC.HE: 66 Gy/33 f/3.5 w							
Horiot et al. (1997)	EORTC 22851	OC, OP, L, NP, O	II–IV	512	4.8	1	N: 70 Gy/35 f/7 w				46[c]	5	Increased LT in arm 2	Benefit of AFRT more prominent in advanced stages
						2	AC.HE.S: 72 Gy/45 f/5 w with 2 w split				59[c]			
Dische et al. (1997) Saunders et al. (2010)	CHART	OC, OP, HP, L, NP, SN	II–IV	918	7	1	N: 66 Gy/33 f/6.5 w			NS[c]		10	More acute mucositis, but less LT in arm 2	
						2	AC.HE: 54 Gy/36 f/1.7 w							
Dobrowsky and Naudé (2000)	V-CHART	OC, OP, HP, L, NP	II–IV	239	4	1	N: 70 Gy/35 f/7 w	NS[c]			NS[c]	4	90% grade ≥3 acute mucositis with AC.HE	LRC reported as crude rates
						2	ACHE: 55.3 Gy/33 f/2.5 w	NS[c]			NS[c]			
						3		Irrelevant						
Fu et al. (2000) Beidler et al. (2014)	RTOG 9003	OC, OP, HP, L	II–IV	1113	14.1	1	N: 70 Gy/35 f/7 w		(1)		NS[c]	5	All AFRT schedules increased AT LT comparable	The study was designed only to compare AFRT arms to arm 1
						2		Irrelevant						
						3	AC.HE.S: 67.2 Gy/42 f/6 w with 2 w split		NS		NS[c]			
						4	AC.CB: 36 Gy/18 f/3.5 w + 36 Gy/24 f/1.5 w.CB		(0.82)		NS[c]			
Poulsen et al. (2001)	TROG 9101	OC, OP, HP, L	III–IV	350	3.9	1	N: 70 Gy/35 f/7 w		NS[c]			3	More acute mucositis, but less LT in arm 2	
						2	AC.HE: 59.4 Gy/33 f/3.5 w							

		Sites	Stage	N		Arm	Regimen				NR	Toxicity	Comments
Ang et al. (2001)	MDACC PORT	OC, OP, HP, L	PORT, "high risk"	151	4.9	1	N: 63 Gy/35 f/7 w				NR	Increased AT and LT in arm 2	Not defined[c] Emphasis on overall radiotherapy and "treatment package" time[c]
						2	AC.CB: 27 Gy/15 f/3 w + 36 Gy/20 f/2 w						
Awwad et al. (2002)	NCI Cairo PORT-2	OC, L, HP	PORT, III–IV	70	NR	1	N: 60 Gy/30 f/6 w			57	3	Increased AT in arm 2	Not defined[c] Emphasis on overall treatment time[c]
						2	AC.HE: 46.2 Gy/33 f/2.4 w			88			
Olmi et al. (2003)	ORO 9301	OP	III–IV	192	6.6	1	N: 66–70 Gy/33–35 f/7 w	NS[c]	NS[c]		2	Lower AT in arm 1	
						2	AC.HE.S: 64–67.2 Gy/40–42 f/6 w with 2 w split						
						3	Irrelevant						
Sanguineti et al. (2005)	Italy multicenter	OC, OP, HP, L	PORT, "high risk"	226	2.6	1	N: 60 Gy/30 f/6 w			NS[c]		Increased AT in arm 2. LT comparable	
						2	AOCB: 49 Gy/25 f/5 w + 7 Gy/5 f in 1. w and 8 Gy/5 f in 5. w(CB)						
Bourhis et al. (2006a)	GORTEC 94-02	OC, OP, HP, L	III–IV	268	6	1	N: 70 Gy/35 f/7 w			19	6	Increased AT and tube feeding in arm 2. LT comparable	
						2	AC.HE: 62–64 Gy/31–32 f/3 w			41			
Daoud et al. (2007)	Sfax	NP	II–IV	154	4.7	1	N: 70 Gy/35 f/7 w			NS[c]	5	Grade 2–3 mucositis and skin fibrosis higher in arm 2	In both arms: induction epirubicin, cisplatin if N2–3
						2	AC.HE.S: 70.4 Gy/44 f/6 w with 1.5 w split						
Ghoshal et al. (2008)	Chandigarh	OP, L, HP	III–IV	290	2	1	N: 66 Gy/33 f/6.5 w		52[c]	55	2	Increased acute mucositis in arm 2	
						2	AC.CB: 45 Gy/25 f/5 w + 22.5 Gy/15 f during last 3 w(CB)		72[c]	74			

(continued)

Table 2 (continued)

Authors (year)	Name or location	Sites	UICC stage[a]	n	Median follow-up (y)	Arm	Radiotherapy	Outcome in % or (HR)[b] OS	PFS	LC	LRC	At y	Grade ≥3 toxicity and QoL[b]	Remarks
Zackrisson et al. (2015) Nyqvist et al. (2016)	ARTSCAN 1	OC, OP, HP, L	III–IV	750	9.1	1	N: 68 Gy/34 f/6.5 w				NS[c]	5	Increased AT and tube feeding in arm 2. LT comparable. Global QoL was significantly inferior at the end of the treatment in arm 2. Some QoL domains continued to be inferior in the following months after RT	p16 prognostic but not predictive
						2	AC.CB: 46 Gy/23 f + 22 Gy/20 f (CB) in 4.4 w							
Miszczyk et al. (2014)	CHA-CHA	OC, OP, HP, L	II–IV	101	1	1	N: 72–74 Gy/36–37 f/7.3 w					NR	Acute mucosal reactions higher in the first 4 weeks of treatment	Not defined[c]
						2	AC.HE.S: 64 Gy/40 f/3 w with 1.2 w split							
Ghosh-Laskar et al. (2016b)	Mumbai	OP, L, HP, O	III–IV	186	4.5	1	N: 66–70 Gy/33–35 f/7 w				NS[c]	5	Lower AT in arm 1 LR comparable	Terminated due to slow accrual
						2	AC.CB: 66–70 Gy/33–35 f/6 w							
						3	Irrelevant							

[a]Nonmetastatic if not otherwise stated

[b]Only differences with $p \leq 0.05$ given, if not stated otherwise

[c]Primary endpoint

AC accelerated fractionation, AFRT altered fractionation, AT acute toxicity, CB concomitant boost, f fractions, HE hyperfractionation, HP hypopharynx, L larynx, LT late toxicity, N normofractionation, NP nasopharynx, NR not reported, NS statistically not significant, O other sites, OC oral cavity, OP oropharynx, PORT post-operative radiotherapy, S split-course, SN sino-nasal, QoL quality of life, y year, w weeks was compared to 80.5 Gy applied to the macroscopic disease in the same time frame of 7 weeks (HE). Without increasing the late toxicities, the primary endpoint of locoregional control significantly improved from 40 to 59% at 5 years. However, no significant improvement in overall survival was observed, which was similar to that shown by previous investigators (Sanchíz et al. 1990), even with lesser total doses (70.4 vs. 66 Gy) of dose escalation (Pinto et al. 1991). A possible explanation may be the less advanced-stage distribution in the EORTC trial compared to those two trials. Details are provided in Table 3.

2.4 Radiation Therapy Oncology Group Trial 9003

As mentioned before, phase III RTOG 7913 and phase I/II RTOG 8313 trials showed the rationale and feasibility of dose escalation via HE without increasing late complications. Just before finishing accrual to 8313, the collaborative group initiated the phase III RTOG 9003 trial with four arms. This trial was designed to compare the locoregional control rates of three well-recognized AFRT schedules to the "standard" N (70 Gy/35 fractions in 7 weeks), but not among each other.

- Arm 1 (N): 70 Gy in 35 fractions over 7 weeks
- Arm 2 (HE): 81.6 Gy in 68 fractions over 7 weeks (University of Florida)
- Arm 3 (split-course AC-HE): 67.2 Gy in 42 fractions over 6 weeks including 2-week split (Massachusetts General Hospital)
- Arm 4 (AC with CB): 36 Gy in 18 fractions over 3.5 weeks followed by 36 Gy in 24 fractions over 1.5 weeks (MD Anderson)

After successfully recruiting 1113 patients between 1986 and 1989, the first results were published in 2000 (Fu et al. 1995). Arms 2 and 4 significantly increased the locoregional control, without any difference in overall survival. All experimental arms showed increased acute toxicities, and only Arm 4 demonstrated significantly increased late toxicities. However, RTOG interpreted them as "prolonged acute effects." Therefore, Arms 2 and 4 were deemed as "similar" in terms of outcome, and since the MD Anderson regimen was more convenient in terms of logistics and costs, it became the standard for future trials, e.g., RTOG 0129. However, the recently published results (Beitler et al. 2014) showed significant improvement in 5-year locoregional control (HR: 0.79) and overall survival (HR: 0.81) with HE versus N, still without hampering the late toxicity profile. However, grade ≥ 3 late toxicities were still associated with Arm 4 ($p = 0.06$), and previously shown statistically significant locoregional control benefit with AC (CB) was lost in 5 years ($p = 0.11$).

There were several reverberations in the RTOG after the publication of these long-term results. In a following editorial, the University of Florida team defended HE and criticized the RTOG for their "biased tendency" toward AC in the past and "downplaying" the toxicity difference in the first published manuscript (Feigenberg et al. 2014). In the same issue, other two authors emphasized that RTOG 9003 was not designed to compare the experimental arms to each other, and through passing years, the AC standard of RTOG changed to DAHANCA anyway (Trotti and Machtay 2014). Subsequently, the MD Anderson team criticized the statistical methodology and reporting in the final manuscript, emphasizing the "marginal benefit" with HE, and questioning its logistical feasibility and its use in the IMRT era (Rosenthal et al. 2015).

2.5 Hypofractionation

Hypofractionation (HO) was investigated in the curative setting of HNSCC many times and was found to increase the late toxicities without any benefit in tumor control or survival compared to N (Weissberg et al. 1982; Overgaard et al. 1989). However, it is still considered as an attractive strategy in special treatment settings, such as where the target volume is relatively small. In such scenarios, four potential advantages of HO

Table 3 Studies comparing normofractionation with hyperfractionation

Authors (year)	Name or location	Sites	UICC stage[a]	n	Median follow-up (y)	Arm	Radiotherapy	OS	PFS	LC	LRC	At y	Grade ≥3 toxicity[b]	Remarks
Marcial et al. (1987)	RTOG 7913	OC, OP, HP, L, SN	III–IV	210	9.5	1	N: 66–73.8 Gy/33–41 f/6.5–8 w					2	AT and LT comparable	Not defined[c]
						2	HE: 60 Gy/50 f/5 w							
Sanchíz et al. (1990)	Barcelona	OC, HP, L, NP, O	III–IV	859	NR	1	N: 60 Gy/30 f/6 w	31	23			5	AT and LT comparable	Not defined[c]
						2	HE: 70.4 Gy/64 f/6.5 w	58	48					
						3		Irrelevant						
Pinto et al. (1991)	Rio	OP	III–IV	103	2.1	1	N: 66 Gy/33/6.5 w	8				NR	AT and LT comparable	Not defined[c]
						2	HE: 70.4 Gy/64 f/6.5 w	27						
Horiot et al. (1992)	EORTC 22791	OP	II–III	356	10.3	1	N: 70 Gy/35 f/7 w				40[c]	5	Increased AT in arm 2. LT comparable	Nodal control was not improved with HE
						2	HE: 80.5 Gy/70 f/7 w				59[c]			
Accrual: 1996–99, unpublished	EORTC 22962	OC, OP, HP, L	II–IV	57[d]	[d]	1	N: 70 Gy/35 f/7 w	Irrelevant				[d]		@: Terminated prematurely due to slow accrual
						2	HE: 80.5 Gy/70 f/7 w							
						3								
						4								
Trotti et al. (2014)	RTOG 9512	T2 glottic L	I	250	7.9	1	N: 70 Gy/35 f/7 w			NS[c]		5	AT and LT comparable	
						2	HE: 79.2 Gy/66 f/6.5 w							
Fu et al. (2000) and Beitler et al. (2014)	RTOG 9003	OC, OP, HP, L	II–IV	1113	14.1	1	N: 70 Gy/35 f/7 w	(1)	(1)		(1)[c]	5	All AFRT schedules increased AT. LT comparable	The study was designed only to compare AFRT arms to arm 1. The improvements for LRC and OS lost their significance when the data is not censored at 5 years
						2	HE: 81.6 Gy/68 f/7 w	(0.81)	(0.78)		(0.79)[c]			
						3		Irrelevant						
						4								

[a]Nonmetastatic if not otherwise stated

[b]Only differences with $p \leq 0.05$ given, if not stated otherwise

[c]Primary endpoint

[d]See remarks

AC, accelerated fractionation, AT acute toxicity, f fractions, HE hyperfractionation, HP hypopharynx, L larynx, LT late toxicity, N normofractionation, NP nasopharynx, NR not reported, NS statistically not significant, O other sites, OC: oral cavity, OP, oropharynx, SN sino-nasal, y year, w weeks are being exploited: first, its logistical, economic benefits due to a significantly lesser number of fractions; second, patient comfort; third, a similar effect of treatment acceleration due to lesser number of fractions; and last but not least, radio-biological therapeutic advantage of HO in slowly proliferating tumors with a relatively lower α/β (e.g., low-grade or in situ early-stage glottic larynx cancer).

With the emergence of modern techniques, HO can be used even in locally advanced HNSCC. In a phase I/II dose escalation study using IMRT on 60 patients with laryngeal/hypopharyngeal prima-ries, the feasibility of HO on macroscopic disease was demonstrated. A combination of induction and concomitant chemotherapy, and an increased total dose of 63–67.2 Gy in 23 fractions, was applied to the macroscopic disease (Gujral et al. 2014). Grade 3 toxicity was 2% and the results indicated a dose-response relationship with increasing local control (68 vs. 75%), locore-gional control (54 vs. 63%), and progression-free (52 vs. 60%) and overall survival (62 vs. 68%), respectively, via increasing total dose.

A different application of HO is to boost the macroscopic disease with stereotactic radiother-apy (SBRT). In a phase I/II trial, 27 patients with locally advanced HPV-negative oropharyngeal cancer were treated with N IMRT and concomi-tant cisplatin to a total dose of 60 Gy, which was then followed by an 8–10 Gy boost in a single fraction. At last follow-up (median: 2.2 years), crude rates of 81–100% locoregional control and 81–93% disease-free survival were achieved, respectively, with 8 and 10 Gy (no statistical comparison). Grade 3 late dysphagia was reported as 15%, and four patients required surgical inter-vention due to hemorrhage (Ghaly et al. 2014). A similar approach from Erasmus MC (Al-Mamgani et al. 2015) is discussed later in this chapter.

2.6 Altered Fractionation for Glottic Larynx Cancer

Generally, potential benefits of a treatment modality are difficult to prove in early-stage HNSCC, mainly because of the need for a large sample size to show a relatively marginal benefit in a disease with a good baseline prognosis. AFRT for the treatment of glottic larynx cancer is an exception to this principle. Two prospective phase III randomized trials compared mild HO versus N in early-stage glottic larynx cancer. Both trials compared N (2 Gy/fraction) with HO (2.25 Gy/fraction), but to different total doses. The first trial (Yamazaki et al. 2006) only included T1 primaries. The patients were ran-domized to either N (60–66 Gy in 30–33 frac-tions over 6–6.5 weeks) or HO (56.25–63 Gy in 25–28 fractions over 5–5.5 weeks). The total dose difference was based on the amount of tumor extension along the vocal cords (lower dose if two-thirds vocal cord involvement or less). Without any difference in acute or chronic toxicities, an improved 5-year local control of 92% versus 77% was in favor of HO arm. The second trial, KROG 0201 (Moon et al. 2013), randomized patients with T1 and T2 tumors sep-arately with different total doses based on T stage. Although showing a trend of improved 5-year local control with HO over N in T1a sub-group (93% vs. 77%, $p = 0.06$), the study was underpowered due to insufficient accrual (156 out of 282 planned, and only 16 T2 cases). No significant difference in toxicity was observed. Ermiş et al. recently summarized the outcome of various retrospective cohorts of early-stage glot-tic larynx cancer patients treated with different HO schedules with fraction sizes ranging from 2.25 to 3.43 Gy (Ermiş et al. 2015). For T1 and T2 disease, 5-year local control rates were reported at 82–95% and 61–81%, respectively.

The positive impact of HE for the treatment of early glottic larynx cancer was also explored in various studies (Garden et al. 2003; Sakata et al. 2008; Chera et al. 2010a). The RTOG 9512 is the only published prospective randomized trial comparing the moderately accelerated HE to con-ventional fractionation in T2 glottic SCC. With a median follow-up of 7.9 years, the 5-year local control was not significantly higher in the HE compared to N arm (78% vs. 70%; $p = 0.14$) (Trotti et al. 2014). Not late, but higher rates of acute toxicities were observed in the HE arm. The authors suggested the usage of the widely accepted HO schedule (2.25 Gy/fraction) due to its effectiveness and convenience.

A recent meta-analysis, done with the above-mentioned three randomized trials, verified the clear benefit of AFRT over N in glottic larynx cancer with a HR of 0.59 (95% CI: 0.43–0.81) (Yamoah et al. 2015). It is also worth to note that the previously discussed DAHANCA 6 trial showed a pronounced positive impact of AC on T1–2 glottic laryngeal primaries ($n = 592$) with a HR of 0.60 (95% CI: 0.41–0.89). These results were based on a median follow-up of 14.5 years, without showing a significant difference in long-term toxicity (Lyhne et al. 2015).

The still widely used RT approach is to treat the whole larynx as a compartment. It is based on the traditional conventional field design, which was established in an era where image guidance in RT was poor. Another reason was the laryngeal displacement due to swallowing during RT, which was later reported to be not a serious concern as previously thought (Van Asselen et al. 2003; Bradley et al. 2011). Nevertheless, this approach has two major consequences: First, it exposes an unnecessary volume of healthy tissue to a high dose (i.e., overtreatment) which may increase the risk of functional loss through inflammation and fibrosis, at the same time depleting the reserves for a future reirradiation if required. Second, the carotid arteries are exposed to a high dose that increases the incidence of stenosis and cerebrovascular events (Dorresteijn et al. 2002; Smith et al. 2008). This problem can be overcome through modified target volumes and IMRT (Chera et al. 2010b). With a technique developed by the Rotterdam group, it is possible to apply 58.08 Gy in 16 fractions just to the involved vocal cord with a significant dose reduction in the vicinity (Kwa et al. 2015). Recently, the clinical results of a prospective study with the primary endpoint of voice quality were reported (Al-Mamgani et al. 2015). Despite short median follow-up of 30 months, the results are impressive: 2-year local control and overall survival of 100% and 90%, respectively, without any grade ≥3 toxicity. When compared with a historical control group, which was treated to the whole larynx (N, 66 at 2 Gy/fraction), single vocal cord irradiation yielded less grade ≥2 acute toxicity (17% vs. 66%, $p < 0.01$) and lower voice-handicap index scores in almost all follow-up visits performed in regular short intervals until 18th month ($p < 0.01$).

In summary, there is level 1 evidence favoring HO and AC for the treatment of early-stage glottic larynx cancer. The possible effect of HO is probably based on its treatment-accelerating effect, rather than the exploitation of the β value (Al-Mamgani et al. 2013a; Lyhne et al. 2016). Nevertheless, it can be safely applied and may be preferred due to its benefits in terms of costs, logistics, and patient comfort. The therapeutic window can be widened with the use of contemporary treatment techniques.

2.7 Altered Fractionation with Intensity-Modulated Radiotherapy

A majority of the clinical trials mentioned throughout this chapter either were done in the pre-IMRT era or contain just some subgroups treated with IMRT. Prospective clinical trials with the focus on AFRT with IMRT started to emerge in the last decade. Data published so far showed its safety, feasibility, and potential advantages. The use of IMRT for HO was discussed in the previous section. Other strategies involve simultaneous integrated boost with dose painting, dose escalation, and testing the feasibility of IMRT in different AFRT schedules. Some examples are provided in Table 4.

3 Comparison Among Different Altered Fractionation Schedules

Although large studies like RTOG 9003 exist, they were not designed to make a head-to-head comparison among AFRT schedules. The highest level of evidence is rather extrapolated from indirect statistical comparisons of accumulated large data, which is discussed further in Sect. 7. In relation to the data

Table 4 Studies with altered fractionation in combination with intensity-modulated radiotherapy

Authors (year)	Name or location	Sites	UICC stage[a]	n	Median follow-up (y)	Arm	Radiotherapy	Systemic agent	Outcome in %							Grade ≥3 toxicity[b]	Remarks
									OS	CSS	PFS	LC	LRC	FFM	at y		
Eisbruch et al. (2010)	RTOG 0022	OP	I–IV	69	2.8	1	AC: 66 Gy/30 f/6 w		96				91[d]		2	Combined highest toxicity not reported. Refer to article for details	IMRT SIB. [c]feasibility @: 100% among non-smokers
Gunn et al. (2010)	Galveston	OP	II–IV	25	3.5	1	HE: 78 Gy/60 f/6 w		70		62		86[c]	76	3	AT: 100% LT: 26%	IMRT SIB
Kao et al. (2011)	Mount Sinai, NY	OC, OP, HP, L, NP, SN.O	III–IV	33	2	1	HE.S: 4 × (15 Gy/10 f/1 w + 1 w split) + 12 Gy/8 f/1 w	Cetuximab, hydroxurea, 5-fluoruracil. Prior induction chemotherapy or surgery allowed	86		69	94	83	79	2	LT: 9%	IMRT SIB
Maguire et al. (2011)	US multicenter	OC, OP, HP, L	III–IV	39	3.1	1	HE: 70 Gy/56 f/5.5 w	Cisplatin	80		82		87		3	38% acute mucositis, 5% dermatitis. 2 LT	IMRT SIB
Cvek et al. (2012	HARTCIB	OC, OP, HP, L	IV	39	0.8	1	AC.HE: 70–75 Gy/50 f/5 w		55				50		1	51% acute mucositis. No LT	IMRT SIB
Gujral et al. (2014)	Royal Marsden	L, HP	III–IV	60	5.9	1	HO: 63–67.2 Gy/28 f/5.5 w	Cisplatin following induction cisplatin, 5-fluorouracil	62–68	75	52–60	68–75	54–63		5	LT: 2%	Dose escalation with IMRT

(continued)

Table 4 (continued)

Authors (year)	Name or location	Sites	UICC stage[a]	n	Median follow-up (y)	Arm	Radiotherapy	Systemic agent	Outcome in %							Grade ≥3 toxicity[b]	Remarks
									OS	CSS	PFS	LC	LRC	FFM	at y		
Songthong et al. (2015)	Bangkok	NP	I–IV	122	1.4	1	N(SEQ): 70 Gy/35 f/7 w	±Cisplatin, 5-fluoruracil							d	AT and LT NS[c]	[c]AT and LT @: at last follow-up (preliminary results)
						2	N(SIB): 70 Gy/33 f/6.5 w	±Cisplatin, 5-fluoruracil									
Ghaly et al. (2014)	New York	OP	III–IV HPV(−)	27	2.2	1	N + HO: 60 Gy/30 f + SRS boost with 8–10 Gy	Cisplatin			81–93		81–100		d		IMRT followed by SRS @: at last follow-up
Al-Mamgani et al. (2015)	Erasmus MC	T1a glottic L	I	30	2.5	1	HO: 58.08 Gy/16 f/3.1 w		90			100			1.5	No AT or LT During 18 months of follow-up, VHI[c] improved compared to baseline and a historical conventional whole larynx irradiation series (n = 131) with 15-year follow-up	

[a]Nonmetastatic if not otherwise stated

[b]Only differences with $p \leq 0.05$ given, if not stated otherwise

[c]Primary endpoint

[d]See remarks

AC accelerated fractionation, AT acute toxicity, f fractions, HE hyperfractionation, HP hypopharynx, HPV Human Papilloma Virus, IMRT intensity modulated radiotherapy, L larynx, LT late toxicity, N normofractionation, NP nasopharynx, NS statistically not significant, O other sites, OC oral cavity, OP oropharynx, S split-course, SEQ sequential boost, SIB simultaneous integrated boost, SN sino-nasal, SRS stereotactic radiosurgery, y year, w weeks about AFRT versus N, the clinical evidence based on the head-to-head comparisons of different AFRT schedules is limited and only available in definitive RT setting. Some examples are provided below.

3.1 Comparison of Different Accelerated Fractionation Schedules

Before completing the two AC trials KBN PO 79 and CAIR, the Polish group started to conduct the CAIR-2 trial, which compared the AC schedules of the previous two trials head to head on 345 patients with stage II–IVB HNSCC. With the primary endpoint of locoregional control, the study demonstrated no significant difference in tumor control, survival, or toxicity rates at 5 years. As the investigators proclaimed, radiation-free weekend was rescued (Skladowski et al. 2013).

3.2 Accelerated Versus Hypofractionation

A phase III randomized trial compared AC (CB) (71.2 Gy in 40 fractions over 4.3 weeks) with HO (60 Gy in 24 fractions over 4.3 weeks) in stage I–III nasopharynx cancer. No primary endpoint was defined. After recruiting 159 patients in 2 years, the study was terminated prematurely due to significantly higher neurological complications with HO (49% vs. 23%) at 5 years. The differences in tumor control or survival were not significant (Teo et al. 2000).

Another phase III randomized trial including 336 stage III–IVB oropharyngeal, laryngeal and hypopharyngeal primaries compared AC-HE (58 Gy in 40 fractions over 4 weeks) to mild HO (50 Gy in 20 fractions over 4 weeks). Despite a trend toward improved survival with AC-HE (40% vs. 30%), none of the outcome parameters, including the primary endpoint locoregional control, were significantly different among trial arms at 5 years. The authors reported significantly increased acute grade ≥3 toxicities with AC-HE (70% vs. 53%). Late toxicities were comparable (Cummings et al. 2007).

3.3 Accelerated Versus Hyperfractionation

Investigators from Skopje randomized 101 patients with stage I–IVB oropharyngeal, laryngeal, and hypopharyngeal primaries into treatment arms with HE (79.2 Gy in 66 fractions over 6.5 weeks) and A (CB) (32.4 Gy in 18 fractions over 3.6 weeks, followed by 39.6 Gy in 24 fractions over 2.4 weeks). The primary endpoint was not defined and the follow-up was short (1.9 years). The study did not demonstrate any significant difference in outcome or toxicity (Krstevska and Crvenkova 2006).

3.4 Hypofractionation with Brachytherapy or Stereotactic Radiotherapy

The Erasmus MC group published their results of T1–2 oropharyngeal cancer cases. Patients were treated with either pulsed-dose brachytherapy (n = 148; 22 Gy in 8 fractions over 24 h) or SBRT (n = 102; 16.5 Gy in 3 fractions over 1 week) boost following 46 Gy N with concomitant cisplatin. Toxicity and quality-of-life scores were comparable with both modalities. Because the brachytherapy was used earlier on, the median follow-up of the brachytherapy cohort was longer than the robotic SBRT cohort: 5.5 versus 3 years (Al-Mamgani et al. 2013b). The authors favored the use of this noninvasive SBRT strategy, mainly based on the fact that it is less labor intensive; and brachytherapy is associated with perioperative and anesthesia-associated complication risks and requires specially trained personnel with hand dexterity. Nevertheless, brachytherapy still remains to be an effective and valid option.

A meta-analysis analyzed the outcome of the low- and intermediate-risk (stages I–III) lip and oral cavity tumors treated with low-dose versus high-dose brachytherapy. With a total number of 607 patients, no significant differences in local control, survival, or late toxicities were detected (Liu et al. 2013).

4 Altered Fractionation with or Without Systemic Therapy

A garden of variety for combining numerous systemic agents and AFRT schedules in the definitive RT setting exists. Although some retrospective data showed the feasibility of combining AFRT and ST (Pehlivan et al. 2009), there is a lack of randomized trials with available results in the PORT setting. Although not being a trial with a question about AFRT, another special remark can be made about the IMCL trial (also known as "Bonner trial"), testing the combination of RT and the monoclonal antibody cetuximab, which inhibits the intracellular downstream activity of the epidermal growth factor, by inhibiting its surface receptor. Over 70% of the patients in both arms were treated with either AC (CB) or HE, which were very well balanced in the control and experimental arms. Despite that, the results favored the combined treatment with cetuximab, which increased the locoregional control (primary endpoint) and overall survival. Grade ≥ 3 acute dermatitis and acneiform rash were significantly increased in the combination arm (Bonner et al. 2006, 2010). The quality of life at 12 months after baseline was comparable between both arms (Curran et al. 2007). However late toxicity was not assessed.

In summary, the trials comparing AFRT with versus without ST demonstrated either an advantage of adding ST therapy to RT or no benefit in terms of tumor control and survival. The cost of this improvement is increased toxicity, mostly in the form of acute side effects (Trotti et al. 2007). Some selected studies are categorized below.

4.1 Accelerated Fractionation with or without Systemic Treatment

Out of six phase III randomized trials, three were positive in terms of improving the primary endpoint when ST was added to AC. Two of these three also showed an improvement in some of the secondary endpoints. All trials with positive results used cytotoxic chemotherapy agents. In one of the three negative trials, cytotoxic agents cisplatin and fluorouracil were used in the experimental arm. The lack of improved progression-free survival (primary outcome) was interpreted by the authors through the excess of early noncancer-related deaths in the ST arm (Bourhis et al. 2006b). Generally, the cytotoxic chemotherapy agents increased the acute toxicities in all of these trials. The other two negative trials had experimental arms using agents to modify the hypoxic tumor environment either with hypoxic cell sensitizer nimorazole or the vasoactive agent nicotinamide combined with carbogen inhalation. On the other hand, it is worth to note that the first trial with nimorazole (IAEA-HypoX) had to be stopped prematurely due to slow accrual ($n = 104/606$), and the latter trial (ARCON) showed a significant improvement in regional control which became sixfold when the hypoxia marker pimonidazole was positive in tumor biopsies. Compared to cytotoxic chemotherapy, these agents did not increase toxicity. Details are provided in Table 5.

4.2 Hyperfractionation with or without Systemic Treatment

Five trials evaluated the potential benefit of ST when added to HE. The RT schedules were pure or impure HE without dose de-escalation. All ST involved cytotoxic chemotherapeutics (cisplatin with or without fluorouracil). Four out of five trials were successful in terms of positive results for primary endpoints, all favoring the addition of chemotherapy. The SAKK 10/94, which was negative in terms of its primary endpoint (progression-free survival), did show significantly improved cause-specific survival, locoregional control, and freedom from metastases. Except for the hematological complications caused by chemotherapy, the toxicities were comparable. Details of those studies are provided in Table 6.

Table 5 Studies investigating the role of systemic therapy when added to accelerated fractionation

Authors (year)	Name or location	Sites	UICC stage[a]	n	Median follow-up (y)	Arm	Radiotherapy	Systemic agent	Outcome in %[b]							Grade ≥3 toxicity[b]	Remarks
									OS	CSS	PFS	LC	LRC	FFM	at y		
Dobrowsky and Naudé (2000)	V-CHART	OC, OP, HP, L, NP	II–IV	239	4	1			Irrelevant							4	Increased acute mucositis in both arms. Acute hematological toxicity exclusive to arm 3.	LRC reported as crude rates
						2	AC.HE: 55.3 Gy/33 f/2.5 w		18[c]				31					
						3	AC.HE: 55.3 Gy/33 f/2.5 w	Mitomycin	32[c]				48					
Staar et al. (2001)	Cologne 95	OP, HP	III–IV	263	4.7	1	AC.CB: 27 Gy/15 f/3 w + 42.9 Gy/26 f/1.5 (CB)	Carboplatin					58[c]		1	Increased AT[i] in arm 1	Prophylactically given G-CSF was a poor prognostic factor (Cox regression), and resulted in reduced LRC (p<0.01)
						2	AC.CB: 27 Gy/15 f/3 w + 42.9 Gy/26 f/1.5 (CB)						44[c]				
Budach et al. (2005, 2015)	ARO 95-06	OC, OP, HP	III–IV	384	8.7	1	AC.CB: 30 Gy/15 f/3 w + 40.6 Gy/29 f/3 w (CB)	Mitomycin 5-fluoruracil	10	39	25		38[c]	48	10	Increased mucositis and dermatitis in arm 2. Increased hematological toxicity in arm 1	Increased toxicity without chemotherapy can be explained by more aggressive RT schedule in arm 2
						2	AC.CB: 14 Gy/7 f/1.5 w + 61.6 Gy/44 f/4.5 w (CB)		9	30	18		26[c]	52			
Ezzat et al. (2005)	NCI Cairo	OC, OP, HP, L	III–IV	40	10.5	1	AC: 68 Gy/34 f/5.5 w		Irrelevant							2	Increased hematological toxicities in arm 3 LT comparable	Not defined[c]
							AC: 68 Gy/34 f/5.5 w	Mitomycin										
Ang et al. (2005) Garden et al. (2008)	RTOG 9914	OC, OP, HP, L	III–IV	84	4.3	1	AC.CB: 30.6 Gy/1.8 Gy f/3.3 w + 41.4 Gy/25 f/2.4 w (CB)	Cisplatin	54				36[c]		4	Overall toxicity 42%	

(continued)

Table 5 (continued)

Authors (year)	Name or location	Sites	UICC stage[a]	n	Median follow-up (y)	Arm	Radiotherapy	Systemic agent	OS	CSS	PFS	LC	LRC	FFM	at y	Grade ≥3 toxicity[b]	Remarks
Bourhis et al. (2011)	GORTEC 96-01	OP, HP, O	IV	109	11.9	1	AC.HE: 64 Gy/32 f/3 w				NS[c]				5	Increased and prolonged grade ≥3 mucositis in arm 1	The lack of survival benefit in favor of the arm 2 was mainly due to the excess of early non-cancer-related death in arm 2.
						2	AC.HE.S: 64 Gy/32 f/5 w with 2 w split	Cisplatin 5-fluoruracil									
Janssens et al. (2012)	ARCON	L	II–IV	345	3.7	1	AC.CB: 44 Gy/22 f/4 w + 24 Gy/11 f/1.1 w(CB)					NS[c]	93 regional		5	No difference in AT or LT	
						2	AC.CB: 44 Gy/22 f/4 w + 24 Gy/11 f/1.1 w(CB)	Nicotinamide Carbogen					86 regional				
Bentzen et al. (2015)	DAHANCA 18	OC, OP, HP, L	III–IV	227	4.6	1	AC: 66–68 Gy/33–34 f/5.5 w	Nimorazole	72		67		80[c]		5	AT: 89%. Tube feeding in acute phase 64%, 6% at 1 year	
Hassan Metwally et al. (2015)	IAEA-HypoX	OC, OP, HP, L	I–IV	104	1.6	1	AC: 66–70 Gy/33–35 f/6 w						NS[c]		[d]	No difference in AT or LT	Stopped due to slow accrual (planned 600) @: at last follow-up
						2	AC: 66–70 Gy/33–35 f/6 w	Nimorazole									

[a]Nonmetastatic if not otherwise stated

[b]Only differences with $p \leq 0.05$ given, if not stated otherwise

[c]Primary endpoint

[d]See remarks

AC accelerated fractionation, AT acute toxicity, CB concomitant boost, f fractions, HE hyperfractionation, HP hypopharynx, L larynx, LT late toxicity, NP nasopharynx NS statistically not significant, O other sites, OC oral cavity, OP oropharynx, S split-course, y year, w weeks

Table 6 Studies investigating the role of systemic therapy when added to hyperfractionation

Authors (year)	Name or location	Sites	UICC stage[a]	n	Median follow-up (y)	Arm	Radiotherapy	Systemic agent	OS	CSS	PFS	LRC	FFM	at y	Grade ≥3 toxicity[b]
Brizel et al. (1998)	Duke 90040	OC, OP, HP, L, NP, SN,O	II–IV	122	7.5	1	HE: 75 Gy/60 f/6 w					44[c]		3	No difference in AT or LT
						2	HE: 70 Gy/56 f/5.5 w	Cisplatin 5-fluorouracil				70[c]			
Jeremic et al. (2000)	Kragujevac	OC, OP, HP, L, O	III–IV	130	6.5	1	HE: 77 Gy/70 f/7 w		49[c]		(0.25)	36	57	5	No difference in AT or LT
						2	HE: 77 Gy/70 f/7 w	Cisplatin	68[c]		(0.46)	50	86		
Huguenin et al. (2004)	SAKK 10/94	OC, OP, HP, L	II–IV	224	9.5	1	HE: 74.4 Gy/62 f/6.5 w			43	NS[c]	32	41	10	No difference in AT or LT
Ghadjar et al. (2012)						2	HE: 74.4 Gy/62 f/6.5 w	Cisplatin		55	NS[c]	40	56		
Bensadoun et al. (2006)	FNCLCC-GORTEC	OP, HP	IV	163	4	1	HE: 75.6–80.4 Gy/63–67 f/6–7 w		20[c]	30	25			2	Acute neutropenia higher in arm 2 LT comparable
						2	HE: 75.6–80.4 Gy/63–67 f/6–7 w	Cisplatin, 5-fluorouracil	38[c]	45	42				
Wendt et al. (1998)	Munich	OC, OP, HP, L	III–IV	298	NR	1	HE.S: 70.2 Gy/38 f/8 w with 2× 1.5 w split		24[c]			17			Increased acute mucositis and dermatitis LT comparable
						2	HE.S: 70.2 Gy/38 f/8 w with 2× 1.5 w split	Cisplatin, 5-fluorouracil	48			36			

[a]Nonmetastatic if not otherwise stated

[b]Only differences with $p \leq 0.05$ given, if not stated otherwise

[c]primary endpoint

AT acute toxicity, f fractions, HE hyperfractionation, HP hypopharynx, L larynx, LT late toxicity, NP nasopharynx, NR not reported; NS statistically not significant, O other sites; OC oral cavity, OP oropharynx, S split-course, SN sino-nasal, y year, w weeks

5   Systemic Therapy with Normofractionated Radiotherapy Versus Radiotherapy Alone with Altered Fractionation

Logistics, treatment effectiveness, and toxicity are important matters of debate, both for AFRT and ST. Therefore, some clinical trials were designed to compare these two strategies. All trials involved AC as AFRT, and platinum-based chemotherapy with or without fluorouracil in their ST + N arms. In terms of disease control and survival, the results either were favoring the ST + N or showed nonsignificant differences among study arms. Three trials, all of them including patients in the definitive RT setting, could show significant improvement in their primary endpoints: one trial with locoregional control and two with progression-free survival. One of these trials demonstrated significantly increased grade ≥ 3 late toxicity in ST + N arm.

Two negative trials in definitive RT setting showed conflicting results concerning toxicities: Rishi et al. from India (Rishi et al. 2013) demonstrated worse treatment compliance and acute grade ≥ 3 toxicities with ST + N, except for mucositis which was higher in AC (CB) arm. Late toxicities and quality of life were also poor with ST + N. Conversely, another negative trial from Thailand (Chitapanarux et al. 2013) showed increased late subcutaneous fibrosis with AFRT alone. Both trials were conducted in the PORT setting and showed comparable toxicities among treatment arms. The investigators of the OCAT trial reported negative results in terms of outcome. The primary endpoint of the p-CAIR-2 trial (locoregional control) was not reported, because the trial was completed with less than the planned number of patients (84/270). Toxicities were comparable. Details are provided in Table 7.

Unfortunately, no results of any prospective randomized trial were published comparing N + ST to HE alone. Two arms of the phase III EORTC 22962 were supposed to answer this question. However, the trial was terminated prematurely due to slow accrual. The previously mentioned trial from Spain (Sanchíz et al. 1990) cannot be considered under this category, since the total dose in the HE-alone arm was 70.4 compared to 60 Gy in N + ST arm. Moreover, it was not clear what the primary endpoint was and whether the study was designed or powered enough to compare those two arms between each other.

6   Systemic Therapy and Radiotherapy, with or without Altered Fractionation

In contrast to the subjects discussed under previous sections, the question whether the modification of the RT schedule can provide further benefit in the concomitant chemo-RT setting for locally advanced HNSCC was investigated in few clinical trials. In the phase II EORTC 22843 trial, 53 patients were randomized to receive either N (70 Gy in 35 fractions over 7 weeks) with concomitant daily cisplatin (6 mg/m^2) or split-course AC-HE (3 times repetition of 24 Gy in 15 fractions over 1 week followed by 2-week split between courses) with concomitant daily cisplatin (10 mg/m^2). The primary endpoint was toxicity. The investigators reported no difference in acute and late toxicity among the two arms (Bartelink et al. 2002).

The phase III GORTEC 99-02 randomized 840 patients into three arms with the primary endpoint as locoregional control. In one of the two arms with chemotherapy (carboplatin and fluorouracil), patients received 70 Gy in 35 fractions over 7 weeks, and in the other arm 70 Gy in 40 fractions over 6 weeks (40 Gy in 20 fractions over 4 weeks followed by 30 Gy in 20 fractions over 2 weeks). At 7 years, the difference in outcome was not significant among the arms. Acute mucositis and feeding tube requirement were higher with AC (CB) + ST than N + ST. Late toxicities were comparable (Bourhis et al. 2012; Tao et al. 2016).

After the first results of RTOG 9003 were published (Fu et al. 1995), AC and HE were deemed equally advantageous over N. The RTOG 0129 trial was then designed by taking

Table 7 Studies comparing radiotherapy alone with altered fractionation versus normofractionation with systemic treatment

Authors (year)	Name or location	Sites	UICC stage[a]	n	Median follow-up (y)	Arm	Radiotherapy	Systemic agent	OS	CSS	PFS	LC	LRC	FFM	at y	Grade ≥3 toxicity and QoL[b]	Remarks
Olmi et al. (2003)	ORO 9301	OP	III–IV	192	6.6	1	AC.HE.S: 64–67.2 Gy/40–42 f/6 w with 2 w split		Irrelevant									Increased late dermatitis, fibrosis, and mucositis in arm 3
						2	N: 66–70 Gy/ 33–35 f/7 w		NS[c]		20				2		
						3		Carboplatin 5-fluorouracil			42						
Bourhis et al. (2012), Tao et al. (2016)	GORTEC 99-02	OC, OP, HP, L, O	III–IV	840	7.7	1	N: 70 Gy/35 f/7 w	Carboplatin 5-fluorouracil			23[c]				7		Acute mucosal toxicity and feeding tube requirement significantly and gradually increased from arm 1 towards 3.
						2		Carboplatin 5-fluorouracil	Irrelevant								
						3	AC.HE: 64.8 Gy/36 f/3.5				20[c]						
Ghosh-Laskar et al. (2016b)	Mumbai	OP, L, HP, O	III–IV	186	4.5	1			Irrelevant								AT comparable among arms 2 and 3. LT comparable	Stopped due to slow accrual
						2	N: 66–70 Gy/33–35 f/7 w	Cisplatin			39		49		5		
						3	AC.CB: 66–70 Gy/33–35 f/6 w				20		27				
Rishi et al. (2013)	Chandigarh	OP	III–IV	216	NR	1	N: 66 Gy/33/6.5 w	Cisplatin			NS[c]				NS		Treatment compliance was superior in arm 2 with less treatment interruptions. AT was higher in arm 1, except for mucositis which was seen more in arm 2. LT was higher in arm 1. QoL was lower in arm 1
						2	AC.CB: 45 Gy/25 f/5 w + 22.5 Gy/15 f during last 3 w(CB)										

(continued)

Table 7 (continued)

Authors (year)	Name or location	Sites	UICC stage[a]	n	Median follow-up (y)	Arm	Radiotherapy	Systemic agent	Outcome in % or (HR)[b]							Grade ≥3 toxicity and QoL[b]	Remarks
									OS	CSS	PFS	LC	LRC	FFM	at y		
Chitapanarux et al. (2013)	Chiang Mai	OC, OP, HP, L	III–IV	85	3.6	1	N: 66 Gy/33/6.5 w	Carboplatin 5-fluorouracil	76				NS[c]		5	Increased acute mucositis, but lower hematological toxicity in arm 2. Higher subcutaneous fibrosis in arm 2	
						2	AC.CB: 40 Gy/20 f/4 w + 30 Gy/20 f/2 w (CB)		63								
Suwinski et al. (2016)	p-CAIR-2	OC, OP	PORT, R0–1	84	NR	1	AC: 63 Gy/35/5 w	Cisplatin				NS[c]			NR	AT comparable	Completed less than planned number of patients (84/270)
						2	N: 63 Gy/35/7 w									
Ghosh-Laskar et al. (2016a)	OCAT	OC	III–IV PORT	700	4.8	1			Irrelevant							Acute mucosal and skin toxicities comparable	
						2	N: 56–60 Gy/ 28–30 f/6	Cisplatin					NS[c]		5		
						3	AC: 56–60 Gy/ 28–30 f/5 w									

[a]Nonmetastatic if not otherwise stated

[b]Only differences with $p \leq 0.05$ given, if not stated otherwise

[c]Primary endpoint

AC accelerated fractionation, AT acute toxicity, CB concomitant boost, f fractions, HE hyperfractionation, HP hypopharynx, L larynx, LT late toxicity, N normofractionation, NP nasopharynx, NR not reported, NS statistically not significant, O other sites, OC oral cavity, OP oropharynx, PORT post-operative radiotherapy, S split-course, QoL quality of life; y year, w weeks the MD Anderson AC (CB) schedule as new standard for AFRT. The trial randomized 743 patients into two arms, both with concomitant cisplatin: N (70 Gy in 35 fractions over 7 weeks with three cycles of cisplatin) versus A (CB) (36 Gy in 18 fractions over 3.5 weeks followed by 36 Gy in 24 fractions over 1.5 weeks with two cycles of cisplatin). At 8 years, no significant difference in overall survival (primary endpoint), any oncological endpoints, or acute and late toxicities was observed. Again, p16 status was shown to be prognostic but not predictive (Nguyen-Tan et al. 2014).

Similar to the above-mentioned observations, the preliminary results of the NPC 0501, which was specifically focusing on nasopharynx cancer, did not demonstrate any benefit of AFRT over N when both RT modalities were combined with one of the three different chemotherapy schedules in a six-armed trial. The only impact of AFRT was increased grade ≥ 3 acute mucositis and dehydration (Lee et al. 2015).

In summary, none of the trials evaluating the impact of AFRT in concomitant chemotherapy setting could demonstrate any added benefit. Nevertheless, it is worth to note that all of them used AC and not HE as AFRT. It is unknown whether the outcome would be different with HE instead of AC.

7   Meta-Analyses

A number of meta-analyses compared different treatment modalities for the treatment of head and neck cancer. In order to provide a general overview, selected articles focusing on AFRT are summarized below. If a meta-analysis has updated results, only the final results are presented. The specific meta-analyses about high- versus low-dose brachytherapy in lip and oral cavity cancers (Liu et al. 2013) and AFRT versus N in early-stage glottic larynx cancer (Yamoah et al. 2015) were discussed previously in the corresponding sections.

Stuschke and Thames (1997) performed four separate meta-analyses to evaluate the potential benefit of HE over N in head and neck, bladder, lung cancer, and malignant gliomas (Blanchard et al. 2011). Only studies published after 1980 were included in their analysis. Four head and neck trials published between 1989 and 1992 were identified. A total number of 1158 patients of various head and neck subsites in locally advanced stages (III–IVB) were included. All of the four studies reported locoregional control, and three of them reported survival. The pooled analysis yielded HRs of 0.35 and 0.48, favoring HE over N for locoregional control and overall survival, respectively.

Budach et al. performed a comprehensive literature search with two separate meta-analyses with the endpoint of overall survival (Budach et al. 2006). Included studies published between 1975 and 2003 with the results of 10,225 patients diagnosed with stage I–IVB head and neck cancer were analyzed. The first analysis evaluated the potential benefit of systemic treatment when added to RT (regardless of N or AFRT), which demonstrated a 12-month prolonged OS benefit with ST. This effect was most prominent when fluorouracil was used (24 months). Interestingly, this result contradicts the results of other meta-analyses (mentioned below), which showed maximum benefit with platinum-based chemotherapy. The second analysis investigated the potential benefit of AC or HF over N without ST. The results showed no benefit for AC over N while favoring HE with 14.2 months of prolonged OS.

The Cochrane Collaboration (Baujat et al. 2010) updated the data of the previously published MARCH individual patient data meta-analysis (Bourhis et al. 2006a): $n = 6515$; inclusion period: 1969–1998; stages: I–IVB, median follow-up: 6 years. At 5 years, absolute locoregional control and overall survival benefits with AFRT were 6.4% and 3.4% (HR: 0.92), respectively. This 5-year absolute overall survival benefit was more prominent (8%) with HE over AC without dose reduction (2%). The benefit of AFRT on local control was more pronounced than that on nodal control as the first site of recurrence, an observation not made in MACH-NC (Pignon et al. 2009). Only HE with increased total dose showed a benefit both on survival and locoregional control. Comparisons of different AFRT schedules indicated a greater survival benefit with HE, whereas for locoregional control, only a nonsignificant trend was reported in favor of HE and AC without total dose reduction. In terms of toxicities, the authors suggested an increased risk with AC without dose reduction. Moreover, the authors emphasized that the 8% survival benefit with HE alone exceeds the 6.5% survival benefit of concomitant chemo-RT reported in MACH-NC.

A mixed treatment network meta-analysis with MACH-NC and MARCH data was performed (Blanchard et al. 2011). The investigators performed indirect comparisons with fixed and random-effect models, using the pooled data ($n = 26,121$; stages: I–IVB) from MACH-NC and MARCH databases, with the aim of using the best outcomes among the following treatment strategies: (1) N; (2) N + ST; (3) AFRT alone; (4) AFRT + ST; (5) N + adjuvant ST; and (6) N + induction ST. With a 94.5% probability, AFRT + ST was found to be the best treatment strategy. The remaining 5.5% probability was assigned to N + ST. When restricted to platinum-based chemotherapy, these probabilities shifted to 81.5% and 18.5%, respectively. With random-effect method, AFRT + ST strategy was the only combination which always yielded HR significantly favoring its use compared to any other treatment strategy. Compared to N, AFRT + ST and N + ST were associated with HR (95% CI) of 0.70 (0.61–0.80) and 0.82 (0.78–0.86), respectively. Presumably, in order to maintain the robustness of the methodology, no further evaluations were performed to investigate the weighted effects of different AFRT schedules.

Yamoah et al. (2015) aimed to provide an extensive systematic review of RT intensification for solid tumors, without focusing solely on head and neck cancer. In their article, they provided two small meta-analyses for head and neck cancer, the first regarding early-stage glottic larynx cancer, and the second about the impact of AFRT in PORT setting. The first has been discussed earlier in the chapter. The latter analysis included four trials and yielded a HR of 0.72 (95% CI: 0.54–0.97) for locoregional control favoring AFRT.

By using their common N arms of the MARCH and MACH-NC data, two meta-analyses were compared indirectly using an adjusted indirect comparison with the main outcome of overall survival ($n = 7708$; stages II–IVB) (Gupta et al. 2015). The overall comparison demonstrated no significant difference between AFRT and N + ST (HR: 1.13, 95% CI: 0.97–1.29). When the different AFRT schedules were compared to N + ST with the random-effect approach, HRs (95% CI) for death were 1.01 for HE (0.89–1.15), 1.22 for AC without dose reduction (0.94–1.59), and 1.22 for AC with dose reduction (1.07–1.30). However, when the fixed-effect approach was used, the HRs (95% CI) for death were 1.10 (0.98–1.22) for HE, 1.18 (1.08–1.28) for AC without dose reduction, and 1.32 (1.18–1.47) for AC with dose reduction. The authors concluded that N + ST and HE were comparable strategies, and advised against the use of any form of AC.

Gupta et al. (2016) performed a systematic review to perform a meta-analysis with randomized controlled trials which directly compared N + ST to AFRT alone. The primary outcome was overall survival. Five randomized trials with a total number of 1117 patients were identified. The results favored N + ST over AFRT. Using fixed-effect models, the HRs (95% CI) for death, disease-free survival, and locoregional control were 0.73 (0.62–0.86), 0.79 (0.68–0.92), and 0.71 (0.59–0.84), respectively. The use of conventionally fractionated radiotherapy (CCRT) was associated with a 27% relative reduction in the risk of mortality compared with AFRT alone. The differences in acute toxicities were nonsignificant. However, odds ratio for grade ≥3 late xerostomia was lower with AFRT: 0.59 (95% CI: 0.37–0.93). As expected, hematological toxicities and nephrotoxicity rates were significantly higher with chemotherapy. In this meta-analysis, there are two points worth emphasis. First, the investigators only included trials which assigned patients to N + platinum-based ST, whereas any form of altered fractionation was allowed. As shown by multiple meta-analyses, platinum-based chemotherapy yields the best outcome. Similarly, AC is known to be a suboptimal AFRT choice. This brings us to the second point: All five trials included in the meta-analysis contained some form of AC (1 AC, 2 AC with CB, 1 AC-HE, and 1 AC-HE with split course). In other words, not the "best of two worlds" were compared, but the suboptimal AFRT was compared with the best concomitant ST. It is clear that the authors were not intentionally biased. This problem stems from the nature of the current landscape of clinical trials conducted so far. In addition, the authors regarded the quality of the analysis as moderate, which requires careful interpretation.

The EORTC 22962 trial would have been the ideal phase III study with four arms, comparing N (70 Gy in 35 fractions) with HE (80.5 Gy in 70 fractions) in 7 weeks with or without cisplatin. Unfortunately, the trial terminated prematurely due to slow accrual after recruiting only 57 patients. Similarly, RTOG 0129 was designed with the MD Anderson AC (CB) schedule. It is unknown what would have happened if the HE arm of the RTOG 9003 was chosen instead of AC.

8 Altered Fractionation for Reirradiation and Palliative Treatment

In cases of recurrent/metastatic head and neck cancer, the life expectancy is poor (Argiris et al. 2004; Vermorken et al. 2008; Ferris et al. 2016). Relative poor prognosis is also expected for secondary primaries emerging in a heavily pretreated area and there are limited therapeutic options for these patients. In a nonmetastatic situation, curative intent should be a first consideration. If salvage surgery is not an option, salvage reirradiation might be a feasible alternative.

8.1 AFRT for Curative Reirradiation

In case of a locoregional recurrence or second primary tumor, salvage surgery is the preferred option (De Crevoisier et al. 2001; Janot et al. 2008), though not always possible, mainly due to unacceptable morbidity or mortality risks. Primary salvage RT offers a moderate chance of

salvage to these patients. Even with the use of IMRT and omission of elective volumes, around one-third of the patients suffer from grade ≥ 3 acute toxicities when N schedules are used. Two-year survival rates are in a range of 28–65%, with around 25% of patients suffering from grade ≥ 3 late toxicities (Langendijk et al. 2006; Chen et al. 2011). Two phase II prospective trials used HE schedules combined with ST. The RTOG 9610 trial included 79 patients, treated up to 60 Gy in 40 fractions over 4 weeks combined with hydroxyurea and fluorouracil. At 2 years, the overall survival was 15%. Grade ≥ 3 acute and late toxicities were 63% (8% toxic deaths) and 9%, respectively (Spencer et al. 2008). RTOG 9911 included 99 patients, treated with split-course HE combined with cisplatin and paclitaxel. Patients received 1.5 Gy twice a day, 5 days every 2 weeks, repeated four times. Overall survival was 26% at 2 years. Grade ≥ 3 acute and late toxicities were 78% (5% toxic deaths) and 37% (4% toxic deaths), respectively (Langer et al. 2007).

Prospective clinical trials investigated the role of SBRT in reirradiation. The dose fractionation schedules are extremely HO. Although no direct statistical comparisons exist, the survival rates seem to be not inferior to N or HE schedules, and the toxicity profiles look counterintuitively better. The last published phase II trial ($n = 50$) demonstrated 6% acute and 6% late grade 3 toxicity rates with 40–44 Gy in five fractions over 2 weeks (Vargo et al. 2015). The same group also published the largest retrospective series so far ($n = 291$). The details of these studies are provided in Table 8. For further reading about SBRT for recurrent HNSCC, two recently published reviews are recommended (Ling et al. 2016a; Quan et al. 2016).

8.2 Altered Fractionation for Palliation

If a curative option is out of discussion, the standard of care for recurrent/metastatic HNSCC is ST. However, these patients may still suffer from local symptoms. For a patient with short life

Table 8 Studies with stereotactic radiotherapy for recurrent or second primary head and neck tumors

Authors (year)	Name or location	Sites	n	Median follow-up (y)	Radiotherapy	Systemic agent	OS	PFS	LC	LRC	FFM	at y	Grade ≥3 toxicity	Remarks
Heron et al. (2009)	Uni. Pittsburgh	OC, OP, L, NP, O	25	NR	25–44 Gy/5 f/2 w		20	0				1	None	Phase I dose escalation trial
Iwata et al. (2012)	Yokohama	SN	51	1.8	20– 41.5 Gy/1–5 f/1 w		67		62			1	23%	
Lartigau et al. (2013)	France multicenter	Mixed	60	1	36 Gy/6 f/2 w	Cetuximab	48	32	42			1	AT + LT (combined): 32%. One grade 5 event	Phase II trial
Vargo et al. (2015)	Univ. Pittsburgh	OC, OP, HP, L, SN, O	50	1.5	40–44 Gy/8 f/1.5 w	Cetuximab	40	33	60[a]	37[a]	71[aa]	1	AT: 6% LT: 6%	Phase II trial a: local and locoregional failure-free survival, respectively aa: distant metastasis-free survival
Ling et al. (2016b)	Univ. Pittsburgh	OC, OP, HP, L, NP, SN, O	291	4.4	Median 44 (range: 16–52.8) Gy/5 (n = 277, remaining 1–13) fractions	Cetuximab (50%)[a]	41 17 11 4					1 3 5 10	AT: 11%, 1 grade 5 LT: 19%, 3% grade 5	Retrospective study a: at the discretion of the treating physician

a, aaSee remarks

AT acute toxicity, *f* fractions, *HP* hypopharynx, *L* larynx, *LT* late toxicity, *NP* nasopharynx, *NR* not reported, *O* other sites, *OC* oral cavity, *OP* oropharynx, *SN* sino-nasal, *y* year, *w* weeks expectancy, palliative RT is a sound option compared to an invasive and potentially mutilating or disabling surgical debulking procedure. In cases of palliative RT, the priorities are short hospital stays, quick symptom alleviation, and comfort with minimal acute toxicity profile. The increased risk of late toxicities may pose a less significant concern.

Split-course RT in the primary curative setting is an outdated concept developed in the 1970s with the aim of reducing the acute toxicity. In order to overcome the "lost dose" caused by the "split" concerning tumor control probability, the total dose was increased. Consequently, late toxicities, which depend on dose per fraction and total dose, increased (Peters et al. 1988). Not only that, locoregional control and survival results were significantly inferior (Overgaard et al. 1988). Currently, there is little use of a detailed discussion of split-course RT with curative intent in its old form. Nevertheless, some of its modern uses for palliative treatment remain attractive. For example, the RTOG 8502 regime, initially developed for pelvic malignancies (Spanos et al. 1994), has become popular for palliation of recurrent and metastatic HNSCC. This schedule (also known as "Quad-Shot") involves the application of at least three cycles of 14.8 Gy in four HO-HE fractions over 2 days, repeated every 4 weeks. The main advantage is its low toxicity profile (9% grade ≥3 toxicity) despite similar efficacy, when compared to other traditional schedules with fraction doses of 2–3 Gy (29–38% grade ≥3 toxicity) (Chen et al. 2008). In a phase II trial, 30 previously untreated patients received a very similar schedule, with the slight difference of 3.5 Gy per fraction instead of 3.7 Gy. Although only 53% of the patients could complete all three fractions, 43% of the patients demonstrated improvement in quality of life. No grade ≥3 toxicity was reported (Corry et al. 2005). Recently, investigators from Memorial Sloan Kettering Cancer Center published the largest series ($n = 75$) with Quad-Shot regimen. This retrospective cohort also included pretreated patients. At the discretion of the treating physician 64% of the patients did not stop their ST

during Quad-Shot course. Grade 2 and 3 toxicities were 28% and 5%, respectively. No grade 3 late toxicity was reported (Lok et al. 2015).

9   Summary and Conclusions

Adding ST to RT or changing the N RT to AFRT improves treatment efficiency. On the other hand, changing the ST + RT schedule from N to AFRT does not improve the outcome, whereas the addition of ST to AFRT increases the therapeutic success. However, no clinical trial evaluated HE within the former strategy, although HE seems to be a better starting point than AC to construct more efficient combined modalities. As presented in the previous sections, platinum-based concomitant chemotherapy and HE is the "best of both worlds." However, no randomized trial directly compared these two strategies. Mixed treatment comparisons suggested that the combination of those strategies could offer the best chance for treatment (Blanchard et al. 2011). However, treatment intensification comes with a price, as shown by GORTEC 99-02 and RTOG 0129, where platinum-based chemotherapy was combined with AC (Trotti et al. 2007).

Today, head and neck oncologists and investigators are reluctant to use AFRT regimens. This might be due to several reasons: clinic- and patient-related logistics, and most probably the toxicity-driven phobia generated by the extremely accelerated regimens tested in 1990s (e.g., CHART schedules). In this context, two other points are also worth noting briefly. First, to our knowledge, no direct cost-effectiveness study was performed between HE, AC, and chemo-RT. Second, the clinical trials are increasingly influenced by the pharmaceutical industry (Devaiah and Murchison 2016a, b), which makes it less likely that AFRT is going to be investigated in the future trials. Actually, there are also potentially attractive uses of AFRT. For example, despite showing a distant metastasis-free survival benefit, induction chemotherapy is not preferred over concomitant chemo-RT. The main reasons are increased chemotherapy-related toxicity, decreased overall treatment compliance, and lack of survival benefit over concomitant chemo-RT (Pignon et al. 2009; Posner et al. 2007; Hitt et al. 2014). A strategy combining induction chemotherapy followed by HE instead of chemo-RT may improve the outcome by not only increasing the distant metastasis-free survival, but also without hampering the locoregional control due to better treatment compliance.

Modern RT techniques offer new avenues to exploit the advantages of AFRT, not only for the primary treatment of treatment-naïve patients, but also in reirradiation and palliative situations. Novel agents, which are at least as effective but less toxic than platinum-compounds, can be combined with contemporary RT techniques to widen the therapeutic window. AFRT, both alone or as part of combined modality with ST, offers many opportunities for head and neck oncologists.

References

Al-Mamgani A, van Rooij PH, Woutersen DP et al (2013a) Radiotherapy for T1-2N0 glottic cancer: a multivariate analysis of predictive factors for the long-term outcome in 1050 patients and a prospective assessment of quality of life and voice handicap index in a subset of 233 patients. Clin Otolaryngol 38:306–312. doi:10.1111/coa.12139

Al-Mamgani A, Van Rooij P, Sewnaik A et al (2013b) Brachytherapy or stereotactic body radiotherapy boost for early-stage oropharyngeal cancer: comparable outcomes of two different approaches. Oral Oncol 49:1018–1024. doi:10.1016/j.oraloncology.2013.07.007

Al-Mamgani A, Kwa SLS, Tans L et al (2015) Single vocal cord irradiation: image guided intensity modulated hypofractionated radiation therapy for T1a glottic cancer: early clinical results. Int J Radiat Oncol Biol Phys 93:337–343. doi:10.1016/j.ijrobp.2015.06.016

Argiris A, Li Y, Forastiere A (2004) Prognostic factors and long-term survivorship in patients with recurrent or metastatic carcinoma of the head and neck. Cancer 101:2222–2229. doi:10.1002/cncr.20640

Bartelink H, Van den Bogaert W, Horiot JC et al (2002) Concomitant cisplatin and radiotherapy in a conventional and modified fractionation schedule in locally advanced head and neck cancer: a randomized phase II EORTC trial. Eur J Cancer 38:667–673. doi:10.1016/S0959-8049(01)00425-7

Baujat B, Bourhis J, Blanchard P et al (2010) Hyperfractionated or accelerated radiotherapy for head and neck cancer. Cochrane Database Syst Rev:CD002026. doi:10.1002/14651858.CD002026

Beitler JJ, Zhang Q, Fu KK et al (2014) Final results of local-regional control and late toxicity of RTOG 9003: a randomized trial of altered fractionation radiation for locally advanced head and neck cancer. Int J Radiat Oncol Biol Phys 89:13–20. doi:10.1016/j.ijrobp.2013.12.027

Bentzen SM, Trotti A (2007) Evaluation of early and late toxicities in chemoradiation trials. J Clin Oncol 25:4096–4103. doi:10.1200/JCO.2007.13.3983

Blanchard P, Hill C, Guihenneuc-Jouyaux C et al (2011) Mixed treatment comparison meta-analysis of altered fractionated radiotherapy and chemotherapy in head and neck cancer. J Clin Epidemiol 64:985–992. doi:10.1016/j.jclinepi.2010.10.016

Blanchard P, Lee A, Marguet S et al (2015) Chemotherapy and radiotherapy in nasopharyngeal carcinoma: an update of the MAC-NPC meta-analysis. Lancet Oncol 16:645–655. doi:10.1016/S1470-2045(15)70126-9

Bonner J, Harari PM, Giralt J et al (2006) Radiotherapy plus cetuximab for squamous-cell carcinoma of the head and neck. N Engl J Med 354:567–578. doi:10.1056/NEJMoa053422

Bonner JA, Harari PM, Giralt J et al (2010) Radiotherapy plus cetuximab for locoregionally advanced head and neck cancer: 5-year survival data from a phase 3 randomized trial, and relation between cetuximab-induced rash and survival. Lancet Oncol 11:21–28. doi:10.1016/S1470-2045(09)70311-0

Bourhis J, Overgaard J, Audry H et al (2006a) Hyperfractionated or accelerated radiotherapy in head and neck cancer: a meta-analysis. Lancet 368:843–854. doi:10.1016/S0140-6736(06)69121-6

Bourhis J, Lapeyre M, Tortochaux J et al (2006b) Phase III randomized trial of very accelerated radiation therapy compared with conventional radiation therapy in squamous cell head and neck cancer: a GORTEC trial. J Clin Oncol 24:2873–2878. doi:10.1200/JCO.2006.08.057

Bourhis J, Sire C, Graff P et al (2012) Concomitant chemoradiotherapy versus acceleration of radiotherapy with or without concomitant chemotherapy in locally advanced head and neck carcinoma (GORTEC 99-02): an open-label phase 3 randomized trial. Lancet Oncol 13:145–153. doi:10.1016/S1470-2045(11)70346-1

Bradley J, Paulson ES, Ahunbay E et al (2011) Dynamic MRI analysis of tumor and organ motion during rest and deglutition and margin assessment for radiotherapy of head-and-neck cancer. Int J Radiat Oncol Biol Phys 81:e803–e812. doi:10.1016/j.ijrobp.2010.12.015

Budach W, Hehr T, Budach V et al (2006) A meta-analysis of hyperfractionated and accelerated radiotherapy and combined chemotherapy and radiotherapy regimens in unresected locally advanced squamous cell carcinoma of the head and neck. BMC Cancer 6:28. doi:10.1186/1471-2407-6-28

Carvalho AL, Nishimoto IN, Califano JA et al (2005) Trends in incidence and prognosis for head and neck cancer in the United States: a site-specific analysis of the SEER database. Int J Cancer 114:806–816. doi:10.1002/ijc.20740

Chen AM, Vaughan A, Narayan S, Vijayakumar S (2008) Palliative radiation therapy for head and neck cancer: toward an optimal fractionation scheme. Head Neck 30:1586–1591. doi:10.1002/hed.20894

Chen AM, Farwell DG, Luu Q et al (2011) Prospective trial of high-dose reirradiation using daily image guidance with intensity-modulated radiotherapy for recurrent and second primary head-and-neck cancer. Int J Radiat Oncol Biol Phys 80:669–676. doi:10.1016/j.ijrobp.2010.02.023

Chera BS, Amdur RJ, Morris CG et al (2010a) T1N0 to T2N0 squamous cell carcinoma of the glottic larynx treated with definitive radiotherapy. Int J Radiat Oncol Biol Phys 78:461–466. doi:10.1016/j.ijrobp.2009.08.066

Chera BS, Amdur RJ, Morris CG et al (2010b) Carotid-sparing intensity-modulated radiotherapy for early-stage squamous cell carcinoma of the true vocal cord. Int J Radiat Oncol Biol Phys 77:1380–1385. doi:10.1016/j.ijrobp.2009.07.1687

Chitapanarux I, Tharavichitkul E, Kamnerdsupaphon P et al (2013) Randomized phase III trial of concurrent chemoradiotherapy vs accelerated hyperfractionation radiotherapy in locally advanced head and neck cancer. J Radiat Res 54:1110–1117. doi:10.1093/jrr/rrt054

Cooper JS, Pajak TF, Rubin P et al (1989) Second malignancies in patients who have head and neck cancer: incidence, effect on survival and implications based on the RTOG experience. Int J Radiat Oncol Biol Phys 17:449–456

Corry J, Peters LJ, D'Costa I et al (2005) The "QUAD SHOT" - A phase II study of palliative radiotherapy for incurable head and neck cancer. Radiother Oncol 77:137–142. doi:10.1016/j.radonc.2005.10.008

Cummings B, Keane T, Pintilie M et al (2007) Five year results of a randomized trial comparing hyperfractionated to conventional radiotherapy over four weeks in locally advanced head and neck cancer. Radiother Oncol 85:7–16. doi:10.1016/j.radonc.2007.09.010

Curran D, Giralt J, Harari PM et al (2007) Quality of life in head and neck cancer patients after treatment with high-dose radiotherapy alone or in combination with cetuximab. J Clin Oncol 25:2191–2197. doi:10.1200/JCO.2006.08.8005

Dakubo GD, Jakupciak JP, Birch-Machin MA et al (2007) Clinical implications and utility of field cancerization. Cancer Cell Int 7:2. doi:10.1186/1475-2867-7-2

De Crevoisier R, Domenge C, Wibault P et al (2001) Full dose reirradiation combined with chemotherapy after salvage surgery in head and neck carcinoma. Cancer 91:2071–2076. doi:10.1002/1097-0142(20010601)91:11<2071::AID-CNCR1234>3.0.CO;2-Z

Devaiah A, Murchison C (2016a) Analysis of 473 US head and neck cancer trials (1996–2014): trends, gaps, and opportunities. Otolaryngol Head Neck Surg 154:309–314. doi:10.1177/0194599815617723

Devaiah A, Murchison C (2016b) Characteristics of NIH- and industry-sponsored head-and-neck cancer clinical trials. Laryngoscope 1–4. doi:10.1002/lary.25942

Dische S, Saunders M, Barrett A et al (1997) A randomized multicentre trial of CHART versus conventional radiotherapy in head and neck cancer. Radiother Oncol 44:123–136. doi:10.1016/S0167-8140(97)00094-7

Dobrowsky W, Naudé J (2000) Continuous hyperfractionated accelerated radiotherapy with/without mitomycin C in head and neck cancers. Radiother Oncol 57:119–124

Dorresteijn LDA, Kappelle AC, Boogerd W et al (2002) Increased risk of ischemic stroke after radiotherapy on the neck in patients younger than 60 years. J Clin Oncol 20:282–288

Ermiş E, Teo M, Dyker KE et al (2015) Definitive hypofractionated radiotherapy for early glottic carcinoma: experience of 55Gy in 20 fractions. Radiat Oncol 10:203. doi:10.1186/s13014-015-0505-6

Feigenberg S, Patel K, Amdur RJ et al (2014) RTOG 9003: the untold story. Int J Radiat Oncol Biol Phys 90:251–252. doi:10.1016/j.ijrobp.2014.04.043

Ferlay J, Shin H-R, Bray F et al (2010) Estimates of worldwide burden of cancer in 2008: GLOBOCAN 2008. Int J Cancer 127:2893–2917. doi:10.1002/ijc.25516

Ferris RL, Blumenschein G, Fayette J et al (2016) Nivolumab for recurrent squamous-cell carcinoma of the head and neck. N Engl J Med. doi:10.1056/NEJMoa1602252

Fu KK, Pajak TF, Marcial V et al (1995) Late effects of hyperfractionated radiotherapy for advanced head and neck cancer: long-term follow-up results of RTOG 83-13. Int J Radiat Oncol Biol Phys 32:577–588. doi:10.1016/0360-3016(95)00080-I

Fu KK, Pajak TF, Trotti A et al (2000) A Radiation Therapy Oncology Group (RTOG) phase III randomized study to compare hyperfractionation and two variants of accelerated fractionation to standard fractionation radiotherapy for head and neck squamous cell carcinomas: first report of RTOG 9003. Int J Radiat Oncol Biol Phys 48:7–16

Garden AS, Forster K, Wong PF et al (2003) Results of radiotherapy for T2N0 glottic carcinoma: does the "2" stand for twice-daily treatment? Int J Radiat Oncol Biol Phys 55:322–328. doi:10.1016/S0360-3016(02)03938-X

Ghaly M, Halthore A, Antone J et al (2014) Dose-escalated stereotactic radiosurgery (SRS) boost for unfavorable locally advanced oropharyngeal cancer: phase I/II trial. Int J Radiat Oncol 90:S122. doi:10.1016/j.ijrobp.2014.05.559

Ghosh-Laskar S, Chaukar D, Deshpande M et al (2016a) Phase III randomized trial of surgery followed by conventional radiotherapy (5 fr/Wk) (Arm A) vs concurrent chemoradiotherapy (Arm B) vs accelerated radiotherapy (6fr/Wk) (Arm C) in locally advanced, stage III and IV, resectable, squamous cell carcinoma oral cavity- oral cavity adjuvant therapy (OCAT): final results (NCT00193843). J Clin Oncol:6004

Good JS, Harrington KJ (2013) The hallmarks of cancer and the radiation oncologist: updating the 5Rs of radiobiology. Clin Oncol 25:569–577. doi:10.1016/j.clon.2013.06.009

Gujral DM, Miah AB, Bodla S et al (2014) Final long-term results of a phase I/II study of dose-escalated intensity-modulated radiotherapy for locally advanced laryngo-hypopharyngeal cancers. Oral Oncol 50:1089–1097. doi:10.1016/j.oraloncology.2014.07.018

Gupta T, Kannan S, Ghosh-Laskar S et al (2015) Concomitant chemoradiotherapy versus altered fractionation radiotherapy in the radiotherapeutic management of loco-regionally advanced head and neck squamous cell carcinoma: an adjusted indirect comparison meta-analysis. Head Neck 37:670–676. doi:10.1002/hed.23661

Gupta T, Kannan S, Ghosh-Laskar S, Agarwal JP (2016) Systematic review and meta-analysis of conventionally fractionated concurrent chemoradiotherapy versus altered fractionation radiotherapy alone in the definitive management of loco-regionally advanced head and neck squamous cell carcinoma. Clin Oncol (R Coll Radiol) 28:50–61. doi:10.1016/j.clon.2015.09.002

Hitt R, Grau JJ, López-Pousa A et al (2014) A randomized phase III trial comparing induction chemotherapy followed by chemoradiotherapy versus chemoradiotherapy alone as treatment of unresectable head and neck cancer. Ann Oncol 25:216–225. doi:10.1093/annonc/mdt46

Hliniak A, Gwiazdowska B, Szutkowski Z et al (2002) A multicentre randomized/controlled trial of a conventional versus modestly accelerated radiotherapy in the laryngeal cancer: influence of a 1-week shortening overall time. Radiother Oncol 62:1–10. doi:10.1016/S0167-8140(01)00494-7

Horiot JC, Le Fur R, N'Guyen T et al (1992) Hyperfractionation versus conventional fractionation in oropharyngeal carcinoma: final analysis of a randomized trial of the EORTC cooperative group of radiotherapy. Radiother Oncol 25:231–241

Horiot JC, Bontemps P, van den Bogaert W et al (1997) Accelerated fractionation (AF) compared to conventional fractionation (CF) improves loco-regional control in the radiotherapy of advanced head and neck cancers: results of the EORTC 22851 randomized trial. Radiother Oncol 44:111–121

Janot F, de Raucourt D, Benhamou E et al (2008) Randomized trial of postoperative reirradiation combined with chemotherapy after salvage surgery compared with salvage surgery alone in head and neck carcinoma. J Clin Oncol 26:5518–5523. doi:10.1200/JCO.2007.15.0102

Krstevska V, Crvenkova S (2006) Altered and conventional fractionated radiotherapy in locoregional control and survival of patients with squamous cell carcinoma of the larynx, oropharynx, and hypopharynx. Croat Med J 47:42–52

Kwa SLS, Al-Mamgani A, Osman S et al (2015) Inter- and intrafraction target motion in highly focused single vocal cord irradiation of T1a larynx cancer patients. Int J Radiat Oncol Biol Phys 93:190–195. doi:10.1016/j.ijrobp.2015.04.049

Langendijk JA, Kasperts N, Leemans CR et al (2006) A phase II study of primary reirradiation in squamous cell carcinoma of head and neck. Radiother Oncol 78:306–312. doi:10.1016/j.radonc.2006.02.003

Langer C, Harris J, Horwitz E et al (2007) Phase II study of low dose Paclitaxel and Cisplatin in combination with split-course concomitant twice-daily reirradiation in recurrent squamoius cell carcinoma of the head and neck: results of RTOG Protocol 9911. J Clin Oncol 25:4800–4805

Lassen P, Eriksen JG, Krogdahl A et al (2011) The influence of HPV-associated p16-expression on accelerated fractionated radiotherapy in head and neck cancer: evaluation of the randomized DAHANCA 6&7 trial. Radiother Oncol 100:49–55. doi:10.1016/j.radonc.2011.02.010

Lee AWM, Tung SY, Chan ATC et al (2011) A randomized trial on addition of concurrent-adjuvant chemotherapy and/or accelerated fractionation for locally-advanced nasopharyngeal carcinoma. Radiother Oncol 98:15–22. doi:10.1016/j.radonc.2010.09.023

Lee AWM, Ngan RKC, Tung SY et al (2015) Preliminary results of trial NPC-0501 evaluating the therapeutic gain by changing from concurrent-adjuvant to induction-concurrent chemoradiotherapy, changing from fluorouracil to capecitabine, and changing from conventional to accelerated radiotherapy. Cancer 121:1328–1338. doi:10.1002/cncr.29208

Ling DC, Vargo JA, Heron DE (2016a) Stereotactic body radiation therapy for recurrent head and neck cancer. Cancer J 22:302–306. doi:10.1097/PPO.0000000000000208

Liu Z, Huang S, Zhang D (2013) High dose rate versus low dose rate brachytherapy for oral cancer--a meta-analysis of clinical trials. PLoS One 8:e65423. doi:10.1371/journal.pone.0065423

Lok BH, Jiang G, Gutiontov S et al (2015) Palliative head and neck radiotherapy with the RTOG 8502 regimen for incurable primary or metastatic cancers. Oral Oncol 51:957–962. doi:10.1016/j.oraloncology.2015.07.011

Lyhne NM, Primdahl H, Kristensen C et al (2015) The DAHANCA 6 randomized trial: effect of 6 vs 5 weekly fractions of radiotherapy in patients with glottic squamous cell carcinoma. Radiother Oncol 117:91–98. doi:10.1016/j.radonc.2015.07.004

Lyhne NM, Johansen J, Kristensen CA et al (2016) Pattern of failure in 5001 patients treated for glottic squamous cell carcinoma with curative intent - A population based study from the DAHANCA group. Radiother Oncol 118:257–266. doi:10.1016/j.radonc.2016.02.006

Marcial VA, Pajak TF, Chang C et al (1987) Hyperfractionated photon radiation therapy in the treatment of advanced squamous cell carcinoma of the oral cavity, pharynx, larynx, and sinuses, using radiation therapy as the only planned modality: (preliminary report) by the Radiation Therapy Oncology. Int J Radiat Oncol Biol Phys 13:41–47

Mohanti BK, Nachiappan P, Pandey RM et al (2007) Analysis of 2167 head and neck cancer patients' management, treatment compliance and outcomes from a regional cancer centre, Delhi, India. J Laryngol Otol 121:49–56. doi:10.1017/S0022215106002751

Moon SH, Cho KH, Chung EJ et al (2013) A prospective randomized trial comparing hypofractionation with conventional fractionation radiotherapy for T1-2 glottic squamous cell carcinomas: results of a Korean Radiation Oncology Group (KROG-0201) study. Radiother Oncol 110:98–103. doi:10.1016/j.radonc.2013.09.016

Mortensen HR, Overgaard J, Specht L et al (2012) Prevalence and peak incidence of acute and late normal tissue morbidity in the DAHANCA 6&7 randomized trial with accelerated radiotherapy for head and neck cancer. Radiother Oncol 103:69–75. doi:10.1016/j.radonc.2012.01.002

Nguyen-Tan PF, Zhang Q, Ang KK et al (2014) Randomized phase III trial to test accelerated versus standard fractionation in combination with concurrent cisplatin for head and neck carcinomas in the Radiation Therapy Oncology Group 0129 trial: long-term report of efficacy and toxicity. J Clin Oncol 32:3858–3866. doi:10.1200/JCO.2014.55.3925

Overgaard J, Hjelm-Hansen M, Johansen LV et al (1988) Comparison of conventional and split-course radiotherapy as primary treatment in carcinoma of the larynx. Acta Oncol 27:147–152. doi:10.3109/02841868809090334

Overgaard J, Hansen HS, Andersen AP et al (1989) Misonidazole combined with split-course radiotherapy in the treatment of invasive carcinoma of larynx and pharynx: report from the DAHANCA 2 study. Int J Radiat Oncol Biol Phys 16:1065–1068

Overgaard J, Hansen HS, Specht L et al (2003) Five compared with six fractions per week of conventional radiotherapy of squamous-cell carcinoma of head and neck: DAHANCA 6 and 7 randomized controlled trial. Lancet (London, England) 362:933–940

Overgaard J, Mohanti BK, Begum N et al (2010) Five versus six fractions of radiotherapy per week for squamous-cell carcinoma of the head and neck (IAEA-ACC study): a randomized, multicentre trial. Lancet Oncol 11:553–560. doi:10.1016/S1470-2045(10)70072-3

Pehlivan B, Luthi F, Matzinger O et al (2009) Feasibility and efficacy of accelerated weekly concomitant boost postoperative radiation therapy combined with concomitant chemotherapy in patients with locally advanced head and neck cancer. Ann Surg Oncol 16:1337–1343. doi:10.1245/s10434-009-0426-4

Peters LJ, Ang KK, Thames HD (1988) Accelerated fractionation in the radiation treatment of head and neck cancer. A critical comparison of different strategies. Acta Oncol 27:185–194. doi:10.3109/02841868809090339

Pignon J-P, le Maître A, Maillard E et al (2009) Meta-analysis of chemotherapy in head and neck cancer (MACH-NC): an update on 93 randomized trials and 17,346 patients. Radiother Oncol 92:4–14. doi:10.1016/j.radonc.2009.04.014

Pinto LH, Canary PC, Araújo CM et al (1991) Prospective randomized trial comparing hyperfractionated versus conventional radiotherapy in stages III and IV oropharyngeal carcinoma. Int J Radiat Oncol Biol Phys 21:557–562. doi:10.1016/0360-3016(91)90670-Y

Posner MR, Hershock DM, Blajman CR et al (2007) Cisplatin and fluorouracil alone or with docetaxel in head and neck cancer. N Engl J Med 357:1705–1715. doi:10.1056/NEJMoa070956

Quan K, Xu KM, Zhang Y et al (2016) Toxicities following stereotactic ablative radiotherapy treatment of locally-recurrent and previously irradiated head and neck squamous cell carcinoma. Semin Radiat Oncol 26:112–119. doi:10.1016/j.semradonc.2015.11.007

Rischin D, Ferris RL, Le Q-T (2015) Overview of advances in head and neck cancer. J Clin Oncol 33:3225–3226. doi:10.1200/JCO.2015.63.6761

Rishi A, Ghoshal S, Verma R et al (2013) Comparison of concomitant boost radiotherapy against concurrent chemoradiation in locally advanced oropharyngeal cancers: a phase III randomized trial. Radiother Oncol 107:317–324. doi:10.1016/j.radonc.2013.05.016

Rosenthal DI, Fuller CD, Peters LJ et al (2015) Final report of radiation therapy oncology group protocol 9003: provocative, but limited conclusions from exploratory analyses. Int J Radiat Oncol Biol Phys 92:715–717. doi:10.1016/j.ijrobp.2015.02.051

Sakata K, Someya M, Hori M et al (2008) Hyperfractionated accelerated radiotherapy for T1, 2 glottic carcinoma. Consideration of time-dose factors. Strahlenther Onkol 184:364–369. doi:10.1007/s00066-008-1819-1

Sanchíz F, Milla A, Torner J et al (1990) Single fraction per day versus two fractions per day versus radiochemotherapy in the treatment of head and neck cancer. Int J Radiat Oncol Biol Phys 19:1347–1350. doi:10.1016/0360-3016(90)90342-H

Saunders MI, Rojas AM, Parmar MKB et al (2010) Mature results of a randomized trial of accelerated hyperfractionated versus conventional radiotherapy in head-and-neck cancer. Int J Radiat Oncol Biol Phys 77:3–8. doi:10.1016/j.ijrobp.2009.04.082

Siegel RL, Miller KD, Jemal A (2015) Cancer statistics, 2015. CA Cancer J Clin 65:5–29. doi:10.3322/caac.21254

Skladowski K, Maciejewski B, Golen M et al (2000) Randomized clinical trial on 7-day-continuous accelerated irradiation (CAIR) of head and neck cancer - report on 3-year tumour control and normal tissue toxicity. Radiother Oncol 55:101–110. doi:10.1016/S0167-8140(00)00139-0

Skladowski K, Maciejewski B, Golen M et al (2006) Continuous accelerated 7-days-a-week radiotherapy for head-and-neck cancer: long-term results of Phase III clinical trial. Int J Radiat Oncol Biol Phys 66:706–713. doi:10.1016/j.ijrobp.2006.05.026

Skladowski K, Hutnik M, Wygoda A et al (2013) Radiation-free weekend rescued! Continuous accelerated irradiation of 7-days per week is equal to accelerated fractionation with concomitant boost of 7 fractions in 5-days per week: report on phase 3 clinical trial in head-and-neck cancer patients. Int J Radiat Oncol Biol Phys 85:741–746. doi:10.1016/j.ijrobp.2012.06.037

Smith GL, Smith BD, Buchholz T et al (2008) Cerebrovascular disease risk in older head and neck cancer patients after radiotherapy. J Clin Oncol 26:5119–5125. doi:10.1200/JCO.2008.16.6546

Spanos WT, Clery M, Perez CA et al (1994) Late effect of multiple daily fraction palliation schedule for advanced pelvic malignancies (RTOG 8502). Int J Radiat Oncol Biol Phys 29:961–967. doi:10.1016/0360-3016(94)90389-1

Spencer SA, Harris J, Wheeler RH et al (2008) Final report of RTOG 9610, a multi-institutional trial of reirradiation and chemotherapy for unresectable recurrent squamous cell carcinoma of the head and neck. Head Neck 30:281–288. doi:10.1002/hed.20697

Suwiński R, Bańkowska-Woźniak M, Majewski W et al (2008) Randomized clinical trial on 7-days-a-week postoperative radiotherapy for high-risk squamous cell head and neck cancer. Radiother Oncol 87:155–163. doi:10.1016/j.radonc.2008.02.009

Tao Y, Aupérin A, Graff P et al (2016) Concurrent chemoradiation therapy versus acceleration of radiation therapy with or without concurrent chemotherapy in locally advanced head and neck carcinoma (GORTEC 99-02): 7-year survival data from a phase 3 randomized trial and prognostic factors. Int J Radiat Oncol Biol Phys 96:E324–E325. doi:10.1016/j.ijrobp.2016.06.1443

Teo PM, Leung SF, Chan AT et al (2000) Final report of a randomized trial on altered-fractionated radiotherapy in nasopharyngeal carcinoma prematurely terminated by significant increase in neurologic complications. Int J Radiat Oncol Biol Phys 48:1311–1322. doi:10.1016/S0360-3016(00)00786-0

Thames HD, Bentzen SM, Turesson I et al (1989) Fractionation parameters for human tissues and tumors. Int J Radiat Biol 56:701–710

Trotti A, Machtay M (2014) RTOG 9003: legacies of a landmark trial. Int J Radiat Oncol Biol Phys 90:253–254. doi:10.1016/j.ijrobp.2014.07.022

Trotti A, Pajak TF, Gwede CK et al (2007) TAME: development of a new method for summarizing adverse events of cancer treatment by the Radiation Therapy Oncology Group. Lancet Oncol 8:613–624. doi:10.1016/S1470-2045(07)70144-4

Trotti A, Zhang Q, Bentzen SM et al (2014) Randomized trial of hyperfractionation versus conventional fractionation in T2 squamous cell carcinoma of the vocal cord (RTOG 9512). Int J Radiat Oncol Biol Phys 89:958–963. doi:10.1016/j.ijrobp.2014.04.041

Van Asselen B, Raaijmakers CPJ, Lagendijk JJW et al (2003) Intrafraction motions of the larynx during radiotherapy. Int J Radiat Oncol Biol Phys 56:384–390. doi:10.1016/S0360-3016(02)04572-8

Vargo JA, Ferris RL, Ohr J et al (2015) A prospective phase 2 trial of reirradiation with stereotactic body radiation therapy plus cetuximab in patients with previously irradiated recurrent squamous cell carcinoma of the head and neck. Int J Radiat Oncol Biol Phys 91:480–8. doi: 10.1016/j.ijrobp.2014.11.023

Vermorken JB, Mesia R, Rivera F et al (2008) Platinumbased chemotherapy plus cetuximab in head and neck cancer. N Engl J Med 359:1116–1127. doi:10.1056/NEJMoa0802656

Weissberg JB, Son YH, Percarpio B et al (1982) Randomized trial of conventional versus high fractional dose radiation therapy in the treatment of advanced head and neck cancer. Int J Radiat Oncol Biol Phys 8:179–185

Yamamoto E, Shibuya H, Yoshimura R et al (2002) Site specific dependency of second primary cancer in early stage head and neck squamous cell carcinoma. Cancer 94:2007–2014. doi:10.1002/cncr.10444

Yamazaki H, Nishiyama K, Tanaka E et al (2006) Radiotherapy for early glottic carcinoma (T1N0M0): results of prospective randomized study of radiation fraction size and overall treatment time. Int J Radiat Oncol Biol Phys 64:77–82. doi:10.1016/j.ijrobp.2005.06.014

Yamoah K, Showalter TN, Ohri N (2015) Radiation therapy intensification for solid tumors: a systematic review of randomized trials. Int J Radiat Oncol Biol Phys 93:737–745. doi:10.1016/j.ijrobp.2015.07.2284

Additional References for Tables

Ang KK, Trotti A, Brown BW et al (2001) Randomized trial addressing risk features and time factors of surgery plus radiotherapy in advanced head-and-neck cancer. Int J Radiat Oncol Biol Phys 51:571–578. doi:10.1016/S0360-3016(01)01690-X

Ang KK, Harris J, Garden AS et al (2005) Concomitant boost radiation plus concurrent cisplatin for advanced head and neck carcinomas: Radiation Therapy Oncology Group Phase II Trial 99-14. J Clin Oncol 23:3008–3015. doi:10.1200/JCO.2005.12.060

Awwad HK, Khafagy Y, Barsoum M et al (1992) Accelerated versus conventional fractionation in the postoperative irradiation of locally advanced head and neck cancer: influence of tumour proliferation. Radiother Oncol 25:261–266. doi:10.1016/0167-8140(92)90245-P

Awwad HK, Lotayef M, Shouman T et al (2002) Accelerated hyperfractionation (AHF) compared to conventional fractionation (CF) in the postoperative radiotherapy of locally advanced head and neck cancer: influence of proliferation. Br J Cancer 86:517–523. doi:10.1038/sj.bjc.6600119

Bensadoun R-JJ, Benezery K, Dassonville O et al (2006) French multicenter phase III randomized study testing concurrent twice-a-day radiotherapy and cisplatin/5-fluorouracil chemotherapy (BiRCF) in unresectable pharyngeal carcinoma: results at 2 years (FNCLCC-GORTEC). Int J Radiat Oncol Biol Phys 64:983–994. doi:10.1016/j.ijrobp.2005.09.041

Bentzen J, Toustrup K, Eriksen JG et al (2015) Locally advanced head and neck cancer treated with accelerated radiotherapy, the hypoxic modifier nimorazole and weekly cisplatin. Results from the DAHANCA 18 phase II study. Acta Oncol 54:1001–1007. doi:10.3109/0284186X.2014.992547

Bourhis J, Lapeyre M, Tortochaux J et al (2011) Accelerated radiotherapy and concomitant high dose chemotherapy in non-resectable stage IV locally advanced HNSCC: results of a GORTEC randomized trial. Radiother Oncol 100:56–61. doi:10.1016/j.radonc.2011.07.006

Brizel DM, Albers ME, Fisher SR et al (1998) Hyperfractionated irradiation with or without concurrent chemotherapy for locally advanced head and neck cancer. N Engl J Med 338:1798–1804. doi:10.1056/NEJM199806183382503

Budach V, Stuschke M, Budach W et al (2005) Hyperfractionated accelerated chemoradiation with concurrent fluorouracil-mitomycin is more effective than dose-escalated hyperfractionated accelerated radiation therapy alone in locally advanced head and neck cancer: final results of the radiotherapy cooperative clinical trials group of the German Cancer Society 95-06 Prospective Randomized Trial. J Clin Oncol 23:1125–1135. doi:10.1200/JCO.2005.07.010

Budach V, Stromberger C, Poettgen C et al (2015) Hyperfractionated accelerated radiation therapy (HART) of 70.6 Gy with concurrent 5-FU/Mitomycin C is superior to HART of 77.6 Gy alone in locally advanced head and neck cancer: long-term results of the ARO 95-06 randomized phase III trial. Int J Radiat Oncol Biol Phys 91:916–924. doi:10.1016/j.ijrobp.2014.12.034

Cvek J, Kubes J, Skacelikova E et al (2012) Hyperfractionated accelerated radiotherapy with concomitant integrated boost of 70-75 Gy in 5 weeks for advanced head and neck cancer: a phase I dose escalation study. Strahlenther Onkol 188:666–670. doi:10.1007/s00066-012-0128-x

Daoud J, Toumi N, Siala W et al (2007) Results of a prospective randomised trial comparing conventional radiotherapy to split-course bifractionated radiation therapy in patients with nasopharyngeal carcinoma. Radiother Oncol 85:17–23. doi:10.1016/j.radonc.2007.01.013

Eisbruch A, Harris J, Garden AS et al (2010) Multi-institutional trial of accelerated hypofractionated intensity-modulated radiation therapy for early-stage oropharyngeal cancer (RTOG 00-22). Int J Radiat Oncol Biol Phys 76:1333–1338. doi:10.1016/j.ijrobp.2009.04.011

Ezzat M, Shouman T, Zaza K et al (2005) A randomized study of accelerated fractionation radiotherapy with and without mitomycin C in the treatment of locally advanced head and neck cancer. J Egypt Natl Canc Inst 17:85–92

Garden AS, Harris J, Trotti A et al (2008) Long-term results of concomitant boost radiation plus concurrent cisplatin for advanced head and neck carcinomas: a phase II trial of the radiation therapy oncology group (RTOG 99-14). Int J Radiat Oncol Biol Phys 71:1351–1355. doi:10.1016/j.ijrobp.2008.04.006

Ghadjar P, Simcock M, Studer G et al (2012) Concomitant cisplatin and hyperfractionated radiotherapy in locally advanced head and neck cancer: 10-year follow-up of a randomized phase III trial (SAKK 10/94). Int J Radiat Oncol Biol Phys 82:524–531. doi:10.1016/j.ijrobp.2010.11.067

Ghoshal S, Goda JS, Mallick I et al (2008) Concomitant boost radiotherapy compared with conventional radiotherapy in squamous cell carcinoma of the head and neck--a phase III trial from a single institution in India. Clin Oncol 20:212–220. doi:10.1016/j.clon.2008.01.011

Ghosh-Laskar S, Kalyani N, Gupta T et al (2016b) Conventional radiotherapy versus concurrent chemoradiotherapy versus accelerated radiotherapy in locoregionally advanced carcinoma of head and neck: results of a prospective randomized trial. Head Neck 38:202–207. doi:10.1002/hed.23865

Gunn GB, Endres EJ, Parker B et al (2010) A phase I/II study of altered fractionated IMRT alone for intermediate t-stage oropharyngeal carcinoma. Strahlenther Onkol 186:489–495. doi:10.1007/s00066-010-2093-6

Hassan Metwally MA, Ali R, Kuddu M et al (2015) IAEA-HypoX. A randomized multicenter study of the hypoxic radiosensitizer nimorazole concomitant with accelerated radiotherapy in head and neck squamous cell carcinoma. Radiother Oncol 116:15–20. doi:10.1016/j.radonc.2015.04.005

Heron DE, Ferris RL, Karamouzis M et al (2009) Stereotactic body radiotherapy for recurrent squamous cell carcinoma of the head and neck: results of a phase I dose-escalation trial. Int J Radiat Oncol Biol Phys 75:1493–1500. doi:10.1016/j.ijrobp.2008.12.075

Huguenin P, Beer KT, Allal A et al (2004) Concomitant cisplatin significantly improves locoregional control in advanced head and neck cancers treated with hyperfractionated radiotherapy. J Clin Oncol 22:4665–4673. doi:10.1200/JCO.2004.12.193

Iwata H, Tatewaki K, Inoue M et al (2012) Salvage stereotactic reirradiation using the CyberKnife for the local recurrence of nasal or paranasal carcinoma. Radiother Oncol 104:355–360. doi:10.1016/j.radonc.2012.01.017

Jackson SM, Weir LM, Hay JH et al (1997) A randomized trial of accelerated versus conventional radiotherapy in head and neck cancer. Radiother Oncol 43:39–46

Janssens GO, Rademakers SE, Terhaard CH et al (2012) Accelerated radiotherapy with carbogen and nicotinamide for laryngeal cancer: results of a phase III randomized trial. J Clin Oncol 30:1777–1783. doi:10.1200/JCO.2011.35.9315

Jeremic B, Shibamoto Y, Milicic B et al (2000) Hyperfractionated radiation therapy with or without concurrent low-dose daily cisplatin in locally advanced squamous cell carcinoma of the head and neck: a prospective randomized trial. J Clin Oncol 18:1458–1464

Johnson CR, Schmidt-Ullrich RK, Arthur DW et al (1995) 42 Standard Once daily versus thrice-daily concomitant boost accelerated superfractionated irradiation for advanced squamous cell carcinoma of the head and neck: preliminary results of a prospective randomized trial. Int J Radiat Oncol 32:162. doi:10.1016/0360-3016(95)97707-8

Kao J, Genden EM, Gupta V et al (2011) Phase 2 trial of concurrent 5-fluorouracil, hydroxyurea, cetuximab, and hyperfractionated intensity-modulated radiation therapy for locally advanced head and neck cancer. Cancer 117:318–326. doi:10.1002/cncr.25374

Lartigau EF, Tresch E, Thariat J et al (2013) Multi institutional phase II study of concomitant stereotactic reirradiation and cetuximab for recurrent head and neck cancer. Radiother Oncol 109:281–285. doi:10.1016/j.radonc.2013.08.012

Lee AWM, Tung SY, Chan ATC et al (2006) Preliminary results of a randomized study (NPC-9902 Trial) on therapeutic gain by concurrent chemotherapy and/or accelerated fractionation for locally advanced nasopharyngeal carcinoma. Int J Radiat Oncol Biol Phys 66:142–151. doi:10.1016/j.ijrobp.2006.03.054

Ling DC, Vargo JA, Ferris RL et al (2016b) Risk of severe toxicity according to site of recurrence in patients treated with stereotactic body radiation therapy for recurrent head and neck cancer. Int J Radiat Oncol Biol Phys 95:973–980. doi:10.1016/j.ijrobp.2016.02.049

Maguire PD, Papagikos M, Hamann S et al (2011) Phase II trial of hyperfractionated intensity-modulated radiation therapy and concurrent weekly cisplatin for stage III and IVa head-and-neck cancer. Int J Radiat Oncol Biol Phys 79:1081–1088. doi:10.1016/j.ijrobp.2009.12.046

Miszczyk L, Maciejewski B, Tukiendorf A et al (2014) Split-course accelerated hyperfractionated irradiation (CHA-CHA) as a sole treatment for advanced head and neck cancer patients-final results of a randomized clinical trial. Br J Radiol 87:20140212. doi:10.1259/bjr.20140212

Nyqvist J, Fransson P, Laurell G et al (2016) Differences in health related quality of life in the randomized ARTSCAN study; accelerated vs. conventional radiotherapy for head and neck cancer. A five year follow up. Radiother Oncol 118:335–341. doi:10.1016/j.radonc.2015.12.024

Olmi P, Crispino S, Fallai C et al (2003) Locoregionally advanced carcinoma of the oropharynx: conventional radiotherapy vs. accelerated hyperfractionated radiotherapy vs. concomitant radiotherapy and chemotherapy--a multicenter randomized trial. Int J Radiat Oncol Biol Phys 55:78–92. doi:10.1016/S0360-3016(02)03792-6

Poulsen MG, Denham JW, Peters LJ et al (2001) A randomized trial of accelerated and conventional radiotherapy for stage III and IV squamous carcinoma of the head and neck: a Trans-Tasman Radiation Oncology Group Study. Radiother Oncol 60:113–122. doi:10.1016/S0167-8140(01)00347-4

Sanguineti G, Richetti A, Bignardi M et al (2005) Accelerated versus conventional fractionated postoperative radiotherapy for advanced head and neck cancer: results of a multicenter phase III study. Int J Radiat

Oncol Biol Phys 61:762–771. doi:10.1016/j.ijrobp.2004.07.682

Songthong AP, Kannarunimit D, Chakkabat C et al (2015) A randomized phase II/III study of adverse events between sequential (SEQ) versus simultaneous integrated boost (SIB) intensity modulated radiation therapy (IMRT) in nasopharyngeal carcinoma; preliminary result on acute adverse events. Radiat Oncol 10:166. doi:10.1186/s13014-015-0472-y

Staar S, Rudat V, Stuetzer H et al (2001) Intensified hyperfractionated accelerated radiotherapy limits the additional benefit of simultaneous chemotherapy - Results of a multicentric randomized German trial in advanced head-and-neck cancer. Int J Radiat Oncol Biol Phys 50:1161–1171. doi:10.1016/S0360-3016(01)01544-9

Stuschke M, Thames HD (1997) Hyperfractionated radiotherapy of human tumors: overview of the randomized clinical trials. Int J Radiat Oncol Biol Phys 37:259–267. doi:10.1016/S0360-3016(96)00511-1

Suwinski R, Wozniak G, Misiolek M et al (2016) Randomized clinical trial on 7-days-a-week postoperative radiotherapy vs concurrent post-operative radiochemotherapy in locally advanced cancer of the oral cavity/oropharynx: a report on acute normal tissue reactions. Br J Radiol 89:20150805. doi:10.1259/bjr.20150805

Wendt TG, Grabenbauer GG, Rödel CM et al (1998) Simultaneous radiochemotherapy versus radiotherapy alone in advanced head and neck cancer: a randomized multicenter study. J Clin Oncol 16:1318–1324

Zackrisson B, Kjellén E, Söderström K et al (2015) Mature results from a Swedish comparison study of conventional versus accelerated radiotherapy in head and neck squamous cell carcinoma - The ARTSCAN trial. Radiother Oncol 117:99–105. doi:10.1016/j.radonc.2015.09.024

Whole-Breast Hypofractionated Radiotherapy

Fernand Missohou, Mark Trombetta, and Jean-Philippe Pignol

Contents

The original version of this chapter was revised. The affiliations of the authors have been updated.

F. Missohou
Division of Radiation Oncology, Institut de Cancérologie de Libreville (ICL), Libreville, Gabon

M. Trombetta (✉)
Allegheny General Hospital, Allegheny Health Network Cancer Institute, Drexel University College of Medicine, Pittsburgh, PA, USA
e-mail: mtrombet@wpahs.org

J.-P. Pignol
Erasmus Medical Center, Rotterdam, The Netherlands
e-mail: j.p.pignol@erasmusmc.nl

Abstract

Breast cancer is the most common malignancy diagnosed in women (http://seer.cancer.gov/statfacts/html/breast.html). Today, with the widespread generalization of mammography, it is most frequently diagnosed at an early stage (Nystrom et al. 2002). The outcomes of those early-stage cancers are excellent, with local control above 98% and a risk of dying of cancer at 5 years below 2% (http://seer.cancer.gov/statfacts/html/breast.html; Strnad et al. 2016). Clinical researches since the 1980s have aimed at optimizing the cosmetic outcome, minimizing the long-term side effects, and reducing the treatment burden. Several randomized clinical trials and meta-analyses have shown that breast-conserving surgery followed by adjuvant radiotherapy (XRT) to the whole breast achieves local control rate and survival equivalent to mastectomy, with the advantage of allowing breast conservation and hence improved quality of life (Fisher et al. 2002; Veronesi et al. 2002; Clark et al. 1996; EBCTCG et al. 2011).

Med Radiol Radiat Oncol (2017)
DOI 10.1007/174_2017_33 © Springer International Publishing AG
Published Online: 26 April 2017

1 Introduction

1.1 Whole-Breast Radiotherapy

Breast cancer is the most common malignancy diagnosed in women (http://seer.cancer.gov/statfacts/html/breast.html). Today, with the widespread generalization of mammography, it is most frequently diagnosed at an early stage (Nystrom et al. 2002). The outcomes of those early-stage cancers are excellent, with local control above 98% and a risk of dying of cancer at 5 years below 2% (http://seer.cancer.gov/statfacts/html/breast.html; Strnad et al. 2016). Clinical researches since the 1980s have aimed at optimizing the cosmetic outcome, minimizing the long-term side effects, and reducing the treatment burden. Several randomized clinical trials and meta-analyses have shown that breast-conserving surgery followed by adjuvant radiotherapy (XRT) to the whole breast achieves local control rate and survival equivalent to mastectomy, with the advantage of allowing breast conservation and hence improved quality of life (Fisher et al. 2002; Veronesi et al. 2002; Clark et al. 1996; EBCTCG et al. 2011).

The 50 Gy in 25 fractions over 5-week dose fractionation regimen used in the NSABP-B06 trial became the most widely accepted "standard" (Fisher et al. 1985). This extended regimen using 2 Gy per fraction was justified by the understanding that on the one hand the normal tissue late side effects were highly sensitive to the fraction size of each treatment, with an alpha/beta value of approximately 3.4 (Whelan et al. 2008; START Trialists' Group et al. 2008a), while the radiosensitivity of breast cancer tumor to fractionation was believed to be low (alpha/beta value of 10). This value is similar to most epithelial tumors including bronchus, cervix, or head and neck tumors (Khan and Haffty 2010; Owen et al. 2006). Also, there have been several reports of horrendous complications following the early experience of hypofractionation, including brachial plexopathy, frozen shoulder, rib fractures, chest wall necrosis, breast fibrosis, or extensive telangiectasia. In 1991, Fletcher summarized those experiences (Table 1) and concluded: "there is overwhelming evidence that fraction size of more than 2 Gy produces unfavorable sequelae, and therefore, despite inconvenience for patients and the taxing of machine time, hypofractionation should not be used" (Fletcher 1991).

1.2 First UK Hypofractionated Multicenter Randomized Clinical Trial

While the radiation oncology community was well aware of the risk of severe and permanent side effects using hypofractionation, large variations in dose fractionation regimens subsisted across and within countries. In the UK, a survey done in 1989 revealed variations between institutes (Rodger 2010). While a large number of centers adopted the NSABP-B06 50 Gy in 25-fraction regimen (Fisher et al. 1985), most centers in the UK and Western Canada used 40–45 Gy in 3 weeks.

Things changed with the discovery from in vitro experiments that the alpha/beta ratio for

Table 1 Preliminary experience of whole-breast hypofractionation irradiation and related complications

Author and institution	Regimen	Complications (%)
Atkins (1964) and Edelman et al. (1965), Columbia- Presbyterian and Washington U	2×12.5 Gy in 1 week	Frozen shoulder, brachial plexopathy, multiple rib fracture
Montague (1968), MD Anderson	6×5 Gy in 3 weeks	Frozen shoulder, brachial plexopathy, chest wall necrosis and fibrosis, multiple rib fracture
Bates (1988), St Thomas Hospital	12×4.44 Gy (3 fractions per week) or 6×6 Gy (2 fractions per week)	Arm edema (30%), severe lung fibrosis (14%), telangiectasia, skin and subcutaneous atrophy, frozen shoulder
Overgaard (1985), Aarhus	2 fractions per week equivalent to 1,345 RET	Moderate to severe fibrosis (50%), telangiectasia (50%), pneumonitis (30%), rib fractures (10%)
Rodger (2010), Glasgow	4.5 Gy $\times$ 10 (3 fractions per week)	Fibrosis and rib fracture

human breast carcinoma cell lines was approximately 4 Gy, and thus as protected by fractionation as normal tissues (Matthews et al. 1989; Steel et al. 1987), which made adherence to a protracted regimen unfounded.

Based on this rationale, the Royal Marsden Hospital and the Gloucestershire Oncology Centre launched a pilot randomized trial comparing three regimens: 50 Gy in 25 fractions, 42.9 Gy in 13 fractions, and 39 Gy in 13 fractions (Yarnold et al. 2005; Owen et al. 2006). The different regimens were all delivered in 5 weeks to keep constant the overall treatment time in the biologically effective dose (BED) calculation. The primary endpoint was breast toxicity and the secondary endpoint was local control. The protocol allowed for regional irradiation, which was delivered in 20% of the patients, and for delivery of an electron boost, which was used in 75% of the patients. The radiation was delivered using a 2-dimensional wedge technique for missing tissue compensation, with the wedge angle defined on a single transverse contour. The dose variation on the central plane was kept between −5% and +7%.

A total of 1410 women were randomized. When comparing the regimens, the shorter 39 Gy in 13 fractions yielded fewer long-term side effect at 10 years with 6.6% marked breast changes and a 27.7% induration rate, compared to 9.8% marked breast changes and a 36.6% induration rate for the 50 Gy in 25-fraction regimen. The 42.9 Gy in 13-fraction regimen did worse in term of long-term side effects and cosmesis (Owen et al. 2006b).

The rates of local recurrence were relatively high but consistent with those reported in this era. Though it was not statistically significant, it was slightly worse for the 39 Gy in 13-fraction regimen. The 5-year local recurrence rates were 7.9% for 50 Gy in 25 fractions, 7.1% for 42.9 Gy in 13 fractions, and 9.1 % for 39 Gy in 13 fractions. The 10-year rates were, respectively, 12.1%, 9.6%, and 14.1% (Owen et al. 2006).

The study allowed an alpha/beta ratio of 3.6 Gy for late breast changes, 3.1 Gy for palpable induration, and 4 Gy for tumor control (Yarnold et al. 2005; Owen et al. 2006). Since the study was not powered to test for noninferiority, three larger confirmatory trials in Canada and the UK followed.

2 Large Multicenter Randomized Trials

2.1 Canadian Hypofractionated Study

From 1993 to 1996 the Ontario Clinical Oncology Group (OCOG) accrued 1234 patients in a multicenter randomized trial comparing whole-breast radiotherapy, 50 Gy in 25 fractions and 5 weeks (612 patients), to 42.5 Gy in 16 treatments and 3.5 weeks (622 patients) (Whelan et al. 2002, 2010). The primary objective was to test for noninferiority in terms of local control between the regimens. Patients with positive nodes, positive margins, primary tumor larger than 5 cm, or a breast separation ≥25 cm were excluded. Also the protocol required limiting the dose distribution heterogeneity to a maximum of 107% of the prescribed dose. At 5 years, the local recurrence rate was equal: 2.8% in the hypofractionated arm and 3.2% in the standard fractionated arm (Whelan et al. 2002), and 6.2% and 6.7%, respectively, at 10 years (Whelan et al. 2010). Both analyses demonstrate the noninferiority of the hypofractionated regimen compared to the standard with 97.5% confidence.

2.2 The UK Multicenter Randomized START A and B Trials

Following the Royal Marsden Hospital and the Gloucestershire Oncology Centre pilot trial, a larger study, the Standardization of Breast Radiotherapy Trial (START) A, was launched in several UK centers from 1998 to 2002 (START Trialists' Group et al. 2008b). It was a noninferiority trial, with a planned sample size of 2000 patients to detect with 80% power a difference of 5% in the local-regional relapse rate between the control arm and two experimental arms (two-sided and $\alpha = 5\%$). A total of 2236 women were accrued and randomized to receive either 50 Gy in 25 fractions, 41.6 Gy in 13 fractions (3.2 Gy per fraction), or 39 Gy in 13 fractions (3 Gy per fraction). Similarly to the pilot trial, all regimens were administered over 5 weeks. Chemotherapy was delivered in 35.5% of the patients, and regional radiation in 14.2%. Of note, 15% of the patients had mastectomy and received chest wall radiotherapy, and 60.6% received a boost. The randomization was stratified by the type of surgery (breast-conserving surgery or mastectomy) and the delivery (or not) of a boost. The 10-year rate of locoregional relapse was 7.4% for the 50 Gy in 25-fraction regimen, compared to 6.3% for the 41.6 Gy in 13-fraction regimen ($p = 0.65$), and 8.8% for the 39 Gy in 13 fractions ($p = 0.41$) (Haviland et al. 2013). The study concluded a noninferiority between the three arms; however since the 39 Gy in 13 fractions had a slightly higher rate of locoregional relapse and the 41.6 Gy in 13 fractions a slightly higher rate of long-term complications, it was decided to fine-tune the optimal hypofractionated regimen.

The START-B was a two-arm randomized trial, selecting an intermediate experimental dose fractionation regimen of 40 Gy in 15 fractions (2.66 Gy per fraction) over 3 weeks, meaning that the treatment was accelerated in the same way as the Canadian trial instead of the START A trial (Haviland et al. 2013). A sample size of 1840 patients was needed to exclude (with 95% power) an increase of 5% in the local-regional relapse rate in the hypofractionated arm (one-sided and $\alpha = 2.5\%$). From January 1999 to December 2002, a total of 2215 women were accrued and randomized to receive either 50 Gy in 25 fractions and 5 weeks or 40 Gy in 15 fractions and 3 weeks. Chemotherapy was delivered in 22.2% of the patients, regional irradiation in 7.3%, postmastectomy chest-wall radiotherapy in 8%, and a boost in 42.6%. The 10-year rate of local relapse was 5.2% for the 50 Gy in 25-fraction regimen, compared to 3.8%, meaning a nonsignificant trend toward a 27% better local control ($p = 0.10$) for the 40 Gy in 15 fractions. Interestingly, the study found a significantly lower rate of distant relapse with the hypofractionation regimen, 12.3% versus 16% for the protracted arm ($p = 0.014$). Also found was a significantly better overall survival, 84.1% versus 80.8%, respectively ($p = 0.042$) (Haviland et al. 2013).

In summary, these four large long-term studies provide Level 1 evidence consistently demonstrating noninferiority (if not a slight superiority) of hypofractionated regimens compared to the classical 50 Gy in 25 fractions.

3 Tolerance and Long-Term Side Effects

3.1 Long-Term Cosmetic and Skin Toxicities

In the Canadian randomized trial, the long-term toxicities were not significantly different in the hypofractionated arm compared to the protracted arm. The rate of excellent to good cosmetic outcomes measured by trained clinical trial nurses using the EORTC cosmetic rating system decreased with time. It was 77.9% for the hypofractionation regimen and 79.2% for the protracted regimen at 5 years, and 69.8% and 71.3%, respectively, at 10 years (Whelan et al. 2002, 2010). Similarly the rate of moderate or marked induration was comparable between arms but increased with time, 6.1% in the protracted arm versus 4.7% with hypofractionation at 5 years, and 10.4% in the protracted arm and 11.9% with hypofractionation at 10 years (Whelan et al. 2002, 2010).

In the UK trials, the tolerance was slightly better for the 39 Gy in 13 fractions and 5-week schedule in the Start A and the 40 Gy in 15 fractions and 3-week regimen in the START B compared to the classical 50 Gy in 25 fractions. The excellent and good cosmetic results at 5 years were 65.9% in the START A and 64.5% in the START B compared to 58.8–59% for the protracted regimen. There were less breast induration, telangiectasia, and breast edema with the hypofractionation schedule (Haviland et al. 2013).

In 2015, the Michigan Radiation Oncology Quality Consortium (MROQC) reported acute toxicity and quality-of-life outcomes for 2309 patients treated between 2011 and 2014 with adjuvant whole-breast radiotherapy, using either a protracted regimen for 75% of them or hypofractionation for 25% (Jagsi et al. 2015). The protracted regimen induced more moist desquamation events (28.5% vs. 6.6%, $p < 0.001$), more patient self-reported moderate to severe pain (41.1% vs. 24.2%, $p = 0.003$), and more fatigue (29.7% vs. 18.9%, $p = 0.02$). The authors concluded that besides the convenience, hypofractionation also improved the immediate experience of radiotherapy, which in the Canadian Breast IMRT trial was also correlated with a reduction in long-term pain, improved cosmesis, and quality of life (Pignol et al. 2016).

3.2 Quality of Life

The MROCQ study also showed a significant increase of physician-reported fatigue using the classical protracted regimen (29.7%, 18.9%; $p = 0.02$) versus hypofractionation (Jagsi et al. 2015). Health-related quality-of-life improvement with hypofractionation was also reported in a Belgian study comparing a protracted regimen with sequential boost over 33 fractions to a hypofractionated regimen with a simultaneous integrated boost (SIB). Treatment was delivered using a TomoTherapy® unit (TomoTherapy, Madison, Wisconsin, USA) using a 15-fraction, 2.8 Gy/fx regimen on the whole breast with a concomitant 0.6 Gy SIB (Versmessen et al. 2012). Patients completed the European Organization for Research and Treatment of Cancer (EORTC) QLQ30 global and BR23 breast module questionnaires at baseline; end of radiotherapy; 3 months; and 1, 2, and 3 years (Jagsi et al. 2015). In both arms, patients experienced a degradation of their global performance status and fatigue at the end of radiotherapy. However, in the hypofractionated arms they recuperated faster on both counts.

3.3 Cardiac Morbidity

One of the main concerns using higher dose per fraction was a potential increase in cardiac morbidity, which often occurs 12–15 years after radiotherapy (McGale et al. 2011). In 2013 Tjessem reported on a Norwegian study including 1107 patients treated between 1975 and 1991 using an ultrahypofractionation regimen delivering 43 Gy in 10 fractions over 5 weeks, twice a week. This regimen was compared to 50 Gy in 20 fractions over 4 weeks in 459 patients treated at the same period. The risk of dying of ischemic heart disease was significantly increased in the ultrahypofractionated group (HR = 2.37, $p = 0.036$) on univariate analysis. On multivariate analysis, the ultrahypofractionated regimen demonstrated borderline difference (HR = 2.9, $p = 0.057$) (Tjessem et al. 2013).

It is however doubtful that with modern radiation techniques, using CT simulation and modern heart-sparing techniques like breath-hold technique, that a significant increase in cardiac morbidity would occur for regimens like the UK 40 Gy in 15 fraction or the Canadian 42.5 Gy in 16-fraction regimens (Lee and Harris 2009). Two studies using the British Columbia registry found no increase in cardiac morbidity for left-sided breast cancer patients treated by either the protracted or the hypofractionated regimen. In the first study, 5334 early-stage breast cancer patients treated between 1990 and 1998 were analyzed by hospital record regarding baseline cardiovascular risk factors. A propensity score model was built to balance cardiac risk factors between 485 patients treated with protracted adjuvant radiotherapy for a left-sided breast cancer compared to 2221 women treated using hypofractionation. The median follow-up was 14.2 years and there was no difference at 15 years in the mortality from cardiac causes (4.8% hypofractionation vs. 4.2% for protracted regimen; $p = 0.74$) (Chan et al. 2015). In another study using the same cohort, Chan reported no difference in hospitalization related to cardiac cause 15 years after radiotherapy (21% hypofractionated vs. 21% protracted) (Chan et al. 2014).

3.4 Impact on Mammography Follow-Up

There were initial concerns that increased breast fibrosis or induration induced by hypofractionation could impact on the reading of mammography or increase the pain of the procedure. However, both in the Canadian and the UK START studies similar or even lower rates of long-term fibrosis were found using hypofractionation (Whelan et al. 2010; Haviland et al. 2013). In addition no mammographic changes were found between those two regimens in terms of architectural distortion, skin thickening, fluid collection, or calcifications at a median follow-up of 4 years. With longer follow-up skin thickening decreased continuously over time (Tian et al. 2016).

4 Unresolved Questions and Absence of Evidence

4.1 Pathology Features

In the long-term report of the Canadian hypofractionation trial, patients with high-grade tumors were found to have a significantly higher hazard ratio of local recurrence with hypofractionation compared to standard fractionation (HR = 3.08, 95% confidence interval 1.22–7.76) (Whelan et al. 2010). However this finding resulted from an unplanned analysis and should be only interpreted as hypothesis generating. This finding was not confirmed in a population-based study from British Columbia. In this study 1335 breast cancer patients had grade 3 infiltrating carcinoma, 252 received 50 Gy in 25 fractions, and 1083 in a hypofractionated regimen. The 10-year local relapse rates were similar in both groups: 6.2% and 6.9%, respectively ($p = 0.99$) (Herbert et al. 2012). Similarly, in a meta-analysis of the START-A and START-B trials and the Royal Marsden Hospital and the Gloucestershire Oncology Centre pilot trial, hypofractionation was not associated with a higher risk of local relapse for grade 3 tumors (Haviland et al. 2013). Hence, it is likely that the finding in the Canadian long-term study was a statistical fluke.

Another challenge is the use of hypofractionation for ductal carcinoma in situ (DCIS) in view of the lack of evidence. From a theoretical standpoint, DCIS is a low-risk disease for which treatment simplification should be warranted and toxicity should be avoided. On the other hand, the clinical sensitivity to fractionation of DCIS is not

well documented and it is difficult to extrapolate findings from invasive cancers, notably the alpha/beta values. However a recent Ontario population-based study reported on 1609 young DCIS patients (median age 56 years) treated between 1994 and 2003 with adjuvant radiotherapy. In this study, 60% of the patients received 50 Gy in 25 fractions, 40% hypofractionation, and 30% a boost dose. A multivariate analysis did not find a difference in local recurrence when the dose fractionation regimen was incorporated in the model, with a nonsignificant but slightly lower hazard ratio for local recurrence at 10 years in favor of the hypofractionated regimen (HR = 0.8, $p = 0.34$) (Lalani et al. 2014).

4.2 Regional Irradiation

In the early hypofractionated regimen from the 1960s, severe long-term complications were reported using regional irradiation, including brachial plexopathy and frozen shoulder. Considering this, there has been an understandable reluctance to use those regimens for locoregional treatments. Budach reported recently a meta-analysis of the four major multicenter randomized trials (Budach et al. 2015) and concluded that further data were needed to recommend hypofractionation when locoregional treatments were indicated. In addition, the German AGO (German Gynecological Oncology Working Group) and the DEGRO (German Society for Radiotherapy and Oncology) groups published guidelines stating "if radiotherapy of the regional lymph nodes is included, conventionally fractionated RT (25–28 fractions)" should be used.

While it is correct that no randomized trials have specifically compared protracted and hypofractionated regimens for locoregional treatment, it is also unlikely that such trials will be done because of the difficulty to define noninferiority in view of the small benefit of regional radiotherapy on regional relapse and overall survival. On the other hand, there is plenty of indirect evidence suggesting that it is safe to use hypofractionation for regional radiotherapy (Caudrelier and Truong 2015). The three UK randomized trials included patients receiving locoregional radiotherapy: 20.6% in the Royal Marsden Hospital and the Gloucestershire Oncology Centre study, 14.2% in the START A, and 7.3% in the START B study. This represents a total of 769 patients (Haviland et al. 2013). Shoulder stiffness and edema of the arm were not more frequent after hypofractionation, and only one case of mild brachial plexopathy symptoms was reported in the highest dose arm of the START A trial using 41.6 Gy in 13 fractions (Haviland et al. 2013). This number remains acceptable as the risk of brachial plexopathy following conventional radiotherapy is estimated to be less than 1% (Holloway et al. 2010). Using various alpha/beta values for brachial plexus radiosensitivity, Haviland reported that even in the worse-case scenario of an α/β of 1 Gy, a dose of 40 Gy in 15 fractions would be equivalent to 48.9 Gy delivered using 2 Gy per fraction and hence equivalent to the classical protracted 50 Gy in 25-fraction regimen (Haviland et al. 2013; Schultheiss 2008).

In regard to the risk of lymphedema, there are many factors other than the fraction size that could contribute to its occurrence, and hypofractionated regimen appears safe. The rate of lymphedema was lower in the hypofractionation arm of the START B (2.8% at 5 years and 4.7% at 10 years), compared to the classical protracted 50 Gy in 25-fraction arm (6% at 5 years and 13.5% at 10 years), though this finding was not statistically significant ($p = 0.21$) (Haviland et al. 2013). Although it was not statistically significant ($p = 0.45$), out of 314 patients receiving regional treatment in the START A trial those receiving the 41.6 Gy in 13-fraction regimen had a higher risk of lymphedema (22.5%) compared to the 50 Gy in 25-fraction regimen (16.3%), and the rate was much lower in the 39 Gy in 13-fraction arm (8.2%) at 10 years postirradiation (Haviland et al. 2013).

4.3 Postmastectomy Radiotherapy (PMRT)

While the Canadian and the UK pilot trial excluded PMRT, both START trials allowed accrual of those patients (Holloway et al. 2010)

such that a total of 513 patients were randomized to receive PMRT using either the classical 50 Gy in 25 fractions or hypofractionation. Post hoc subgroup analyses of the combined hypofractionated regimens versus the control groups for locoregional control showed no effect of the type of primary surgery (Haviland et al. 2013).

Another experience using hypofractionation after PMRT was reported from the Christchurch experience on 133 patients, showing excellent local control at 5 years of 97.6% and only 10.7% long-term grade 2 skin toxicity (Ko et al. 2015). There are, however, no good data regarding the impact of hypofractionation on the long-term results after breast reconstruction.

4.4 Sequential or Simultaneous Integrated Boost

The delivery of a boost is a well-known factor for increased delayed skin side effects and poorer cosmetic outcomes, especially when other comorbidities are present including diabetes mellitus (Ciammella et al. 2014). In the Canadian trial, the use of a boost dose was not allowed. However, in the three UK trials, a boost was permitted and randomization was stratified on boost delivery to ensure that the arms were balanced. In the pilot UK study, 74.5% of the patients received a boost, while 60.6% in the START A and 42.6% in the START B received a boost (Holloway et al. 2010). The boost was decided before randomization and consisted of a sequential tumor bed dose of 10 Gy in five fractions. In the meta-analysis of the START trials, the delivery of a boost did not modify the risk of normal tissue late effects between treatment arms (Haviland et al. 2013). Another study from British Columbia reported Breast Cancer Treatment Outcome Scale (BCTOS) questionnaire responses from 312 survivors, which showed that protracted treatment with boost had a slightly worse self-reported cosmetic outcome ($p = 0.02$) and worse pain experience ($p < 0.001$) (Chan et al. 2016).

A more controversial issue is the use of a simultaneous integrated boost (SIB) with hypofractionated radiotherapy since the increase of the dose per fraction becomes significant. Lessons learned from the UK pilot and START trials show that very small changes in the dose fractionation regimen can lead to significant differences in clinical outcomes (Haviland et al. 2013). There are several small trials reporting on the use of SIB in combination with hypofractionation; however most are lacking power and maturity to conclude whether or not the association is safe. In the early publication of the German ELAS trial, 151 patients received whole-breast radiotherapy: 40 Gy in 16 fractions (2.5 Gy per fraction) with a SIB of 0.5 Gy per fraction to the tumor bed totaling 48.0 Gy in 16 fractions (3 Gy per fraction). The reported early tolerance was excellent; however in this Phase II trial, patients were only evaluated for acute toxicity during radiotherapy while those side effects generally peaked 1–2 weeks after the end of radiotherapy (Dellas et al. 2014; Pignol et al. 2008). A comparative study with simultaneous and sequential boost with longer follow-up is necessary before concluding on this issue. In the meantime, caution should be recommended as this dose fractionation schedule may well result in an increase in late side effects (Budach et al. 2015).

4.5 Techniques for Patients with Expected Large-Dose Distribution Heterogeneity

Similarly to the issue of SIB, patients with large breasts present dose "hot-spot" areas in the breast receiving a significantly higher dose than prescribed. This generally occurs in the inframammary fold, the axillary tail, or the parasternal area when the breast incident central axis separation exceeds 25 cm. Those patients may therefore be at a higher risk to develop acute and delayed side effects. There were legitimate concerns in the Canadian study such that patients with breast separation exceeding 25 cm were not eligible (Whelan et al. 2002). However this was not the case in the UK trials where 14.3% and 17.2% of the patients had "large" breasts in the START A and START B trials, respectively,

corresponding to a total of 476 large-breasted patients (Haviland et al. 2013). In his meta-analysis Haviland did not find a detrimental effect for larger breasts in terms of moderate to marked physician-assessed breast changes between the hypofractionated arms and the classical 50 Gy in 25-fraction regimen. On the contrary, he reported a slight but nonsignificant protective effect using hypofractionation with a hazard ratio of 0.91 [range 0.72–1.15] (Haviland et al. 2013).

Since the inception and maturation of the four large trials on hypofractionation, several new radiation techniques have been proposed and successfully tested to reduce the breast dose distribution heterogeneity. These techniques include breast IMRT and prone breast irradiation (Vicini et al. 2002; Grann et al. 2000). For breast IMRT, a series of field-in-field segments are defined based on a sagittal dose distribution in a plane perpendicular to the beam axis. The segments are then weighted to keep the dose distribution heterogeneity within ±5% or better. This technique significantly reduces acute moist desquamation by 35%, a side effect that is associated with acute and long-term mastalgia, as well as long-term telangiectasia and fibrosis (Pignol et al. 2008, 2016; Donovan et al. 2007; Mukesh et al. 2013). Similarly for large-breasted patients, the use of a prone treatment position reduces the breast separation and hence the hot spots in the axillary tail and the parasternal area. When used in combination with breast IMRT, the impact on the dose distribution homogeneity is quite spectacular. There is recent evidence from a Belgium Phase III trial that this has a large and significant clinical impact with a threefold reduction in the occurrence of moist desquamation ($p = 0.04$) (Mulliez et al. 2013).

A lesson learned from the UK trials, and especially from the START A study, is that a slight decrease in the dose per fraction with hypofractionation can have a measurable clinical impact. So it is reasonable to assume that breast IMRT and/or prone technique for large-breasted patients can improve long-term tolerance using hypofractionation since they reduce the dose distribution hot spots (Holloway et al. 2010).

4.6 Chemotherapy

There are also concerns about potential increased long-term toxicities using combined or sequential hypofractionated radiotherapy and chemotherapy. In an analysis of factors associated with poorer tolerance of accelerated partial breast irradiation, Wazer reported that the use of Adriamycin-based chemotherapy was significantly associated with an increase in high-grade skin toxicity, fat necrosis, and suboptimal cosmetic outcome (Wazer et al. 2006). However it is important to bear in mind that, for accelerated partial breast irradiation, the dose fractionation regimen was 3.4 Gy delivered twice daily over 5 consecutive days up to a total dose of 34 Gy combined with the implicit large dose distribution heterogeneity associated with HDR brachytherapy. So it is unlikely that this finding may apply to whole-breast hypofractionation as in the UK or Canadian trials.

A total of 1617 patients received adjuvant chemotherapy in the four large hypofractionation trials (13.9% in the pilot UK trial, 35.5% in the START A, 22.2% in the START B, and 11% in the Canadian trial) (Holloway et al. 2010). In post hoc analyses of the combined hypofractionation and control arms of the UK trials, the treatment effect between groups was not different accounting for adjuvant chemotherapy on locoregional relapse, or for the incidence of normal tissue side effects including breast shrinkage, induration, edema, or telangiectasia (Haviland et al. 2013). It should be noted, however, that the chemotherapy regimens used in the 1990s were much less toxic than the ones used today where most regimens include high-dose anthracycline or taxanes. Several reports evaluated and did not suggest an increased risk of pneumonitis and brachial plexopathy when a taxane is used with radiotherapy (Ellerbroek et al. 2003; Yu et al. 2004). Therefore it is unlikely that this finding may change using hypofractionation.

Similarly, trastuzumab was not clinically available at the time of the UK and Canadian trials. However, trastuzumab can be safely delivered after or concurrently with radiotherapy and it is unlikely that a small change in the size of the dose per radiotherapy fraction may generate significant cardiac morbidity (Halyard et al. 2009). However in the absence of evidence it is logical to cautiously respect mean heart dose constraints if trastuzumab will be administered concomitantly with hypofractionated radiotherapy (Darby et al. 2013).

4.7 Ultrahypofractionation

Beyond those hypofractionated regimens delivered in 3 weeks, there have been several attempts to shrink further the whole-breast radiotherapy schedule to a single week. At the time of the writing of this chapter, the still ongoing FAST-Forward clinical trial designed as a three-arm Phase III trial is testing a 1-week course of whole-breast radiotherapy after surgery for early breast cancer delivering either 27 or 26 Gy in 5 daily fractions, compared to the UK standard 40 Gy in 15 fractions over 3 weeks (Brunt et al. 2016). The primary endpoint for the trial is local recurrence, and the secondary endpoints are the occurrence of acute and late side effects. While the 5-year results are expected in 2017, the results of two substudies reporting on acute toxicity for patients accrued between 2011 and 2013 were published in 2016 (Brunt et al. 2016). The need of two substudies came from the use of two different scales, the Radiation Therapy Oncology Group (RTOG) criteria in the first study and the National Cancer Institute Common Terminology Criteria for Adverse Effects (NCI-CTCAE v 4.03) for the second study. The first scale tends to overestimate acute toxicity as it includes edema, a side effect that is frequent after surgery and hence nonspecific to breast radiotherapy. After discussion with the data safety monitoring committee and the trial steering committee, it was agreed that the RTOG scale may not be the most appropriate scoring system and a second substudy was designed. Effectively the rate of grade 3 or higher toxicity was different in the two studies: 13.6% and 0% for the 40 Gy in 15-fraction arm; 9.8% and 2.4% for the 27 Gy in 5 fractions; and 5.8% and 0% for the 26 Gy in 5-fraction regimen using the RTOG or the NCI-CTCAE criteria, respectively (Brunt et al. 2016).

There have also been historical series of ultra-hypofractionation, mainly from France, aiming at reducing the burden of radiation treatment for elderly patients (Kirova et al. 2009; Ortholan et al. 2005; Courdi et al. 2006). This was felt justified for patients with limited life expectancy having difficulty attending long courses of daily treatment in a cancer center, and the assumption that delayed side effects may be less of a concern for such patients. Those series used the radiobiological time-dose-fractionation (TDF) equivalence of a single dose of 6.5 Gy delivered once weekly as compared to a dose of 10 Gy delivered in five daily fractions of 2 Gy. The whole breast received a total dose of 32.5 Gy over 5 weeks, with or without a boost of two or three additional fractions in case of exclusive radiotherapy.

Between 1995 and 1999 at the Institut Curie, 317 women aged 70 or higher with a T1 or T2 breast cancer were randomized after breast-conserving surgery to receive radiotherapy (either 32.5 Gy in 5 weekly fractions or the standard 50 Gy in 25 daily fractions) (Kirova et al. 2009). At a median follow-up of 93 months, similar 7 years of local recurrence-free survival (93% vs. 91% for the standard vs. the hypofractionated regimen, respectively), cause-specific survival (93% vs. 87%), and metastasis-free survival (92% vs. 93%) were reported. This study did not report on long-term tolerance of this regimen (Kirova et al. 2009).

A similar regimen of 32.5 Gy in 5 weekly fractions of 6.5 Gy was used for a cohort of 150 elderly patients (median age 78 years) treated in Nice, France, between 1987 and 1999. Patients were mainly T1 and T2 stage but 34% were also node positive (Ortholan et al. 2005). These patients underwent either breast-conserving surgery in 71.5% of the cases or a mastectomy in 28.5%. After a median follow-up of 65 months, 45% of patients presented with delayed side effects (mainly grade 1 or 2) and those reactions were higher if a boost dose was delivered. The rate of local recurrence was only 2.3% (Ortholan et al. 2005). The main drawback of this retrospective study is the lack of blinding and lack of standardization of late side effect capture. One of the authors of the present chapter has contributed

to the follow-up clinic of those patients and, although this is not statistically represented, many patients developed major breast shrinkage.

4.8 Adoption of the Hypofractionation Regimen

Despite the existence of four very-well-designed multicenter randomized controlled trials with blinded assessment and long-term outcomes showing noninferiority (if not an overt trend toward better outcomes) using hypofractionation, the adoption of those regimens has been surprisingly slow.

In an Australian study of 5880 patients in New South Wales published in 2016, 55% received the classical protracted regimen over 5 weeks and 45% received hypofractionation. A logistic regression analysis to determine the factor associated with a lack of adoption of hypofractionation found that the treatment facility and the individual radiation oncologist were the main factors determining the use of the 5-week regimen, suggesting that physician individual preference subordinated the overwhelming clinical evidence (Delaney et al. 2016). Similarly, the Michigan Radiation Oncology Quality Consortium reported on a study of 1477 patients receiving adjuvant radiotherapy between 2011 and 2013. Among them, 913 had a T1 or T2 tumor and were node negative, and were treated with breast-conserving surgery followed by radiotherapy. Only 283 patients (31%) received a hypofractionation regimen. Hypofractionation was less likely for patients younger than 50 years of age ($p < 0.007$), patients with large separation ($p = 0.002$), and postchemotherapy ($p < 0.001$), once again demonstrating a selection bias (Jagsi et al. 2014).

Conclusion

There is solid level 1 evidence based on long-term outcomes including four randomized trials showing that hypofractionation should be the standard after breast-conserving surgery for most early-stage breast cancers. Meta-analysis of START-A and the START pilot trial provided an adjusted alpha/beta value for locoregional relapse of 3.5 Gy (95% CI 1.2–5.7 Gy) (Haviland et al. 2013). In regard to long-term side effects, an alpha/beta value for change in breast appearance at 5 years of 3.6 Gy (95% CI 1.8–5.4 Gy) and of 3.1 Gy for palpable breast induration (95% CI 1.8–4.4 Gy) was calculated from the pilot UK trial (Yarnold et al. 2005).

Despite the following factors that may limit adoption of hypofractionation, there is no evidence that young age, tumor grade, DCIS, regional radiotherapy, use of a prone technique, and large breast separation (as long as the $V_{107\%}$ is minimized to practically less than 2 cm³) should prevent a patient to receive this more convenient regimen.

On the other hand while there is no evidence of any risk using hypofractionation for patients treated with chemotherapy, caution should be recommended for patients receiving concomitant radiotherapy-chemotherapy. Similarly, hypofractionation may not be used when a high-dose boost is prescribed on a large volume using SIB. Finally, more mature-quality data are needed to conclude the safety and efficacy of the ultrahypofractionation regimen delivering the radiotherapy in a single week.

References

cancer.gov. http://seer.cancer.gov/statfacts/html/breast.html. Accessed 11 Oct 2016

Atkins HL (1964) Massive dose technique radiation therapy of inoperable carcinoma of the breast. Am J Roentgenol 91:80

Bates TD (1988) The 10-year results of a prospective trial of post-operative radiotherapy delivered 3 fractions per week versus 2 fractions per week in breast carcinoma. Br J Radiol 61:625–630

Brunt AM, Wheatley D, Yarnold J et al (2016) Acute skin toxicity associated with a 1-week schedule of whole breast radiotherapy compared with a standard 3-week regimen delivered in the UK FAST-Forward Trial. Radiother Oncol 120:114–118

Budach W, Bölke E, Matuschek C (2015) Hypofractionated radiotherapy as adjuvant treatment in early breast cancer. A review and meta-analysis of randomized controlled trials. Breast Care 10:240–245. doi:10.1159/000439007

Caudrelier JM, Truong PT (2015) Role of hypofractionated radiotherapy in breast locoregional radiation. Cancer Radiother 19:241–247. doi:10.1016/j.canrad.2015.02.012

Chan EK, Woods R, McBride ML et al (2014) Adjuvant hypofractionated versus conventional whole breast radiation therapy for early-stage breast cancer: long-term hospital-related morbidity from cardiac causes. Int J Radiat Oncol Biol Phys 88:786–792. doi:10.1016/j.ijrobp.2013.11.243

Chan EK, Woods R, Virani S et al (2015) Long-term mortality from cardiac causes after adjuvant hypofractionated vs. conventional radiotherapy for localized left-sided breast cancer. Radiother Oncol 114:73–78. doi:10.1016/j.radonc.2014.08.021

Chan EK, Tabarsi N, Tyldesley S et al (2016) Patient-reported long-term cosmetic outcomes following short fractionation whole breast radiotherapy with boost. Am J Clin Oncol 39:473–478. doi:10.1097/COC.0000000000000084

Ciammella P, Podgornii A, Galeandro M et al (2014) Toxicity and cosmetic outcome of hypofractionated whole-breast radiotherapy: predictive clinical and dosimetric factors. Radiat Oncol 9:97. doi:10.1186/1748-717X-9-97

Clark RM, Whelan T, Levine M et al (1996) Randomized clinical trial of breast irradiation following lumpectomy and axillary dissection for node-negative breast cancer: an update. Ontario Clinical Oncology Group. J Natl Cancer Inst 88:1659–1664

Courdi A, Ortholan C, Hannoun-Lévi JM et al (2006) Long-term results of hypofractionated radiotherapy and hormonal therapy without surgery for breast cancer in elderly patients. Radiother Oncol 79:156–161

Darby SC, Ewertz M, McGale P et al (2013) Risk of ischemic heart disease in women after radiotherapy for breast cancer. N Engl J Med 368:987–998. doi:10.1056/NEJMoa1209825

Delaney GP, Gandhidasan S, Walton R et al (2016) The pattern of use of hypofractionated radiation therapy for early-stage breast cancer in New South Wales, Australia, 2008 to 2012. Int J Radiat Oncol Biol Phys 96:266–272. doi:10.1016/j.ijrobp.2016.05.016

Dellas K, Vonthein R, Zimmer J, ARO Study Group et al (2014) Hypofractionation with simultaneous integrated boost for early breast cancer: results of the German multicenter phase II trial (ARO-2010–01). Strahlenther Onkol 190:646–653

Donovan E, Bleakley N, Denholm E et al (2007) Randomized trial of standard 2D radiotherapy (RT) versus intensity modulated radiotherapy (IMRT) in patients prescribed breast radiotherapy. Radiother Oncol 82:254–264

Early Breast Cancer Trialists' Collaborative Group (EBCTCG), Darby S, McGale P et al (2011) Effect of radiotherapy after breast-conserving surgery on 10-year recurrence and 15-year breast cancer death: meta-analysis of individual patient data for 10,801 women in 17 randomised trials. Lancet 378:1707–1716

Edelman AH, Holtz S, Powers WE (1965) Radiotherapy for inoperable carcinoma of the breast. Am J Roentgenol 9:585

Ellerbroek N, Martino S, Mautner B et al (2003) Breast-conserving therapy with adjuvant paclitaxel and radiation therapy: feasibility of concurrent treatment. Breast J 9:74–78

Fisher B, Bauer M, Margolese R et al (1985) Five-year results of a randomized trial comparing total mastectomy and segmental mastectomy with or without radiation in the treatment of breast cancer. N Engl J Med 312:665–673

Fisher B, Anderson S, Bryant J et al (2002) Twenty-year follow-up of a randomized trial comparing total mastectomy, lumpectomy, and lumpectomy plus irradiation for the treatment of invasive breast cancer. N Engl J Med 347(16):1233–1241

Fletcher GH (1991) Hypofractionation: lessons from complications. Radiother Oncol 20:10–15

Grann A, McCormick B, Chabner ES et al (2000) Prone breast radiotherapy in early-stage breast cancer: a preliminary analysis. Int J Radiat Oncol Biol Phys 47:319–325

Halyard MY, Pisansky TM, Dueck AC et al (2009) Radiotherapy and adjuvant trastuzumab in operable breast cancer: tolerability and adverse event data from the NCCTG Phase III Trial N9831. J Clin Oncol 27:2638–2644. doi:10.1200/JCO.2008.17.9549

Haviland JS, Owen JR, Dewar JA et al (2013) The UK Standardization of Breast Radiotherapy (START) trials of radiotherapy hypofractionation for treatment of early breast cancer: 10-year follow-up results of two randomized controlled trials. Lancet Oncol 14:1086–1094. doi:10.1016/S1470-2045(13)70386-3

Herbert C, Nichol A, Olivotto I et al (2012) The impact of hypofractionated whole breast radiotherapy on local relapse in patients with Grade 3 early breast cancer: a population-based cohort study. Int J Radiat Oncol Biol Phys 82(5):2086–2092

Holloway CL, Panet-Raymond V, Olivotto I (2010) Hypofractionation should be the new 'standard' for radiation therapy after breast conserving surgery. Breast 19:163–167. doi:10.1016/j.breast.2010.03.002

Jagsi R, Griffith KA, Heimburger D et al (2014) Choosing wisely? Patterns and correlates of the use of hypofractionated whole-breast radiation therapy in the state of Michigan. Int J Radiat Oncol Biol Phys 90:1010–1016. doi:10.1016/j.ijrobp.2014.09.027

Jagsi R, Griffith KA, Boike TP et al (2015) Differences in the acute toxic effects of breast radiotherapy by fractionation schedule: comparative analysis of physician-assessed and patient-reported outcomes in a large multicenter cohort. JAMA Oncol 1:918–930. doi:10.1001/jamaoncol.2015.2590

Khan A, Haffty B (2010) Hypofractionation in adjuvant breast radiotherapy. Breast 19:168–171

Kirova YM, Campana F, Savignoni A et al (2009) Breast-conserving treatment in the elderly: long-term results of adjuvant hypofractionated and normofractionated radiotherapy. Int J Radiat Oncol Biol Phys 75:76–81. doi:10.1016/j.ijrobp.2008.11.005

Ko DH, Norriss A, Harrington CR et al (2015) Hypofractionated radiation treatment following mastectomy in early breast cancer: the Christchurch experience. J Med Imaging Radiat Oncol 59:243–247. doi:10.1111/1754-9485.12242

Lalani N, Paszat L, Sutradhar R et al (2014) Long-term outcomes of hypofractionation versus conventional radiation therapy after breast-conserving surgery for ductal carcinoma in situ of the breast. Int J Radiat Oncol Biol Phys 90:1017–1024. doi:10.1016/j.ijrobp.2014.07.026

Lee LJ, Harris JR (2009) Innovations in radiation therapy (RT) for breast cancer. Breast 18:S103–S111. doi:10.1016/S0960-9776(09)70284-X

Matthews JH, Meeker BE, Chapman JD (1989) Response of human tumor cell lines in vitro to fractionated irradiation. Int J Radiat Oncol Biol Phys 16:133–138

McGale P, Darby SC, Hall P et al (2011) Incidence of heart disease in 35,000 women treated with radiotherapy for breast cancer in Denmark and Sweden. Radiother Oncol 100:167–175. doi:10.1016/j.radonc.2011.06.016

Montague ED (1968) Experience with altered fractionation in radiation therapy of breast cancer. Radiology 90:962–966

Mukesh MB, Barnett GC, Wilkinson JS et al (2013) Randomized controlled trial of intensity-modulated radiotherapy for early breast cancer: 5-year results confirm superior overall cosmesis. J Clin Oncol 31:4488–4495

Mulliez T, Veldeman L, van Greveling A et al (2013) Hypofractionated whole breast irradiation for patients with large breasts: a randomized trial comparing prone and supine positions. Radiother Oncol 108:203–208. doi:10.1016/j.radonc.2013.08.040

Nystrom L, Andersson I, Bjurstam N et al (2002) Long-term effects of mammography screening: updated overview of the Swedish randomized trials. Lancet 359:909–919

Ortholan C, Hannoun-Lévi JM, Ferrero JM et al (2005) Long-term results of adjuvant hypofractionated radiotherapy for breast cancer in elderly patients. Int J Radiat Oncol Biol Phys 61:154–162

Overgaard M (1985) The clinical implications of nonstandard fractionation. Int J Radiat Oncol Biol Phys 11:1225–1226

Owen JR, Ashton A, Bliss JM et al (2006) Effect of radiotherapy fraction size on tumour control in patient with early-stage breast cancer after local tumour excision: long-term results of randomized trial. Lancet Oncol 7:467–471

Pignol JP, Olivotto I, Rakovitch E et al (2008) A multicenter randomized trial of breast intensity-modulated radiation therapy to reduce acute radiation dermatitis. J Clin Oncol 26:2085–2092. doi:10.1200/JCO.2007.15.2488

Pignol JP, Truong P, Rakovitch E et al (2016) Ten years results of the Canadian breast intensity modulated radiation therapy (IMRT) randomized controlled trial.

Radiother Oncol. doi:10.1016/j.radonc.2016.08.021. [Epub ahead of print]

Rodger A (2010) Should fewer fractions be the new standard for postoperative radiotherapy in patients with early breast cancer? Breast 19:157–158. doi:10.1016/j.breast.2010.03.006

Schultheiss TE (2008) The radiation dose-response of the human spinal cord. Int J Radiat Oncol Biol Phys 71:1455–1459

START Trialists' Group, Bentzen SM, Agrawal RK et al (2008b) The UK Standardization of Breast Radiotherapy (START) Trial A of radiotherapy hypofractionation for treatment of early breast cancer: a randomized trial. Lancet Oncol 9:331–341. doi:10.1016/S1470-2045(08)70077-9

START Trialists' Group, Bentzen SM, Agrawal RK, Aird EG et al (2008a) The UK Standardization of Breast Radiotherapy (START) Trial B of radiotherapy hypofractionation for treatment of early breast cancer: a randomized trial. Lancet 371:1098–1107

Steel GG, Deacon JM, Duchesne GM et al (1987) The dose-rate effect in human tumour cells. Radiother Oncol 9:299–310

Strnad V, Ott OJ, Hildebrandt G, Groupe Européen de Curiethérapie of European Society for Radiotherapy and Oncology (GEC-ESTRO) et al (2016) 5-year results of accelerated partial breast irradiation using sole interstitial multicatheter brachytherapy versus whole-breast irradiation with boost after breast-conserving surgery for low-risk invasive and in-situ carcinoma of the female breast: a randomized, phase 3, non-inferiority trial. Lancet 387:229–238. doi:10.1016/S0140-6736(15)00471-7

Tian S, Paster LF, Kim S et al (2016) Comparison of mammographic changes across three different fractionation schedules for early-stage breast cancer. Int J Radiat Oncol Biol Phys 95:597–604. doi:10.1016/j.ijrobp.2016.01.056

Tjessem KH, Johansen S, Malinen E et al (2013) Long-term cardiac mortality after hypofractionated radiation

therapy in breast cancer. Int J Radiat Oncol Biol Phys 87:337–343. doi:10.1016/j.ijrobp.2013.05.038

Veronesi U, Cascinelli N, Mariani L et al (2002) Twenty-year follow-up of a randomized study comparing breast-conserving surgery with radical mastectomy for early breast cancer. N Engl J Med 347(16):1227–1232

Versmessen H, Vinh-Hung V, Van Parijs H et al (2012) Health-related quality of life in survivors of stage I–II breast cancer: randomized trial of post-operative conventional radiotherapy and hypofractionated tomotherapy. BMC Cancer 12:495. doi:10.1186/1471-2407-12-495

Vicini FA, Sharpe M, Kestin L et al (2002) Optimizing breast cancer treatment efficacy with intensity-modulated radiotherapy. Int J Radiat Oncol Biol Phys 54:1336–1344

Wazer DE, Kaufman S, Cuttino L et al (2006) Accelerated partial breast irradiation: an analysis of variables associated with late toxicity and long-term cosmetic outcomes after high dose rate interstitial brachytherapy. Int J Radiat Oncol Biol Phys 64:489–495

Whelan T, MacKenzie R, Julian J et al (2002) Randomized trial of breast irradiation schedules after lumpectomy for women with lymph node-negative breast cancer. J Natl Cancer Inst 94:1143–1150

Whelan TJ, Kim DH, Sussman J (2008) Clinical experience using hypofractionated radiation schedules in breast cancer. Semin Radiat Oncol 18:257–264

Whelan TJ, Pignol JP, Levine MN et al (2010) Long-term results of hypofractionated radiation therapy for breast cancer. N Engl J Med 362:513–520. doi:10.1056/NEJMoa0906260

Yarnold J, Ashton A, Bliss J et al (2005) Fractionation sensitivity and dose response of late adverse effects in the breast after radiotherapy for early breast cancer: long-term results of a randomized trial. Radiother Oncol 75:9–17

Yu TK, Whitman GJ, Thames HD et al (2004) Clinically relevant pneumonitis after sequential paclitaxel-based chemotherapy and radiotherapy in breast cancer patients. J Natl Cancer Inst 96:1676–1681

Accelerated Partial Breast Irradiation

Jean-Philippe Pignol, Nienke Hoekstra,
Fernand Missohou, and Mark Trombetta

Contents

The original version of this chapter was revised. The affiliations of the authors have been updated.

J.-P. Pignol (✉) • N. Hoekstra
Department of Radiation Oncology, Erasmus MC Cancer Institute, Rotterdam, The Netherlands
e-mail: j.p.pignol@erasmusmc.nl

F. Missohou
Department of Radiation Oncology, Libreville, Gabon

M. Trombetta
Allegheny General Hospital, Allegheny Health Network Cancer Institute, Drexel University College of Medicine, Pittsburgh, PA, USA

1 Background

Rarely since the introduction of breast conserving therapy in the 80's has the breast radiation oncology community been so passionately divided and arguing for the introduction of a new concept as for accelerated partial breast irradiation (APBI). The idea looks *a priori* counter intuitive – limiting the concept of clinical target volume (CTV) and hence the irradiated volume within anatomical breast boundaries. The passion in published opinions possibly comes from a strange mix of financial interest, competition between techniques and the extensive use of patient's advertisements and press releases instead of clinical (Smith et al. 2012; Khan et al. 2012). It is striking that in 2016 two articles reviewing the best available evidences, one by Vicini et al. and the other from the Cochrane Library (Vicini et al. 2016; Hickey et al. 2016), had exactly opposite conclusions. The former concluded that *"Four contemporary trials with over 2000 patients comparing APBI and whole breast irradiation (WBI) have been published and demonstrate*

Med Radiol Radiat Oncol (2017)
DOI 10.1007/174_2017_96, © Springer International Publishing AG
Published Online: 01 September 2017

no differences in the rates of local/regional recurrence or survival though long-term follow-up is limited to one study. In addition, reductions in the rates of acute and chronic toxicity and improvements in cosmetic outcome were noted in two of these trials." The later concluded that *"It appeared that local recurrence and 'elsewhere primaries' (new primaries in the ipsilateral breast) are increased with PBI/APBI (the difference was small), but we found no evidence of detriment to other oncological outcomes. It appeared that cosmetic outcomes and some late effects were worse with PBI/APBI but its use was associated with less acute skin toxicity".* There is one things most expert would agree on, it is that almost 25 years after the first mention of partial breast irradiation by Bethune in the Journal of the National Medical Association (Bethune 1991), evidences are now emerging that the APBI paradigm is safe for highly selected patients. This chapter will review a selection of the available evidences.

2 History of APBI

2.1 First Mention

The first mention of APBI was described in the pioneering hypothesis of Bethune in the Journal of the National Medical Association in 1991 (Bethune 1991), when he questioned the need for whole-breast irradiation, in the light of a series of facts including the following:

- In patients treated with partial mastectomy and radiation, ipsilateral breast recurrences were roughly 1% per year, with half or more of the relapses occurring in the close vicinity of the surgical bed.
- The majority of early recurrence, within 2 years, tends to occur at the site of the primary, while later recurrence tends to occur elsewhere in the breast.
- After 10 years, patients have a 5% risk of contralateral breast cancer, and hence a rate similar to the rate of recurrence far from the surgical bed.

So in his provocative view, treating the whole breast to prevent recurrences far from the surgical bed may as well justify treating both breasts, and he recommended treating the tumor with an adequate margin that he set at 2 cm (Bethune 1991).

2.2 The William Beaumont Experience

The William Beaumont Hospital was one of the first centers to test this concept based on their experience using brachytherapy for radiation boost with multi-catheter brachytherapy (Vicini et al. 1997a). In March 1993, the team started a prospective clinical trial using low-dose-rate (LDR) brachytherapy in 60 women with infiltrating ductal carcinoma (IDC) less than 3 cm, clear margin over 2 mm, no extensive in situ carcinoma, less than 3 nodes positive, and clear postoperative mammograms (Vicini et al. 1997b). The catheters were placed either perioperatively (30%) or postoperatively (70%) with a minimum of three planes. ^{125}I seeds were used as LDR sources and temporarily placed inside the catheters. A dose of 50 Gy over 96 h (0.52 Gy/h) was delivered as an in-patient procedure over 4 days to the seroma with an additional 2 cm margin. The choice of this short half-lived isotope was based on radioprotection arguments (Vicini et al. 1993). In 1997, Vicini reported the early outcomes after a median follow-up of 20 months (Vicini et al. 1997b). The tolerance was excellent, with mainly a transient erythema followed by temporary hyperpigmentation on the catheter entries as the most frequent acute side effect. Four patients (6.7%) developed mild infections of the breast 2 and 4 months post-implant, and the cosmetic results were estimated as good or excellent in all cases.

Later the team shifted to ^{192}Ir high-dose-rate (HDR) brachytherapy, and in 2003 Vicini reported mature data on a cohort of 199 patients treated in three different prospective trials (Vicini et al. 2003a). Out of those, 120 patients (60%) were treated with LDR brachytherapy and 79 patients were treated with HDR brachytherapy delivering either 32 Gy in eight fractions of

4 Gy for 71 patients or 34 Gy in ten fractions of 3.6 Gy for eight patients. Most patient were 40 years or older, had an infiltrating ductal carcinoma (178 patients) or DCIS (21 patients), tumor diameter less than 3 cm with negative resection margins of at least 2 mm, and negative lymph nodes. Lobular and extensive in situ carcinomas were excluded. Those patients were randomly matched 1:1 according to age, tumor size, lymph node status, hormone receptor status, and use of tamoxifen to a cohort of 709 patients treated with whole-breast radiotherapy. After a median follow-up of 65 months, the rate of local recurrence was similar at 1% in the APBI and the WBI-matched arm ($p = 0.65$). There was also no difference in the rate of regional failure, overall survival, or cause-specific survival (Vicini et al. 2003a).

Following this publication, the brachytherapy technique evolved toward balloon-based catheter treatment, which greatly simplified the procedure being placed either intraoperatively or after the final pathology report was obtained (Edmundson et al. 2002; Keisch and Arthur 2005). The balloon was initially single lumen but evolved toward multiple lumen catheters enabling the user to fine-tune the dose distribution especially with regard to the skin and chest wall doses (Brown et al. 2009). The balloon technique was evaluated through a Registry maintained by the American Society of Breast Surgeons (ASBS) (Shah et al. 2013a).

Finally the William Beaumont team developed, in 2000, the concept of external beam 3D conformal radiotherapy (3D-CRT), which has the advantage of enabling a more global use of APBI in centers without an active brachytherapy program (Vicini et al. 2003b). A first 3D conformal radiotherapy (3D-CRT) APBI Phase I/II study was performed on 31 patients between 2000 and 2002. Patient eligibility was similar to the brachytherapy trials. The prescribed dose was 38.5 Gy in ten fractions twice daily on 5 consecutive days and separated by at least 6 h for most patients. The target coverage as reflected by the V_{95}, which is the proportion of the planned target volume (PTV) receiving at least 95% of the prescribed dose, was 100% on average. No patient had

significant acute skin side effects and t technique was further evaluated in the RTOG 0319 clinical trial. Between 2003 and 2004, 58 patients were accrued and the acute tolerance was reported in 2005, with only one patient (2%) developing a grade 3 skin toxicity (Vicini et al. 2005).

Based on those results, the National Surgical Adjuvant Breast and Bowel Project (NSABP) and the Radiation Therapy Oncology Group (RTOG) designed a large multicenter randomized clinical trial comparing whole-breast irradiation of 50 Gy in 25 treatments, with an optional boost of 10 or 16 Gy, to partial irradiation using either multi-catheter or balloon brachytherapy delivering 34 Gy in ten fractions twice daily or 3D-CRT delivering 38.5 Gy also in ten fractions twice daily (http://www.nsabp.pitt.edu/B-39. asp). Eligible patients included unifocal invasive or in situ breast adenocarcinoma of less than 3 cm in diameter, with negative excision margins, less than 3 nodes positive, and a clearly identifiable seroma of less than 30% of the breast volume. The primary endpoint was the time of in-breast tumor recurrence as a primary event, and secondary endpoints include the distant disease-free interval, recurrence-free survival, and overall survival. Between 2005 and 2015, 4216 patients were accrued in the study and the final data collection for primary outcome measure is scheduled in 2018.

2.3 Other Early Initiatives

There have been several other APBI initiatives outside the extensive William Beaumont experience. Between 1997 and 2000, 100 women from 11 institutions in the USA were enrolled in the Phase II RTOG 95-17 study to receive brachytherapy APBI with either 45 Gy in 3.5–5 days using stranded ^{125}I seeds LDR or 34 Gy in ten fractions twice daily using HDR. In 2006, with a medium follow-up of 2.7 years, White reported the tolerance for 33 patients treated with LDR and 66 patients treated with HDR brachytherapy (White et al. 2016). Though the number could not be statistically compared due to the small overall cohort size, the rate of Grade 3 or 4 toxicity was 3% in the HDR group and 9% in the LDR group. After a median follow-up of 12 years, the 10-year rate of cumulative local recurrence was 6.2% out of 98 evaluable patients (95% confidence interval 1.4–11.1%).

In Europe, between 1996 and 1998, 45 patients with unifocal invasive ductal carcinoma grade I or II, a diameter 2 cm or less, clear margins, and pN0-1 were treated with HDR brachytherapy delivering 36.4 Gy in seven fractions at the Budapest National Institute of Oncology in a Phase I–II protocol. After a median follow-up of 57 months, the rate of local failure was 4.4%, the rate of regional recurrence was 6.7%, and the rate of distant failure was also 6.7% (Polgár et al. 2002). Based on those results, the study was converted into a Phase III study randomizing 258 patients to receive WBI 50 Gy in 25 fractions (130 patients) or APBI (128 patients). For 88 patients, APBI was delivered using multi-catheter brachytherapy, while for 40 patients it was delivered using electron partial breast irradiation 50 Gy in 25 fractions (Polgár et al. 2013). After a median follow-up of 10 years, the actuarial rate of local recurrence was 5.9% in the APBI arm and 5.1% in the WBI arm ($p = 0.77$). This pioneer work from Hungary was followed by studies done in Barcelona and Florence (Rodríguez et al. 2013; Livi et al. 2015).

2.4 Single-Fraction Treatments

While brachytherapy and external beam radiotherapy techniques significantly reduce the treatment burden for patients, they are still delivered over several days, and in the case of twice-daily fractions require the patient to spend a significant amount of time at the hospital. Several initiatives have tried to reduce the number of treatments to the strict minimum of a single fraction; either intraoperatively or postoperatively.

In 1998, the University College London tested a new form of intraoperative irradiation using a 50 kV X-ray generator. A single dose of 20 Gy was delivered using an applicator of various sizes to the surface of the resection margin, and the dose typically attenuated to 5–7 Gy at 1 cm depth (Vaidya et al. 2001). This pilot study was followed by the TARGIT-A Phase III protocol, which (between 2000 and 2012) accrued 2228 patients from 28 institutions to receive either WBI or intraoperative treatment (Vaidya et al. 2016). The details of the techniques and the results of the trial are described in the next section.

Also in the field of intraoperative radiotherapy (IORT), between 2000 and 2007, the European Institute of Oncology of Milan randomized 1305 patients with tumors less than 2.5 cm in diameter to receive WBI delivering 50 Gy in 25 fractions or a single dose of 21 Gy IORT using a 6–9 MeV electron beam (Veronesi et al. 2013).

In regard to single-fraction radiotherapy delivered postoperatively, a technique similar to permanent seed implant prostate brachytherapy was developed in 2006 and evaluated for breast cancers through two Phase I–II trials, and further as a Registry trial in Canada (Pignol et al. 2006, 2015).

3 Techniques and Protocols

3.1 Brachytherapy

Brachytherapy is the oldest of all APBI techniques and the one for which the best evidence is available to date. Before 2000, the technique was tested using multi-catheter implantation and a temporary LDR source, in a technique similar to the one used to boost radiation dose after WBI (Vicini et al. 1997b; White et al. 2016). Later the majority of institutions switched to ^{192}Ir HDR brachytherapy, while Canadian teams kept using LDR sources as permanent implants. In 2015 the rate of utilization of brachytherapy for APBI was 11% in patients older than 50 who had undergone breast-conserving surgery (Smith et al. 2015).

Multi-catheter brachytherapy involves a dedicated workflow, including (1) CT simulation, (2) target volume segmentation contouring and expansion, (3) pre-implant planning to decide on the implantation geometry and fulfill dose distribution and homogeneity constraints, (4) the implantation itself under general anesthesia, (5) a post-implant CT simulation, (6) the calculation of a new dose distribution and optimization, (7) the delivery of several fractions of HDR twice daily over 4–7 days, and (8) catheter removal.

To simplify the HDR workflow, balloon catheters were introduced in 2000 after FDA approval (Edmundson et al. 2002). This catheter greatly simplified the workflow as it can be inserted during surgery or during a surgical follow-up appointment. There is no need for pre-implant CT planning, dosimetry, or implantation in the operating room steps. The procedure simply involves (after catheter placement) a CT simulation, followed by dosimetry and treatment, which is the same number of steps as for standard external beam radiotherapy. Using a single catheter, the dose distribution is less uniform with a reported mean dose homogeneity index ($DHI = \dfrac{V100 - V150}{V100}$) of 0.77 for the balloon vs. 0.93 for multi-catheter brachytherapy (Edmundson et al. 2002). The target coverage is, however, improved with a minimum dose to 90% of the target volume (D_{90}) of 90% compared to 69.8% with multiple catheters. The release of the balloon catheter boosted the adoption of brachytherapy APBI (Keisch and Arthur 2005; Smith et al. 2015). As of 2016, over 50,000 patients in the USA have been treated with the MammoSite® (Hologic Inc, Marlborough, Massachusetts, USA) (http://www.mammosite.com/physicians/radiation-therapy/faq.cfm). Yet patients were often treated outside of standardized guidelines early on, including patients with positive surgical margins, tumors larger than 3 cm, nodal positivity, or lobular features (Shah et al. 2013a). This may explain why in the American Society of Breast Surgeons MammoSite® Registry actuarial recurrence rate was 3.8% at 5 years, and 5.5% at 7 years. The balloon brachytherapy is associated with a 30% risk of permanent seroma, with about a third being symptomatic, and with a 9.6% risk of infection (Shah et al. 2013a; Gitt

et al. 2016). To enable the dose distribution fine-tuning and enable a reduction of the skin and chest wall doses, multilumen balloon catheters were proposed in 2009 (Brown et al. 2009). Despite the fact that the actual introduction was delayed; as of 2012 multilumen balloon catheters have been more frequently used than single-lumen balloons (Huo et al. 2016). Beyond the dosimetric advantage, there are financial incentives to use the multilumen balloon that may explain this rapid adoption.

For permanent breast seed implants (PBSI), patients are seen and offered the technique during the radiotherapy consult after the surgical scar is healed and when the final pathology report is available (Pignol et al. 2006). The patient is sent for a CT simulation using a standard radiotherapy protocol and it is only after the target volume has been identified and contoured that the patient is informed if they can receive PBSI. If the implant is deemed not suitable or challenging, the patient is redirected to standard WBI using the CT simulation for planning. There is hence minimal impact on the patient's workflow, scheduling, and experience. The permanent seed implant procedure is realized under light sedation and local freezing. This enables discharging the patient on the same day, and a return to normal activity the following day. The implant starts with the accurate placement of a grooved fiducial needle which is attached to a template to immobilize the seroma cavity, realizing a procedure very similar to prostate LDR brachytherapy. Compared to HDR brachytherapy, the breast seed implant utilization of operating room time is minimal and this technique has minimal impact on other brachytherapy programs, e.g., prostate or cervix HDR, which sometime conflict with a technique requiring the patient to be treated twice daily over several days. In 2015, the results of a prospective cohort of 134 early-stage breast cancer patients accrued in three consecutive clinical trials were reported (Pignol et al. 2015). Eligible patients were older than 50, had an infiltrating ductal carcinoma (91%) or DCIS (9%) of less than 3 cm in diameter with clear margin over 2 mm, were without lymphovascular infiltration, and were node negative. With a median follow-up of 63 months, the actuarial rate of ipsilateral breast local recurrence was 1.2%, which was not statistically different than the theoretical estimate of 1.5% after WBI based on risk calculation using nomograms ($p = 0.23$) for respective infiltrating ductal carcinoma and ductal carcinoma in situ recurrence after WBI.

3.2 Intraoperative APBI

Between 2000 and 2012, the TARGIT multi-center randomized controlled clinical trial accrued 3451 patients from 33 institutions in 11 countries (Vaidya et al. 2016). Eligible patients included women 45 years old or older, diagnosed with a unifocal infiltrating ductal carcinoma of less than 3.5 cm in diameter. Patients were initially randomized for the IORT procedure for 1140 patients, or conventional WBI for 1158 patients arm. In 2004 the protocol was amended to allow the participation of centers delivering the IORT procedure after the final pathology result was known and a second surgery performed to reopen the scar. An additional 1153 patients were included. In the "pre-pathology" cohort, patients with close margins received adjuvant WBI after the IORT procedure, which was considered as a radiation boost (Vaidya et al. 2016).

For the TARGIT trial, the IORT procedure uses low-energy X-rays emitted from a 50 kV generator inside a spherical applicator of various sizes, ranging from 1.5 to 5 cm in diameter. After lumpectomy, the surgeon chooses the applicator that tightly fits into the surgical cavity and uses a purse ring suture to close the skin. To avoid skin necrosis around the suture, a tungsten ring shield is sometimes used. A dose of 20 Gy is prescribed at the surface of the applicator, and delivered in 30–45 min depending on the applicator diameter (Vaidya et al. 2001).

In 2016, Vaidya published the trial outcomes in a 221-page detailed report, and about one-third of the patients had a median follow-up of more than 5 years (Vaidya et al. 2016). The local recurrence rate for patients treated with WBI was 1.3% and, despite it was 2.5 times higher, the recurrence rate in the IORT arm at 3.3% was estimated non-inferior since it did not reach the non-inferiority threshold set at 2.5% ($p < 0.001$ for non-inferiority). The patients had the same overall survival, respectively, 1.9% in the WBI arm and 2.6% in the IORT arm.

At the European Institute of Oncology in Milan, the IORT technique was performed using a Linac to deliver 6–9 MeV electrons directly to the lumpectomy cavity at the time of surgery (Veronesi et al. 2013). Patients were treated after being enrolled in a randomized clinical trial, and between 2000 and 2007, a total of 1305 patients aged 48 or older with early-stage breast cancer less than 2.5 cm in diameter had accrued. Half of the patients received adjuvant WBI 50 Gy in 25 fractions followed by a boost of 10 Gy, and the other half the electron IORT delivering 21 Gy on the 90% isodose. The study design was an equivalence trial and hence two sided, and the randomization was blocked on tumor size. After a median follow-up of 5 years there was significantly more ipsilateral breast recurrence in the WBI arm [4.4%] compared to the IORT arm [0.4% (HR = 9.3, $p < 0.001$)], and more regional recurrence [1% compared to 0.3% ($p = 0.03$)], but no difference in overall survival (HR = 1.1, $p = 0.59$) (Veronesi et al. 2013). In the discussion, Veronesi pointed out the very low rate of local recurrence in the WBI arm at 0.4%, which is quite uncommon, and pointed out the fact that in the APBI arm the patients were relatively unselected and hence many had high-risk features. For those patients the risk of local relapse was significantly higher, including 20% patients with grade 3 tumors that had a local relapse rate of 11.9% at 5 years, 13% with lesions larger than 4 cm that had a local relapse rate of 10.9%, 7% with triple-negative breast cancer and a local relapse rate of 19%, and 5% with four nodes positive or more that had a local relapse rate of 15%. This study emphasizes the challenge of treating patients with radiotherapy without having available the full pathology picture.

3.3 External Beam Radiotherapy and Radiosurgery

Following the initial William Beaumont experience and the RTOG 0319 Phase I–II trial, 3D-CRT APBI was tested as one of the three techniques in the experimental arm of the NSABP-B39 multicenter randomized controlled trial (http://www.nsabp.pitt.edu/B-39.asp). It was also tested as the sole APBI technique in the Canadian RAPID trial (Olivotto et al. 2013). A higher dose per fraction is used for 3D-CRT external beam radiotherapy APBI compared to HDR brachytherapy (38.5 Gy in ten fractions vs. 34.0 Gy in ten fractions). However since the dose distribution homogeneity is much improved in 3D conformal radiotherapy, the bulk of the PTV eventually receives a lower dose compared to brachytherapy. Efficiency outcomes in terms of local control are still pending at the time of writing this chapter for the NSABP-B39 and the RAPID trials, and it is unknown if non-inferiority is achieved using external beam radiotherapy APBI vs. WBI. There are however several smaller studies that have reported efficiency outcomes suggesting so. In 2013, Rodriguez reported the outcome of the Barcelona randomized trial on 102 patients older than 60, with early-stage breast cancer treated using 3D-CRT APBI 37 Gy in 10 fractions twice daily or WBI 48 Gy in 24 fractions of 2 Gy with or without an additional boost (Rodríguez et al. 2013). At 5 years there was no recurrence in either arms. In 2015, Livi reported the result of the Florence prospective randomized controlled trial that accrued 520 patients older than 40 years with invasive ductal carcinoma or DCIS early-stage breast cancers (Livi et al. 2015). Patients were randomized to receive either APBI (30 Gy in 5 fractions of 6 Gy over 2 weeks) or WBI delivering 50 Gy in 25 fractions followed by a boost of 10 Gy in 5 fractions. After a median follow-up of 5 years, the local recurrence rate was 1.5% in both arms, while the acute ($p < 0.001$) and late tolerance ($p = 0.004$) as well as the cosmetic results ($p = 0.045$) were better in the APBI arm (Livi et al. 2015). In 2016, Horst reported outcomes on the Stanford prospective cohort of 141 patients aged 60 or older, with invasive ductal carcinomas (61%) or pure DCIS (36%) of less than 2.5 cm in diameter and node negative. Patients received 3D-CRT APBI delivering 38.5 Gy in ten fractions twice daily. With a median follow-up of more than 5 years, the local recurrence rates were similar at 0.9%. The cosmetic outcome was judged good to excellent in 95% of the cases (Horst et al. 2016).

3.4 Highly Conformal Techniques and Radiosurgery

Several teams have explored improved conformal techniques and radiosurgery for APBI, with the aim of reducing the amount of normal tissue irradiated. In 2016, the team at the San-Giovanni-Addolorata Hospital in Rome reported on helical tomotherapy to deliver 38.5 Gy in ten daily fractions using the NSABP-B39 contouring guidelines and constraints. Using the EORTC cosmetic rating system, excellent cosmetic outcomes were found at 5 years for all 111 patients treated between 2010 and 2013. Also, no local recurrences were found after a median FU of 34 months (De Paula et al. 2016).

In regard to robotic radiosurgery very preliminary results of a pilot study on ten patients were reported by Obayomi-Davies from the Georgetown University Hospital in Washington, DC (Obayomi-Davies et al. 2016). A total of 10 patients received a dose of 30 Gy in five daily fractions of 6 Gy. The clinical target volume was tracked using four gold fiducial markers implanted around the surgical cavity with the Synchrony® system (Accuray LLC, Sunnyvale, California, USA). Tracking was doable in 100% of the fractions, so the CTV-to-PTV margin expansion was reduced to 5 mm. Left-sided breast patients received a low heart dose with a maximum of 30% of the heart receiving 1.5 Gy or more. The lung dose was also small, with only 3% of the ipsilateral lung receiving 9 Gy or more.

More recently, a dedicated radiosurgery device, GammaPod® (Xcision Medical Systems, Columbia, Maryland, USA), for partial breast irradiation has been proposed. It is based on the same principle as the Gamma Knife® (Elekta Inc, Stockholm, Sweden) with a suction cup immobilizing the breast while the patient is treated in prone position. A total of 36 ^{60}Co sources are cross firing using a rotating collimator to generate non-coplanar conical arcs (Yu et al. 2013). There are no clinical outcomes available published at the time of writing this chapter.

4   Volume and Constraints

4.1   Breast Cancer with Limited Extent

In 2001 Faverly introduced the concept of breast carcinoma of limited extent (BCLE) corresponding to tumors with no additional invasive carcinoma, ductal carcinoma in situ, or lymphatic emboli beyond 1 cm from the edge of the invasive mass, which corresponded to the recommended distance of resection beyond the tumor index for lumpectomy (Faverly et al. 2001). In a series of 296 consecutive patients treated with mastectomy in Nijmegen between 1980 and 1986, 135 had a tumor less than 4 cm in largest diameter, without skin or fascia involvement, were purely of ductal subtype, had good-quality mammograms, and did not had previous surgery of the breast. For each patient, the mastectomy specimen was frozen and cut in 5 mm thickness slices. The extent of the tumor was evaluated calculating the distance between the edge of the tumor and additional micro foci of invasive or DCIS. In 72 patients (53%), no tumor was found beyond 1 cm. Looking at the factors associated with an a priori identification of BCLE, mammography alone was an inefficient tool to identify BCLE. The absence of calcification or density beyond the edge of the tumor index was found on univariate and multivariate analysis, the best predictor of BCLE ($p < 0.001$), but the rate of false negative remained high at 35%. The rate of false negatives dropped to 11% when pathology criteria, including free margins of 2 cm, absence of

lymphovascular infiltration, or DCIS, were added. In his conclusion Faverly proposed the following criteria for BCLE: a tumor detected by mammography without calcification or density outside the main tumor mass, a resection-free margin of at least 1 cm from the last microscopic foci, and negative postoperative mammography (Faverly et al. 2001). The Faverly study demonstrated on the one hand that mammography is not adequate to identify BCLE and that a full set of clinical and pathology factors are needed to identify tumors with limited extension in the breast. On the other hand, this study is frequently cited in the APBI literature to define the 2 cm threshold beyond the dominant mass as being the safety margin to cover cancer microscopic extension for patients eligible for APBI.

4.2   Clinical Target Volume

The rule of thumb for breast-conserving therapy is to have a surgery procedure with a 1 cm resection margin beyond the edge of the tumor mass, and the radiotherapy-ensuring treatment of the remaining 1 cm where microscopic disease may be present. This 1 cm margin corresponds to the clinical target volume (CTV) expansion (Strnad et al. 2015). In reality surgical margins are rarely uniform and there is a consensus for infiltrating ductal carcinoma that a margin negative at ink is enough and that a 2 mm margin from ink is also sufficient for DCIS (Moran et al. 2014; Morrow et al. 2016). Two recipes are used to define the CTV margins, one from the GEC-ESTRO group and the other one from the NSABP group (http://www.nsabp.pitt.edu/B-39.asp; Strnad et al. 2015). In the GEC-ESTRO study the "total safety margin" after breast-conserving surgery is defined as the sum of the existing surgical resection margins in each direction plus an added radiation safety margin (Strnad et al. 2015). Since the total safety margin is set at 2 cm around the tumor index, limited to 5 mm below skin and on the fascia pectoralis, the size of the radiation

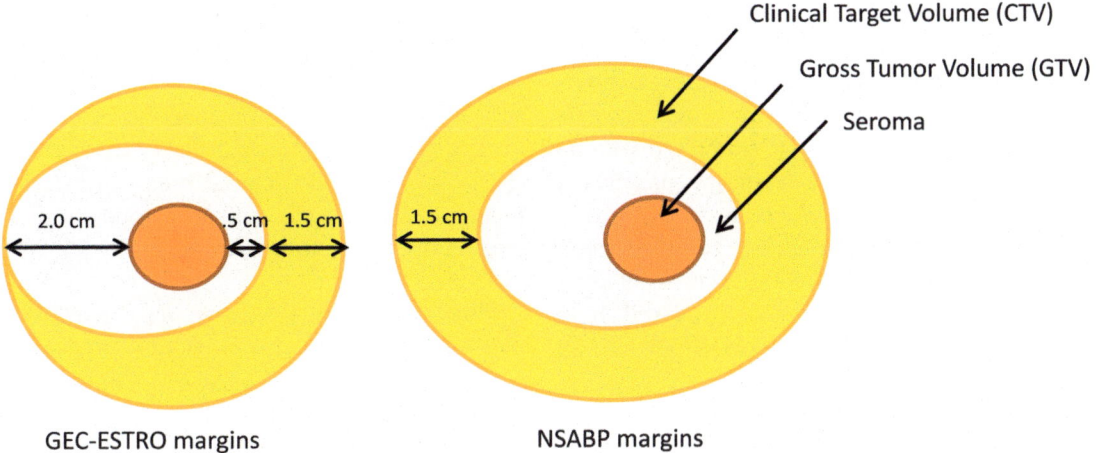

Fig. 1 Definition of the clinical target volume in the GEC-ESTRO and the NSABP studies. The GEC-ESTRO uses a "total safety margin" that is equal to 2 cm, while the NSABP proposes a uniform expansion of 1.5 cm around the lumpectomy cavity

safety margins outside the seroma is 2 cm minus the size of the surgical margin for each direction. In the NSABP study the CTV expansion is simplified adding a 1.5 cm margin in all directions around the lumpectomy cavity, and also limiting the expansion 5 mm under the skin and on the fascia pectoralis (http://www.nsabp.pitt.edu/B-39.asp 2017). Figure 1 summarizes those guidelines, and it shows that the NSABP simplification also implies that the treated volume is larger.

4.3 Planning Target Volume

To account for geographical uncertainties, the volume is expanded into a planning target volume (PTV). The size of this expansion is technique and protocol dependent.

In the NSABP study, for 3D-CRT APBI, a 1 cm margin limited to 5 mm under the skin and to the fascia pectoralis is added around the CTV to create the PTV creating a total margin of 2.5 cm beyond the lumpectomy cavity. For the multi-catheter brachytherapy technique, no margin is added, such that the PTV equals the CTV. For balloon brachytherapy the expansion around the seroma for the CTV is set at 1 cm, and no further expansion is required for the PTV (http://www.nsabp.pitt.edu/B-39.asp). In the 3D-CRT arm of the RAPID trial the expansion for the CTV beyond the surgical cavity was 1 cm, with an additional 1 cm to create the PTV (Olivotto et al. 2013). In the GEC-ESTRO guidelines no additional margin is recommended in case of multi-catheter brachytherapy if the seroma is clearly visible or identifiable. But in case of doubt, an additional margin of 0.5–1 cm is recommended (Strnad et al. 2015).

Interestingly, not all studies recommend a constraint on the "absolute volume" for the PTV but instead on a "relative volume." In the partial breast irradiation arm of the Canadian RAPID study and the 3D-CRT arm of the NSABP-B39 study, the volume receiving at least 95% of the prescribed dose (V_{95}) must be less than 35% of the breast volume. Yet, the absolute breast volume can vary significantly between patients. In the Canadian breast IMRT study the median breast size was 950 cc ranging from 214 to 2890 cc (Pignol et al. 2008). Using the threshold of 35% on this cohort, 60% of the patients would have a volume of 300 cc or more receiving the full dose, and 18% of them a volume of 500 cc or more. This may be excessive for a hypofractionated technique. The GEC-ESTRO guidelines however recommend avoiding absolute CTV volumes larger than 250 cc to prevent complications (Strnad et al. 2015). A similar absolute threshold is used for permanent breast seed implant studies (Pignol et al. 2006).

4.4 Constraints

Relatively similar constraints for critical structures are recommended across the various studies. In the NSABP-B39 study, the volume of the heart receiving 5% of the prescribed dose (V_5) should be less than 40% for left breast tumors and less than 5% for right-sided cancers (http://www.nsabp.pitt.edu/B-39.asp). Also, less than 15% of the ipsilateral lung should receive more than 30% of the prescribed dose, and the contralateral lung less than 5%. The contralateral breast and the thyroid should receive less than 3% of the prescribed dose.

For multi-catheter brachytherapy, additional constraints are required to limit excessive dose heterogeneity in the treated volume. First, the volumes receiving more than 150% (V_{150}) and 200% (V_{200}) of the prescribed dose are limited to 70 cc and 20 cc, respectively. Second, the dose homogeneity index, which is the ratio

$$DHI = \frac{V100 - V150}{V100}, \text{ should be above } 75\%.$$

5 Evidence and Guidelines

5.1 Level 1 Evidence of APBI Efficacy

There is high-quality Level 1 evidence supporting the use of APBI, with currently 5-year outcomes from several randomized clinical trials. The oldest randomized trial was performed at the National Institute of Oncology in Prague. Between 1998 and 2004, it accrued 258 patients with T1-0 grade 1–2 infiltrating ductal carcinoma and negative margins, excluding lobular carcinoma and extensive in situ carcinoma (Polgár et al. 2013). Patients were randomized to receive either WBI 50 Gy in 25 fractions (130 patients) or APBI using either multi-catheter interstitial high-dose-rate (HDR) brachytherapy delivering 36.4 Gy in 7 fractions (88 patients) or electron external beam 50 Gy in 25 fractions (40 patients). After a median follow-up

of 10 years, there was no difference in the actuarial rates of local recurrence, 5.1% WBI compared to 5.9% with APBI ($p = 0.77$); overall survival (80% vs. 82%); cancer-specific survival (94% vs. 92%); or disease-free survival (85% vs. 84%). The partial-breast arm had a higher proportion of excellent or good cosmetic outcomes, 81%, compared to 63% with WBI ($p < 0.01$).

The strongest evidence to date supporting APBI is the results of the GEC-ESTRO multicenter randomized controlled trial (Strnad et al. 2016). Between 2004 and 2009, a total of 1184 patients were randomized to receive WBI (50 Gy in 25 fractions) +/− a boost of 10 Gy in 551 patients, or multi-catheter brachytherapy delivering 32 Gy in eight fractions twice daily or 30.3 Gy in seven fractions also twice daily in 633 patients. Eligible patients were 40 years or older, with an infiltrating carcinoma or ductal carcinoma in situ (DCIS) of 3 cm maximum diameter, clear resection margins of at least 2 mm for infiltrating ductal carcinoma and 5 mm for DCIS or lobular carcinoma, absence of lymphovascular infiltration, and node negative. In 2016 Strnad reported non-inferior rate of cumulative incidence of local control of 1.44% with APBI, compared to 0.92% for WBI ($p = 0.42$) (Strnad et al. 2016).

The efficiency of IORT was evaluated in the TARGIT and ELIOT trials, with the first one reporting non-inferiority and the other one an increased risk of local relapse (Vaidya et al. 2016; Veronesi et al. 2013). Finally there are two large multicenter randomized controlled trials for which efficiency results have not yet been reported, the NSABP-B39 and the RAPID trials which are both testing 3D-CRT in the experimental treatment arm.

Looking at the available evidence, it appears that the brachytherapy APBI studies, using either multi-catheter or PBSI, have very low rate of local recurrence, in the range of 1–2% at 5 years. Intraoperative techniques or balloon brachytherapy consistently have higher local recurrence rate at 5 years, above 3–4%. The early results on single-center studies for external beam radiotherapy are similar to multi-catheter brachytherapy, and the results of larger randomized trials are pending to fully conclude on the efficiency of 3D-CRT.

5.2 Level 1 Evidence on APBI Tolerance

Ott reported in 2016 the early tolerance outcomes of the GEC-ESTRO study (Ott et al. 2016). Out of 1328 patients accrued in the study 1186 were analyzable. Lower acute grade 3 toxicities were found in the brachytherapy APBI arm compared to external beam, 7% vs. 0.2%, respectively ($p < 0.001$), and also lower rates of breast infections (0% vs. 0.2%). APBI also had much lower incidence of low-grade acute skin toxicity [21% vs. 86% ($p < 0.001$)], but 20% of the patients had a hematoma after brachytherapy. Interestingly the same number of patients experienced pain in each arm, 26% compared to 29% ($p = 0.23$).

Strnad reported late side effect outcomes on a subset of 969 patients reaching the 5-year follow-up mark (Strnad et al. 2016). The risk of severe grade 2–3 skin or subcutaneous side effects was not significantly different in the APBI arm (3.2% and 7.6%, respectively) compared to the WBI arm, 5.6% and 6.3%, respectively. It is important to note that in the brachytherapy arm the maximum skin dose was restricted to 70% of the prescribed dose (Strnad et al. 2016).

In a retrospective analysis of 1034 patients treated between 2000 and 2013 at the Ohio State University, Wobb compared the long-term tolerance between 545 patients receiving brachytherapy and 489 treated with WBI (Wobb et al. 2015). For WBI the dose distribution homogeneity was maximized using field-in-field IMRT, and the brachytherapy was delivered using interstitial multi-catheters in 40% and a strut or balloon applicator in 60%. A much larger proportion of patients received adjuvant chemotherapy in the WBI group compared to the APBI group [70% vs. 15%, respectively ($p < 0.001$)] and the median follow-up was longer for APBI compared to WBI, 6.7 vs. 3.9 years, respectively ($p < 0.001$). Brachytherapy induced more seromas of grade 2 or higher (14.4% vs. 2.9%, $p < 0.001$), more painful fat necrosis (10.2% vs. 3.6%, $p < 0.001$), more induration/fibrosis grade 2 or higher (23.2% vs. 5.7%, $p < 0.001$), and more telangiectasia grade 2 or higher (12.3% vs. 2.1%, $p < 0.001$). WBI induced more hyperpigmentation (14.5% vs. 5.8%, $p < 0.001$).

Regarding 3D-CRT, the early results of cosmetic outcome from the RAPID trial were reported in 2013 (Olivotto et al. 2013). In this study, women aged 40 years or older were randomized to receive either WBI delivering either 42.5 Gy in 16 fractions or 50 Gy in 25 fractions with a boost depending on institutional guideline or 3D-CRT 38.5 Gy in 10 fractions twice daily without boost. Between 2006 and 2011 a total of 2135 patients were enrolled. After a median follow-up of 36 months the cosmetic results were significantly worse with APBI. With half of the patients reaching the 3-year mark, the proportion of poor and fair cosmetic results evaluated by nurses was 29% using APBI compared to 17% with WBI ($p < 0.001$). When evaluated by patients, 26% compared to 18% rated the same grade, respectively ($p = 0.002$), and when evaluated by a panel of experts reviewing photographs the rate was 35% compared to 17% ($p < 0.001$) (Olivotto et al. 2013).

There are no clinical data assessing the long-term risk in regard to cardiovascular morbidity or secondary cancers for APBI. There are however several dosimetry studies on limited amounts of patients showing a reduction of dose to the heart (Chan et al. 2015; Lettmaier et al. 2011) and the lung. However, those studies used standard treatment planning to evaluate scattered dose far outside the beam, which is unreliable. Also, the Chan study focused on the left anterior descending artery which, in the WBI technique used in his institute, is included in the treatment volume (Chan et al. 2015). The results were hence artificially biased toward APBI. Another experimental study reported by Merino evaluated the mean heart dose for various APBI techniques (Merino Lara et al. 2014). An external beam radiotherapy regimen of 50 Gy in 25 fractions yielded the highest mean heart dose of 2.99 Gy for a typical average breast volume. This translated into a relative increase in cardiac morbidity of 22% following the Darby model (Darby et al. 2013). In contrast 3D-CRT APBI reduced the mean heart dose to 0.5 Gy, which translates into a negligible increased relative risk of 1%. HDR brachytherapy induced a mean heart dose of 1.5 Gy, translating into an increased risk of 4%. In regard to secondary cancers, Donovan estimated the lifetime increased risk of secondary cancer using the BEIR-VII model and dose measured on an anthropomorphic phantom irradiated with WBI, breast IMRT, or 3D-CRT APBI (Donovan et al. 2012). He found little dependence by technique on the lifetime risk that remained very low. In regard to HDR brachytherapy, it is important to note that there was a 70% increased risk of secondary cancers in the partial breast irradiation arm compared to WBI in the randomized GEC-ESTRO study (Strnad et al. 2016).

5.3   Guidelines

Several consensus guidelines have been published for the selection of patients eligible for APBI, and many have been recently updated. The most conservative remains the American Society for Radiation Oncology (ASTRO) consensus statement on APBI. The 2017 update defines as "suitable" patients to receive APBI outside clinical trial those aged 50 or older, treated with breast-conserving surgery for an infiltrating ductal carcinoma less than 2 cm, with margins of at least 2 mm, node negative, hormone receptors positive, and absence of lymphovascular infiltration. Are also eligible patients with a low or intermediate DCIS less than 2.5 cm diagnosed on mammogram and with clear margins equal to or larger than 3 mm (Correa et al. 2017).

The GEC-ESTRO and the American Brachytherapy Society (ABS) guidelines published in 2009 and 2013, respectively, are more flexible (Polgár et al. 2010; Shah et al. 2013b). The age threshold is the same but tumors up to 3 cm are eligible, the hormone receptor status is indifferent, and the size of negative margins is not specified. Patients should also have negative nodes and should not have lymphovascular infiltration. The GEC-ESTRO guidelines also exclude patients receiving neoadjuvant chemotherapy.

The American Society of Breast Surgeons (ASBS) guidelines were updated in 2011 and are very similar to the ABS guidelines, though more flexible in regard to age. Eligible patients are 45 or older for invasive ductal carcinoma, but 50 or older for DCIS (Shah et al. 2013b). In those published guidelines, the tumor grade and the biological subtype are not included in the selection criteria but lobular carcinoma is always excluded.

6   Economics

6.1   Patient Selection

In developed countries with the generalization of screening mammography, the vast majority of women are diagnosed at an early stage, and the overall survival has dramatically improved (Peto et al. 2000). The SEER database shows that in the era of mammography detection, 60% of breast cancers are diagnosed at an early stage (node negative) (https://seer.cancer.gov/statfacts/html/breast.html). More early-stage patients means more patients eligible for APBI. Manyam calculated the proportion of eligible patients for various breast techniques on a selected cohort of 108,484 early-stage breast cancers from the SEER database (Manyam et al. 2016). A total of 41.2% of those early-stage and therefore 24.7% of newly diagnosed breast cancers were eligible for APBI using the old ASTRO guidelines, but 89.7% were eligible using the GEC-ESTRO guidelines, corresponding to 53.8% of newly diagnosed breast cancers. Besides eligibility based on pathology criteria, not all patients can receive APBI because of technical issues, comorbidities, or patient's preference issues. In any case, since breast cancer often represents one of the largest proportions of patients referred to a radiotherapy center, this implies significant impact on the patient's workflow organization and possible large cost saving or spending.

The number of patients treated with APBI is increasing. Using data from the National Cancer Data Base (NCDB), Shaitelman identified 399,705 women treated between 2004 and 2011 for nonmetastatic breast cancers (Shaitelman et al. 2016). She found an increased use of APBI from 4% to about 10% during this period. In addition, APBI was used in 14.8% of the cases for patients in the "suitable" category of the ASTRO guidelines. In terms of technique, the majority of patients were treated with brachytherapy (82%), and less by external beam radiotherapy. The use of IORT remained confidential.

6.2 Cost-Effectiveness

Several studies have reported on the cost of APBI, and a few have done a cost-effectiveness analysis (Greenup et al. 2012). Most studies used Medicare reimbursement schemes, which limits their findings to the US medical system and may not represent the true societal cost of the technique since the Medicare codes sometimes under- or overestimate some care components. Using micro-costing, Schutzer compared the cost of WBI delivering 50 Gy in 25 fractions to balloon-based brachytherapy APBI delivering 10 fractions over 5 days in the USA (Schutzer et al. 2016). He found relatively similar cost, $5333 for WBI, including 56% personnel costs and 44% for space and equipment, compared to $6941 for brachytherapy APBI, including 51% personnel cost, 6% for space and equipment, and 43% for consumables.

A recent study from Canada using activity-based costing and a Markov analysis to account for downstream costs, utilities, and probabilities adapted from the literature shows that HDR brachytherapy is the most expensive technique ($14,400) compared to permanent breast seed implants ($8700), and compared to WBI ($6200). Interestingly, looking at who pays what, the author found that the patient's share of the cost is larger for WBI compared to HDR, which is larger than PBSI, since protracted treatment has a significant impact on transportation, homecare, and work (McGuffin et al. 2017).

Conclusions

This review demonstrates plenty of evidence supporting the use of APBI as a treatment option for well-selected patients outside of clinical trials. Among the multiple techniques available, brachytherapy has a very high rate of local control: between 1 and 2% at 5 years. Balloon brachytherapy or IORT seems to have a slightly higher rate of local recurrence: between 3 and 4% at 5 years. The local control rates of 3D-CRT are promising but results from large multicenter randomized trials are needed to formally conclude such. In terms of treatment convenience, protocols using one fraction per day are promising and treatments in a single fraction are possible using intraoperative or permanent breast seed implants.

References

Bethune WA (1991) Partial breast irradiation for early breast cancer. J Natl Med Assoc 83:768. 800–808

Brown S, McLaughlin M, Pope K et al (2009) Initial radiation experience evaluating early tolerance and toxicities in patients undergoing accelerated partial breast irradiation using the Contura® Multi-Lumen Balloon breast brachytherapy catheter. Brachytherapy 8:227–233

Chan TY, Tan PW, Tan CW et al (2015) Assessing radiation exposure of the left anterior descending artery, heart and lung in patients with left breast cancer: a dosimetric comparison between multi-catheter accelerated partial breast irradiation and whole breast external beam radiotherapy. Radiother Oncol 117:459–466

Correa C, Harris EE, Leonardi MC et al (2017) Accelerated partial breast irradiation: executive summary for the update of an ASTRO evidence-based consensus statement. Pract Radiat Oncol 7:73–79

Darby SC, Ewertz M, McGale P et al (2013) Risk of ischemic heart disease in women after radiotherapy for breast cancer. N Engl J Med 368:987–998

De Paula U, D'Angelillo RM, Barbara R et al (2016) Once daily accelerated partial breast irradiation: preliminary results with helical tomotherapy. Anticancer Res 36:3035–3039

Donovan EM, James H, Bonora M et al (2012) Second cancer incidence risk estimates using BEIR VII models for standard and complex external beam radiotherapy for early breast cancer. Med Phys 39:5814–5824

Edmundson GK, Vicini FA, Chen PY et al (2002) Dosimetric characteristics of the MammoSite RTS, a new breast brachytherapy applicator. Int J Radiat Oncol Biol Phys 52:1132–1139

Faverly DR, Hendriks JH, Holland R (2001) Breast carcinomas of limited extent: frequency, radiologic-pathologic characteristics, and surgical margin requirements. Cancer 91:647–659

Gitt A, Böse-Ribeiro H, Nieder C et al (2016) Treatment results of MammoSite catheter in combination with whole-breast irradiation. Anticancer Res 36:355–360

Greenup RA, Camp MS, Taghian AG et al (2012) Cost comparison of radiation treatment options after lumpectomy for breast cancer. Ann Surg Oncol 19:3275–3281

Hickey BE, Lehman M, Francis DP et al (2016) Partial breast irradiation for early breast cancer. Cochrane Database Syst Rev 7:CD007077

https://seer.cancer.gov/statfacts/html/breast.html. Accessed 28 Feb 2017.

http://www.mammosite.com/physicians/radiation-therapy/faq.cfm. Accessed 28 Feb 2017

http://www.nsabp.pitt.edu/B-39.asp. Accessed 28 Feb 2017

Horst KC, Fasola C, Ikeda D et al (2016) Five-year results of a prospective clinical trial investigating accelerated partial breast irradiation using 3D conformal radiotherapy after lumpectomy for early stage breast cancer. Breast 28:178–183

Huo J, Giordano SH, Smith BD et al (2016) Contemporary toxicity profile of breast brachytherapy versus external beam radiation after lumpectomy for breast cancer. Int J Radiat Oncol Biol Phys 94:709–718

Keisch M, Arthur DW (2005) Current perspective on the MammoSite® Radiation Therapy System—a balloon breast brachytherapy applicator. Brachytherapy 4:177–180

Khan AJ, Vicini FA, Arthur D (2012) Brachytherapy vs whole-breast irradiation for breast cancer. JAMA 308:567

Lettmaier S, Kreppner S, Lotter M et al (2011 Aug) Radiation exposure of the heart, lung and skin by radiation therapy for breast cancer: a dosimetric comparison between partial breast irradiation using multicatheter brachytherapy and whole breast teletherapy. Radiother Oncol 100(2):189–194

Livi L, Meattini I, Marrazzo L et al (2015) Accelerated partial breast irradiation using intensity-modulated radiotherapy versus whole breast irradiation: 5-year survival analysis of a phase 3 randomized controlled trial. Eur J Cancer 51:451–463

Manyam BV, Tendulkar R, Cherian S et al (2016) Evaluating candidacy for hypofractionated radiation therapy, accelerated partial breast irradiation, and endocrine therapy after breast conserving surgery: a surveillance epidemiology and end results (SEER) analysis. Am J Clin Oncol. Epub ahead of print

McGuffin M, Merino T, Keller B et al (2017) Who should bear the cost of convenience? A cost-effectiveness analysis comparing external beam and brachytherapy radiotherapy techniques for early stage breast cancer. Clin Oncol 29:e57–e63

Merino Lara TR, Fleury E, Mashouf S et al (2014) Measurement of mean cardiac dose for various breast irradiation techniques and corresponding risk of major cardiovascular event. Front Oncol 4:284

Moran MS, Schnitt SJ, Giuliano AE et al (2014) Society of Surgical Oncology-American Society for Radiation Oncology consensus guideline on margins for breast-conserving surgery with whole-breast irradiation in stages I and II invasive breast cancer. J Clin Oncol 32:1507–1515

Morrow M, Van Zee KJ, Solin LJ et al (2016) Society of Surgical Oncology-American Society for Radiation Oncology-American Society of Clinical Oncology consensus guideline on margins for breast-conserving surgery with whole-breast irradiation in ductal carcinoma in situ. J Clin Oncol 34:4040–4046

Obayomi-Davies O, Kole TP, Oppong B et al (2016) Stereotactic accelerated partial breast irradiation for early-stage breast cancer: rationale, feasibility, and early experience using the CyberKnife radiosurgery delivery platform. Front Oncol 6:129

Olivotto IA, Whelan TJ, Parpia S et al (2013) Interim cosmetic and toxicity results from RAPID: a randomized trial of accelerated partial breast irradiation using three-dimensional conformal external beam radiation therapy. J Clin Oncol 31:4038–4045

Ott OJ, Strnad V, Hildebrandt G et al (2016) GEC-ESTRO multicenter phase 3-trial: accelerated partial breast irradiation with interstitial multi-catheter brachytherapy versus external beam whole breast irradiation: early toxicity and patient compliance. Radiother Oncol 120:119–123

Peto R, Boreham J, Clarke M et al (2000) UK and USA breast cancer deaths down 25% in year 2000 at ages 20–69 years. Lancet 355:1822

Pignol JP, Keller B, Rakovitch E et al (2006) First report of a permanent breast [103]Pd seed implant as adjuvant radiation treatment for early-stage breast cancer. Int J Radiat Oncol Biol Phys 64:176–181

Pignol JP, Olivotto I, Rakovitch E et al (2008) Multicenter randomized trial of breast intensity-modulated radiation therapy to reduce acute radiation dermatitis. J Clin Oncol 26:2085–2092

Pignol JP, Caudrelier JM, Crook J et al (2015) Report on the clinical outcomes of permanent breast seed implant for early-stage breast cancers. Int J Radiat Oncol Biol Phys 93:614–621

Polgár C, Sulyok Z, Fodor J et al (2002) Sole brachytherapy of the tumor bed after conservative surgery for T1 breast cancer: five-year results of a phase I-II study and initial findings of a randomized phase III trial. J Surg Oncol 80:121–128

Polgár C, Van Limbergen E, Pötter R et al (2010) Patient selection for accelerated partial-breast irradiation (APBI) after breast conserving surgery: recommendations of the Groupe European de Curietherapie-European Society for Therapeutic Radiology and Oncology (GEC-ESTRO) breast cancer working group based on clinical evidence (2009). Radiother Oncol 94:264–273

Polgár C, Fodor J, Major T et al (2013) Breast-conserving therapy with partial or whole breast irradiation: ten-year results of the Budapest randomized trial. Radiother Oncol 108:197–202

Rodríguez N, Sanz X, Dengra J et al (2013) Five-year outcomes, cosmesis, and toxicity with 3-dimensional conformal external beam radiation therapy to deliver accelerated partial breast irradiation. Int J Radiat Oncol Biol Phys 87:1051–1057

Schutzer ME, Arthur DW, Anscher MS et al (2016) Time-driven activity-based costing: a comparative cost analysis of whole-breast radiotherapy versus balloon-based brachytherapy in the management of early-stage breast cancer. J Oncol Pract 12:e584–e593. doi:10.1200/JOP.2015.008441

Shah C, Badiyan S, Ben Wilkinson J et al (2013a) Treatment efficacy with accelerated partial breast irradiation (APBI): final analysis of the American Society of Breast Surgeons MammoSite® breast brachytherapy registry trial. Ann Surg Oncol 20:3279–3285

Shah C, Vicini F, Wazer DE et al (2013b) The American Brachytherapy Society consensus statement for accelerated partial breast irradiation. Brachytherapy 12:267–277

Shaitelman SF, Lin HY, Smith BD et al (2016) Practical implications of the publication of consensus guidelines by the American Society for Radiation Oncology: Accelerated Partial Breast Irradiation and the National Cancer Data Base. Int J Radiat Oncol Biol Phys 94:338–348

Smith GL, Xu Y, Buchholz TA et al (2012) Association between treatment with brachytherapy vs whole-breast irradiation and subsequent mastectomy, complications, and survival among older women with invasive breast cancer. JAMA 307:1827–1837

Smith GL, Huo J, Giordano SH et al (2015) Utilization and outcomes of breast brachytherapy in younger women. Int J Radiat Oncol 93:91–101

Strnad V, Hannoun-Levi JM, Guinot JL et al (2015) Recommendations from GEC ESTRO Breast Cancer Working Group (I): target definition and target delineation for accelerated or boost Partial Breast Irradiation using multi-catheter interstitial brachytherapy after breast conserving closed cavity surgery. Radiother Oncl 115(3):342–348

Strnad V, Ott OJ, Hildebrandt G et al (2016) 5-year results of accelerated partial breast irradiation using sole interstitial multi-catheter brachytherapy versus whole-breast irradiation with boost after breast-conserving surgery for low-risk invasive and in-situ carcinoma of the female breast: a randomized, phase 3, non-inferiority trial. Lancet 387:229–238

Vaidya JS, Baum M, Tobias JS et al (2001) Targeted intraoperative radiotherapy (Targit): an innovative method of treatment for early breast cancer. Ann Oncol 12:1075–1080

Vaidya JS, Wenz F, Bulsara M et al (2016) An international randomized controlled trial to compare TARGeted Intraoperative radioTherapy (TARGIT) with conventional postoperative radiotherapy after breast-conserving surgery for women with early-stage breast cancer (the TARGIT-A trial). Health Technol Assess 20:1–188

Veronesi U, Orecchia R, Maisonneuve P et al (2013) Intraoperative radiotherapy versus external radiotherapy for early breast cancer (ELIOT): a randomized controlled equivalence trial. Lancet Oncol 14:1269–1277

Vicini F, White J, Gustafson G et al (1993) The use of iodine-125 seeds as a substitute for iridium-192 seeds in temporary interstitial breast implants. Int J Radiat Oncol Biol Phys 27:561–566

Vicini FA, Horwitz EM, Lacerna MD et al (1997a) Long-term outcome with interstitial brachytherapy in the management of patients with early-stage breast cancer treated with breast-conserving therapy. Int J Radiat Oncol Biol Phys 37:845–852

Vicini FA, Chen PY, Fraile M et al (1997b) Low-dose-rate brachytherapy as the sole radiation modality in the management of patients with early-stage breast cancer treated with breast-conserving therapy: preliminary results of a pilot trial. Int J Radiat Oncol Biol Phys 38:301–310

Vicini FA, Kestin L, Chen P et al (2003a) Limited-field radiation therapy in the management of early-stage breast cancer. J Natl Cancer Inst 95:1205–1210

Vicini FA, Remouchamps V, Wallace M et al (2003b) Ongoing clinical experience utilizing 3D conformal external beam radiotherapy to deliver partial-breast irradiation in patients with early-stage breast cancer treated with breast-conserving therapy. Int J Radiat Oncol Biol Phys 57:1247–1253

Vicini F, Winter K, Straube W et al (2005) A phase I/II trial to evaluate three-dimensional conformal radiation therapy confined to the region of the lumpectomy cavity for Stage I/II breast carcinoma: initial report of feasibility and reproducibility of Radiation Therapy Oncology Group (RTOG) Study 0319. Int J Radiat Oncol Biol Phys 63:1531–1537

Vicini F, Shah C, Tendulkar R et al (2016) Accelerated partial breast irradiation: an update on published Level I evidence. Brachytherapy 15:607–615

White J, Winter K, Kuske RR et al (2016) Long-term cancer outcomes from study NRG oncology/RTOG 9517: a phase 2 study of accelerated partial breast irradiation with multi-catheter brachytherapy after lumpectomy for early-stage breast cancer. Int J Radiat Oncol Biol Phys 95:1460–1465

Wobb JL, Shah C, Jawad MS et al (2015) Comparison of chronic toxicities between brachytherapy-based accelerated partial breast irradiation and whole breast irradiation using intensity modulated radiotherapy. Breast 24:739–744

Yu CX, Shao X, Zhang J et al (2013) GammaPod®—a new device dedicated for stereotactic radiotherapy of breast cancer. Med Phys. 40:051703

Lung Cancer

Mauro Loi and J.J. Nuyttens

Contents

M. Loi • J.J. Nuyttens (✉)
Erasmus Medical Center,
Rotterdam, The Netherlands
e-mail: j.nuyttens@erasmusmc.nl

1   Introduction

Non-small-cell lung cancer (NSCLC), the most common cause of cancer death worldwide, is amenable to surgery in patients with early or localized disease (approximately 15–20% of cases) (Shields 1993). Surgical resection of stage I (T1–2, N0) NSCLC yields satisfying outcome results with 5-year survival rates of 60–70%, and remains at present the golden standard in this population. Nevertheless its use is restricted to compliant, medically fit patients (Naruke et al. 1988; Mountain 1997; Adebonojo et al. 1999). Patients refusing surgery or deemed medically inoperable due to comorbidities, who despite impaired life expectancy would ultimately die of cancer progression in more than half of cases if no specific cancer treatment is performed (McGarry et al. 2002), have been treated with nonsurgical therapies such as standard fractionated radiotherapy, with disappointing results (Dosoretz et al. 1992). Optimal tumor control might be obtained by adequate dose escalation, though at the expense of increased toxicity with traditional radiotherapy techniques and schedules (Rosenzweig et al. 2005). Moreover, irradiation of lung lesions must also take into account tumor motion during the breathing cycle that can result, during expiration and deep inspiration, in excursions up to 3 cm as a function of tumor location and

Med Radiol Radiat Oncol (2017)
DOI 10.1007/174_2017_34 © Springer International Publishing AG
Published Online: 03 May 2017

respiratory pattern (Seppenwoolde et al. 2002). Since wide margins would be needed to cover the presumed range of motion, detection of tumor position during the treatment course may contribute to maintain acceptable treatment volumes, thus reducing exposure of healthy lung to radiation damage. Therefore improvement in dose delivery and in target recognition became of primary interest in radiation research during the last decade, pushing toward development of stereotactic body radiotherapy (SBRT) as a valuable option in this setting. In a pivotal work comparing four-dimensional SBRT with three-dimensional conformal radiotherapy, an increase up to 75% in mean biological dose was possible without significant additional dose to the organs at risk, in particular lung (Prevost et al. 2008). Data from retrospective series of unresectable patients showed promising local control rates of 80–100% (Onishi et al. 2004; van der Voort et al. 2009; Lagerwaard et al. 2008; Grills et al. 2010) and overall survival rates of 40–80% at 3 years (Simone et al. 2013), in particular when biologically effective dose (BED) superior to 100 Gy is delivered (Onishi et al. 2004). It is also noteworthy that overall survival was comparable to surgery in SBRT patients when treatment groups were adjusted for variables (age, comorbidities, etc.) that might lead to a selection bias (Palma et al. 2011; Soldà et al. 2013). However, no direct comparison is available at present since the two phase III trials; STARS (StereoTActic Radiotherapy vs. Surgery) and ROSEL (Radiosurgery Or Surgery for operable Early stage non-small-cell Lung cancer) comparing SBRT to surgical resection were prematurely closed due to low accrual (Chang et al. 2015). These favorable results are achieved by modern image-guided radiotherapy systems that combine high-dose delivery with accurate treatment guidance by integration of linear accelerators with medical imaging devices like Cone-Beam CT, MegaVoltage CT (Tomotherapy®: Accuray Inc., Sunnyvale, California, USA) or X-ray tubes (CyberKnife®; Accuray Inc., Sunnyvale, California, USA). In this chapter, a summary of methods to minimize the impact of tumor motion and clinical aspects of SBRT in the treatment of primary lung tumors is discussed.

2 Technical Aspects of Lung SBRT

2.1 Simulation

Precise delineation of patient anatomy is mandatory for SBRT. Simulation CT should be performed in the treatment position with or without a vacuum mattress to minimize the motion of the patient (Fig. 1). The treatment planning CT scan is made with intravenous contrast, usually with a wide-bore multi-slice computed tomography (CT) simulator. The use of 4-D CT scans, exhale or inhale CT scan combined or not combined with a contrast-enhanced planning CT scan, depends on the radiation technique.

The patient is scanned from his teeth to the middle of his abdomen (a minimum of 10–15 cm above and below the treatment field margins) in order to adequately cover the target and the organs at risk. Trans-axial imaging has a slice thickness of 1.5–3 mm.

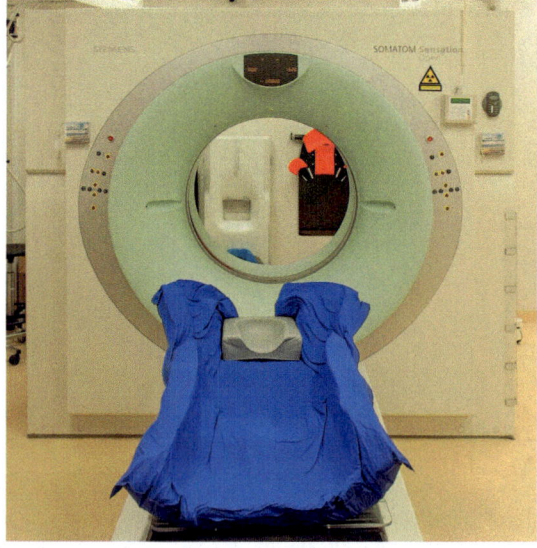

Fig. 1 Vacuum mattress used for positioning during CT simulation

2.2 Tumor Motion Control

Following recommendations from the International Commission on Radiation Units and Measurements (ICRU) (Purdy 2004), treatment margins should encompass (Fig. 2):

- Delineation of tumor as seen on primary image set is called the gross tumor volume (GTV).
- GTV plus expansion to areas susceptible to microscopic involvement is the clinical tumor volume (CTV).
- Internal target volume (ITV) incorporates the CTV plus an internal margin (IM) that accounts for respiratory motion.
- A further security margin (to compensate for setup error and intrafraction patient movement) is added to build the planning target volume (PTV).

The aim of tumor motion control techniques is to reduce the target volume, and consequently the dose to the organs at risk without compromising adequate tumor coverage.

2.3 Real-Time Tumor Tracking

The CyberKnife Synchrony System® is the most widespread tumor-tracking system that allows correction for respiratory motion by repositioning the radiation beam according to tumor position in function of the breathing cycle. CyberKnife® is a frameless radiotherapy unit composed by a 6 MV linear accelerator installed on a robotic arm possessing six degrees of freedom (Chang and Adler 2001) (Fig. 3). The CyberKnife® is equipped with an imaging system consisting of 2 X-ray sources mounted on the ceiling of the treatment platform paired with amorphous silicon detectors to acquire live orthogonal digital radiographic images of the tumor, or tumor-localizing surrogates such as the skull, spine, or fiducial markers. First, the patient is placed in supine position on the treatment couch and allowed to breathe normally: initial alignment is made by the X-ray image guidance system. A correlation model is set up by the Synchrony System® between an external signal related to respiratory movements from three light-emitting diodes (LEDs) on the patient's chest or belly and tumor (or fiducial

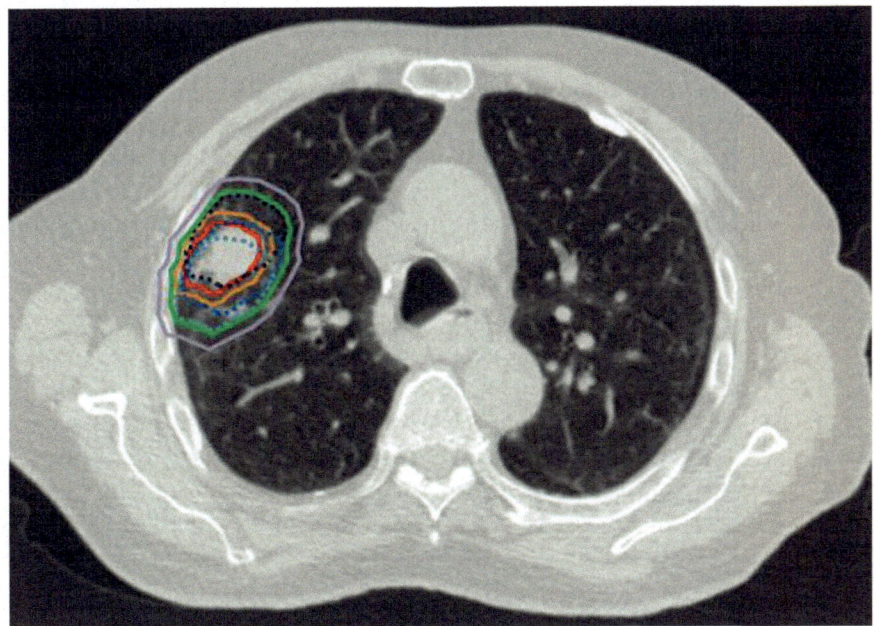

Fig. 2 Volumes of treatment according to ICRU. *Red*: GTV. *Orange*: CTV. *Dashed lines* represent tumor position on different phases of respiratory motion on 4D or forced respiration CT: the sum of all tumor positions in the breathing cycle accounts for the IM. *Green*: ITV. *Violet*: PTV

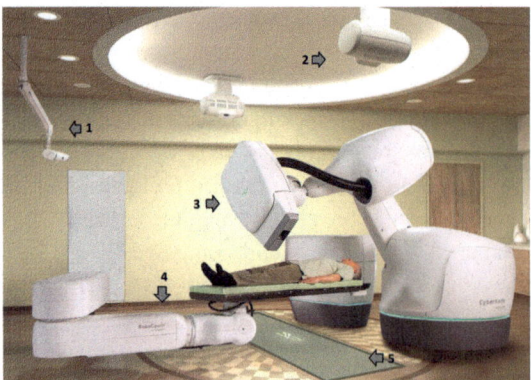

Fig. 3 The CyberKnife radiosurgery system: (*1*) Synchrony camera; (*2*) X-ray sources; (*3*) linear accelerator mounted on robot; (*4*) robotic arm connected to treatment couch: (*5*) X-ray flat panel detectors. Courtesy of Accuray Inc. (Sunnyvale, CA)

markers) position reconstructed by autosegmentation on approximately eight X-ray image pairs at different phases of the breathing cycle: by coupling LED motion to tumor motion the CyberKnife® can perform continuous tumor tracking resulting in clinical submillimeter accuracy, real-time beam correction, and thus possibility to significantly reduce PTV (Murphy 2004; Casamassima et al. 2006). The correlation model is updated throughout the fraction course with regular acquisition of new X-ray images, rebuilding the model if the correlation error is larger than 5 mm (Adler et al. 1997; Nuyttens and van de Pol 2012; Sayeh et al. 2007). Focusing on target identification, tumor recognition can be obtained by two methods:

- X-sight® lung system (Accuray Inc., Sunnyvale, California, USA), based on the contrast between tumor and surrounding lung tissue, thereby removing the need to implant fiducial markers in particular for peripheral tumors larger than 15 mm in all axes detectable on orthogonal X-ray projections (Bahig et al. 2013). Despite its availability since 2006, few reports are available (Bibault et al. 2012).
- Use of fiducial markers: a minimum of three fiducial markers (implanted within 6 cm of the lesion and separated by ≤2 cm distance) is required to acquire both translation and rotation data. Despite extensive literature and a wide range of techniques available to place markers (percutaneous, bronchoscopic with or without electromagnetic navigation,

intravascular insertion), the procedure can result in iatrogenic complications and delay in treatment concerning reliability. The risk of fiducial migration requiring repositioning should be taken into account during evaluation (Nuyttens and van de Pol 2012).

2.4 CT-Based Internal Tumor Volume

A CT-based ITV is built by using different methods. The ITV should be preferably delineated on 4D CT by contouring the GTV on the primary image set (usually acquired in the expiratory phase) and registering the outline on image sets acquired on other phases of the breathing cycle to create a cumulative target encompassing all the possible tumor positions. To improve the efficiency, postprocessing tools like the maximum intensity projection (MIP) allow one to reduce the multiple 4D CT image sets to a single data set where each voxel corresponds to the maximum intensity detected (Underberg et al. 2005). However, the main limitation of this technique is that 4D CT represents only a sample of the patient breathing; therefore it does not take into account variations in respiratory patterns during the treatment sessions. If 4D CT is not available, an ITV can be generated based on breath-hold CT images by combining GTVs outlined on two image sets (acquired at the end of the expiration and at the end of the inspiration, respectively) on an extended temporal CT scan, in order to cover the entire path of the tumor along the entire breathing cycle (Barnes et al. 2001).

2.5 Forced Shallow Breathing with Abdominal Compression

A diaphragm control device, consisting of an abdominal plate and a screw attached to a rigid stereotactic body frame, can be used to reduce tumor motion by exerting a pressure on the upper abdomen (Fig. 4). The combination of shallow breathing and consequent reduction of tumor motion, combined with correct patient immobilization by the stereotactic frame, allows a margin reduction from CTV to PTV (Guckenberger et al. 2007a; Jensen et al. 2008; Hansen et al. 2006; Song et al. 2009).

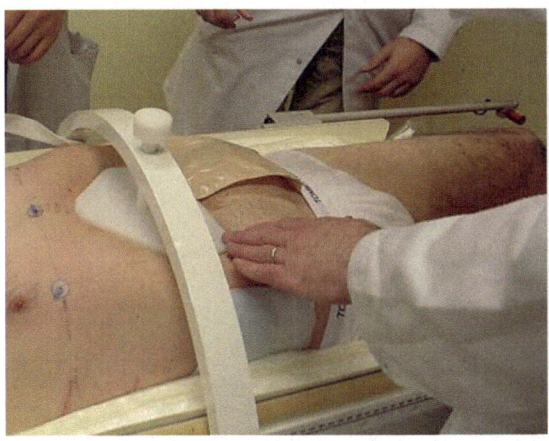 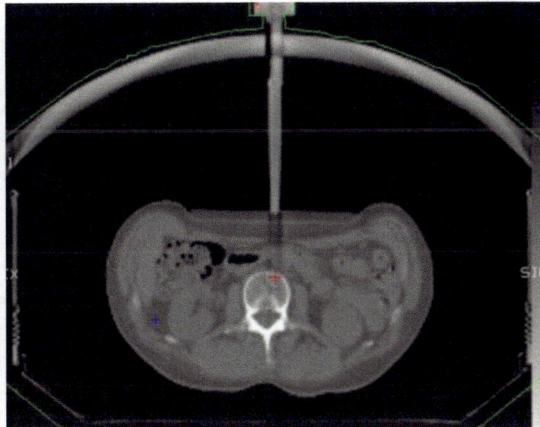

Fig. 4 Abdominal compression positioning for SBRT treatment: exterior (*left*) and CT (*right*) view

2.6 Breath-Hold Methods

In the deep inspiration breath-hold technique (DIBH), treatment is simulated, planned, and delivered during breath-holding at nearly 100% of the vital capacity. Lung inflation is monitored through a spirometer while nasal breathing is prevented by a nose clip (Wong et al. 1999; Rosenzweig et al. 2000; Mah et al. 2000). In the self-gated DIBH modality, the patient is taught, after a training session, to signal when he or she attains the correct inspiration level to start the treatment. Self-gated DIBH decreased the percent of lung volume receiving 20 Gy (V20) from 12.8 to 8.8% with GTV-to-PTV margin reduction (Barnes et al. 2001). However, breath-holding techniques require compliance of the patients and active participation of the therapist and may be poorly tolerated (Jiang 2006).

2.7 Respiratory Gating Methods

Several devices have been developed to monitor patient breathing, allowing radiotherapy administration only during a selected time window corresponding to a phase of the respiratory cycle. Among them, the real-time position management respiratory gating system (RPM) consists of two reflective markers placed on the patient's trunk. The marker motion, corresponding to the breathing pattern of the patient, is analyzed by software that triggers the CT and linac according to a predefined gate (Hara et al. 2002; Shirato et al. 2000a, b; Giraud et al. 2006). This modality is well tolerated by patients with poor lung function, but inconsistencies

between the PTV and the external respiratory surrogates have been reported (Hunjan et al. 2010).

2.7.1 Treatment Planning

The planning CT is transferred to the treatment planning system (TPS). The tumor and organs at risk (OAR) are then contoured. The gross tumor volume (GTV) is contoured using the lung window. Margins to the GTV are added depending on the radiation technique (as previously described). The OAR consist of both lungs, esophagus, heart, and spinal cord. Usually, inverse treatment planning is used and the number of beams varies between 7 and 15 using conventional 3D techniques or up to 150 beams using stereotactic radiotherapy with the CyberKnife®. According to the major phase II prospective trials RTOG 0813 and 0915 [41–42], requirements for an SBRT plan are the following:

- An isodose prescription between ≥60% and <90% of the maximum dose providing 95% PTV coverage; 99% of the target volume (PTV) receives a minimum of 90% of the prescription dose.
- Tissue receiving ≥105% of the prescription dose must be restricted to the PTV (high-dose spillage), and should not exceed 15% of the PTV volume. Maximum dose must be comprised between 111.11 and 166.67%.
- Conformity index (CI), defined as the ratio of the volume of the reference isodose to the PTV volume, should be inferior to 1.2.
- Dose constraint must be met according to the chosen dose and fractionation schedules (Table 1).

Table 1 Dose constraints used in relevant prospective trials

	RTOG 0236	JCOG0403	ROSEL		RTOG 0813	RTOG 0915		LUNGTECH	STARS	
Schedule	60 Gy/3 fr	40 Gy/4 fr	60 Gy/3 fr	60 Gy/5 fr	60 Gy/5 fr	34 Gy/1 fr	48 Gy/4 fr	60 Gy/8 fr	Peripheral: 60 Gy/3 fr	Central: 60 Gy/4 fr
Lung	$V20 \leq 10\%$	MLD < 18.0 Gy V15 < 25% V20 < 20%	V20<10%	V20<10%	$V12.5<1500$ cm^3 $V13.5<1000$ cm^3	$V7<1500$ cm^3 $V7.4<1000$ cm^3	$V11.6<1500$ cm^3 $V12.4<1000$ cm^3	–	V20Gy<20% V10Gy<30% V5Gy<50%	V20Gy<20% V10Gy<30% V5Gy<50%
Spinal cord	D_{max} 18 Gy	D_{max} 25 Gy	D_{max} 18 Gy	D_{max} 25 Gy	Dmax 30 Gy $V13.5<0.5$ cm^3	Dmax 14 Gy $V7 < 1.2$ cm^3	Dmax 26 Gy $V13.6 < 1.2$ cm^3	D_{max} 32 Gy	D_{max} 18 Gy	D_{max} 25 Gy $V20<1$ cm^3 $V15<10$ cm^3
Esophagus	D_{max} 27 Gy	$V40<1$ cm^3 $V35<10$ cm^3	D_{max} 24 Gy	D_{max} 27 Gy	D_{max} 105%PTV $V27.5 < 5$ cm^3	Dmax 15.4 Gy $V11.9 < 5$cm^3	Dmax 30 Gy $V18.8 < 5$ cm^3	D_{max} 40 Gy	D_{max} 27 Gy	D_{max} 50 Gy $V35<1$ cm^3 $V30<10$ cm^3
Brachial plexus	D_{max} 24 Gy	–	D_{max} 24 Gy	D_{max} 27 Gy	$D_{max} < 32$ Gy $V30<3$ cm^3	Dmax 17.5 Gy $V14<3$ cm^3	Dmax 27.2 Gy $V23.6<3$ cm^3	D_{max} 38 Gy	D_{max} 24 Gy	D_{max} 40 Gy $V35 < 1$ cm^3 $V30 < 10$cm^3
Trachea/bronchi	D_{max}30 Gy	$V40<10$ cm	D_{max} 30 Gy	D_{max}32 Gy	D_{max} 105%PTV $V18 < 4$ cm^3	Dmax 20.2 Gy $V10.5<4$ cm^3	Dmax 34.8 Gy $V15.6 < 4$ cm^3	D_{max} 44 Gy	D_{max} 30 Gy	D_{max} 50 Gy $V35 < 1$ cm^3 $V30 < 10$ cm^3
Chest wall/ribs	–	–	–	–	Dmax 32 Gy $V30 < 10$ cm^3	Dmax 30 Gy $V22 < 1$ cm^3	Dmax 40 Gy $V32 < 1$ cm^3	–	$V35 < 1$cm^3 $V30 < 10$ cm^3	–
Heart	D_{max}30 Gy	–	D_{max} 24 Gy	D_{max} 27 Gy	Dmax <105%PTV $V32 < 15$ cm^3	Dmax 22 Gy $V16 < 15$ cm^3	Dmax 34 Gy $V28 < 15$ cm^3	–	D_{max} 30 Gy	D_{max} 50 Gy $V40 < 1$ cm^3 $V35 < 10$ cm
Vessels	–	$V40 < 1$ cm^3 $V35 < 10$ cm^3	–	–	D_{max} 105%PTV $V47 < 10$ cm^3	Dmax 37 Gy $V31 < 10$ cm^3	Dmax 49 Gy $V43 < 10$ cm^3	–	–	D_{max} 50 Gy $V40 < 1$ cm^3 $V35 < 10$ cm
Skin	D_{max} 24 Gy	$D_{max}<40$ Gy	V20 < 10%	V20 < 10%	Dmax 32 Gy $V32 < 10$ cm^3	Dmax 26 Gy $V23 < 10$ cm^3	Dmax 36 Gy $V17.6 < 10$ cm^3	–	$V35 < 1$ cm^3 $V30 < 10$ cm^3	$V40 < 1$ cm^3 $V35 < 10$ cm^3 $V30 < 100$ cm^3

3 Lung SBRT in Clinical Practice

3.1 Treatment Regimens and Outcome Results

Initial experiences favored single-fraction schedules. Whyte et al. reported feasibility of a single fraction of 15 Gy in a phase I clinical trial (Whyte et al. 2003). Subsequent experiences (Hara et al. 2002; Le et al. 2006) demonstrated the safety and improved efficacy of doses up to 30 Gy in a single fraction (2-year local control rate of 83% compared to 52% for doses less than 30 Gy) (Hara et al. 2002). Nevertheless, the applicability to larger tumors has been questioned (Hof et al. 2007), leading to the emergence of multiple-fractions schedules. Pivotal experiences of dose escalation performed at the University of Indiana showed that dose escalation from 24 Gy in three fractions up to 60 Gy in three fractions was feasible and effective in medically inoperable early-stage NSCLC patients, resulting in an 87% overall response rate to treatment (Timmerman et al. 2003). Onishi et al., in a Japanese multicenter study enrolling 245 stage I NSCLC patients treated by different SBRT schedule, stressed the importance of the delivery of a biologic effective dose (BED) ≥ 100 Gy resulting in superior 2-year local failure rates (8.1% vs. 26.4%, p <0.01) and 3-year overall survival in operable patients (88.4% vs. 69.4%, $p < 0.05$) (Onishi et al. 2004) (Fig. 5).

These results supported the use, as a standard of treatment, of biologically effective schedules with three fractions of 17–20 Gy for peripheral lesions, resulting in 2-year local control of 93% and 2-year overall survival between 58 and 91% according to patient stratification for age and comorbidities (see Table 2) (van der Voort van Zyp et al. 2009; Lagerwaard et al. 2008; Verstegen et al. 2011; Xia et al. 2006; Nagata et al. 2005; Ng et al. 2008; Nyman et al. 2006; Chang et al. 2008; Taremi et al. 2012; Ricardi et al. 2010; Haasbeek et al. 2011; Nuyttens et al. 2012; Fakiris et al. 2009; Baumann et al. 2009; Senthi et al. 2012). However these dosing schedules might result in a higher incidence (Bral et al. 2011) and grade

(Song et al. 2009; Timmerman et al. 2006) of toxicity when delivered to central lesions located <2 cm from the trachea, mainstem bronchus, main bronchi, or esophagus (Timmerman et al. 2006). By increasing the number of fractions and reducing the fractional dose, some groups have reported successful treatment of central lung tumors with minimal complications (Chang et al. 2008; Chi et al. 2010), but reduction of toxicity might come at the expense of impaired local control (Chi et al. 2010; Onimaru et al. 2003). Other authors, however, have reported the ability to deliver doses corresponding to a BED ≥ 100 Gy, resulting in the combination of adequate tumor control and low toxicity (Lagerwaard et al. 2008). Haasbeek et al. reported results from 63 patients with central lung lesions who were treated with eight fractions of 7.5 Gy, showing a 3-year local control rate of 92.6%, and 3-year overall survival rate of 64.3% (Haasbeek et al. 2011). The NRG-RTOG 0813 study, a prospective trial on 110 medically inoperable and centrally located NSCLC undergoing a dose-escalating five-fraction SBRT schedule ranging from 10 to 12 Gy/fractions, showed encouraging preliminary results with acceptable toxicity at the highest dose level (range 11.5–12 Gy/fraction) and outcome data comparable to results in peripheral lesions (2-year overall survival 70.2–72.7%) (Timmerman et al. 2010). LungTech, a European prospective study, is currently enrolling inoperable centrally located NSCLC patients eligible for SBRT (7.5 Gy × 8 fractions). The primary endpoint is local progression-free survival at 3 years (Adebahr et al. 2015). It is noteworthy that single-fractionation SBRT is enjoying a renewed interest following the publication of early data from the RTOG 0915 trial, comparing 34 Gy in one fraction to a regimen of 48 Gy given in four daily 12 Gy fractions (Videtic et al. 2015). The NCT00843726 trial, comparing single-fraction 30 Gy SBRT to a 60 Gy three-fraction regimen, is also currently ongoing.

Additionally, comparative studies between lobar resection and SBRT in operable patients have been published. Despite limitations related to the retrospective design and/or to selection bias in the repartition between the two options (due to

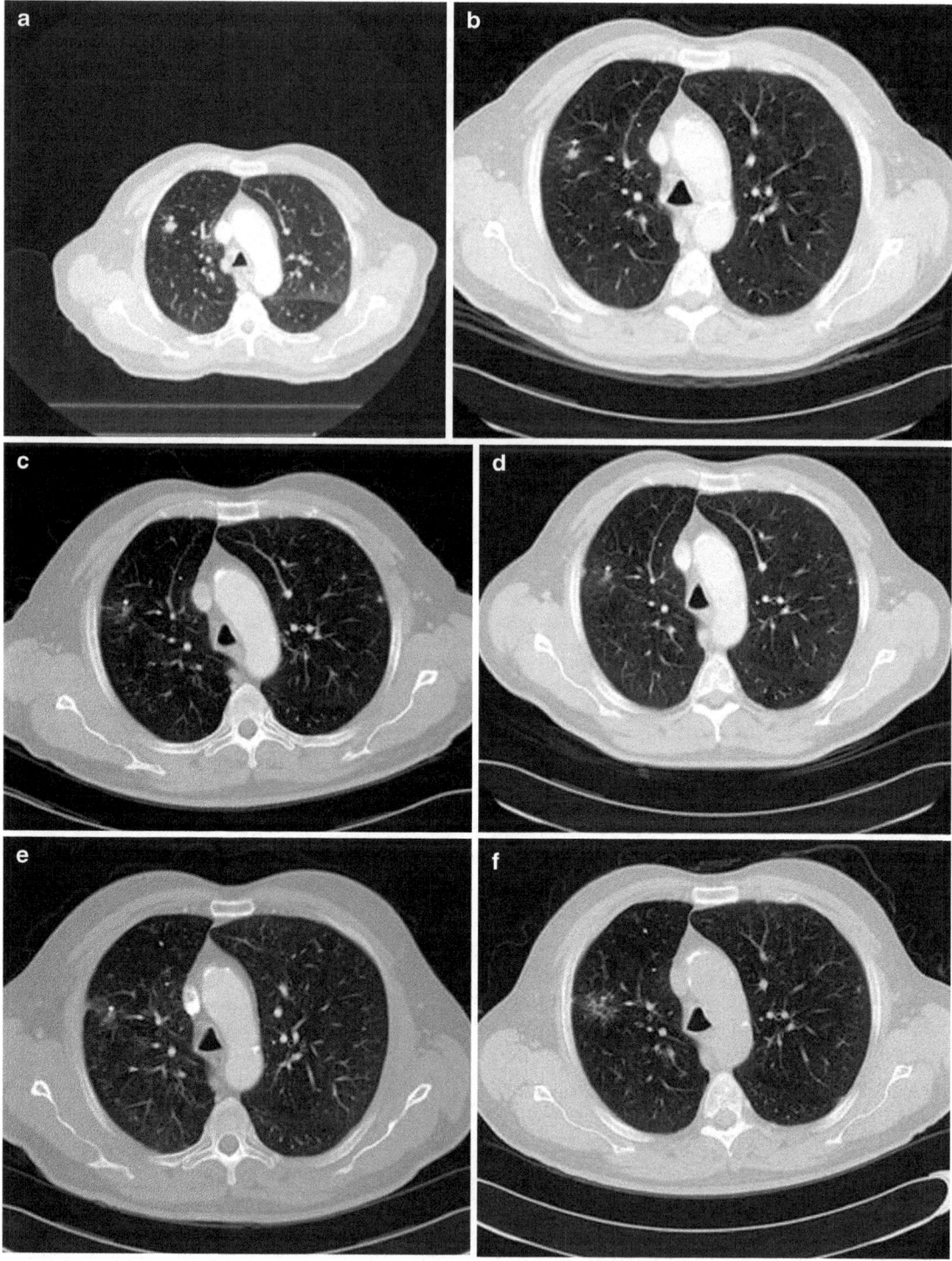

Fig. 5 Stereotactic radiotherapy of stage I non-small-cell lung cancer: pretreatment CT (**a**) and assessment of efficacy at 3, 6, 12, 24, 36, 48, and 60 months (**b–h**)

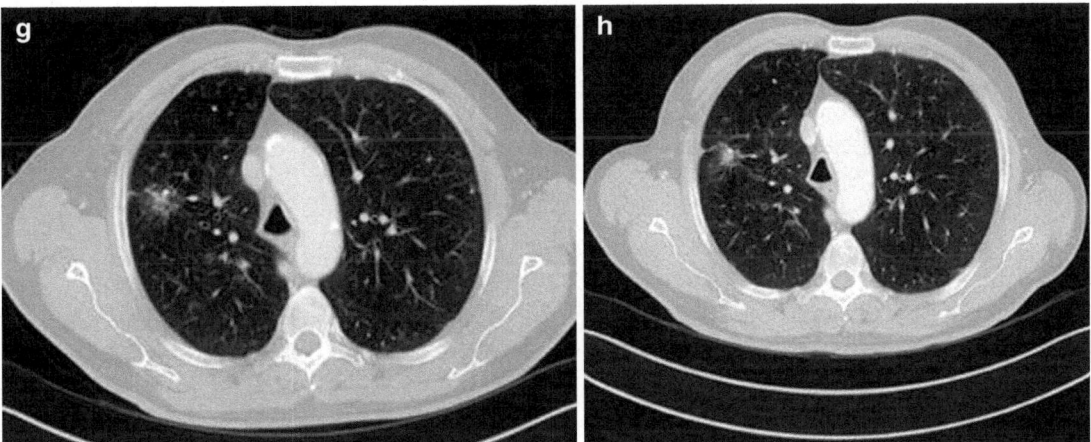

Fig. 5 (continued)

Table 2 Outcome results of selected studies according to treatment schedule

Study	Type	Year	Location	Schedule	No. of patients	LC	OS
Hara et al. (2002)	Retrospective	2002	Central and peripheral	20–30/1 fr	23	1-year LC: 63–88%	–
Timmerman et al. (2003)	Prospective phase I	2002	Central and peripheral	24-60 Gy/3 fr	37	83.7%	–
Onishi et al. (2004)	Retrospective	2004	Central and peripheral	18–75 Gy/1–25 fr	245	5-year LC: 86.5%	3-year OS: 56%
							5-year OS: 47%
Nagata et al. (2005)	Prospective phase I/II	2005	Central and peripheral	48 Gy/4 fr	45	5-year LC: 71–95%	5-year OS: 72–83%
Le et al. (2006)	Prospective phase I	2006	Central and peripheral	15–30 Gy/1 fr	21	1-year LC:67%	1-year OS: 85%
Xia et al. (2006)	Prospective phase I/II	2006	Central and peripheral	50 Gy/10 fr	43	3-year LC: 95%	3-year OS: 78%
Nyman et al. (2006)	Retrospective	2006	Central and peripheral	45 Gy/3 fr	45	5-year LC: 80%	5-year OS: 30%
Hof et al. (2007)	Retrospective	2007	Central and peripheral	19–30 Gy/1 fr	42	1-year LC: 89.5%	–
						2-year LC: 67.9%	
Lagerwaard et al. (2008)	Retrospective	2008	Central and peripheral	60 Gy/3 fr	206	2-year LC: 97.0%	1-year OS: 81%
				60 Gy/5 fr			2-year OS: 64%
				60 Gy/8 fr			
Ng et al. (2008)	Retrospective	2008	Central and peripheral	45 Gy/3 fr 54 Gy/4 fr	20	2-year LC: 94.7%	2-year OS: 77.6%
Chang et al. (2008)	Retrospective	2008	Central and peripheral	40–50 Gy/4 fr	27	1-year LC: 88.8%	–
van der Voort et al. (2009)	Retrospective	2009	Central and peripheral	45 Gy/3 fr	70	2-year LC: 78%	2-year OS: 62%
				60 Gy/3 fr		2-year LC: 96%	
Fakiris et al. (2009)	Prospective phase II	2009	Central and peripheral	60–66 Gy/3 fr	70	3-year LC: 88.1%	3-year OS: 42.7%
							3-year DSS: 81.7%

Table 2 (continued)

Study	Type	Year	Location	Schedule	No. of patients	LC	OS
Baumann et al. (2009)	Prospective phase II	2009	Central and peripheral	45 Gy/3 fr	57	3-year LC: 92%	3-year OS: 60%
Ricardi et al. (2010)	Prospective	2010	Central and peripheral	45 Gy/3 fr	62	3-year LC: 87.8%	3-year OS: 57.1%
							3-year DSS: 72.5%
Timmerman et al. (2010)	Prospective phase II	2010	Central and peripheral	54 Gy/3 fr	59	3-year LC: 97.6%	3-year OS: 55.8%
Verstegen et al. (2011)	Retrospective	2011	Central and peripheral	60 Gy/3 fr	591	3-year LC: 90.4–91.2%	3-year OS: 53.7–55.4%
				60 Gy/5 fr			
				60 Gy/8 fr			
Haasbeek et al. (2011)	Retrospective	2011	Central	60 Gy/8 fr	63	3-year LC: 92.6%	3-year OS: 64.3%
Taremi et al. (2012)	Retrospective	2012	Central and peripheral	54–60 Gy/3 fr	108	4-year LC: 92%	4-year OS: 30%
				48 Gy/4 fr			4-year DSS: 77%
				50–60 Gy/8–10 fr			
Senthi et al. (2012)	Retrospective	2012	Central and peripheral	54–60 Gy/3–8 fr	676	5-year LC: 89.5%	–

age, tumor location, and comorbidities), a consistent tendency toward noninferiority in terms of local control and overall survival after adjustment for outcome-related variables was observed (Palma et al. 2011; Soldà et al. 2013; Robinson et al. 2013; Varlotto et al. 2013; Verstegen et al. 2013; Shirata et al. 2012; Shirvani et al. 2012; Crabtree et al. 2010). It is controversial whether SBRT might replace surgery as the "gold standard" in the future. Advocates of surgical resection claim that only an operative assessment can rule out the extent of disease and the presence of occult nodal involvement due to insufficient accuracy of PET-CT staging and pretherapeutic biopsy (Paravati et al. 2014), while SBRT experts report a low incidence of nodal relapse after radiotherapy and scarce impact of histological assessment on outcome (Verstegen et al. 2011, 2013). Concerning toxicity, SBRT showed lower treatment-related mortality adjusted to age and minor respiratory function degradation compared to surgery (Palma et al. 2011; Soldà et al. 2013), while evaluation of cost-effectiveness showed contradictory results according to the different methodology (Puri et al. 2012; Shah et al. 2013). These considerations led to the approval of two phase III prospective trials: the STARS trial (StereoTActic Radiotherapy vs. Surgery) comparing CyberKnife® lung SBRT with lobectomy and the ROSEL trial (Radiosurgery Or Surgery for operable Early stage non-small-cell Lung cancer), allocating patients to SBRT or surgery. Unfortunately both studies were prematurely closed due to low accrual. However, a pooled analysis of the two trials performed by Chang et al. suggested a survival benefit for SBRT (overall survival at 3 years 95% vs. 79%, HR: 0.14) possibly related to reduction in perioperative mortality (Chang et al. 2015).

3.2 Toxicity

3.2.1 Pulmonary Toxicity

Lung toxicity is a mostly asymptomatic occurrence in patients undergoing SBRT requiring medical therapy in less than 10% of cases (Guckenberger et al. 2007b), but grade ≥ 3 toxicity may account for up to 5% of cases in historical trials (Timmerman et al. 2010; Videtic et al. 2015) (Fig. 6). Conversely, recognition of radiation-related lung injury is complicated by the coexistence of confounding medical conditions like COPD, heart failure, and susceptibil-

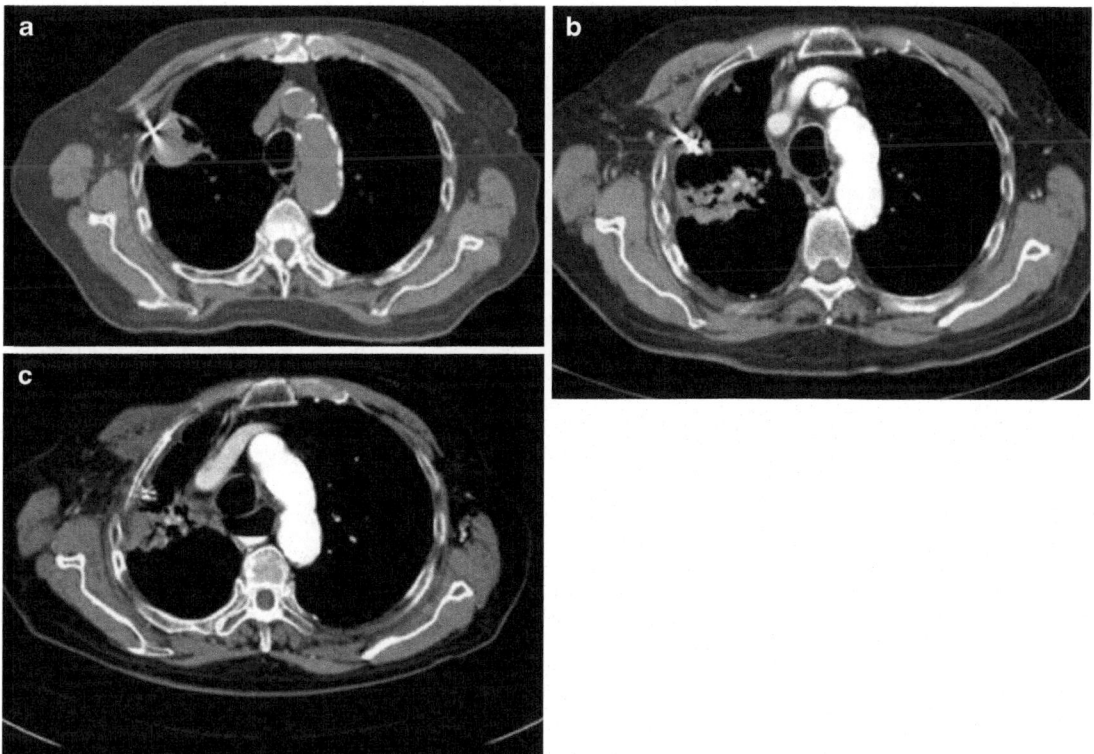

Fig. 6 Chest computed tomography images showing radiation pneumonitis following lung stereotactic radiotherapy. (**a**) pretreatment imaging of planned target lesion. (**b**) CT at 3 months: patchy opacity with air bronchogram in the irradiated lung. (**c**) CT at 6 months: evolution to fibrosis with airspace consolidation and volume loss

ity to infection due to immune deficit (Kocak et al. 2005). Initial works showed a strong correlation between mean lung dose (MLD) and onset of lung toxicity (Borst et al. 2009). Barriger et al. reported a significant reduction of the incidence of radiation pneumonitis for an MLD ≤4 Gy and V20 ≤4% in patients receiving 60 Gy in three fractions (Barriger et al. 2012). Transient decline in pulmonary function has been observed, but the impact of prior functional test values is unclear (Stephans et al. 2009). Concerning late toxicity, partial or complete bronchial stenosis can occur as a consequence of irradiation after a median delay of 20 months (Song et al. 2009). Most authors agree that Dmax is a major predictor of bronchial stricture (Miller et al. 2005). Nevertheless, it has been reported that dose correlation with bronchial sequelae is influenced by both irradiated volume and diameter of the pretreated bronchial

structure, with an increased susceptibility to radiation damage for segmental bronchi (Duijm et al. 2016).

3.2.2 Esophageal Toxicity

Careful evaluation of the dose received by the esophagus is mandatory due to the risk of severe, but seldom fatal (Le et al. 2006), radiation toxicity. An estimated incidence of 13% grade ≥2 toxicity has been reported in patients treated by SBRT, with a correlation between onset of toxicity and proximity to the PTV (Modh et al. 2014). Nevertheless dosimetric analysis is flawed by the heterogeneity of irradiation schedules and nonradiation-related variables (concurrent or prior chemotherapy, interindividual sensitivity, comorbidities) that hamper an accurate modelization; therefore proposed constraints vary among different author. Stephans et al. reported absence of late toxicity for Dmax ≤50 Gy and

D1cm^3 < 45 Gy in patients treated with 50 Gy in five fractions (Stephans et al. 2014). Considering fractionation, Wu et al. reported a risk of toxicity onset inferior to 20% with a Dmax of 52.9 Gy BED10, and a D5cm^3 of 26.3 Gy BED10 (Wu et al. 2014). In a recent dose-response model proposed by our institution on a series of 57 patients treated with CyberKnife®, a D1cm^3 of 32.9 and 50.7 Gy and a Dmax of 43.4 and 61.4 Gy correlated with a TD50 for grade 2 and grade 3 toxicities, respectively, for 5-fraction equivalent doses using an $\alpha/\beta = 3$ [87]. It is noteworthy that a 20 Gy difference between TD50 for grade 2 and grade 3 toxicities emerged in different studies (Stephans et al. 2014; Nuyttens et al. 2016).

3.2.3 Cardiac Toxicity

Radiation-induced heart injury has been postulated in three studies investigating lung SBRT. Haasbeek reported five cases of fatal heart failure in patients treated with SBRT for central lesions, while three acute cardiac events (two pericarditis and one myocardial infarction) were observed by Modh et al. (Haasbeek et al. 2011; Modh et al. 2014). One case of acute pericarditis occurred in the retrospective series by Milano et al. (Milano et al. 2009). On the other hand, while a strong dose-correlation between prior radiotherapy and heart-related morbidity has been established in patients treated by standard fractionation for breast cancer (Darby et al. 2013), Nishimura et al. did not record any cardiac events in patients receiving a dose >25 Gy in five fractions (Nishimura et al. 2014).

3.2.4 Chest Wall Toxicity

Rib fracture may occur in up to 23% patients after a mean delay of 21.2 months following the completion of SBRT (Nambu et al. 2011). The risk of fracture correlates to the maximum dose and high-dose volume parameters like V10, V20, V30, and V40 (Asai et al. 2012). However, chest wall pain may arise in the absence of radiologically documented rib fracture. Though compounded in most studies as a single category, chest wall pain might represent a stand-alone independent radiation-related event whose physiopathology is not well understood and may be related to underlying sub-

clinical rib injury or neuropathic etiology. Obesity is a risk factor for chest wall pain, with almost a twofold incidence in subjects with BMI ≥29 (27% vs. 13%, respectively; $p = 0.01$) (Welsh et al. 2011). Exposure of >30 cm^3 of the chest wall to 30 Gy irradiation in three to five fraction was predictive of chest wall pain in one-third of cases (Dunlap et al. 2010). Bongers et al. reported that patients with chest wall pain had larger treatment volumes and shorter tumor-chest wall distances, whereas patients with rib fractures had larger tumor diameters and treatment volumes (Bongers et al. 2011), corroborating the hypothesis of two distinct clinical entities.

3.2.5 Brachial Neuropathy

Brachial plexopathy is an infrequent toxicity that may result from neurological damage following treatment of apical lesions. In a study by Forquer et al., the 2-year incidence of brachial plexopathy was 46% vs. 8% ($p = 0.04$) for patients receiving ≥26 Gy in three fractions to the brachial plexus (Forquer et al. 2009). In a study by Chang et al., the onset of brachial neuropathy was limited to patients receiving a Dmax > 35 Gy and V30 > 0.2 cm^3 (Chang et al. 2014) following SBRT using a 50 Gy in four-fraction schedule.

Conclusions

Stereotactic radiotherapy emerged as a valuable option in the treatment of early-stage tumors in the lung, with excellent local control and encouraging survival rates, with acceptable toxicity. Different techniques have been developed to control the motion of the tumor. When treating central tumors, adapted dose schedules are advocated to prevent severe toxicity. Prospective comparative trials are needed to establish the place of SBRT in the clinical management of operable patients.

References

Adebahr S, Collette S, Shash E et al (2015) LungTech, an EORTC phase II trial of stereotactic body radiotherapy for centrally located lung tumours: a clinical perspective. Br J Radiol 88:20150036

Adebonojo SA, Bowser AN et al (1999) Impact of revised stage classification of lung cancer on survival: a military experience. Chest 115:1507–1513

Adler JR Jr, Chang SD, Murphy MJ et al (1997) The Cyberknife®: a frameless robotic system for radiosurgery. Stereotact Funct Neurosurg 69:124–128

Asai K, Shioyama Y, Nakamura K et al (2012) Radiation-induced rib fractures after hypofractionated stereotactic body radiation therapy: risk factors and dose-volume relationship. Int J Radiat Oncol Biol Phys 84:768–773

Bahig H, Campeau MP, Vu T et al (2013) Predictive parameters of CyberKnife fiducial-less (XSight Lung) applicability for treatment of early non-small cell lung cancer: a single-center experience. Int J Radiat Oncol Biol Phys 87:583–589

Barnes EA, Murray BR, Robinson DM et al (2001) Dosimetric evaluation of lung tumor immobilization using breath hold at deep inspiration. Int J Radiat Oncol Biol Phys 50:1091–1098

Barriger RB, Forquer JA, Brabham JG et al (2012) A dose-volume analysis of radiation pneumonitis in non-small cell lung cancer patients treated with stereotactic body radiation therapy. Int J Radiat Oncol Biol Phys 82:457–462

Baumann P, Nyman J, Hoyer M et al (2009) Outcome in a prospective phase II trial of medically inoperable stage I non-small-cell lung cancer patients treated with stereotactic body radiotherapy. J Clin Oncol 27(20):3290–3296

Bibault JE, Prevost B, Dansin E et al (2012) Image-guided robotic stereotactic radiation therapy with fiducial-free tumor tracking for lung cancer. Radiat Oncol 7:102

Bongers EM, Haasbeek CJ, Lagerwaard FJ et al (2011) Incidence and risk factors for chest wall toxicity after risk-adapted stereotactic radiotherapy for early-stage lung cancer. J Thorac Oncol 6:2052–2057

Borst GR, Ishikawa M, Nijkamp J et al (2009) Radiation pneumonitis in patients treated for malignant pulmonary lesions with hypofractionated radiation therapy. Radiother Oncol 91:307–313

Bral S, Gevaert T, Linthout N et al (2011) Prospective, risk-adapted strategy of stereotactic body radiotherapy for early-stage non-small-cell lung cancer: results of a phase II trial. Int J Radiat Oncol Biol Phys 80:1343–1349

Casamassima F, Cavedon C, Francescon P et al (2006) Use of motion tracking in stereotactic body radiotherapy: evaluation of uncertainty in off-target dose distribution and optimization strategies. Acta Oncol 45:943–947

Chang SD, Adler JR (2001) Robotics and radiosurgery—the cyberknife. Stereotact Funct Neurosurg 76:204–208

Chang JY, Balter PA, Dong L et al (2008) Stereotactic body radiation therapy in centrally and superiorly located stage I or isolated recurrent non-small-cell lung cancer. Int J Radiat Oncol Biol Phys 72:967–971

Chang JY, Li QQ, Xu QY et al (2014) Stereotactic ablative radiation therapy for centrally located early stage or isolated parenchymal recurrences of non-small cell lung cancer: how to fly in a "no fly zone". Int J Radiat Oncol Biol Phys 88:1120–1128

Chang JY, Senan S, Paul MA et al (2015) Stereotactic ablative radiotherapy versus lobectomy for operable stage I non-small-cell lung cancer: a pooled analysis of two randomised trials. Lancet Oncol 16:630–637

Chi A, Liao Z, Nguyen NP et al (2010) Systemic review of the patterns of failure following stereotactic body radiation therapy in early-stage non-small-cell lung cancer: clinical implications. Radiother Oncol 94:1–11

Crabtree TD, Denlinger CE, Meyers BF et al (2010) Stereotactic body radiation therapy versus surgical resection for stage I non-small cell lung cancer. J Thorac Cardiovasc Surg 140:377–386

Darby SC, Ewertz M, McGale P et al (2013) Risk of ischemic heart disease in women after radiotherapy for breast cancer. N Engl J Med 368:987–998

Dosoretz DE, Katin MJ, Blitzer PH et al (1992) Radiation therapy in the management of medically inoperable carcinoma of the lung: results and implications for future treatment strategies. Int J Radiat Oncol Biol Phys 24:3–9

Duijm M, Schillemans W, Aerts JG et al (2016) Dose and volume of the irradiated main bronchi and related side effects in the treatment of central lung tumors with stereotactic radiotherapy. Semin Radiat Oncol 26:140–148

Dunlap NE, Cai J, Biedermann GB et al (2010) Chest wall volume receiving >30 Gy predicts risk of severe pain and/or rib fracture after lung stereotactic body radiotherapy. Int J Radiat Oncol Biol Phys 76:796–801

Fakiris AJ, McGarry RC, Yiannoutsos CT et al (2009) Stereotactic body radiation therapy for early-stage non-small-cell lung carcinoma: four-year results of a prospective phase II study. Int J Radiat Oncol Biol Phys 75:677–682

Forquer JA, Fakiris AJ, Timmerman RD et al (2009) Brachial plexopathy from stereotactic body radiotherapy in early-stage NSCLC: dose-limiting toxicity in apical tumor sites. Radiother Oncol 93:408–413

Giraud P, Yorke E, Ford EC et al (2006) Reduction of organ motion in lung tumors with respiratory gating. Lung Cancer 51:41–51

Grills IS, Mangona VS, Welsh R et al (2010) Outcomes after stereotactic lung radiotherapy or wedge resection for stage I non-small-cell lung cancer. J Clin Oncol 28:928–935

Guckenberger M, Wilbert J, Meyer J et al (2007a) Is a single respiratory correlated 4D-CT study sufficient for evaluation of breathing motion? Int J Radiat Oncol Biol Phys 67:1352–1359

Guckenberger M, Heilman K, Wulf J et al (2007b) Pulmonary injury and tumor response after stereotactic body radiotherapy (SBRT): results of a serial follow-up CT study. Radiother Oncol 85:435–442

Haasbeek CJ, Lagerwaard FJ, Slotman BJ et al (2011 Dec) Outcomes of stereotactic ablative radiotherapy for centrally located early-stage lung cancer. J Thorac Oncol 6(12):2036–2043

Hansen AT, Petersen JB, Hoyer M (2006) Internal movement, set-up accuracy and margins for stereotactic body radiotherapy using a stereotactic body frame. Acta Oncol 45:948–952

Hara R, Itami J, Kondo T et al (2002) Stereotactic single high dose irradiation of lung tumors under respiratory gating. Radiother Oncol 63:159–163

Hof H, Muenter M, Oetzel D et al (2007) Stereotactic single-dose radiotherapy (radiosurgery) of early stage nonsmall-cell lung cancer (NSCLC). Cancer 110:148–155

Hunjan S, Starkschall G, Prado K et al (2010) Lack of correlation between external fiducial positions and internal tumor positions during breath-hold CT. Int J Radiat Oncol Biol Phys 76:1586–1591

Jensen HR, Hansen O, Hjelm-Hansen M et al (2008) Inter- and intrafractional movement of the tumour in extracranial stereotactic radiotherapy of NSCLC. Acta Oncol 47:1432–1437

Jiang SB (2006) Radiotherapy of mobile tumors. Semin Radiat Oncol 16:239–248

Kocak Z, Evans ES, Zhou SM et al (2005) Challenges in defining radiation pneumonitis in patients with lung cancer. Int J Radiat Oncol Biol Phys 62:635–638

Lagerwaard FJ, Haasbeek CJ, Smit EF et al (2008) Outcomes of risk-adapted fractionated stereotactic radiotherapy for stage I non-small-cell lung cancer. Int J Radiat Oncol Biol Phys 70:685–692

Le QT, Loo BW, Ho A et al (2006) Results of a phase I dose-escalation study using single-fraction stereotactic radiotherapy for lung tumors. J Thorac Oncol 1:802–809

Mah D, Hanley J, Rosenzweig KE et al (2000) Technical aspects of the deep inspiration breath-hold technique in the treatment of thoracic cancer. Int J Radiat Oncol Biol Phys 48:1175–1185

McGarry RC, Song G, des Rosiers P et al (2002) Observation-only management of early stage, medically inoperable lung cancer: poor outcome. Chest 121:1155–1158

Milano MT, Chen Y, Katz AW et al (2009) Central thoracic lesions treated with hypofractionated stereotactic body radiotherapy. Radiother Oncol 91:301–306

Miller KL, Shafman TD, Anscher MS et al (2005) Bronchial stenosis: an underreported complication of high-dose external beam radiotherapy for lung cancer? Int J Radiat Oncol Biol Phys 61:64–69

Modh A, Rimner A, Williams E et al (2014) Local control and toxicity in a large cohort of central lung tumors treated with stereotactic body radiation therapy. Int J Radiat Oncol Biol Phys 90:1168–1176

Mountain CF (1997) Revisions in the international system for staging lung cancer. Chest 111:1710–1717

Murphy MJ (2004) Tracking moving organs in real time. Semin Radiat Oncol 14:91–100

Nagata Y, Takayama K, Matsuo Y et al (2005) Clinical outcomes of a phase I/II study of 48 Gy of stereotactic body radiotherapy in 4 fractions for primary lung cancer using a stereotactic body frame. Int J Radiat Oncol Biol Phys 63:1427–1431

Nambu A, Onishi H, Aoki S, Koshiishi T et al (2011) Rib fracture after stereotactic radiotherapy on follow-up thin-section computed tomography in 177 primary lung cancer patients. Radiother Oncol 6:137

Naruke T, Goya T, Tsuchiya R et al (1988) Prognosis and survival in resected lung carcinoma based on the new international staging system. J Thorac Cardiovasc Surg 96:440–447

Ng AW, Tung SY, Wong VY (2008) Hypofractionated stereotactic radiotherapy for medically inoperable stage I non-small cell lung cancer—report on clinical outcome and dose to critical organs. Radiother Oncol 87:24–28

Nishimura S, Takeda A, Sanuki N et al (2014) Toxicities of organs at risk in the mediastinal and hilar regions following stereotactic body radiotherapy for centrally located lung tumors. J Thorac Oncol 9:1370–1376

Nuyttens JJ, van de Pol M (2012 Sep) The CyberKnife® radiosurgery system for lung cancer. Expert Rev Med Devices 9(5):465–475

Nuyttens JJ, van der Voort van Zyp NC, Praag J et al (2012) Outcome of four-dimensional stereotactic radiotherapy for centrally located lung tumors. Radiother Oncol 102:383–387

Nuyttens JJ, Moiseenko V, McLaughlin M et al (2016) Esophageal dose tolerance in patients treated with stereotactic body radiation therapy. Semin Radiat Oncol 26:120–128

Nyman J, Johansson KA, Hulten U (2006) Stereotactic hypofractionated radiotherapy for stage I non-small cell lung cancer—mature results for medically inoperable patients. Lung Cancer 51:97–103

Onimaru R, Shirato H, Shimizu S et al (2003) Tolerance of organs at risk in small-volume, hypofractionated, image-guided radiotherapy for primary and metastatic lung cancers. Int J Radiat Oncol Biol Phys 56:126–135

Onishi H, Araki T, Shirato H et al (2004) Stereotactic hypofractionated high-dose irradiation for stage I non-small cell lung carcinoma: clinical outcomes in 245 subjects in a Japanese multiinstitutional study. Cancer 101:1623–1631

Palma D, Visser O, Lagerwaard FJ et al (2011) Treatment of stage I NSCLC in elderly patients: a population-based matched-pair comparison of stereotactic radiotherapy versus surgery. Radiother Oncol 101:240–244

Paravati AJ, Johnstone DW, Seltzer MA et al (2014) Negative predictive value (NPV) of FDG PET-CT for nodal disease in clinically node-negative early stage lung cancer (AJCC 7th ed T1-T2aN0) and identification of risk factors for occult nodal (pN1-N2) metastasis: implications for SBRT. Transl Cancer Res 3:313–319

Prevost JB, Voet P, Hoogeman M et al (2008) Four-dimensional stereotactic radiotherapy for early stage non-small cell lung cancer: a comparative planning study. Technol Cancer Res Treat 7:27–34

Purdy JA (2004) Current ICRU definitions of volumes: limitations and future directions. Semin Radiat Oncol 14:27–40

Puri V, Crabtree TD, Kymes S et al (2012) A comparison of surgical intervention and stereotactic body radiation therapy for stage I lung cancer in high-risk patients: a decision analysis. J Thorac Cardiovasc Surg 143:428–436

Ricardi U, Filippi AR, Guarneri A et al (2010) Stereotactic body radiation therapy for early stage non-small cell lung cancer: results of a prospective trial. Lung Cancer 68:72–77

Robinson CG, DeWees TA, El Naqa IM et al (2013) Patterns of failure after stereotactic body radiation therapy or lobar resection for clinical stage I non-small-cell lung cancer. J Thorac Oncol 8:192–201

Rosenzweig KE, Hanley J, Mah D et al (2000) The deep inspiration breath-hold technique in the treatment of inoperable non-small-cell lung cancer. Int J Radiat Oncol Biol Phys 48:81–87

Rosenzweig KE, Fox JL, Yorke E et al (2005) Results of a phase I dose-escalation study using three-dimensional conformal radiotherapy in the treatment of inoperable nonsmall cell lung carcinoma. Cancer 103:2118–2127

Sayeh S, Wang J, Main WT et al (2007) Respiratory motion tracking for robotic radiosurgery. In: Urschel HC Jr, Kresl JJ, Luketich JD, Papiez L, Timmerman RD (eds) Robotic radiosurgery: treating tumors that move with respiration. Springer, Berlin, pp 15–29

Senthi S, Lagerwaard FJ, Haasbeek CJ, Slotman BJ et al (2012) Patterns of disease recurrence after stereotactic ablative radiotherapy for early stage non-small-cell lung cancer: a retrospective analysis. Lancet Oncol 13:802–809

Seppenwoolde Y, Shirato H, Kitamura K et al (2002) Precise and real-time measurement of 3D tumor motion in lung due to breathing and heartbeat, measured during radiotherapy. Int J Radiat Oncol Biol Phys 53:822–834

Shah A, Hahn SM, Stetson RL, Friedberg JS, Pechet TT, Sher DJ (2013) Cost-effectiveness of stereotactic body radiation therapy versus surgical resection for stage I non-small cell lung cancer. Cancer 119:3123–3132

Shields TW (1993) Surgical therapy for carcinoma of the lung. Clin Chest Med 14:121–147

Shirata Y, Jingu K, Koto M et al (2012) Prognostic factors for local control of stage I non-small cell lung cancer in stereotactic radiotherapy: a retrospective analysis. Radiat Oncol 7:182

Shirato H, Shimizu S, Kitamura K et al (2000a) Four-dimensional treatment planning and fluoroscopic real-time tumor tracking radiotherapy for moving tumor. Int J Radiat Oncol Biol Phys 48:435–442

Shirato H, Shimizu S, Kunieda T et al (2000b) Physical aspects of a real-time tumor-tracking system for gated radiotherapy. Int J Radiat Oncol Biol Phys 48:1187–1195

Shirvani SM, Jiang J, Chang JY et al (2012) Comparative effectiveness of 5 treatment strategies for early-stage non-small cell lung cancer in the elderly. Int J Radiat Oncol Biol Phys 84:1060–1070

Simone CB 2nd, Wildt B, Haas AR et al (2013) Stereotactic body radiation therapy for lung cancer. Chest 143:1784–1790

Soldà F, Lodge M, Ashley S et al (2013) Stereotactic radiotherapy (SABR) for the treatment of primary non-small cell lung cancer systematic review and comparison with a surgical cohort. Radiother Oncol 109:1–7

Song SY, Choi W, Shin SS et al (2009) Fractionated stereotactic body radiation therapy for medically inoperable stage I lung cancer adjacent to central large bronchus. Lung Cancer 66:89–93

Stephans KL, Djemil T, Reddy CA et al (2009) Comprehensive analysis of pulmonary function test (PFT) changes after stereotactic body radiotherapy (SBRT) for stage I lung cancer in medically inoperable patients. J Thorac Oncol 4:838–844

Stephans KL, Djemil T, Diaconu C et al (2014) Esophageal dose tolerance to hypofractionated stereotactic body radiation therapy: risk factors for late toxicity. Int J Radiat Oncol Biol Phys 90:197–202

Taremi M, Hope A, Dahele M et al (2012) Stereotactic body radiotherapy for medically inoperable lung cancer: prospective, single-center study of 108 consecutive patients. Int J Radiat Oncol Biol Phys 82:967–973

Timmerman R, Papiez L, McGarry R et al (2003) Extracranial stereotactic radioablation: results of a phase I study in medically inoperable stage I non-small cell lung cancer. Chest 124:1946–1955

Timmerman R, McGarry R, Yiannoutsos C et al (2006) Excessive toxicity when treating central tumors in a phase II study of stereotactic body radiation therapy for medically inoperable early-stage lung cancer. J Clin Oncol 24:4833–4839

Timmerman R, Paulus R, Galvin J et al (2010) Stereotactic body radiation therapy for inoperable early stage lung cancer. JAMA 303:1070–1076

Underberg RW, Lagerwaard FJ, Slotman BJ et al (2005) Use of maximum intensity projections (MIP) for target volume generation in 4D-CT scans for lung cancer. Int J Radiat Oncol Biol Phys 63:253–260

Varlotto J, Fakiris A, Flickinger J et al (2013) Matched-pair and propensity score comparisons of outcomes of patients with clinical stage I non-small cell lung cancer treated with resection or stereotactic radiosurgery. Cancer 119:2683–2691

Verstegen NE, Lagerwaard FJ, Haasbeek CJ et al (2011) Outcomes of stereotactic ablative radiotherapy following a clinical diagnosis of stage I NSCLC: comparison with a contemporaneous cohort with pathologically proven disease. Radiother Oncol 101:250–254

Verstegen NE, Oosterhuis JW, Palma DA et al (2013) Stage I-II non-small-cell lung cancer treated using either stereotactic ablative radiotherapy (SABR) or lobectomy by video-assisted thoracoscopic surgery (VATS): outcomes of a propensity score-matched analysis. Ann Oncol 24:1543–1548

Videtic GM, Hu C, Singh AK et al (2015) A randomized phase 2 study comparing 2 stereotactic body radiation therapy schedules for medically inoperable patients with stage I peripheral non-small cell lung cancer: NRG Oncology RTOG 0915 (NCCTG N0927). Int J Radiat Oncol Biol Phys 93:757–764 van der Voort van Zyp NC, Prevost JB et al (2009) Stereotactic radiotherapy with real-time tumor tracking for non-small cell lung cancer: clinical outcome. Radiother Oncol 91:296–300

van der Voort N, van Zyp NC, Prevost JB et al (2009) Stereotactic radiotherapy with real-time tumor tracking for non-small cell lung cancer: clinical outcome. Radiother Oncol 91:296–300

Welsh J, Thomas J, Shah D et al (2011) Obesity increases the risk of chest wall pain from thoracic stereotactic body radiation therapy. Int J Radiat Oncol Biol Phys 81:91–96

Whyte RI, Crownover R, Murphy MJ et al (2003) Stereotactic radiosurgery for lung tumors: preliminary report of a phase I trial. Ann Thorac Surg 75:1097–1101

Wong JW, Sharpe MB, Jaffray DA et al (1999) The use of active breathing control (ABC) to reduce margin for breathing motion. Int J Radiat Oncol Biol Phys 44:911–919

Wu AJ, Williams E, Modh A et al (2014) Dosimetric predictors of esophageal toxicity after stereotactic body radiotherapy for central lung tumors. Radiother Oncol 112:267–271

Xia T, Li H, Sun Q, Wang Y et al (2006) Promising clinical outcome of stereotactic body radiation therapy for patients with inoperable stage I/II non-small-cell lung cancer. Int J Radiat Oncol Biol Phys 66:117–125

Alternate Fractionation for Hepatic Tumors

Alejandra Méndez Romero, Thomas B. Brunner,
Alexander V. Kirichenko, Wolfgang A. Tomé,
Yun Liang, Nathan Ogden, and Ben J.M. Heijmen

Contents

The original version of this chapter was revised. The
affiliations of the authors have been updated.

A. Méndez Romero (✉) • B. J. M. Heijmen
Erasmus Medical Center, Rotterdam, The Netherlands
e-mail: a.mendezromero@erasmusmc.nl

T. B. Brunner
Freiburg University Medical Center, Freiburg, Germany

A. V. Kirichenko • Y. Liang
Department of Radiation Oncology, Allegheny Health
Network Cancer Institute, Pittsburgh, PA, USA

W. A. Tomé
Albert Einstein College of Medicine, Montefiore
Medical Center, Bronx, New York, NY, USA

N. Ogden
Department of Radiology, Allegheny Health Network
Cancer Institute, Pittsburgh, PA, USA

1   A Historical Perspective to Liver Radiotherapy

Historically, the liver was thought to be an organ unsuitable for radical doses needed to treat primary or secondary tumors. This determination was made in the time where only 2D treatment planning was available (Ingold et al. 1965; Wharton et al. 1973). However, the consequent interpretation of liver toxicities with 3D-conformal radiotherapy with the use of dose–volume histograms allowed us to describe the normal tissue complication probability (NTCP) characteristics of the liver, an organ with a parallel tissue structure which is reflected in a high "volume effect parameter," $n = 0.69$ (Jackson et al. 1995). The data underlying the NTCP modeling came from a series of 79 patients including nine patients that developed clinical radiation hepatitis. All of the patients with radiation hepatitis, also called radiation-induced liver disease (RILD), had whole-liver radiation with doses of at least 37 Gy in conventional fractionation. On the other hand, patients who had partial liver radiotherapy to much higher doses did not develop RILD. Subsequently, a phase I trial of escalated focal liver radiation and concurrent hepatic artery fluorodeoxyuridine (FUdR) was conducted for patients with unresectable intrahepatic malignancies (Dawson et al. 2000). Twenty-seven patients had hepatobiliary cancer and 16 colorectal liver metastases. This trial employed a dose per fraction of 1.5 Gy twice daily with concomitant intra-arterial FUdR during the first 4 weeks of radiotherapy. Continuous-infusion FUdR required placement of a percutaneous brachial artery catheter to deliver a dose of 0.2 mg/kg/d. The trial was designed to be isotoxic and to escalate radiation dose in cases where the target volumes were small enough to allow dose escalation according to the above-described NTCP model. This resulted in a median radiotherapy dose of 58.5 Gy with a range from 28.5 to 90 Gy. Of note, the median tumor size was as large as $10 \times 10 \times 8$ cm. The dose to the stomach and duodenum was restricted to a maximum of 68 Gy in 1.5 Gy fractions. Twenty-five patients were assessable for response evaluation achieving 16 partial and 1 complete response. Intriguingly, improved progression-free and overall survival depended on multivariate analysis on escalated dose. There was only one incidence of late liver toxicity, namely one patient suffering a reversible grade 3 RILD.

Due to the favorable results of the phase I trial, a consecutive phase II trial was conducted to validate the good tolerance of this therapy and to test the hypothesis of improved local control and survival (Ben-Josef et al. 2005). A total of 128 patients were included

with liver metastases (LM), cholangiocarcinoma (CCC), and hepatocellular carcinoma (HCC) with 46, 47, and 35 patients, respectively. Chemoradiotherapy was performed as in the preceding phase I trial (Dawson et al. 2000). The primary endpoint, overall survival (OS), was superior compared to controls for all three entities (median OS time 15.2 vs. 9; 13.3 vs. 9; 17.2 vs. 8 months, respectively) with a median OS time for all patients of 15.2 months. Disease-specific survival for the three entities was superior compared to controls for the entities in the same order of naming ($p = .014$, $p = .0008$, $p = .0001$). The median dose of 60.7 Gy was a significant predictor of survival with a median OS of 18.4 vs. 15.2 months above and below the median. Intriguingly, patients with doses in the upper quartile, i.e., ≥ 75 Gy, survived significantly longer (23.9 vs. 14.9 months, $p = .01$) than patients below that dose, pointing to a continuous improvement of OS at doses above the median. Similarly, progression-free survival (PFS) was longer for patients treated with ≥ 75 Gy (20.7 vs. 10.9 months, $p = .05$). High-grade toxicities were observed in 30% of the patients and these were GI ulceration and bleeding in 5%, RILD in 4%, and catheter-related problems in 3%. There was one grade 5 toxicity of RILD. The authors acknowledged the challenges of this regimen requiring radiotherapy and arterial catheter continuous chemotherapy anticipating hypofractionation as an option for modification.

Due to the high incidence of primary liver tumors in Asia, especially HCC, many reports on radiotherapy for hepatic tumors emanate from that continent. Almost all of these series did not use concomitant chemotherapy. Below is a summary of the recently published retrospective experience with single fractions that are lower than current typical doses used for stereotactic body radiation therapy (SBRT) (<5 Gy). A group from the Korea University

Medical Center analyzed their experience of 45 patients with both HCC and portal vein thrombosis (PVT) (Rim et al. 2012). The median dose was 61.2 Gy in five single doses per week of 1.8–2.5 Gy delivered with a 3D-planned technique. The PVT close to HCC in contrast-enhanced CT (CECT) was contoured and treated in addition to the HCC lesions as were enlarged lymph nodes >1 cm in the short axis diameter. Motion and positioning uncertainty was taken into account by a 1–1.5 cm expansion margin from CTV to PTV. Total dose (TD) was ≥60 Gy in 87% and lowest TD prescribed was 55 Gy. One-year OS was 52% in this poor prognosis cohort with PVT. Overall response rate was 62% and therapy was well tolerated with only 2% of toxicities ≥grade 3. In multivariate analysis, PVT response, CLIP staging, and Okuda staging were significant for OS. This was reflected in the difference of 1-year OS of 28 PVT responders and 27 nonresponders of 64% vs. 28% ($p = .003$). Median OS was 14 months for all patients.

In a similarly sized series of 44 patients with HCC reported by a group from Taiwan, the overall response rate was almost identical, namely 61% after 3D-planned radiotherapy with 1.8 Gy per fraction (Liu et al. 2004). Total dose ranged from 39.6 to 60 Gy (median 50.4 Gy). A PVT was present in 14/44 patients, of which 6 responded in the absence of any toxicity >grade 2. Interestingly, the dose of radiotherapy was prognostic ($p = .013$) as was PVT ($p = .006$). For patients with PVT, the 2-year OS was only 8% compared to 55% for patients without PVT. Patients with PVT had a median OS of 10 months compared to 14 months without as found by Rim et al., which might be due to the lower total dose given (Rim et al. 2012).

A group from the Kyung Hee University Center in Seoul reported their results on 25 and 22 patients with HCC treated from 2008 to 2011/2013, respectively (Kong et al. 2013; Kong and Hong 2015). The majority of their patients were treated with 50 Gy in 2.5 Gy daily doses (range: dose per fraction 2–4 Gy, total dose 40–60 Gy). Three-quarters of the patients were Child-Pugh (CP) stage A, and the remainder of patients was stage Child Pugh B. One-third of patients had PVT. The first publication of the group focused on survival and the second on response. Median OS was 14 months and both the 1-year and 2-year OS rate was 86%. Child-Pugh stage, as well as PVT, was prognostically significant. The second report on 39 lesions in 25 patients specifically reported the time course of response which was 15%, 72%, and 87% after 3, 6, and 9 months, respectively, among 92% responding lesions with a median time to objective response of 4 months. The authors recommended continuing restaging for at least 9 months to fully detect responses. The local recurrence rate was 12% at 12 months in this series with moderate total dose. A further report from the same group restricting analysis to 20 patients with 33 lesions treated with helical tomotherapy at the same radiotherapy doses showed a local recurrence rate of 30% at 2 years (Jung et al. 2014a).

A more hypofractionated approach was taken at the University of Freiburg where 13 patients with Klatskin tumors received a total dose of 40–48 Gy prescribed according to the International Commission on Radiation Units and Measurements (ICRU) guidelines given in 4 Gy fractions delivered every other day (Momm et al. 2010). This dose corresponds to a biologically effective dose (BED_{10}) of 67.2 Gy_{10}. Treatment was performed using a vacuum positioning device and abdominal compression including 4D imaging to detect respiratory motion. The imaging was used to derive an internal target volume (ITV) that was isotropically expanded to generate the PTV. The aim of this approach was to achieve a higher dose delivered within a relatively short time and to maintain a low level of toxicity of the organs at risk (OARs), especially the duodenum as this dose is equivalent to 67.2 Gy in 2 Gy fractions for the duodenum (EQD2₃). Only one patient had ≥grade 3 acute toxicity (nausea). Importantly, no major late side effects were observed, especially no late gastrointestinal side effects. Five patients had cholangitis during therapy needing dose reductions in two patients (32 Gy, 39 Gy). Local control at 1 year was 78% and median OS 33.5 months in this retrospective series. Since the publication of this small series, the technique has been improved, using a simultaneous integrated protection (SIP) technique to keep doses to the duodenum low in small volumes of overlap (PTV_{SIP}) while increasing the dose in the dominant PTV (PTV_{dom}) far from critical OARs delivering 12 × 5.0–5.5 Gy and a BED_{10} of 102.3 Gy (Brunner et al. 2016).

Recently, a similar approach was reported from the MDACC in 79 retrospectively identified patients with inoperable intrahepatic cholangiocarcinoma (IHCC) with a median tumor size of 8 cm ranging up to 17 cm (Tao et al. 2016). The group used a central SIB of 75 Gy in 15 fractions or 100 Gy in 25 fractions and also relied on a SIP technique to protect adjacent OARs. Median dose per fraction was 2 Gy in the subgroup of 60 patients with a BED_{10} ≤80.5 Gy and 4 Gy in the 19 patients with BED_{10} >80.5 Gy. At a median follow-up of 33 months the median OS was 30 months and 3-year OS rate of 44%. In line with the trials discussed up to this point, BED was statistically significant for OS being 73% (BED_{10} >80.5 Gy) vs. 38% (BED_{10} ≤80.5 Gy) at 3 years (p = .017). At the same time, local control at 3 years was significantly improved with higher doses 78% vs. 45% (p = .04). Regarding toxicity, no RILD was reported. Two patients were hospitalized ≤90 days after completion of radiotherapy, one due to stent occlusion and the

other due to tumor progression. There were two patients with one having gastric bleeding ≤90 days after the end of radiotherapy and the other with radiation pneumonitis after treatment of lung metastases. Bile duct stenosis was seen in seven patients (9%) at a median time of 10 months (range 2–33 months) after radiotherapy. These patients had stent (re)placements. It was not always possible to discriminate tumor progression (four patients in field, two patients elsewhere in the liver) from therapy-related toxicity in these cases. In these seven patients the maximum dose to the bile duct ranged from 34 Gy in 14 fractions to 75 Gy in 25 fractions (EQD2₃ and EQD2₂ 90 and 93.75 Gy).

In summary, the pioneering work of the Michigan group kicked off a new era of hepatic radiotherapy. This work successfully defined safe doses to the liver in cases where sufficient spared liver volume and adequate liver function exist. Long-term local control can be achieved for both primary and secondary liver tumors. This was a prerequisite to develop hypofractionation and SBRT schedules for these indications. At the same time it could also be demonstrated that conventionally fractionated radiotherapy is a valid therapeutic option to treat targets in the liver safely.

2 Role of SBRT Within the Treatment Algorithms for Liver Tumors and Indications for SBRT

2.1 Liver Metastases

In the Western hemisphere, primary liver cancer is rare compared to liver metastases, whereas in Asia the opposite is true especially for regions in the Far East. In Europe and Northern America only 2% of the tumors in the noncirrhotic liver are primary liver tumors whereas 98% are secondary tumors arising from other primary sites

(Goodman 2007). In cirrhotic livers, more than three-quarters of malignant neoplasms are primary liver cancers, predominantly hepatocellular carcinoma (HCC). Hepatocellular carcinoma is the most common primary liver tumor type followed by CCC.

In general systemic therapy is the preferred treatment for most patients with liver metastases, but patients with a limited number of metastases and with favorable histology should be considered for surgical resection or nonsurgical ablation (Lo et al. 2010; Mendez Romero and Hoyer 2012; Simmonds et al. 2006; Wong et al. 2010). Patients with liver metastases referred for SBRT are generally those who are ineligible for surgery and are often ineligible for radiofrequency ablation (Goodman et al. 2010, 2016; Lee et al. 2009; Mendez Romero et al. 2006; Scorsetti et al. 2015a; Stintzing et al. 2010).

The largest group of patients treated with SBRT consists of patients with liver metastases from primary colorectal cancer. Nevertheless, many studies have also included patients having metastases from other primaries such as breast, nonsmall-cell lung cancer, ovary, and melanoma (Goodman et al. 2016; Mendez Romero et al. 2006; Ambrosino et al. 2009; Meyer et al. 2016; van der Pool et al. 2010). Ideally, if extrahepatic disease is present in these patients, it should be limited and potentially treatable (Goodman et al. 2010, 2016; Ambrosino et al. 2009; van der Pool et al. 2010; Rusthoven et al. 2009). A Karnofsky performance status ≥70% or an ECOG scale ≤2 is often recommended (Goodman et al. 2010, 2016; Mendez Romero et al. 2006; Meyer et al. 2016; Rusthoven et al. 2009).

There is no clear cutoff value for the number and size of liver metastases that can be treated with SBRT, although most studies include patients with one to five lesions (Goodman et al. 2010, 2016; Scorsetti et al. 2015a; Ambrosino et al. 2009; Meyer et al. 2016; van der Pool et al. 2010; Rusthoven et al. 2009; Rule et al. 2011; Vautravers-Dewas et al. 2011) measuring up to 5 or 6 cm (Goodman 2007; Goodman et al. 2010; Scorsetti et al. 2015a; Stintzing et al. 2010; Ambrosino et al. 2009; van der Pool et al. 2010) (Table 1).

Table 1 Treatment outcomes of SBRT for liver metastases

Author	Design	Primary tumor	Number of patients	Scheme	2 year local control	2 year overall survival (%)	Toxicity[a]
Rusthoven et al. (2009)	P (Phase I–II)	Mixed	47	3 × 12–20 Gy	92%	30	1 Gr 3 soft tissue
Lee et al. (2009)	P (Phase I)	Mixed	68	6 × 4.6–10 Gy	Not reported (ly 71%)	39	1 Gr 4 Duodenal bleed and 1 Gr 5 bowel obstruction (tumor progression) 1 Gr 4 small bowel obstruction (hernia) 3 Gr 3 thrombocytopenia 2 Gr 3 liver enzymes 2 Gr 3transient esophagitis/gastritis

(continued)

Table 1 (continued)

Author	Design	Primary tumor	Number of patients	Scheme	2 year local control	2 year overall survival (%)	Toxicity[a]
Rule et al. (2011)	P (Phase I)	Mixed	27	3 × 10 Gy	56%	50	None
				5 × 10 Gy	89%	67	
				5 × 12 Gy	100%	56	
Vautravers-Dewas et al. (2011)	R	Mixed	42	4 × 10 Gy	86%	48	1 Gr 3 epidermitis 1 cirrhotic hepatic failure
				3 × 15 Gy			
Scorsetti et al. (2015a)	P (Phase II)	Colorectal	42	3 × 25 Gy	91%	65	None
Meyer et al. (2016)	P (Phase I)	Mixed	14	1 × 35–40 Gy	100%	78	None
Goodman et al. (2016)	R	Mixed	81	3 × 12–20 Gy	91%	69	4 Gr 3–5 hepatic (1 gr 3, 2 gr 4, 1 gr5)
				4 × 8 Gy			
				5 × 6–10 Gy			
Méndez Romero (doi:10.1016/j.rp or.2016.10.003)	R	Colorectal	40	3 × 12.5 Gy	74%	69	2 Gr 3 liver enzymes (GGT)
				3 × 16.75 Gy	90%	81	1 transient Gr 3 asthenia
							1 Gr 3 portal hypertension (after 2 SBRT)
							1 Gr 3 biliary tree dilatation (centrally located lesion)

[a]Toxicity: Grade 3–5 reported

P prospective, *R* retrospective, *GGT* gamma glutamyl transferase

2.2 Hepatocellular Carcinoma

There are several classifications of HCC such as TNM/AJCC staging, Cancer of the Liver Italian Program (CLIP), and Model of End Stage Liver Disease-Score (MELD); however the Barcelona Clinic Liver Cancer (BCLC) is the most commonly used classification and forms the backbone for therapeutic algorithms (European Association for the Study of the Liver, European Organisation for Research and Treatment of Cancer 2012). Surgery is the preferred therapeutic approach in stages BCLC 0 and A. Thermoablation (RFA) is considered as an alternative for surgical resection as is liver transplantation. In the intermediate stage of BCLC B, transarterial catheter embolization (TACE) is the mainstay of therapy. Advanced stage, BCLC C, is generally considered to be adequately treated with sorafenib, a VEGF inhibitor. At terminal stage, BCLC D, best supportive care is reasonable.

To date, radiotherapy is not (yet) mapped on this treatment algorithm. Therefore, it is of high importance for radiation oncologists to treat as many patients as possible on prospective clinical trials to increase the evidence (Klein and Dawson 2013; Mendez Romero and de Man 2016).

Generally, CP A is the best indication for SBRT in HCC. Treatment of patients with CP B stage led to more hepatic toxicities with frequent temporary deteriorations of Child scores by 1–2 points (Table 2). Although there is no clear limit for the tumor size or number that can be treated with SBRT, most groups included patients with a maximum lesion size of ≤5 cm (Goodman et al. 2010; Iwata et al. 2010; Kimura et al. 2015; Louis

Table 2 Treatment outcomes of SBRT for hepatocellular carcinoma

Author	Design	Number of patients	CP score	Diameter (cm)*	Fractionation	1 year local control	Median survival	Toxicity
Mendez Romero et al. (2006)	P	5 2 1	A B N.A.	4.7	3–5 × 5–12 Gy	75%	22	1 lethal liver failure
Tse et al. (2008)	P	31	A	173 cm³**	6 × 4–9 Gy	65%	11.7	8 grade 3 liver enzyme elevations, 1 lethal pulmonary embolism, 1 tumor–duodenal connection
Jang et al. (2013)	R	74	A B	3	3 × 11–20 Gy	87% at 2 years	63% at 2 years	5 GI toxicity grade 3 6 CTP elevation >2
Huang et al. (2012)	R	23 4 1	A B C	4.4	10 × 4.5 Gy 18–20 × 2.5 Gy 18–20 × 1.8 Gy	87.6%	23	1 grade 3 gastric ulcer
Bae et al. (2013)	R	18 2	A B	≤3 cm (80%) 3–5 cm (20%)	5 × 10 Gy	85%	100% at 1 year	No grade 3 toxicities
Jung et al. (2013)	R	68 24	A B	8.6 × cm³	3–4 × 10–20 Gy	92% at 3 years		6 patients grade 3 RILD
Wahl et al. (2016)	R	57 24 2	A B C	<2 cm (48%) 2–3 cm (26%) 3–5 cm (23%) >5 cm (3.7%)	3–5 × 6–10 Gy	97.4%	74% at 1 year	1 RILD, 1 GI bleeding 1 worsening ascites
Andolino et al. (2011)	R	36 24	A B	3.1 cm	3–5 × 8–16 Gy	90% at 2 years	48% at 2 years	20% CTP progression
Bibault et al. (2013)	R	66 9	A B	3.7 cm	3 × 8–15 Gy	89.8	15	5 liver decompensations 1 grade 4 gastric ulcer 3 grade 2 duodenal ulcers
Huertas et al. (2015)	R	76 11	A B	2.4 cm	3 × 15 Gy	99%	82% at 1 year	1 grade 5 hematemesis 2 grade >3 gastric ulcers

(continued)

Table 2 (continued)

Author	Design	Number of patients	CP score	Diameter (cm)*	Fractionat ion	1 year local control	Median survival	Toxicity
Scorsetti et al. (2015b)	R	23	A	4.8 cm	3 × 16–25 Gy	86%	18	7 grade >3 liver enzyme elevations
		20	B		6 × 6–10 Gy			
Seo et al. (2010)	R	34	A	40.5 mL**	3 × 11–12 Gy	79%	32	1 grade 3 soft tissue toxicity
		4	B		4 × 10 Gy			
Kwon et al. (2010)	R	38	A	15.4 cm³''	3 × 10–13 Gy	72%	93% at 1 year	1 radiation induced hepatic failure
		4	B					
Takeda et al. (2014)	R	14	A	1.9–7 cm	5–7 × 5–10 Gy	100%	100%	1RILD
		2	B					
Price et al. (2012)	R	14	A	Max 6 cm	3–5 × 8–16 Gy	97%	77%	20% CTP worsening
		12	B					
Kang et al. (2012)	P	41	A	2.9 cm	3 × 14–20 Gy	94% at 2 years	68.7 at 2 years	3 grade 3 GI toxicity
		6	B					2 grade 4 gastric ulcers
Weiner et al. (2016)	P	12	A, B	Ca. 5 cm	5 × 8–11 Gy	91%	38% at 1 year	9 CTP decline
								2 grade 5 hepatic failure
Que et al. (2014)	R	22	A	11.4 cm	5 × 5.2–8 Gy	55.6%	11	1 grade 3 liver enzyme elevation
		2	B					
Bujold et al. (2013)	P	102	A	7.2 cm	6 × 4–9 Gy	88%	17	6 grade > 3 liver failure
		None	B					2 grade > 3 liver failure
								1 grade 5 cholangitis
								16 grade > 3 liver enzyme elevations
Culleton et al. (2014)	P/R	29	B	5.1 cm	5–15 fractions 19.7–46.8 Gy‡	N.A.	7.9	63% CTP decline > 2 points 5 grade 3 thrombocytopenia
								3 > grade 3 elevation of liver enzymes
Gkika (submitted)	R	27	A	7 cm	3–12 × 4–15 Gy	88%	9	4 liver decompensation
		19	B					1 grade 3 GI-bleed
								1 cholangitis
								1 necrotic abscess

P prospective, *R* retrospective, *CP* Child-Pugh score

et al. 2010; Sanuki et al. 2014; Su et al. 2016), ≤6 cm (Andolino et al. 2011; Cardenes et al. 2010), or <10 cm (Kang et al. 2012; Seo et al. 2010). Patients with 1–3 nodules are often treated, but again no cutoff value has been established (Kimura et al. 2015; Sanuki et al. 2014; Su et al. 2016; Andolino et al. 2011). In this fragile patient population, tumor size and number that can be treated with SBRT are very dependent on the nontumoral liver volume that can be spared.

Many series reporting on SBRT as definitive therapy include patients with BCLC scores A, B, and C (Kimura et al. 2015; Sanuki et al. 2014; Su et al. 2016; Andolino et al. 2011; Kang et al. 2012; Bibault et al. 2013; Bujold et al. 2013; Park et al. 2013). Studies using SBRT in a pretransplant setting include mainly patients with BCLC A and B scores, and sometimes even with BCLC D due to Child-Pugh C cirrhosis (Andolino et al. 2011; Facciuto et al. 2012; Katz et al. 2011; O'Connor et al. 2012; Sandroussi et al. 2010). In these series, patients with vascular invasion or extrahepatic metastases (BCLC C) are often excluded.

2.3 Cholangiocarcinoma

The second most common primary liver tumor is cholangiocarcinoma. The anatomy of the bile duct is important for the pathology of cholangiocarcinoma because the following subsites need to be discriminated: intrahepatic cholangiocarcinoma (IHCC), extrahepatic cholangiocarcinoma (EHCC), and gallbladder cancer (GBC). Extrahepatic cholangiocarcinoma commonly is subdivided into proximal (hilar or Klatskin) tumors and distal tumors (Benavides et al. 2015), and is usually detected much earlier than IHCC because of jaundice as a clinical symptom. This often allows surgical treatment which is the only curative therapy of all subtypes of cholangiocarcinoma. The only exception is hilar EHCC that may prevent resection due to infiltration of the right and left hepatic ducts as well as the hepatic artery and portal vein which all are in close proximity to each other in the hepatic hilum (Khan et al. 2012). Gallbladder cancer should also be regarded as a distinct entity as it is often detected by coincidence at gallbladder resection and then requires, in certain conditions, adjuvant or additive therapy which is not a typical indication for SBRT. Both nonresectable IHCC and hilar cholangiocarcinoma are commonly treated with gemcitabine- and cisplatin-based chemotherapy (Valle et al. 2010).

A role for SBRT in the treatment of cholangiocarcinoma is not currently well defined. Various groups have tried to use SBRT to deliver high doses of irradiation to control disease locally. Most published studies are retrospective in nature and the majority of them report on intrahepatic tumors (Table 3). Treatment has been delivered as a definitive therapy for primary or recurrent tumors in patients who are ineligible for resection, although it has also been adminis-

Table 3 Treatment outcomes of SBRT for cholangiocarcinoma

Author	Design	Location	Lesion number	Fraction number	Total dose	1 year local control (%)	Median survival	Toxicity[a]
Kopek et al. (2010)	R	EHCC	26	3	45	85	10.6	6 ulcerations
		IHCC	1					3 stenosis
Tse et al. (2008)	P	IHCC	10	6	28–48	65	15	1 biliary obstruction
								1 bowel obstruction
Goodman et al. (2010)	P	IHCC	5	1	18–30	77	28.6	None
Polistina et al. (2011)	R	EHCC	10	3	30	80	35.5	1 ulceration
								2 stenosis
Ibarra et al. (2012)	R	IHCC	11	3	22–50	55.5	11	3 patients Grade 3

(continued)

Table 3 (continued)

Author	Design	Location	Lesion number	Fraction number	Total dose	1 year local control (%)	Median survival	Toxicity[a]
Barney et al. (2012)	R	IHCC	6	3–5	45–60	100	15.5	1 Grade 3 biliary stenosis,
		EHCC	4					1 Grade 5 liver failure
Momm et al. (2010)	R	EHCC	13	10–12	32–56	78	33.5	1 Grade 3 5 cholangitis
Jung et al. (2014b)	R	IHCC	33	1–5	15–60	85	10	6 Grade 3
		EHCC	25					(ulceration, cholangitis, stenosis Perforation)
Mahadevan et al. (2015)	R	IHCC	31	3–5	24–45	88	17	4 Grade 3
		EHCC	11					(ulceration, cholangitis, abscess)
Weiner et al. (2016)	P	IHCC	12	5	40–55	91[§]	13.2	1 hepatic failure[§] 1 biliary stricture
Sandier (in press)	R	IHCC	6	5	40	78%	15.7	5 Grade ≥ 3
		EHCC	25					
Gkika (submitted)	R	IHCC	16	3–12	21–66	77%	14	3 Grade ≥ 3
		EHCC	24					

[a]Toxicity: Late toxicity reported

P prospective, *R* retrospective, *OS* overall survival, *IHCC* intrahepatic cholangiocarcinoma, *EHCC* extrahepatic cholangiocarcinoma

tered after surgery with positive margins (Mahadevan et al. 2015). The ECOG performance status of patients treated in these trials was usually 0–2, although patients with ECOG 3 have also been treated (Jung et al. 2014b). Extension of the disease varied between the studies, with many patients presenting a locally advanced stage with enlarged/positive lymph nodes, and even with metastases (Momm et al. 2010; Tao et al. 2016; Mahadevan et al. 2015; Jung et al. 2014b; Barney et al. 2012; Kopek et al. 2010; Polistina et al. 2011; Tse et al. 2008). Most studies have not proposed a limit on the number of lesions or their maximum diameter, with only one trial proposing a maximum diameter (≥6 cm) as an exclusion criterion (Polistina et al. 2011). One experience with SBRT in the pretransplant setting has been published by the University of Michigan, Ann Arbor (Welling et al. 2014). This retrospective pilot study analyzed data from 12 patients with unresectable perihilar cholangiocarcinoma and negative lymph nodes who had undergone neoadjuvant therapy with SBRT followed by capecitabine until liver transplantation.

3 Treatment Preparation:

3.1 Three- and Four-Dimensional Contrast-Enhanced Computed Tomography Scan (3D-CT; 4D-CT) Simulation for Liver SBRT

Ablative hypofractionated stereotactic body radiotherapy for liver tumors warrants accurate assessment of the treatment target set in motion by respiration. This can be achieved in a number of ways including fluoroscopy, "slow" CT, and typically helical "fast" 4D-CT. With the latter technique a combination of free-breathing CT and 4D-CT images corresponding to different phases of the respiratory cycle is obtained. The software then selects phase-specific images defined by the user to produce a series of CT axial images of the target position throughout the respiratory cycle. For SBRT planning, the patient is positioned supinely on the flat table top in a custom-molded immobilization device such as a vacuum bag, with arms up extended above the head. The patient will then be asked to breathe freely or to hold their breath during the contrast-enhanced 3D-CT used to accurately delineate the gross tumor volume (GTV). This is followed immediately by helical 4D-CT to assess tumor/surrogates, breathing motion, and internal target volume (ITV) if needed. There are several commercial motion-monitoring systems available to capture respiratory phases during 4D-CT, including respiratory airflow, position of an infrared marker on the abdominal surface, or placement of pressure sensors on the abdominal wall.

3.2 Motion-Monitoring Systems

The Anzai Respiratory Gating System® (Siemens Inc, Concord, California, USA) utilizes a pressure sensor load cell to detect external respiratory motion pressure change in real time. It consists of a fixation belt which is used to position a pressure transducer at a patient's upper abdomen. The respiratory abdominal motion signal (both amplitude and phase) detected by the pressure sensor is amplified and then evaluated by the Anzai® software. The system includes two kinds of pressure transducers (low/high) with different sensitivities for patients with shallow vs. deep respiration amplitudes, as well as four differently sized fixation belts used to compensate for varying abdominal circumferences of patients (Li et al. 2006).

Another respiratory gating system, RPM® (Varian Inc, Palo Alto, California, USA), used for the 4D-CT scanner is based on an infrared camera to detect motion of external markers, placed on a fixation pad on the abdomen, between the sternum and umbilicus. The RPM® system measures the motion of two markers which are illuminated by infrared-emitting diodes surrounding the camera and records both the amplitude and phase of the external respiratory signal in real time (Li et al. 2006; Glide-Hurst et al. 2013).

There are other motion-monitoring systems that are specific to certain treatment systems,

e.g., Accuray Cyberknife Synchrony® (Accuray, LLC, Sunnyvale, California, USA) and Novalis BRAINLAB ExacTrac® (BRAINLAB, Munich, Germany).

3.3 Motion Management to Compensate Respiratory-Induced Liver Tumor Motion During Radiotherapy

A major issue in liver SBRT is predominantly breathing-induced target motion during treatment delivery. There are various techniques currently in clinical use or that have been proposed to explicitly compensate for respiratory-induced tumor motion. These techniques can be broadly separated into four categories: direct abdominal compression, treatment under breath hold, respiratory gating, and tumor tracking with dedicated treatment devices (Guckenberger et al. 2012; Jiang et al. 2008; Keall et al. 2006). They are summarized here:

(a) Direct abdominal compression: Employing a pressure plate against the abdomen in a reproducible fashion to force the patient to breathe shallowly, thereby reducing normal breathing and decreasing maximum displacement during respiration. A study by Heinzerling et al. showed that it roughly reduced tumor motion from 12–16 mm (free-breathing) to 5–11 mm (compression), and a significant difference in the control of both superior-inferior (SI) and overall motion of tumors was seen with the application of compression (Heinzerling et al. 2008).

(b) Breath-holding technique: The beam is only on when the patient is holding their breath: the diaphragmatic motion is limited. There have been several techniques developed, e.g., deep inspiration breath-hold (DIBH) (Boda-Heggemann et al. 2016) and active breathing control (ABC) (Dawson et al. 2005). Some methods may be uncomfortable for some patients which limits applicability. It also increases treatment time which causes the potential of patient movement.

(c) Respiratory gating: Turning the beam on and off in conjunction with the normal respiratory cycle. Free breathing gating strategies have typically been used during end expiration, which occupies the majority of the breathing cycle. This approach therefore allows for the application of large doses during the gating phase. Compared to the breath-holding technique, the patient is under less stress. There is residual motion within the gating window and there exist baseline shifts. Furthermore, gating increases treatment time. Due to quasiperiodic motion of the liver and its partially nonrigid behavior, internal fiducial markers are regarded as the gold standard when delivering high radiation doses to malignant liver lesions. The procedure is invasive, which may cause side effects, specifically in patients with hepatic cirrhosis, with peritoneal and subcapsular hemorrhage and needle track seeding of cancer cells as major concerns. External markers minimize the burden on patients but the correlation between marker and tumor position may be doubtful (Jiang et al. 2008; Keall et al. 2006).

(d) Tumor tracking with dedicated treatment devices, shifts dynamically the radiation dose to follow the moving tumor during free breathing. The advantage of 4D-RT is its promise of sparing additional normal tissue by synchronizing the radiation with the moving target in real time, while its disadvantage is that implantation of surrogates is invasive.

3.4   PET/CT Simulation

PET/CT simulation is a joint effort between the nuclear medicine and radiation oncology departments. The immobilization vacuum bag is custom-made in the radiation oncology department. The radiation therapists then accurately set up patients in the nuclear medicine department with a customized vacuum bag in the treatment position utilizing external laser lights and a flat table support needed for the radiotherapy setup. PET utilizes 18F-fluorodeoxyglucose (FDG) to visualize the glucose metabolism, which is typically increased in metastatic cancer. The hybrid spiral PET/CT scan is acquired when the patient is in the radiation treatment position capturing both metabolic activity and precise anatomic localization in a single imaging procedure. PET/CT has demonstrated improved accuracy of tar-

get localization on a dedicated hybrid PET/CT scanner as opposed to the procedures that fuse PET and CT scans acquired on separate scanners (Li and Xiao 2013; Pan and Mawlawi 2008). One of the challenges of PET/CT for target delineation is the impact of respiratory organ motion on the image quality in a free-breathing patient. Four-dimensional PET/CT is one of the strategies to minimize the impact of respiratory motion-related image degradation (Chi and Nguyen 2014; Nehmeh et al. 2004). However, due to its complexity and prolonged acquisition time, which impacts on patient comfort and increases the potential for patient movement, it has not been widely used. Since PET/CT images are acquired over prolonged period of time (usually 20 min), it should be noted that they may serve as a surrogate of tumor motion volume, especially in cases when the target is not clearly defined on 4D-CT due to the fade of the contrast.

3.5   Diagnostic Imaging of Hepatocellular Carcinoma

HCC and associated premalignant lesions have imaging characteristics with sufficient specificity to provide confident diagnosis and staging without the need for tissue sampling (Bruix and Sherman 2005). All clinical practice guidelines recommend multiphasic CT and MR with extracellular contrast as first-line diagnostic tools (European Association for the Study of the Liver, European Organisation for Research and Treatment of Cancer 2012; Bruix and Sherman 2011; Kudo 2010; Omata et al. 2010). Ultrasound is often utilized for initial surveillance of patients with cirrhosis and viral hepatitis (Kudo 2010; Omata et al. 2010).

3.5.1   Premalignant Hepatocellular Lesions

HCC typically arises through progressive dedifferentiation of phenotypically abnormal nodules, most often in the background of cirrhosis and cirrhotic nodules, although some variants of HCC can arise from a background of steatohepatitis. These premalignant lesions include regenerative cirrhotic nodules and low- and high-grade dysplastic nodules. It should be noted that HCC can develop without identifiable histologic precursors, known as "de novo" hepatocarcinogenesis.

(a) *Cirrhotic nodules* are seen as innumerable, well-defined regions of cirrhotic parenchyma surrounded by scar tissue. They are most often 1–15 mm in diameter, and if greater than 10 mm are described as "large cirrhotic nodules" or "large regenerative nodules." These nodules are usually indistinguishable from one another. Relative to background parenchyma, cirrhotic nodules are often isoattenuating/isointense on unenhanced CT and MR imaging. Cirrhotic nodules that have undergone relatively early architectural changes can demonstrate T1 hyperintensity and T2 hypointensity, similar to dysplastic nodules described below.

(b) *Dysplastic nodules* are classified as either low-grade or high-grade dysplastic nodules. Both types are typically iso- or hypoattenuating in arterial, portal, and delayed phase imaging due to loss of portal triad architecture and lack of neoarterialization early on. They typically exhibit T1 hyperintensity and T2 iso- or hypointensity on MR imaging. As hepatocarcinogenesis progresses, dysplastic nodules may begin to develop neoarterialization and associated hyperenhancement. These are signs of high-grade dysplastic nodules, and can resemble HCC. However in contrast to HCC, high-grade dysplastic nodules will not demonstrate contrast washout or capsular enhancement. Either of these features, if seen in conjunction with arterial hyperenhancement, is diagnostic of HCC. Dysplastic nodules are more likely to demonstrate iso- or hypoenhancement due to portal triad architectural changes that include loss of hepatic arterial and portal venous blood supply.

3.5.2 Diagnosis of Hepatocellular Carcinoma

The imaging principles of HCC are essentially identical between CT and MR. Several hallmark characteristics are seen on both of these imaging modalities, as detailed below, enabling imaging-based diagnosis of HCC with near-100% positive predictive value (Forner et al. 2008; Hatfield et al. 2008). HCC is often divided into "early" and "progressed" HCC. Early HCC is an incipient stage of hepatocar-

cinogenesis, gradually replacing parenchyma and neighboring portal tracts and central veins without destroying these structures. Progressed HCC is an overtly malignant lesion which displaces or destroys adjacent parenchyma, able to invade blood vessels and metastasize. See Figs. 1 and 2 for examples of the major imaging characteristics of HCC.

(a) *Arterial phase hyperenhancement* is defined as arterial phase enhancement that is unequivocally greater than background parenchymal enhancement. This feature is caused by neoarterialization of hepatocarcinogenesis. When a hyperenhancing hepatic lesion is seen in combination with either contrast washout or capsule enhancement, a diagnosis of HCC can be made with high confidence. However, when seen on its own, arterial phase hyperenhancement is nonspecific and can be seen in earlier stages of hepatocarcinogenesis (including cirrhotic and dysplastic nodules), as well as in other benign lesions such as benign perfusion alterations, small hemangiomas, small focal nodular hyperplasia (FNH)-like lesions, atypical cases of focal or confluent fibrosis, IHCC, and small hypervascular metastases.

(b) *Washout* is defined as the temporal reduction of HCC enhancement relative to surrounding liver from an earlier to a later phase, resulting in portal venous hypoenhancement. The mechanism is likely multifactorial, including reduced intratumoral portal venous blood supply, early venous drainage, progressive enhancement of background parenchyma, and intrinsic hypoattenuation/hypointensity. Similar to arterial phase hyperenhancement, washout on its own is a nonspecific finding for HCC. However, in cirrhotic patients, the combination of arterial phase hyperenhancement and lesion washout is 100% specific for HCC in lesions greater than 2 cm, and approximately 90% specific for HCC in lesions measuring 1.0–1.9 cm. This feature combination is rarely seen in IHCC. In the general population without a specific risk for HCC, the differential includes hypervascular metastases, hepatocellular adenoma, and other lesions.

(c) *Capsule appearance* is defined as the appearance of a peripheral rim of smooth hyperen-

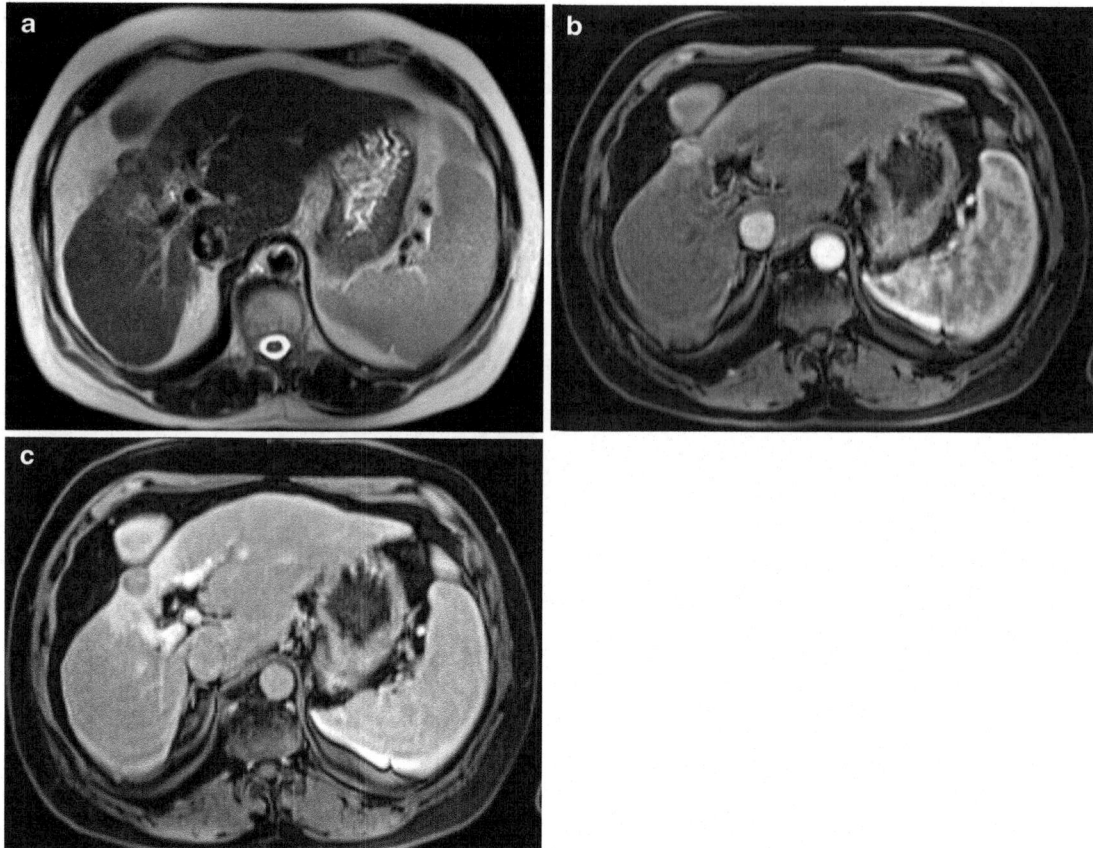

Fig. 1 These images show the MR characteristics of a biopsy-proven HCC. In (**a**) T2-weighted HASTE images show heterogeneous T2 signal. In (**b**) T1-weighted images acquired 20 s after contrast injection show arterial phase enhancement. The images of (**c**) were obtained 40 s after contrast injection demonstrated contrast washout, enhancing tumor capsule and surrounding coronal enhancement, all characteristic of progressed HCC

hancement in the portal venous or delayed phase. This feature is usually more conspicuous in the delayed phase compared to the portal venous phase. The capsule appearance is attributed to slow flow within intracapsular vessels as well as contrast retention within the extravascular connective tissue of the capsule. This imaging feature is frequently associated with progressed HCC, but rarely with early HCC or dysplastic or cirrhotic nodules. Therefore, the imaging presence of the enhancing capsule is an important predictor of progressed HCC, particularly when seen in combination with other features such as arterial phase hyperenhancement. This finding should be interpreted carefully, as some small IHCCs peripherally enhance in all phases, which can be misinterpreted as capsule enhancement. However, this enhancement tends to peak in the arterial phase rather than the later phases, as seen in HCC. Disruption of the capsule by tumor suggests infiltration of the surrounding tissue, and may indicate poor prognosis. Some HCCs demonstrate infiltrative rather than expansive growth. These have poorly defined boundaries without capsules.

(d) *Extracapsular extension* is the formation of satellite nodules. This is frequently seen with large progressed HCCs, and represents intrahepatic metastases within the venous drainage area of the primary tumor. These often appear as multiple subcentimeter nodules outside of the tumor margins, but usually within 2 cm of the same margin. By definition, each satellite nodule represents a progressed lesion, and

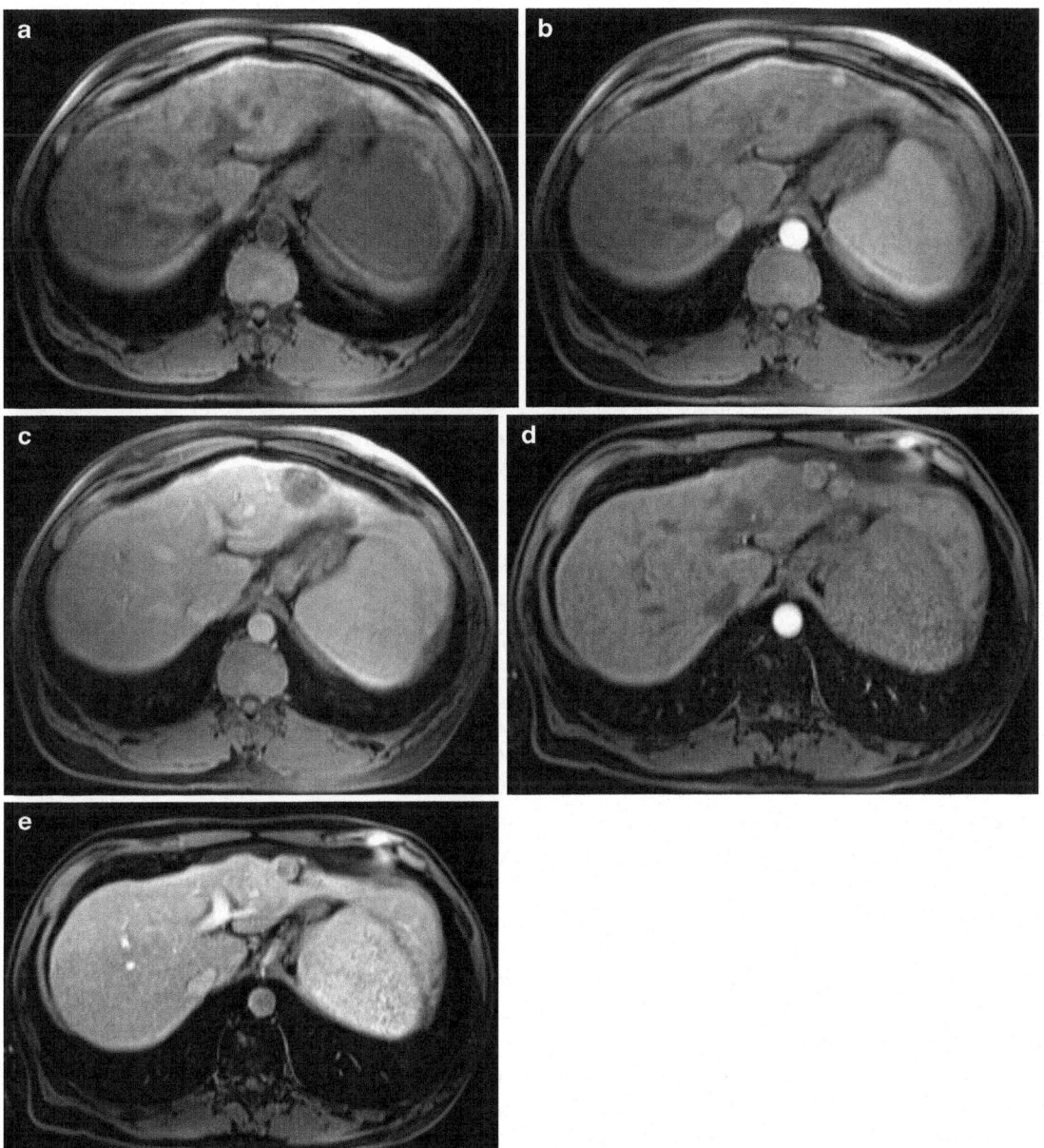

Fig. 2 T1-weighted contrast-enhanced images of a biopsy-proven HCC precontrast (**a**), 20 s postcontrast (**b**), and 40 s postcontrast (**c**). The arterial-phase enhancing nodule in (**b**) is contained within a larger nodule which is only apparent on (**c**) as a hypoenhancing mass with the contrast washout. This is an example of nodule-in-nodule architecture. The smaller nodule demonstrates early arterial hyperenhancement with washout, consistent with neoarterialization during progression of hepatocarcinogenesis. The larger nodule demonstrates an early arterial isoenhancement and late arterial hypoenhancement, consistent with the lower grade HCC. With the nodule-in-nodule architecture, these findings suggest focal high-grade progression within a lower grade early HCC. (**d** and **e**) (20 and 40 s postcontrast) show the same lesion 16 months later, now demonstrating mosaic architecture, early arterial enhancement with washout, and coronal enhancement representing classical findings for progressed HCC

each typically demonstrates arterial hyperenhancement which would be atypical for small, primary precursor lesions. These lesions are nonspecific, and can also be seen with IHCC.

(e) *Macrovascular invasion*, also known as "tumor thrombus," is the macroscopic infiltration of vasculature by the tumor. Differentiation from bland thrombus is critical, as macrovascular invasion precludes surgical treatment options such as resection or liver transplantation, while the presence of bland thrombus may alter the surgical approach but does not necessarily exclude surgery. This can manifest as arterial-enhancing neovessels within an occluded vein, appearing as thin or punctate hyperenhancing "threads and streaks" within a portal or hepatic venous thrombus.

(f) *Intralesional fat* is the presence of fat within a lesion greater than that of background parenchyma and is manifested as signal loss between in- and out-of-phase T1-weighted imaging. Lesions containing fat appear hypoattenuating on CT, but this is nonspecific. This finding is very rare in non-HCC hepatic malignancy, and the presence of intralesional fat can help exclude ICC. This is generally associated with early HCC versus progressed HCC. Except in the steatohepatitic variant of HCC, this finding is generally a good prognostic indicator, and may be associated with longer time to progression and less risk of metastasis.

(g) *Corona enhancement* is defined as a transient zone or rim of enhancement in the late arterial or early portal venous phase, fading to isoenhancement in later phases. During hepatocarcinogenesis, venous drainage of the lesion evolves from drainage via hepatic veins (in cirrhotic or dysplastic nodules and early HCC) to sinusoids (unencapsulated, progressed HCC) to portal venules (encapsulated, progressed HCC). The sinusoids and portal venules of progressed HCC communicate with the surrounding perinodular hepatic parenchyma and give the appearance of early enhancement of the surrounding parenchyma. The corona may be circumferential or eccentric to the lesion, and may blend into the lesion in the arterial phase. The presence of coronal enhancement is associated with microvascular invasion, and poor prognosis. Metastatic satellite nodules and local recurrences often occur within the corona zone. Some authors recommend that corona enhancement areas are included in surgical resection margins or ablation zones.

(h) *Nodule-in-nodule architecture* suggests the emergence of progressed HCC within a dysplastic nodule or early HCC. This can appear as an area of arterial phase hyperenhancement within an iso- or a hypoenhancing nodule, or an area of T2 hyperintensity within a T2 hypointense nodule. The surrounding nodule usually represents more well-differentiated tissue. This may also be seen in parent nodules containing more fat or iron, or iron-sparing nodules in a background of iron-laden parenchyma. Foci of fat- or iron-sparing within an otherwise fat- or iron-laden nodule are suspicious for local progression.

4 Planning for Liver SBRT: Coplanar Vs. Noncoplanar Treatments

Currently, both coplanar and noncoplanar beam setups are being used for liver SBRT. Generally, in coplanar treatment volumetric arc therapy (VMAT) is applied, while noncoplanar setups can be provided with a conventional linear accelerator or a robotic Cyberknife® treatment unit. The Cyberknife® features noncoplanar treatment without treatment couch translation and rotation, minimizing the risk of undesired intra-fraction patient and tumor displacement. With the Synchrony® tumor tracking system, margins can be further minimized.

Systematic comparison of coplanar vs. noncoplanar treatment plan quality requires an algorithm for beam angle optimization (BAO). To avoid bias in treatment technique comparison, it is also highly desirable that treatment plans are generated fully automatically, i.e., without the usual manual trial-and-error tweaking of parameters in a treatment planning system (TPS). At Erasmus MC, development and evaluation of those algorithms has been a research topic since the 1990s. Woudstra et al. developed the "cycle" algorithm for BAO with open, wedged, and segmented IMRT fields (Woudstra and Storchi 2000). With cycle, new beam directions were sequentially added to the plan. For this purpose all feasible directions were temporarily added to the current plan in order to select the optimal new direction to be included.

de Pooter et al. extended cycle with a feature for nonisotropic beam penumbra margin optimization for SBRT, and used it to investigate treatment planning for liver SBRT (de Pooter et al.

2006). For eight liver SBRT patients, the clinical plan was compared with automatically generated coplanar and noncoplanar plans, containing open fields with optimized penumbra margins. Manual plan generation took 1–2 days per patient while no workload was involved in automatic plan generation (1–2-h computation time for a computer). Both the noncoplanar and the coplanar automatically generated plans were of substantially higher quality than the clinically applied, manually generated plans. The most favorable therapeutic ratio was obtained with the automatically generated noncoplanar plans. In a separate study, cycle was used to compare PTV dose prescription at the 65% isodose with prescription at 80% isodose for metastatic liver tumors (de Pooter et al. 2007). To this purpose, for both prescription doses, noncoplanar plans were automatically generated for 15 patients, aiming at the maximum achievable PTV dose without violating imposed constraints. On average, the 65% strategy was superior, but for a limited number of patients dose prescription at 80% was more favorable. Using cycle, Heijmen et al. (Heijmen et al. 2007) demonstrated that biological optimization of noncoplanar liver SBRT based on generalized

equivalent uniform dose (gEUD) cost functions was, on average, superior to conventional strategies with a 65 or 80% isodose that closely surrounds the PTV, with exceptions of a limited number of patients that seemed to benefit more from one of the latter strategies. de Pooter et al. compared 10-beam coplanar and noncoplanar IMRT plans with optimized beam directions with a reference coplanar, 11-beam, equi-angular IMRT plan (de Pooter et al. 2008). All IMRT plans were manually generated with a commercial TPS, but optimal beam directions for the ten-beam IMRT plans were established with cycle. For this purpose, cycle was used to automatically generate optimal 3D-CRT plans for ten-beam coplanar and noncoplanar treatments with optimized beam directions. Using IMRT with optimized coplanar setups, the PTV dose could be enhanced by ~5% compared to equi-angular treatment, without violating planning constraints. For optimized noncoplanar treatment this increase was ~30%, clearly demonstrating the advantage of noncoplanar treatment. Moreover, de Pooter demonstrated that the enhancement in PTV dose resulting from noncoplanar treatment was similar for 3D-CRT and for IMRT (Fig. 3). In other words, also when

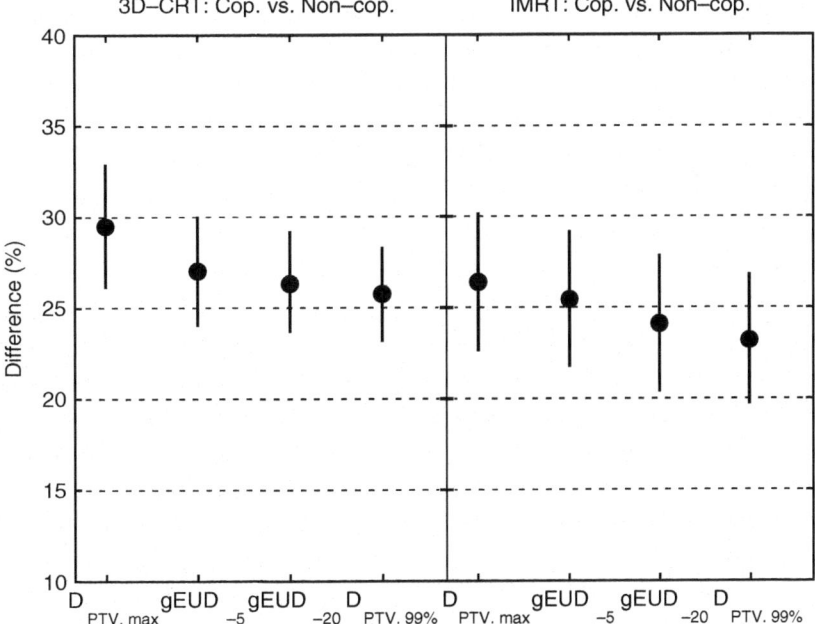

Fig. 3 Patient group mean differences for the PTV dose parameters DPTV, max, gEUD (−5), gEUD (−20), and DPTV, 99% between optimized coplanar and noncoplanar beam setups for 3D-CRT and IMRT plans

treating with IMRT, it remains important to use optimized noncoplanar beam setups instead of a coplanar approach.

A disadvantage of IMRT plan generation in the study by de Pooter et al. is the sequential optimization of beam angles and beam profiles and the manual generation of IMRT plans (de Pooter et al. 2008). Furthermore, "optimal" beam configurations were established for 3D-CRT without a guarantee for optimality for IMRT. Recently, we have developed a novel algorithm, designated "iCycle," for fully automated and integrated beam angle and IMRT optimization (Breedveld et al. 2009, 2012; Leinders et al. 2013; Rossi et al. 2012; Sharfo et al. 2015; Voet et al. 2012, 2013a). In several studies we have demonstrated superiority in quality of automatically generated iCycle plans compared to the conventional interactive trial-and-error planning (Sharfo et al. 2016; Voet et al. 2013b, 2014). Currently, all VMAT and IMRT plans for head-and-neck cancer, cervical cancer, prostate cancer, and advanced lung cancer patients in our department are fully automatically generated.

In a recent study, iCycle has been used for detailed investigations on noncoplanar IMRT and coplanar VMAT in SBRT for liver metastases (Sharfo et al. n.d.). All plans were generated fully automatically. Compared to VMAT, all 15 patients in this study benefitted from 25-beam noncoplanar treatment (25-NCP) in terms of OAR sparing. For three patients, adequate PTV coverage without OAR constraint violation was not achievable with VMAT, while proper coverage could be obtained with noncoplanar treatment due to enhanced OAR avoidance. The authors also proposed a novel treatment approach, designated VMAT+, involving addition of <5 IMRT beams with computer-optimized noncoplanar orientations to VMAT. With VMAT+ the maximum achievable tumor BED was equal to that of 25-NCP. Conversely, VMAT resulted in a lower tumor BED in five patients (reduction 27–48 Gy). Compared to VMAT, VMAT+ also yielded significant dose reductions in OARs. Treatment times with VMAT+ were on average only enhanced by 4.1 min compared to 8.4 min for VMAT. Improvements in OAR sparing with 25-NCP, compared to VMAT+, were generally

modest and/or statistically insignificant, while delivery times of 25-NCP were on average 20.6 min longer. It was concluded that VMAT+ was equivalent to time-consuming treatment with 25 noncoplanar beams in terms of achievable tumor BED and OAR sparing. Moreover, VMAT+ was superior to VMAT in terms of tumor BED, OAR sparing, and intermediate-dose spillage, with only a minor increase in delivery time.

Recent studies from other groups confirm superiority of noncoplanar beam setups in liver SBRT. Dong et al. demonstrated the dosimetric benefit of the novel 4π noncoplanar delivery technique (Dong et al. 2013). To achieve superior plan quality, between 14 and 22 noncoplanar beams were required, at the cost of prolonged treatment delivery times. Woods et al. demonstrated that the 4π technique allowed for a clinically relevant dose escalation with the intention to improve local tumor control in liver SBRT (Woods et al. 2016).

Recently, novel treatment units have been proposed featuring in-room MR guidance for enhanced soft-tissue contrast compared to kV or MV image guidance (Lagendijk et al. 2014; Mutic and Dempsey 2014). The role of these units for liver SBRT needs to be investigated in future studies. As described above, noncoplanar treatment is advantageous in liver SBRT, while the novel machines with MR guidance can only be used for coplanar treatment. Perhaps, the lack of noncoplanar beams could be compensated with smaller CTV-PTV margins due to the MR guidance. However, currently applied implanted fiducials already allow liver SBRT with small CTV-PTV margins (Seppenwoolde et al. 2011; Wunderink et al. 2008, 2010), especially when used in combination with breath-hold treatment, gating, or tumor tracking with a Cyberknife®. For noncoplanar treatment, Molinelli et al. used automated planning to investigate the potential impact of margin reduction in liver SBRT on the therapeutic ratio (Molinelli et al. 2008). A similar approach could be followed to compare coplanar treatment with an MR-guided approach vs. a noncoplanar treatment at a linac or Cyberknife.

To summarize, the systematic studies presented above clearly demonstrate superior plan quality in liver SBRT for optimized noncoplanar beam setups compared to coplanar treatment like VMAT. However, a disadvantage of many-beam noncoplanar treatment is prolonged treatment time. This can be avoided with the VMAT+ approach, adding a few optimized noncoplanar beams to VMAT. The role of recently proposed in-room MR guidance for liver SBRT needs systematic investigation. It is unknown whether the MR guidance can compensate for the limitation of only coplanar treatment, and whether it can compete with high-accuracy image guidance based on implanted fiducials combined with kV imaging.

5 Using Bio-Effect Measures to Evaluate the Effectiveness and Safety of a Liver SBRT Treatment Plan

One way to evaluate the possible biological effect of liver SBRT treatment plans in terms of their potential local tumor control and their potential normal tissue effects is to convert their associated dose distributions to biologically normalized dose distributions. Using biologically normalized distributions, bio-effect measures can then be calculated to rank and compare liver SBRT treatment plans. Examples of such bio-effect measures are the biologically equivalent dose (BED), equivalent dose (EQD), effective volume v_{eff} of an organ at risk being irradiated to a reference EQD, and equivalent uniform dose (EUD).

BED formalizes the conversion of doses delivered using any fractionation scheme to their biologically effective level delivered at an ultralow-dose rate, the only parameter needed for this conversion being the α/β- ratio for the biological endpoint studied:

$$\text{BED} = nd\left(1 + \frac{d}{\alpha/\beta}\right) - \frac{\lambda}{\alpha}\left(T - T_k\right)$$

In this expression, n denotes the number of fractions, d is the dose per fraction, and the α/β-ratio has the usual meaning and has to be chosen appropriately for the biological endpoint studied

(Fowler 1989). The proliferation term in the above expression contains the radiation sensitivity α and the three parameters T_p, T_k, and T. T denotes the overall length of treatment in days including weekends, and Tp denotes the proliferation rate, which is defined as $\lambda \equiv \ln(2)/T_{\text{eff}}$, where T_{eff} denotes the effective doubling time of the clonogenic cells in days. T_k denotes the kickoff time, which represents any delay in the start of rapid clonogenic cell repopulation in response to radiation treatment after treatment has started. As pointed out above, when using BED all fractionation schemes are converted to a dose fraction schedule of infinitesimal fraction size delivered continuously over an infinitely long time. This is good for standardization purposes, but means that the standard fractionation scheme to which all doses are converted is ultralow radiation therapy, producing BED values that are very different from the dose levels used in standard treatment schedules.

In order to reference the biological effectiveness of a dose distribution for which the dose fractionation scheme is varied to a standard fractionation schedule, the concept of equivalent dose (EQD) was introduced (Withers et al. 1983). EQD is defined as the total dose, given in reference dose fractions, that has the same biological effect as the actual dose fractionation schedule under consideration. EQD is given by

$$\text{EQD} = nd\left(\frac{\alpha/\beta + d}{\alpha/\beta + d_{\text{ref}}}\right) \quad (1)$$

In this expression, n denotes the number of fractions, d the dose per fraction for the liver SBRT fractionation schedule under consideration, and d_{ref} is the per fraction for the reference fractionation schedule from which the modeled normal tissue complication data was derived, where the alpha/beta ratio has to be chosen as is appropriate for the organ and endpoint at risk being studied. Essentially, when using EQD one reconverts BED values back to biologically equi-effective doses delivered at the reference dose per fraction that was used in derivation of the normal tissue complication probability (NTCP) model one would like to use.

For "*serial*" organs, the risk of incurring a complication is strongly influenced by high-dose regions and hot spots, and therefore the maximum EQD received by such an organ will strongly correlate with NTCP. On the other hand, for a "*parallel*" organ the risk of developing a complication depends on the dose distribution throughout the organ at risk rather than the high dose to a small area within the organ at risk. Therefore, for "*parallel*" organs the mean EQD received by the organ strongly correlates with NTCP. For this reason one is interested in the mean EQD when considering "parallel" organs. The mean EQD is defined as follows:

$$EQD_{mean} = \sum_{i=1}^{N_b} v_i EQD_i \qquad (2)$$

where

$$EQD_i = nd_i \left(\frac{\alpha / \beta + d_i}{\alpha / \beta + d_{ref}} \right) \text{ and } \sum_{i=1}^{N_b} v_i = 1 \quad (3)$$

In the above expression N_b denotes the total number of dose bins in the differential DVH being converted to an EQD-DVH, EQD_i the EQD for the i-th dose bin, n the total number of fractions, di the dose per fraction in the i-th dose bin, and v_i the partial volume associated with the i-th dose bin. In particular, Dawson et al. (2006) have proposed the use of a iso-NTCP dose escalation strategy for liver SBRT in which the risk level for RILD is set not to exceed 5% for either liver metastases or primary liver cancer using the Lyman-Kutcher-Burman NTCP model (D_{50} (metastases)=48.5 Gy, D_{50} (primary liver cancer)=39.8 Gy, n=0.97, m=0.12) for RILD derived from the University of Michigan experience of treating liver cancer using a dose per fraction of d_{ref}=1.5 Gy. The NTCP model is given by

$$NTCP(EQD_{ref}, v_{eff}) = \frac{1}{\sqrt{2\pi}} \int_{-\infty}^{t} \exp(-x^2 / 2) dx$$
$$(4)$$

with

$$t = \frac{EQD_{ref} v_{eff}^n - EQD_{50}}{m \ EQD_{50}} \qquad (5)$$

and

$$v_{\mathit{eff}} = \sum_i v_i \left(\frac{EQD_i}{EQD_{ref}} \right)^{\frac{1}{n}} \text{ where} \sum_i v_i = 1 \quad (6)$$

Here, EQD_{ref} is the prescription dose for the intended liver SBRT schedule converted to EQD using an α/β-ratio equal to 2.5 Gy and a d_{ref}=1.5 Gy (cf. (Dawson et al. 2006)). Note that for n=1, we see from Eqs. (3) and (6) that

$$v_{eff} = \sum_i v_i \left(\frac{EQD_i}{EQD_{ref}} \right) = \frac{1}{EQD_{ref}} \sum_i v_i EQD_i$$
$$= \left(\frac{EQD_{mean}}{EQD_{ref}} \right) \qquad (7)$$

Since n=0.97 for RILD, Eqs. (4) and (5) can be rewritten using the identity $EQD_{mean} = EQD_{ref} v_{eff}$ (cf. Eq. (7) above) as follows:

$$NTCP(EQD_{mean}) = \frac{1}{\sqrt{2\pi}} \int_{-\infty}^{t} \exp(-x^2 / 2) dx,$$
$$(8)$$

with

$$t = \frac{EQD_{mean} - EQD_{50}}{m \ EQD_{50}} \qquad (9)$$

To simplify the process of selecting an appropriate prescription dose based on iso-NTCP (Dawson et al. 2006), developed tables and graphs of v_{eff} and corresponding prescription doses. Based on the observation made above in Eqs. (8) and (9) this process was further simplified in RTOG 1112 to the use of liver mean dose as the primary constraint. The use of an iso-NTCP prescription strategy should be preferred if there is no significant tumor dose–response over the dose range the iso-NTCP paradigm is to be employed or if the toxicity guarded against is so severe that its occurrence would negate the possible positive effect of increased local tumor control by intensifying the dose schedule beyond a given NTCP threshold. In particular, Ohri et al. (2014) in their meta-analysis of available liver SBRT studies that reported local control data at 1 year, 2 years, and 3 years following treatment found no dose–response for primary liver cancer and only a very shallow one for liver metastases over the investigated BED range of 60 Gy_{10}–180 Gy_{10}.

Lastly, in order to describe the radiobiological effect of a liver SBRT dose distribution on the tumor volume the EUD concept proposed by (Niemierko 1997) can be employed. EUD has been defined as the dose that when applied uniformly to a tumor volume will have the same biological effect (i.e., local control) as the inhomogeneous DVH for the tumor volume from which it has been derived (cf. (Rim et al. 2012)). Niemierko (1997) has put forward various expressions for EUD. Kavanagh et al. (Kavanagh et al. 2003) have used the simplest model for EUD proposed by (Niemierko 1997),

$$\text{EUD} = 2\text{Gy}\frac{\ln\left(\sum_{i=1}^{N}v_i\text{SF}_2^{\frac{D_i}{2}}\right)}{\ln(\text{SF}_2)}, \quad (10)$$

to rank and describe the radiobiologic effect of SBRT dose distributions. As one can see from the above expression, in order to calculate the EUD for a particular treatment plan one needs a differential DVH for the tumor volume, an α/β-ratio describing the biological end point in question, and a value for SF_2 (surviving fraction of clonogens after a 2 Gy fraction). (Niemierko 1997) has shown that EUD depends only weakly on SF_2 and the alpha/beta ratio; hence one can work with generic values for SF_2 the alpha/beta ratio when using EUD for plan evaluation. For tumors a generic value for the alpha/beta ratio is 10 Gy, while a generic value for SF_2 for a moderately radiation sensitive tumor is 0.48 (Suit et al. 1992).

To summarize, the bio-effect measures discussed above can be used in the evaluation of the effectiveness and safety of liver SBRT dose distributions. In particular, the EUD concept can be used to rank competing treatment plans in terms for their expected tumor effect, while the BED and EQD concept can be used to evaluate the biological effectiveness of different dose fraction schemes. It must be understood that a dose distribution giving a desired prescription dose has different biological effect both in terms of expected normal tissue com-plications and possibly tumor effect depending upon what fractionation schedule is employed (Suit et al. 1992; Fowler et al. 2004).

Lastly, it is emphasized that the bio-effect measures discussed above are only models whose input parameters need to be further studied and understood; hence they should only be used as a guide in the assessment of the potential efficacy and safety of a liver SBRT treatment plan. As more and more clinical data becomes available these models will need to be refined and updated.

6 Treatment Outcomes

6.1 Liver Metastases

After the delivery of high-radiotherapy doses to liver metastases, high local control rates have been reported at 2 years, with most values lying around 90%. Table 1 presents results from prospective and retrospective studies after SBRT for liver metastases (Goodman et al. 2016; Lee et al. 2009; Scorsetti et al. 2015a; Meyer et al. 2016; Rusthoven et al. 2009; Rule et al. 2011; Vautravers-Dewas et al. 2011). Several trials showed a significant relationship between dose and local control (Rule et al. 2011; Chang et al. 2011; McCammon et al. 2009; Wulf et al. 2006). An SBRT working group was organized by the American Association for Physics in Medicine (AAPM) to investigate the chance of tumor control related to various dose fractionation schemes for primary and metastatic liver tumors; this found that, in liver metastases, local control was significantly better after the delivery of high biologically effective doses >100 Gy_{10} (Ohri et al. 2014).

A relationship between local control and size or volume of the metastases was suggested in two trials in which univariate analysis showed local control to be lower in tumors with a diameter >3 cm or a volume ≥75.2 mL (Lee et al. 2009; Rusthoven et al. 2009). However, other studies did not demonstrate such a relationship (Scorsetti et al. 2015a; Ambrosino et al. 2009; van der Pool et al. 2010; Vautravers-Dewas et al. 2011).

The different rates of overall survival found between studies may have resulted from different inclusion criteria, probably resulting in the selection of patients with differing degrees of intra- and extra-hepatic disease (Chang et al. 2011).

In order to avoid toxicity in the treatment of liver metastases, it is recommended that liver function is adequate and that a sufficient liver volume (700 cm^3) is irradiated under a certain dose (15 Gy in three fractions) (Schefter et al. 2005). The presence of cirrhosis is unusual in patients with liver metastases. To be able to deliver high doses of radiation to the tumor without jeopardizing the luminal organs, it might also be advisable to keep a small distance between the two. Toxicity will be limited by complying with internationally established dose constraints for the liver and other surrounding organs. Although grade ≥3 toxicity is uncommon, there have been episodes of hepatic toxicity (Goodman et al. 2010; Hoyer et al. 2006), elevation of liver enzymes (Lee et al. 2009; Mendez Romero et al. 2006), transient gastritis/esophagitis (Lee et al. 2009), portal hypertension, and asthenia (Mendez Romero et al. 2006). Similarly, there have been reports of isolated cases of soft-tissue toxicity and chronic chest pain (Rusthoven et al. 2009; Vautravers-Dewas et al. 2011; Scorsetti et al. 2013).

To investigate RFA and SBRT as a salvage treatment for colorectal liver metastases in a single institution, a German group compared the outcomes of 30 patients treated with SBRT with those of the same number of patients treated with RFA matched for the size and number of metastases. Although 1- and 2-year local control rates did not differ significantly, local disease-free survival was found significantly in favor of SBRT (Stintzing et al. 2013).

6.2   Hepatocellular Carcinoma

There are a number of challenges for radiotherapy for HCC such as late presentation, concurrent liver disease, difficulties of diagnosis at imaging, contouring uncertainties, liver toxicity, and luminal gastrointestinal toxicity. However, strategies exist for all of these to overcome such barriers. Conventionally fractionated radiotherapeutic regimens are described at the beginning of this chapter, and here the focus will be on SBRT.

SBRT was used for the first time to treat HCC in 1991 by Blomgren et al. (Blomgren et al. 1995) and since then a large number of prospective and retrospective studies have reported the outcome of SBRT on HCC as shown in Table 2 (Mendez Romero et al. 2006; Andolino et al. 2011; Kang et al. 2012; Seo et al. 2010; Bibault et al. 2013; Bujold et al. 2013; Tse et al. 2008; Bae et al. 2013; Culleton et al. 2014; Huang et al. 2012; Huertas et al. 2015; Jang et al. 2013; Jung et al. 2013; Kwon et al. 2010; Price et al. 2012; Que et al. 2014; Scorsetti et al. 2015b; Takeda et al. 2014; Wahl et al. 2016; Weiner et al. 2016). A common feature of all studies on SBRT in HCC with good hepatic tolerance is careful consideration of adequate protection of sufficient non-PTV liver volume. Dose constraints for liver volumes such as protection of 700 mL of the liver below EQD of about 30 Gy using an alpha/beta ratio = 2 Gy are of high importance and some centers prefer to use software to calculate the effective volume treated (v_{eff}) with a NTCP algorithm to avoid RILD. Additionally, it is necessary to take into account Child stages. Generally, Child A is the best indication for SBRT in HCC. Treatment of patients with Child B stage led to more hepatic toxicities with frequent temporary deteriorations of Child scores by 1–2 points. Another risk factor for hepatic toxicity is active hepatitis B, and it is necessary to first start effective antiviral treatment before SBRT is safe to be initiated.

Most series used 3–6 fractions of SBRT at doses that usually were below BED = 100 Gy$_{10}$ that is considered to be necessary to achieve good local control for liver metastasis as well as for lung metastasis with SBRT. Nevertheless, local control rates for HCC typically ranged between 75 and 95% across the series with such radiotherapy doses pointing to better radiosensitivity of HCC compared to secondary liver tumors. It is also necessary to stress that some series reported treatment of very large lesions with a good toxicity profile if liver and GI dose constraints were adequately respected. Due to the frequent proximity of lesions to bowel structures, strategies to protect the duodenum and the stomach were developed which appear to allow safe treatment (Brunner et al. 2016; Tao et al. 2016). However, all of the dose constraints and risk factors for toxicity that were named above have to be carefully taken into account to minimize the risk for toxicities especially to the liver and bowel. Most of the hitherto reported studies are retrospective and therefore they need to be interpreted with caution. Recently, a phase I trial tried to combine SBRT with concurrent sorafenib which was however not successful due to a high rate of gastrointestinal toxicities and also deterioration of the liver function including a loss of liver volume and function after SBRT (Brade et al. 2016; Pollom et al. 2015; Swaminath et al. 2016).

In addition to the above-reported studies on definitive treatment, SBRT has also been used to bridge patients to transplantation. This was especially the case when other local therapies were not suitable (Al Hamad et al. 2009). A prospective SBRT phase II trial included 23 patients of 60 who were treated with SBRT and subsequently underwent transplantation with a 2-year survival of 96% (Andolino et al. 2011). In general, prospective and retrospective studies followed by transplantation did not report an increased risk of toxicities intraoperatively or after transplantation.

6.3 Cholangiocarcinoma

Over the past decade a number of studies have demonstrated that SBRT can achieve good local control rates for IHCC and Klatskin tumors. Prolonged survival in early studies prompted the analysis of dose–response relationship that now has been demonstrated (Tao et al. 2016; Crane et al. 2002; Shinohara et al. 2008). Table 3 summarizes the literature on SBRT in cholangiocarcinoma (Momm et al. 2010; Goodman et al. 2010; Mahadevan et al. 2015; Jung et al. 2014b; Barney et al. 2012; Kopek et al. 2010; Polistina et al. 2011; Tse et al. 2008; Weiner et al. 2016; Ibarra et al. 2012). Similar to HCC, cholangiocarcinoma is locally controlled in 70–90% of the patients with SBRT doses that range in the same area as for HCC, i.e., often below a BED of 100 Gy_{10} that

appears to be necessary to control liver metastases. As the disease is less frequent than HCC most series comprise patient numbers below a total of 30. It is difficult to compare survival between the different series because they contain very heterogeneous stages and both IHCC and EHCC. This explains the wide range of median OS times between 11 and 35 months. Median OS times above 30 months have only been reported for EHCC that usually have smaller tumor volumes compared to IHCC. Hepatic toxicities after SBRT for cholangiocarcinoma are less frequent because usually there is no underlying cirrhosis that additionally compromises liver function. Cholangitis is the most important toxicity-hampering treatment and is also a cause of death. However, cholangitis is often not therapy related (excluding stenting as a radical therapy). Stenting which is often necessary allows bacteria from the gut to ascend into the bile duct and leads frequently to cholangitis. The latter aspect may be one of the reasons why SBRT can more often be administered in full compared to chemoradiotherapy, where chemotherapy-induced neutropenia in combination with cholangitis may be fatal. Bile duct stenosis as a late effect of SBRT is something that has been discussed in the literature but no clear dose-toxicity relationship has been established so far (Tao et al. 2016). Stenting of larger bile ducts often provides an efficient way to treat such complications. As generally for upper abdominal SBRT, GI toxicity has certainly to be considered and adequate sparing of the duodenum and stomach is of high importance to avoid ulceration, bleeding, and perforation. We recommend the use of more fractionated SBRT schedules to cope with the challenges to achieve both local control and low rates of toxicity (Tao et al. 2016; Brunner and Seufferlein 2016).

7 Radiographic Follow-Up

There is no standardized imaging protocol available for assessment of tumor response after SBRT due to limited studies describing radiological alterations after liver SBRT.

Radiographic evaluation of posttreatment tumor changes is currently performed with traditional Response Evaluation Criteria in Solid Tumors (RECIST), based on tumor size. Nevertheless, available data suggest that tumor size response on follow-up imaging is not a reliable test for interpretation, and could be misleading as SBRT target volume goes beyond the tumor margins (Price et al. 2012).

In addition to the tumor size, the parameter of tumor enhancement was added for HCC in order to determine the presence of an active tumor versus treatment-related alterations such as necrosis. This is reflected in a modified mRECIST and EASL (European Association for Study of the Liver) response criteria to liver SBRT (Eisenhauer et al. 2009; Kim et al. 2015; Lencioni and Llovet 2010). However, contrast enhancement within the target site after completion of SBRT has to be interpreted with understanding of a contrast "halo"

formation at the periphery of treatment volume that correlates with radiation-induced histopathologic alterations (Sanuki-Fujimoto et al. 2010), specifically with veno-occlusive disease (Olsen et al. 2009). The contrast enhancement of normal liver parenchyma around the target site has been described in all irradiated patients by 6 months after SBRT (Rusthoven et al. 2009; Brook et al. 2015; Lock et al. 2016). It appears by 3 months, peaks at 6 months, and nearly disappears after 9 months. Awareness of these postradiation changes helps to differentiate a normal halo from a recurrence or progression of disease (Fig. 4).

There are no standardized guidelines available on timing and frequency of posttreatment imaging after SBRT. We perform follow-up imaging at 3-, 6-, 9-, and 12-month intervals for the first year and at intervals of 6 months after 1 year.

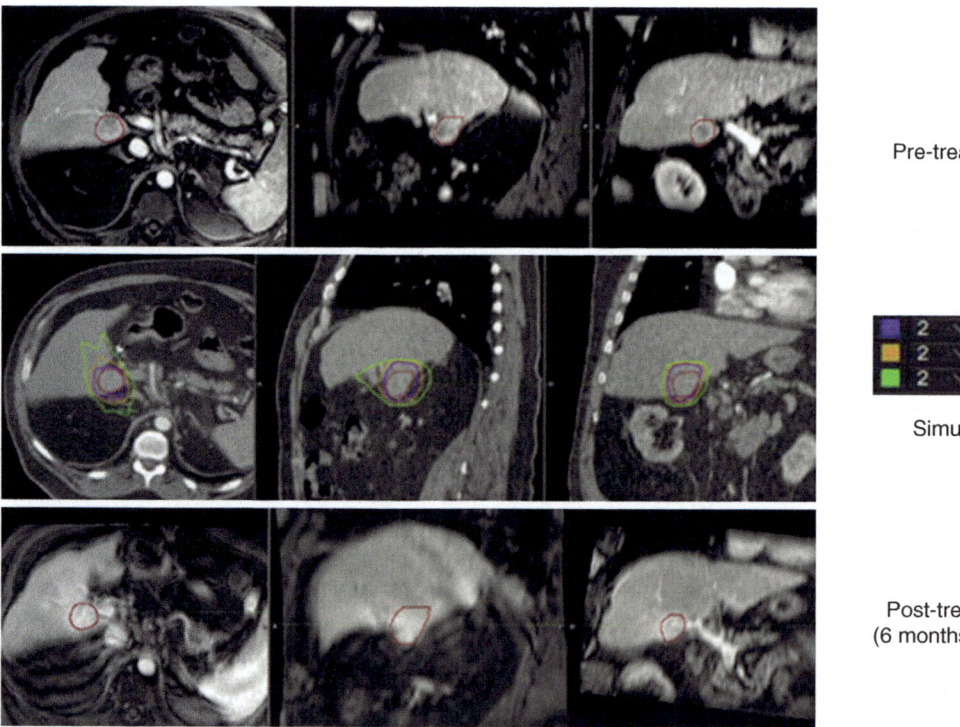

Fig. 4 Patient with a solitary hepatocellular carcinoma and Child-Pugh B cirrhosis completed liver SBRT to 45 Gy in five fractions as a bridging therapy prior to liver transplant. MRI scan (*upper* panel) demonstrates a 2.5 cm tumor with contrast washout outlined in red as gross target volume (GTV). Middle panel represents CT simulation images of the same patient with isodose lines encompassing GTV. Patient received liver transplant in 6 months after completion of SBRT with pretransplant MRI demonstrating diffuse contrast enhancement within the GTV in the absence of contrast washout (*lower* panel). Pathologic assessment of the explanted liver demonstrates tumor downsizing to 0.3 cm with active fibrotic reaction of surrounding hepatic parenchyma

References

Al Hamad AA, Hassanain M, Michel RP et al (2009) Stereotactic radiotherapy of the liver: a bridge to transplantation stereotactic radiotherapy of the liver: a bridge to transplantation. Technol Cancer Res Treat 8(6):401–405

Ambrosino G, Polistina F, Costantin G et al (2009) Image-guided robotic stereotactic radiosurgery for unresectable liver metastases: preliminary results. Anticancer Res 29(8):3381–3384

Andolino DL, Johnson CS, Maluccio M et al (2011) Stereotactic body radiotherapy for primary hepatocellular carcinoma. Int J Radiat Oncol Biol Phys 81(4):e447–e453

Bae SH, Kim MS, Cho CK et al (2013) Feasibility and efficacy of stereotactic ablative radiotherapy for Barcelona Clinic Liver Cancer-C stage hepatocellular carcinoma. J Korean Med Sci 28(2):213–219

Barney BM, Olivier KR, Miller RC et al (2012) Clinical outcomes and toxicity using stereotactic body radiotherapy (SBRT) for advanced cholangiocarcinoma. Radiat Oncol 7:67

Benavides M, Anton A, Gallego J et al (2015) Biliary tract cancers: SEOM clinical guidelines. Clin Transl Oncol 17(12):982–987

Ben-Josef E, Normolle D, Ensminger WD et al (2005) Phase II trial of high-dose conformal radiation therapy with concurrent hepatic artery floxuridine for unresectable intrahepatic malignancies. J Clin Oncol 23(34):8739–8747

Bibault JE, Dewas S, Vautravers-Dewas C et al (2013) Stereotactic body radiation therapy for hepatocellular carcinoma: prognostic factors of local control, overall survival, and toxicity. PLoS One 8(10):e77472

Blomgren H, Lax I, Naslund I et al (1995) Stereotactic high dose fraction radiation therapy of extracranial tumors using an accelerator. Clinical experience of the first thirty-one patients. Acta Oncol 34(6):861–870

Boda-Heggemann J, Knopf AC, Simeonova-Chergou A et al (2016) Deep inspiration breath hold-based radiation therapy: a clinical review. Int J Radiat Oncol Biol Phys 94(3):478–492

Brade AM, Ng S, Brierley J et al (2016) Phase 1 trial of sorafenib and stereotactic body radiation therapy for hepatocellular carcinoma. Int J Radiat Oncol Biol Phys 94(3):580–587

Breedveld S, Storchi PR, Heijmen BJ (2009) The equivalence of multi-criteria methods for radiotherapy plan optimization. Phys Med Biol 54(23):7199–7209

Breedveld S, Storchi PR, Voet PW et al (2012) iCycle: integrated, multicriterial beam angle, and profile optimization for generation of coplanar and noncoplanar IMRT plans. Med Phys 39(2):951–963

Brook OR, Thornton E, Mendiratta-Lala M et al (2015) CT imaging findings after stereotactic radiotherapy for liver tumors. Gastroenterol Res Pract 2015:126245

Bruix J, Sherman M (2005) Management of hepatocellular carcinoma. Hepatology 42(5):1208–1236

Bruix J, Sherman M (2011) Management of hepatocellular carcinoma: an update. Hepatology 53(3):1020–1022

Brunner TB, Seufferlein T (2016) Radiation therapy in cholangiocellular carcinomas. Best Pract Res Clin Gastroenterol 30(4):593–602

Brunner TB, Nestle U, Adebahr S et al (2016) Simultaneous integrated protection: a new concept for high-precision radiation therapy. Strahlenther Onkol 192(12):886–894

Bujold A, Massey CA, Kim JJ et al (2013) Sequential phase I and II trials of stereotactic body radiotherapy for locally advanced hepatocellular carcinoma. J Clin Oncol 31(13):1631–1639

Cardenes HR, Price TR, Perkins SM et al (2010) Phase I feasibility trial of stereotactic body radiation therapy for primary hepatocellular carcinoma. Clin Transl Oncol 12(3):218–225

Chang DT, Swaminath A, Kozak M et al (2011) Stereotactic body radiotherapy for colorectal liver metastases: a pooled analysis. Cancer 117(17):4060–4069

Chi A, Nguyen NP (2014) 4D PET/CT as a strategy to reduce respiratory motion artifacts in FDG-PET/CT. Front Oncol 4:205

Crane CH, Macdonald KO, Vauthey JN et al (2002) Limitations of conventional doses of chemoradiation for unresectable biliary cancer. Int J Radiat Oncol Biol Phys 53(4):969–974

Culleton S, Jiang H, Haddad CR et al (2014) Outcomes following definitive stereotactic body radiotherapy for patients with Child-Pugh B or C hepatocellular carcinoma. Radiother Oncol 111(3):412–417

Dawson LA, McGinn CJ, Normolle D et al (2000) Escalated focal liver radiation and concurrent hepatic artery fluorodeoxyuridine for unresectable intrahepatic malignancies. J Clin Oncol 18(11):2210–2218

Dawson LA, Eccles C, Bissonnette JP et al (2005) Accuracy of daily image guidance for hypofractionated liver radiotherapy with active breathing control. Int J Radiat Oncol Biol Phys 62(4):1247–1252

Dawson LA, Eccles C, Craig T (2006) Individualized image guided iso-NTCP based liver cancer SBRT. Acta Oncol 45(7):856–864

Dong P, Lee P, Ruan D et al (2013) 4pi non-coplanar liver SBRT: a novel delivery technique. Int J Radiat Oncol Biol Phys 85(5):1360–1366

Eisenhauer EA, Therasse P, Bogaerts J et al (2009) New response evaluation criteria in solid tumours: revised RECIST guideline (version 1.1). Eur J Cancer 45(2):228–247

European Association for the Study of the Liver, European Organisation for Research and Treatment of Cancer (2012) EASL-EORTC clinical practice guidelines: management of hepatocellular carcinoma. J Hepatol 56(4):908–943

Facciuto ME, Singh MK, Rochon C et al (2012) Stereotactic body radiation therapy in hepatocellular carcinoma and cirrhosis: evaluation of radiological and pathological response. J Surg Oncol 105(7):692–698

Forner A, Vilana R, Ayuso C et al (2008) Diagnosis of hepatic nodules 20 mm or smaller in cirrhosis: Prospective validation of the noninvasive diagnostic criteria for hepatocellular carcinoma. Hepatology 47(1):97–104

Fowler JF (1989) The linear-quadratic formula and progress in fractionated radiotherapy. Br J Radiol 62(740):679–694

Fowler JF, Tome WA, Fenwick JD et al (2004) A challenge to traditional radiation oncology. Int J Radiat Oncol Biol Phys 60(4):1241–1256

Glide-Hurst CK, Schwenker SM, Ajlouni M et al (2013) Evaluation of two synchronized external surrogates for 4D CT sorting. J Appl Clin Med Phys 14(6):4301

Goodman ZD (2007) Neoplasms of the liver. Mod Pathol 20(Suppl 1):S49–S60

Goodman KA, Wiegner EA, Maturen KE et al (2010) Dose-escalation study of single-fraction stereotactic body radiotherapy for liver malignancies. Int J Radiat Oncol Biol Phys 78(2):486–493

Goodman BD, Mannina EM, Althouse SK et al (2016) Long-term safety and efficacy of stereotactic body radiation therapy for hepatic oligometastases. Pract Radiat Oncol 6(2):86–95

Guckenberger M, Richter A, Boda-Heggemann J et al (2012) Motion compensation in radiotherapy. Crit Rev Biomed Eng 40(3):187–197

Hatfield MK, Beres RA, Sane SS et al (2008) Percutaneous imaging-guided solid organ core needle biopsy: coaxial versus noncoaxial method. Am J Roentgenol 190(2):413–417

Heijmen B, de Pooter JA, Mendez Romero A, et al (2007) Computer generation of fully non-coplanar plans for SBRT of liver tumours based on gEUD optimisation. In: Proceedings of the XVth International Conference on the use of Computers in Radiation Therapy, Toronto, 2007. pp 333–337

Heinzerling JH, Anderson JF, Papiez L et al (2008) Four-dimensional computed tomography scan analysis of tumor and organ motion at varying levels of abdominal compression during stereotactic treatment of lung and liver. Int J Radiat Oncol Biol Phys 70(5):1571–1578

Hoyer M, Roed H, Traberg HA et al (2006) Phase II study on stereotactic body radiotherapy of colorectal metastases. Acta Oncol 45(7):823–830

Huang WY, Jen YM, Lee MS et al (2012) Stereotactic body radiation therapy in recurrent hepatocellular carcinoma. Int J Radiat Oncol Biol Phys 84(2):355–361

Huertas A, Baumann AS, Saunier-Kubs F et al (2015) Stereotactic body radiation therapy as an ablative treatment for inoperable hepatocellular carcinoma. Radiother Oncol 115(2):211–216

Ibarra RA, Rojas D, Snyder L et al (2012) Multicenter results of stereotactic body radiotherapy (SBRT) for non-resectable primary liver tumors. Acta Oncol 51(5):575–583

Ingold JA, Reed GB, Kaplan HS et al (1965) Radiation Hepatitis. Am J Roentgenol Radium Therapy, Nucl Med 93:200–208

Iwata H, Shibamoto Y, Hashizume C et al (2010) Hypofractionated stereotactic body radiotherapy for primary and metastatic liver tumors using the Novalis image-guided system: preliminary results regarding efficacy and toxicity. Technol Cancer Res Treat 9(6):619–627

Jackson A, Ten Haken RK, Robertson JM et al (1995) Analysis of clinical complication data for radiation hepatitis using a parallel architecture model. Int J Radiat Oncol Biol Phys 31(4):883–891

Jang WI, Kim MS, Bae SH et al (2013) High-dose stereotactic body radiotherapy correlates increased local control and overall survival in patients with inoperable hepatocellular carcinoma. Radiat Oncol 8:250

Jiang SB, Wolfgang J, Mageras GS (2008) Quality assurance challenges for motion-adaptive radiation therapy: gating, breath holding, and four-dimensional computed tomography. Int J Radiat Oncol Biol Phys 71(1 Suppl):S103–S107

Jung J, Yoon SM, Kim SY et al (2013) Radiation-induced liver disease after stereotactic body radiotherapy for small hepatocellular carcinoma: clinical and dose-volumetric parameters. Radiat Oncol 8:249

Jung J, Kong M, Hong SE (2014a) Conventional fractionated helical tomotherapy for patients with small to medium hepatocellular carcinomas without portal vein tumor thrombosis. Onco Targets Ther 7:1769–1775

Jung DH, Kim MS, Cho CK et al (2014b) Outcomes of stereotactic body radiotherapy for unresectable primary or recurrent cholangiocarcinoma. Radiat Oncol J 32(3):163–169

Kang JK, Kim MS, Cho CK et al (2012) Stereotactic body radiation therapy for inoperable hepatocellular carcinoma as a local salvage treatment after incomplete transarterial chemoembolization. Cancer 118(21):5424–5431

Katz AW, Chawla S, Qu Z et al (2011) Stereotactic hypofractionated radiation therapy as a bridge to transplantation for hepatocellular carcinoma: clinical outcome and pathologic correlation. Int J Radiat Oncol Biol Phys 83(3):895–900

Kavanagh BD, Timmerman RD, Benedict SH et al (2003) How should we describe the radiobiologic effect of extracranial stereotactic radiosurgery: equivalent uniform dose or tumor control probability? Med Phys 30(3):321–324

Keall PJ, Mageras GS, Balter JM et al (2006) The management of respiratory motion in radiation oncology report of AAPM Task Group 76. Med Phys 33(10):3874–3900

Khan SA, Davidson BR, Goldin RD et al (2012) Guidelines for the diagnosis and treatment of cholangiocarcinoma: an update. Gut 61(12):1657–1669

Kim MN, Kim BK, Han KH et al (2015) Evolution from WHO to EASL and mRECIST for hepatocellular carcinoma: considerations for tumor response assessment. Expert Rev Gastroenterol Hepatol 9(3):335–348

Kimura T, Aikata H, Takahashi S et al (2015) Stereotactic body radiotherapy for patients with small hepatocellular carcinoma ineligible for resection or ablation therapies. Hepatol Res 45(4):378–386

Klein J, Dawson LA (2013) Hepatocellular carcinoma radiation therapy: review of evidence and future opportunities. Int J Radiat Oncol Biol Phys 87(1):22–32

Kong M, Hong SE (2015) Optimal follow-up duration for evaluating objective response to radiotherapy in patients with hepatocellular carcinoma: a retrospective study. Chin J Cancer 34(2):79–85

Kong M, Hong SE, Choi WS et al (2013) Treatment outcomes of helical intensity-modulated radiotherapy for unresectable hepatocellular carcinoma. Gut Liver 7(3):343–351

Kopek N, Holt MI, Hansen AT et al (2010) Stereotactic body radiotherapy for unresectable cholangiocarcinoma. Radiother Oncol 94(1):47–52

Kudo M (2010) Real practice of hepatocellular carcinoma in Japan: conclusions of the Japan Society of Hepatology 2009 Kobe Congress. Oncology 78(Suppl 1):180–188

Kwon JH, Bae SH, Kim JY et al (2010) Long-term effect of stereotactic body radiation therapy for primary hepatocellular carcinoma ineligible for local ablation therapy or surgical resection. Stereotactic radiotherapy for liver cancer. BMC Cancer 10:475

Lagendijk JJ, Raaymakers BW, van Vulpen M (2014) The magnetic resonance imaging-linac system. Semin Radiat Oncol 24(3):207–209

Lee MT, Kim JJ, Dinniwell R et al (2009) Phase I study of individualized stereotactic body radiotherapy of liver metastases. J Clin Oncol 27(10):1585–1591

Leinders SM, Breedveld S, Mendez Romero A et al (2013) Adaptive liver stereotactic body radiation therapy: automated daily plan reoptimization prevents dose delivery degradation caused by anatomy deformations. Int J Radiat Oncol Biol Phys 87(5):1016–1021

Lencioni R, Llovet JM (2010) Modified RECIST (mRECIST) assessment for hepatocellular carcinoma. Semin Liver Dis 30(1):52–60

Li J, Xiao Y (2013) Application of FDG-PET/CT in radiation oncology. Front Oncol 3:80

Li XA, Stepaniak C, Gore E (2006) Technical and dosimetric aspects of respiratory gating using a pressure-sensor motion monitoring system. Med Phys 33(1):145–154

Liu MT, Li SH, Chu TC et al (2004) Three-dimensional conformal radiation therapy for unresectable hepatocellular carcinoma patients who had failed with or were unsuited for transcatheter arterial chemoembolization. Jpn J Clin Oncol 34(9):532–539

Lo SS, Teh BS, Mayr NA et al (2010) Stereotactic body radiation therapy for oligometastases. Discov Med 10(52):247–254

Lock M, Malayeri AA, Mian OY et al (2016) Computed tomography imaging assessment of postexternal beam radiation changes of the liver. Future Oncol 12(23):2729–2739

Louis C, Dewas S, Mirabel X et al (2010) Stereotactic radiotherapy of hepatocellular carcinoma: preliminary results. Technol Cancer Res Treat 9(5):479–487

Mahadevan A, Dagoglu N, Mancias J et al (2015) Stereotactic Body Radiotherapy (SBRT) for intrahepatic and hilar cholangiocarcinoma. J Cancer 6(11):1099–1104

McCammon R, Schefter TE, Gaspar LE et al (2009) Observation of a dose-control relationship for lung and liver tumors after stereotactic body radiation therapy. Int J Radiat Oncol Biol Phys 73(1):112–118

Mendez Romero A, de Man RA (2016) Stereotactic body radiation therapy for primary and metastatic liver tumors: from technological evolution to improved patient care. Best Pract Res Clin Gastroenterol 30(4):603–616

Mendez Romero A, Hoyer M (2012) Radiation therapy for liver metastases. Curr Opin Support Palliat Care 6(1):97–102

Mendez Romero A, Wunderink W, Hussain SM et al (2006) Stereotactic body radiation therapy for primary and metastatic liver tumors: a single institution phase i-ii study. Acta Oncol 45(7):831–837

Meyer JJ, Foster RD, Lev-Cohain N et al (2016) A phase I dose-escalation trial of single-fraction stereotactic radiation therapy for liver metastases. Ann Surg Oncol 23(1):218–224

Molinelli S, de Pooter J, Mendez-Romero A et al (2008) Simultaneous tumour dose escalation and liver sparing in Stereotactic Body Radiation Therapy (SBRT) for liver tumours due to CTV-to-PTV margin reduction. Radiother Oncol 87(3):432–438

Momm F, Schubert E, Henne K et al (2010) Stereotactic fractionated radiotherapy for Klatskin tumours. Radiother Oncol 95(1):99–102

Mutic S, Dempsey JF (2014) The ViewRay system: magnetic resonance-guided and controlled radiotherapy. Semin Radiat Oncol 24(3):196–199

Nehmeh SA, Erdi YE, Pan T et al (2004) Quantitation of respiratory motion during 4D-PET/CT acquisition. Med Phys 31(6):1333–1338

Niemierko A (1997) Reporting and analyzing dose distributions: a concept of equivalent uniform dose. Med Phys 24(1):103–110

O'Connor JK, Trotter J, Davis GL et al (2012) Long-term outcomes of stereotactic body radiation therapy in the treatment of hepatocellular cancer as a bridge to transplantation. Liver Transpl 18(8):949–954

Ohri N, Jackson A, Mendez-Romero A et al (2014) Local control following stereotactic body radiotherapy for liver tumors: a preliminary report of the AAPM Working Group for SBRT. Int J Radiat Oncol Biol Phys 90(1):S52

Olsen CC, Welsh J, Kavanagh BD et al (2009) Microscopic and macroscopic tumor and parenchymal effects of liver stereotactic body radiotherapy. Int J Radiat Oncol Biol Phys 73(5):1414–1424

Omata M, Lesmana LA, Tateishi R et al (2010) Asian Pacific Association for the study of the liver consensus recommendations on hepatocellular carcinoma. Hepatol Int 4(2):439–474

Pan T, Mawlawi O (2008) PET/CT in radiation oncology. Med Phys 35(11):4955–4966

Park JH, Yoon SM, Lim YS et al (2013) Two-week schedule of hypofractionated radiotherapy as a local salvage treatment for small hepatocellular carcinoma. J Gastroenterol Hepatol 28(10):1638–1642

Polistina FA, Guglielmi R, Baiocchi C et al (2011) Chemoradiation treatment with gemcitabine plus stereotactic body radiotherapy for unresectable, non-metastatic, locally advanced hilar cholangiocarcinoma. Results of a five year experience. Radiother Oncol 99(2):120–123

Pollom EL, Deng L, Pai RK et al (2015) Gastrointestinal toxicities with combined antiangiogenic and stereotactic body radiation therapy. Int J Radiat Oncol Biol Phys 92(3):568–576

van der Pool AE, Mendez Romero A, Wunderink W et al (2010) Stereotactic body radiation therapy for colorectal liver metastases. Br J Surg 97(3):377–382

de Pooter JA, Mendez Romero A, Jansen WP et al (2006) Computer optimization of noncoplanar beam setups improves stereotactic treatment of liver tumors. Int J Radiat Oncol Biol Phys 66(3):913–922

de Pooter JA, Wunderink W, Mendez Romero A et al (2007) PTV dose prescription strategies for SBRT of metastatic liver tumours. Radiother Oncol 85(2):260–266

de Pooter JA, Mendez Romero A, Wunderink W et al (2008) Automated non-coplanar beam direction optimization improves IMRT in SBRT of liver metastasis. Radiother Oncol 88(3):376–381

Price TR, Perkins SM, Sandrasegaran K et al (2012) Evaluation of response after stereotactic body radiotherapy for hepatocellular carcinoma. Cancer 118(12):3191–3198

Que JY, Lin LC, Lin KL et al (2014) The efficacy of stereotactic body radiation therapy on huge hepatocellular carcinoma unsuitable for other local modalities. Radiat Oncol 9:120

Rim CH, Yang DS, Park YJ et al (2012) Effectiveness of high-dose three-dimensional conformal radiotherapy in hepatocellular carcinoma with portal vein thrombosis. Jpn J Clin Oncol 42(8):721–729

Rossi L, Breedveld S, Heijmen BJ et al (2012) On the beam direction search space in computerized non-coplanar beam angle optimization for IMRT-prostate SBRT. Phys Med Biol 57(17):5441–5458

Rule W, Timmerman R, Tong L et al (2011) Phase I dose-escalation study of stereotactic body radiotherapy in patients with hepatic metastases. Ann Surg Oncol 18(4):1081–1087

Rusthoven KE, Kavanagh BD, Cardenes H et al (2009) Multi-institutional phase I/II trial of stereotactic body radiation therapy for liver metastases. J Clin Oncol 27(10):1572–1578

Sandroussi C, Dawson LA, Lee M et al (2010) Radiotherapy as a bridge to liver transplantation for hepatocellular carcinoma. Transpl Int 23(3):299–306

Sanuki N, Takeda A, Oku Y et al (2014) Stereotactic body radiotherapy for small hepatocellular carcinoma: a retrospective outcome analysis in 185 patients. Acta Oncol 53(3):399–404

Sanuki-Fujimoto N, Takeda A, Ohashi T et al (2010) CT evaluations of focal liver reactions following stereotactic body radiotherapy for small hepatocellular carcinoma with cirrhosis: relationship between imaging appearance and baseline liver function. Br J Radiol 83(996):1063–1071

Schefter TE, Kavanagh BD, Timmerman RD et al (2005) A phase I trial of stereotactic body radiation therapy (SBRT) for liver metastases. Int J Radiat Oncol Biol Phys 62(5):1371–1378

Scorsetti M, Arcangeli S, Tozzi A et al (2013) Is stereotactic body radiation therapy an attractive option for unresectable liver metastases? A preliminary report from a phase 2 trial. Int J Radiat Oncol Biol Phys 86(2):336–342

Scorsetti M, Comito T, Tozzi A et al (2015a) Final results of a phase II trial for stereotactic body radiation therapy for patients with inoperable liver metastases from colorectal cancer. J Cancer Res Clin Oncol 141(3):543–553

Scorsetti M, Comito T, Cozzi L et al (2015b) The challenge of inoperable hepatocellular carcinoma (HCC): results of a single-institutional experience on stereotactic body radiation therapy (SBRT). J Cancer Res Clin Oncol 141(7):1301–1309

Seo YS, Kim MS, Yoo SY et al (2010) Preliminary result of stereotactic body radiotherapy as a local salvage treatment for inoperable hepatocellular carcinoma. J Surg Oncol 102(3):209–214

Seppenwoolde Y, Wunderink W, Wunderink-van Veen SR et al (2011) Treatment precision of image-guided liver SBRT using implanted fiducial markers depends on marker-tumour distance. Phys Med Biol 56(17):5445–5468

Sharfo AW, Voet PW, Breedveld S et al (2015) Comparison of VMAT and IMRT strategies for cervical cancer patients using automated planning. Radiother Oncol 114(3):395–401

Sharfo AW, Breedveld S, Voet PW et al (2016) Validation of fully automated VMAT plan generation for library-based plan-of-the-day cervical cancer radiotherapy. PLoS One 11(12):e0169202

Sharfo AWM, Dirkx MLP, Breedveld S, Méndez Romero A, Heijmen BJM (n.d.) VMAT plus a few computer-optimized non-coplanar IMRT beams (VMAT+)—a novel treatment strategy tested for liver SBRT. Radioth Oncol (accepted for publication)

Shinohara ET, Mitra N, Guo M et al (2008) Radiation therapy is associated with improved survival in the adjuvant and definitive treatment of intrahepatic cholangiocarcinoma. Int J Radiat Oncol Biol Phys 72(5):1495–1501

Simmonds PC, Primrose JN, Colquitt JL et al (2006) Surgical resection of hepatic metastases from colorectal cancer: a systematic review of published studies. Br J Cancer 94(7):982–999

Stintzing S, Hoffmann RT, Heinemann V et al (2010) Frameless single-session robotic radiosurgery of liver metastases in colorectal cancer patients. Eur J Cancer 46(6):1026–1032

Stintzing S, Grothe A, Hendrich S et al (2013) Percutaneous radiofrequency ablation (RFA) or robotic radiosurgery

(RRS) for salvage treatment of colorectal liver metastases. Acta Oncol 52(5):971–977

Su TS, Liang P, Lu HZ et al (2016) Stereotactic body radiation therapy for small primary or recurrent hepatocellular carcinoma in 132 Chinese patients. J Surg Oncol 113(2):181–187

Suit H, Skates S, Taghian A et al (1992) Clinical implications of heterogeneity of tumor response to radiation therapy. Radiother Oncol 25(4):251–260

Swaminath A, Knox JJ, Brierley JD et al (2016) Changes in liver volume observed following sorafenib and liver radiation therapy. Int J Radiat Oncol Biol Phys 94(4):729–737

Takeda A, Sanuki N, Eriguchi T et al (2014) Stereotactic ablative body radiotherapy for previously untreated solitary hepatocellular carcinoma. J Gastroenterol Hepatol 29(2):372–379

Tao R, Krishnan S, Bhosale PR et al (2016) Ablative radiotherapy doses lead to a substantial prolongation of survival in patients with inoperable intrahepatic cholangiocarcinoma: a retrospective dose response analysis. J Clin Oncol 34(3):219–226

Tse RV, Hawkins M, Lockwood G et al (2008) Phase I study of individualized stereotactic body radiotherapy for hepatocellular carcinoma and intrahepatic cholangiocarcinoma. J Clin Oncol 26(4):657–664

Valle J, Wasan H, Palmer DH et al (2010) Cisplatin plus gemcitabine versus gemcitabine for biliary tract cancer. N Engl J Med 362(14):1273–1281

Vautravers-Dewas C, Dewas S, Bonodeau F et al (2011) Image-guided robotic stereotactic body radiation therapy for liver metastases: is there a dose response relationship? Int J Radiat Oncol Biol Phys 81(3):e39–e47

Voet PW, Breedveld S, Dirkx ML et al (2012) Integrated multicriterial optimization of beam angles and intensity profiles for coplanar and noncoplanar head and neck IMRT and implications for VMAT. Med Phys 39(8):4858–4865

Voet PW, Dirkx n, Breedveld S et al (2013a) Automated generation of IMRT treatment plans for prostate cancer patients with metal hip prostheses: comparison of different planning strategies. Med Phys 40(7):701–704

Voet PW, Dirkx ML, Breedveld S et al (2013b) Toward fully automated multicriterial plan generation: a prospective clinical study. Int J Radiat Oncol Biol Phys 85(3):866–872

Voet PW, Dirkx ML, Breedveld S et al (2014) Fully automated volumetric modulated arc therapy plan generation for prostate cancer patients. Int J Radiat Oncol Biol Phys 88(5):1175–1179

Wahl DR, Stenmark MH, Tao Y et al (2016) Outcomes after stereotactic body radiotherapy or radiofrequency ablation for hepatocellular carcinoma. J Clin Oncol 34(5):452–459

Weiner AA, Olsen J, Ma D et al (2016) Stereotactic body radiotherapy for primary hepatic malignancies—report of a phase I/II institutional study. Radiother Oncol 121(1):79–85

Welling TH, Feng M, Wan S et al (2014) Neoadjuvant stereotactic body radiation therapy, capecitabine, and liver transplantation for unresectable hilar cholangiocarcinoma. Liver Transpl 20(1):81–88

Wharton JT, Delclos L, Gallager S et al (1973) Radiation hepatitis induced by abdominal irradiation with the cobalt 60 moving strip technique. Am J Roentgenol Radium Therapy, Nucl Med 117(1):73–80

Withers HR, Thames HD Jr, Peters LJ (1983) A new isoeffect curve for change in dose per fraction. Radiother Oncol 1(2):187–191

Wong SL, Mangu PB, Choti MA et al (2010) American Society of Clinical Oncology 2009 clinical evidence review on radiofrequency ablation of hepatic metastases from colorectal cancer. J Clin Oncol 28(3):493–508

Woods K, Nguyen D, Tran A et al (2016) Viability of noncoplanar VMAT for liver SBRT as compared to coplanar VMAT and beam orientation optimized 4pi IMRT. Adv Radiat Oncol 1(1):67–75

Woudstra E, Storchi PR (2000) Constrained treatment planning using sequential beam selection. Phys Med Biol 45(8):2133–2149

Wulf J, Guckenberger M, Haedinger U et al (2006) Stereotactic radiotherapy of primary liver cancer and hepatic metastases. Acta Oncol 45(7):838–847

Wunderink W, Mendez-Romero A, de Kruijf W et al (2008) Reduction of respiratory liver tumor motion by abdominal compression in stereotactic body frame, analyzed by tracking fiducial markers implanted in liver. Int J Radiat Oncol Biol Phys 71(3):907–915

Wunderink W, Mendez-Romero A, Seppenwoolde Y et al (2010) Potentials and limitations of guiding liver stereotactic body radiation therapy set-up on liver-implanted fiducial markers. Int J Radiat Oncol Biol Phys 77(5):1573–1583

Stereotactic Body Radiotherapy with Functional Treatment Planning in Hepatocellular Carcinoma

Alexander Kirichenko, Eugene J. Koay,
Shaakir Hasan, and Christopher Crane

Contents

Abstract

Hepatocellular carcinoma (HCC) is the fastest growing cause of cancer-related death in the United States, and considered an aggressive tumor with mean survival estimated between 6 and 20 months (El-Serag, NEJM 365:1118–1127, 2011). The choice of curative liver resection is limited by the presence of hepatic cirrhosis in 90% of patients, and the most appropriate therapy for HCC has historically been hepatic transplantation with 5-year survival rate of up to 85%. However, only 10% of patients are eligible for surgery (Fortune et al., J Clin Gastroenterol 47:S37–S42, 2013). We discuss functional treatment planning for patients with hepatic cirrhosis and HCC and present an argument in favor of liver SBRT as a viable option.

The original version of this chapter was revised. The affiliations of the authors have been updated.

A. Kirichenko (✉) • S. Hasan
Department of Radiation Oncology,
Allegheny Health Network Cancer Institute,
Pittsburgh, PA, USA
e-mail: Alexander.Kirichenko@ahn.org

E. J. Koay
MD Anderson Cancer Center, Houston, TX, USA

C. Crane
Memorial Sloan Kettering Cancer Center, New York, NY, USA

1 Introduction

SBRT for unresectable hepatoma provides local control rates in the range of 75–100% with low toxicity (Klein and Dawson 2013). It can be applied for tumor downsizing or as bridging therapy for patients awaiting liver transplantation (Katz et al. 2012; Kirichenko et al. 2016) or used in combination with trans-arterial hepatic chemo-embolization (TACE) for more advanced tumors (Meng et al. 2009). As more data indicate the efficacy and curative potential of SBRT for patients with HCC, there is a

Med Radiol Radiat Oncol (2017)
DOI 10.1007/174_2017_42, © Springer International Publishing AG
Published Online: 07 April 2017

greater need to optimize therapy. It has been demonstrated that patients with more advanced hepatic cirrhosis are at a much higher risk of developing radiation-induced liver disease (RILD) than patients with hepatic tumors in the absence of cirrhosis (Cheng et al. 2002, 2004; Liang et al. 2006; Andolino et al. 2011; Xu et al. 2006).

Lawrence et al. demonstrated the impact of nondosimetric biologic parameters on RILD with a tolerance dose of 50% of the hepatic volume (TD_{50}) for patients with primary versus metastatic hepatic malignancy of 39.8 Gy and 45.8 Gy, respectively (Lawrence et al. 1992). Multiple data indicate that the severity of hepatic cirrhosis in patients with HCC undergoing three-dimensional conformal radiotherapy (3D-CRT) directly correlates with the incidence of lethal RILD (Cheng et al. 2002, 2006; Liang et al. 2006; Andolino et al. 2011; Mendez-Romero et al. 2006; Bujold et al. 2013; Lasley et al. 2015). Therefore, it is advisable to estimate the dynamics of Child-Pugh score changes after completion of liver SBRT to grade the prognosis of RILD in cirrhotic patients (Guha and Kavanagh 2011). The Child-Pugh score employs five clinical measures of liver disease. Each measure is scored 1–3, with 3 indicating most severe derangement (Table 1) (Cholongitas et al. 2005).

Another scoring system for assessment of the severity of liver disease in cirrhotic patients is a Model for End-Stage Liver Disease or MELD score. The MELD system uses the patient's values for serum bilirubin, serum creatinine, and the international normalized ratio for prothrombin time (INR) to predict survival. It is calculated according to the following formula (Kamath and Kim 2007):

$$MELD = 3.78 \times \ln[\text{serum bilirubin (mg/dL)}] + 11.2 \times \ln[\text{INR}] + 9.57 \times \ln[\text{serum creatinine (mg/dL)}] + 6.43$$

This scoring system is preferred by the United Network for Organ Sharing (UNOS) and Eurotransplant in determining survival prognosis based on the severity of hepatic dysfunction in prioritizing allocation of liver transplants instead of the Child-Pugh score (Wiesner et al. 2003). A MELD score ≥9 is a threshold measure of a patient's mortality and decreased long-term survival (Teh et al. 2005; Cucchetti et al. 2006). In our practice we use both MELD and Child-Pugh scores to assess the dynamics of liver function following SBRT in patients with HCC.

Higher sensitivity of cirrhotic livers to irradiation could be linked to active proliferation of fibrotic tissue with loss of hepatic functional reserve characterized by combined function of hepatocytes and nonparenchymal cells residing along hepatic sinusoids (Kupffer cells, endothelial cells, stellate, and pit cells). As a result, cirrhotic liver volume obtained from 3D-CRT may not adequately represent functional hepatic parenchyma and CT-based dose volume constraints applied to noncirrhotic livers may be inappropriate. Therefore, prediction of RILD by the normal tissue complication probability (NTCP) model for patients with advanced cirrhosis can be underestimated (Xu et al. 2006).

Preoperative assessment of hepatic functional reserve is one of the most important issues in resection of primary hepatic tumors. Functional imaging modalities, such as single-photon emission hepatic computed tomography (SPECT) with ^{99m}Tc-galactosyl serum albumin (^{99m}Tc-GSA) and magnetic resonance imaging with gadolinium-ethoxybenzyl-diethylenetriamine pentaacetic acid (E-DTPA), provide visualization of hepatic functional remnants in cirrhotic livers prior to surgery and allow selecting patients for safe hepatic resection (Schneider 2004).

Recent data indicate feasibility of this approach for radiotherapy planning. Imaging of a

Table 1 Child-Pugh (C-P)[a] hepatic function scoring system

Measure	1 point	2 points	3 points
Total bilirubin, μmol/L (mg/dL)	<34 (<2)	34–50 (2–3)	>50 (>3)
Serum albumin, g/dL	>3.5	2.8–3.5	<2.8
Prothrombin time prolongation	<4.0	4.0–6.0	>6.0
Ascites	None	Mild (or suppressed with medication)	Moderate to severe (or refractory)
Hepatic encephalopathy	None	Grades I–II	Grades III–IV

[a]Child-Pugh A score range = 5–6, C-P B = 7–9, C-P C = 10–15

hepatocyte mass with ^{99m}Tc-GSA SPECT helped to direct radiation beams during 3D-CRT in combination with transcatheter arterial chemo-embolization (TACE) for bulky HCC with portal vein tumor thrombus (Shirai et al. 2010).

Emerging but limited data exist on functional planning of stereotactic liver radiotherapy in cirrhotic patients utilizing ^{99m}Tc-sulfur colloid hepatic SPECT/CT. ^{99m}Tc-sulfur colloid is a known, FDA-approved diagnostic radiopharmaceutical that is selectively taken up by nonparenchymal hepatic Kupffer cell masses in proportion to sinusoidal blood flow (Everson et al. 2012; Hoefs et al. 1997; Zuckerman et al. 2003). When irradiated, Kupffer cells release oxygen radicals, tumor necrosis factor, and interleukins 1 and 6 which are responsible for early apoptosis of hepatocytes, delayed periportal fibrosis, and sinusoidal congestion—all characteristics of RILD (Christiansen et al. 2004; Tello et al. 2008; Seong et al. 2000). Furthermore, selective depletion of Kupffer cells with gadolinium chloride prior to whole-liver irradiation significantly reduces the production of reactive cytokines and protects animals against acute RILD with marked decrease in liver enzymatic activity, hepatocyte apoptosis, and micronucleus formation (Du et al. 2010).

Evolving data on ^{99m}Tc-sulfur colloid SPECT/CT treatment planning with conformal avoidance of hepatic Kupffer cell masses highlight a reduction in hepatic toxicity compared to conventional 3D-CRT-based treatment planning. Notably, the reduced hepatotoxicity risk with functional treatment planning appears to only benefit those with advanced cirrhosis, as they are at greatest risk for RILD (Lasley et al. 2015). We previously demonstrated a 43% reduction ($p < 0.001$) in the amount of functional liver volume defined on ^{99m}Tc-sulfur colloid SPECT/CT as a percentage of predicted liver volume in Child–Pugh B patients; however no such difference was observed for patients with Child–Pugh A cirrhosis or noncirrhotic patients (Kirichenko et al. 2016; Logan et al. 2016). Conversely, SPECT/CT studies that quantified the intensity of radioactive colloid uptake described little to no variation within the Child-Pugh A group of patients compared to noncirrhotic control group (Bowen et al. 2016). Despite hepatic Kupffer cell volume loss defined on [99m]

Tc-sulfur colloid SPECT in patients with advanced cirrhosis, optimal radiation beam placement with 3D-CT/SPECT planning permitted mean dose reduction to residual functionally active hepatic parenchyma while decreasing the percentage of predicted functional liver volume receiving threshold irradiation. There was no incidence of RILD, grade 3 or higher hepatic toxicity, or accelerated liver failure in HCC patients with advanced cirrhosis who completed liver SBRT with ablative doses utilizing ^{99m}Tc-sulfur colloid 3D-SPECT/CT functional treatment planning (Kudithipudi et al. 2016; Kirichenko et al. 2016). Other studies demonstrated accelerated hepatic failure only when dose to the functionally active volumes on ^{99m}Tc-sulfur colloid SPECT/CT exceeded predicted functional liver volume thresholds (Logan et al. 2016; Shirai et al. 2014). The outcomes in these studies compare favorably to prospective trials evaluating SBRT in HCC without functional treatment planning, where the incidence of grade 3 or higher hepatotoxicity ranges between 5 and 36% (Mendez-Romero et al. 2006; Lasley et al. 2015; Tse et al. 2008).

We have adapted these functional imaging principles in a prospective Phase I trial of fractionated SBRT for patients with impaired liver function and liver tumors (NCT02626312). Rather than using 3–6 fractions, as described above, the study is evaluating the safety of fractionated radiotherapy in 15 or 25 fractions in this patient population at high risk of developing RILD. We use the same techniques of immobilization and daily image guidance that are used for SBRT. The principles of using SPECT/CT to define functional liver volumes were incorporated into this trial, using the general ideas that were described above. The results of this prospective evaluation of the technique are anticipated within 2 years.

2   Conclusion

Recent independent retrospective studies have shown that functional treatment planning with SPECT/CT as an emerging technique warrants validation in prospective trials in an effort to improve the therapeutic ratio and broaden selection of cirrhotic patients with hepatic malignancies for liver SBRT.

3   Special Methodology Addendum

Below is the methodology behind optimal avoidance of functional liver parenchyma defined on SPECT/CT in an effort to irradiate hepatocellular carcinoma in patients with advanced cirrhosis safely and effectively.

3.1   SPECT/CT Rigid Image Registration Based on Surface Fiducials

At the time of simulation, patients are immobilized in custom-molded vacuum bag (Vac-Lok MEDTEC, Orange City, Iowa, USA) in the supine position with arms extended overhead and

nine radiopaque "BBs" (IZI Medical Products, Owings Mills, Maryland, USA) are affixed to the patient's surface laterally and anteriorly at three different axial planes located along the thorax and abdomen, with middle plan at the level of the liver (Gayou et al. 2012).

A free-breathing helical CT with 3 mm thick slices is acquired with intravenous contrast in the radiation oncology department. Next, the patient is sent to the nuclear medicine department for SPECT scanning and injected intravenously with 5.5–6.5 mCi of ^{99m}Tc-sulfur colloid approximately 30 min prior to the SPECT scan. Radioactive SPECT markers (RM) ($\sim$10 μCi of ^{99m}Tc each) are placed at the location of each BB.

The patient treatment position is reproduced on a flat table top of the SPECT scanner by radiation therapists. The 3D-SPECT volumetric image

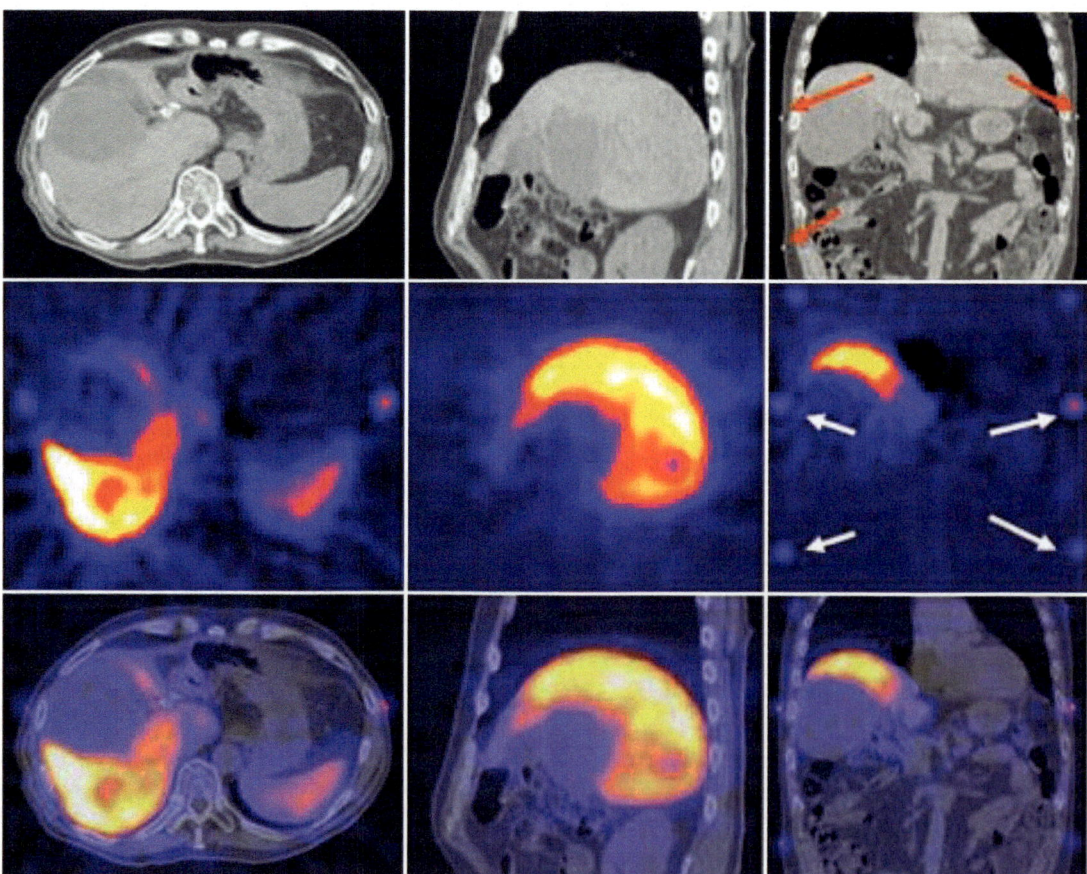

Fig. 1 Point-based registration of functional SPECT to the treatment-planning CT using MIM-Maestro multi-modality software (MIM Software Inc., Cleveland, Ohio, USA) Radiopaque "BBs" is seen on CT images (*red arrows—upper panel*) with corresponding superimposed radioactive markers on SPECT images (*white arrows—mid-panel*). *Lower panel* demonstrates fused SPECT/CT images used for 3D-SPECT/CT functional treatment planning

with 4.42 mm pixel size and 4.42 mm slice thickness are acquired on a dual-head Millennium VG Gamma Camera (GE Healthcare, Chalfont St. Giles, UK) in an approximately 20-min session. No attenuation correction is used. A point-based rigid image registration is performed between SPECT and CT images. Initially, the user selects a minimum of three points that are unambiguously identified on both image sets. The correlation between markers on SPECT and CT images then assists the software registration of the two images by minimizing the average distance between the corresponding markers using translational and rotational degrees of freedom (Fig. 1).

Figure 2 shows fused CT/SPECT images of the liver for noncirrhotic (top) and cirrhotic (bottom) patients. Noncirrhotic patients with normal liver function (control group) have diffuse, homogeneous uptake and distribution of ^{99m}Tc-sulfur colloid with the functional liver volume (FLV-SPECT) matching the liver volume on CT (LV-CT). HCC patients with various degrees of hepatic cirrhosis have sequestration and retraction of functionally active liver parenchyma with residual FLV-SPECT often smaller compared to the anatomical liver volume derived from CT.

3.2 Treatment Planning and Dose Constraints

Gross tumor volume (GTV) is contoured on the contrast-enhanced free-breathing CT followed by helical 4D-CT to assess the internal target volume (ITV) from individual datasets of axial CT images obtained during different phases of the respiratory cycles. An additional 3–5 mm margin is added to create a planning target volume (PTV). The SBRT dose is prescribed to the isodose line encompassing the PTV (generally >90% isodose line), allowing up to 20% hot-spot dose to the target volume. Functional hepatic parenchyma is reflected by areas of uptake on SPECT/3DCT and contoured as "residual functional liver volume." Liver dose constraints are imposed exclusively on residual functional liver volume.

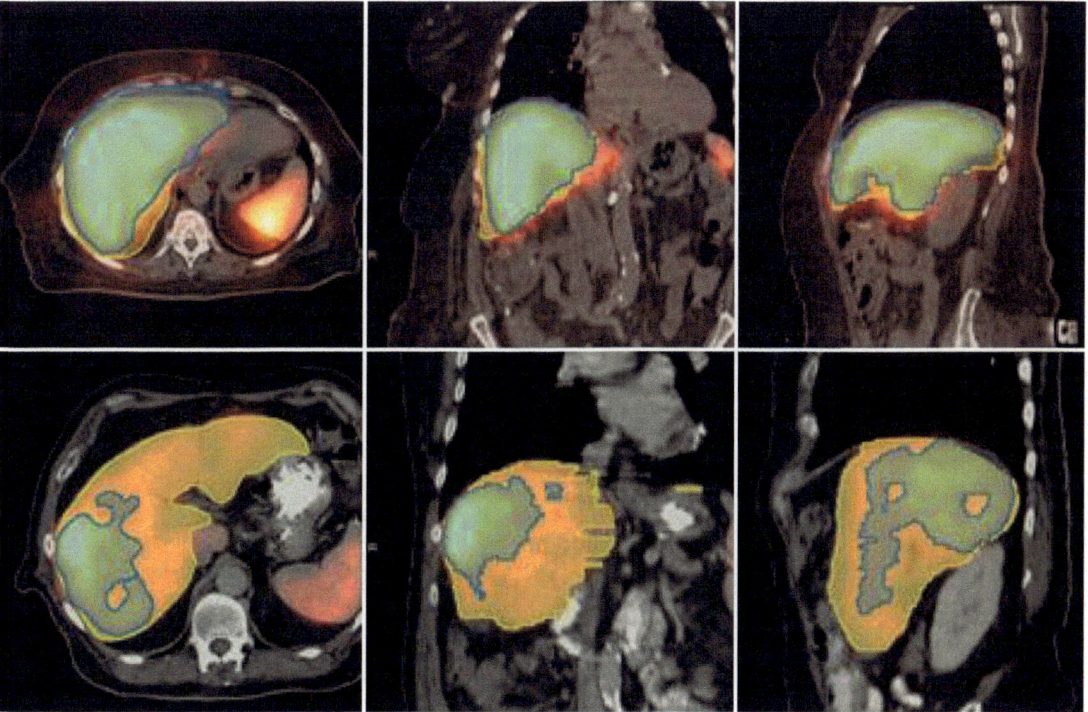

Fig. 2 (from *left* to *right*). Axial, coronal, and sagittal fused SPECT/CT liver images for noncirrhotic (*top*) and cirrhotic (*bottom*) patients. CT-defined anatomical liver contours are shown in *yellow*, while the SPECT-defined functional liver is shown in *blue*

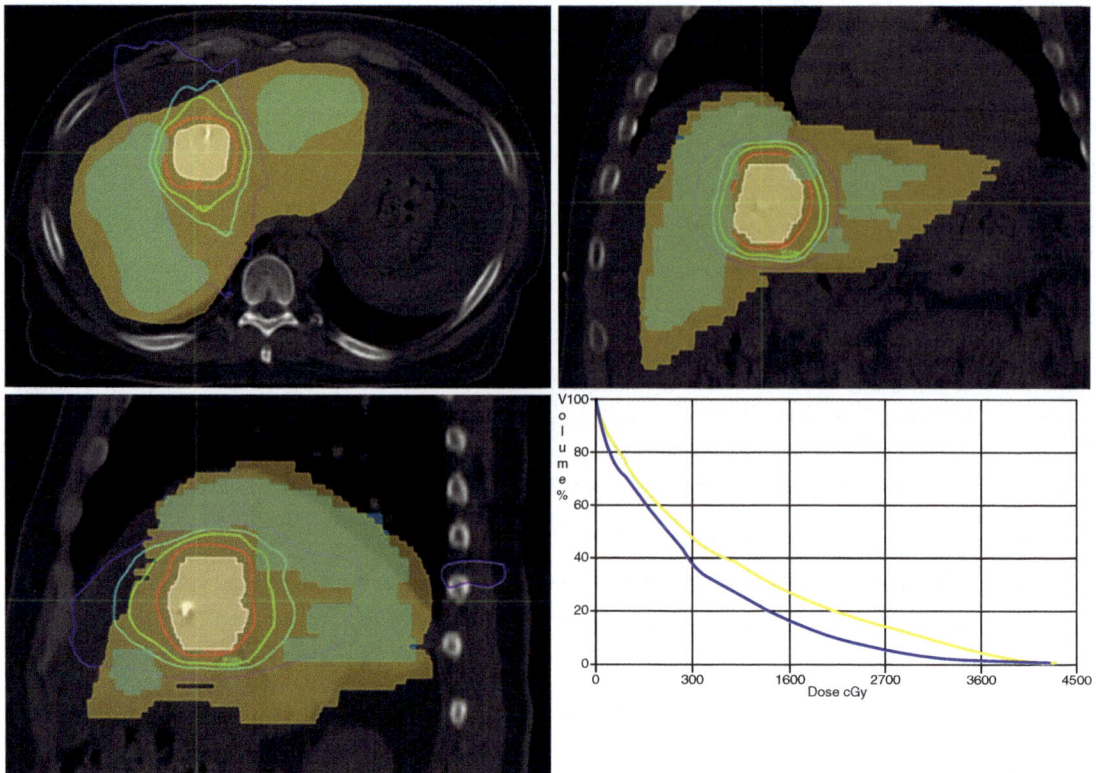

Fig. 3 Representative CT/SPECT treatment planning images with dose distribution for a patient with Child–Pugh B cirrhosis. Functional liver contoured on 99mTc-sulfur colloid SPECT (FLV-SPECT; *blue color wash*) and anatomic liver volume contoured on CT (LV-CT; *yellow color wash*). There is 52% FLV-SPECT loss compared to LV-CT. Forty Gy in four fractions prescribed to the periphery of the internal target volume (*white color wash*) with selective avoidance of FLV-SPECT pursuing the goal to keep ≥600 cc of FLV-SPECT (30% predicted) at ≤16 Gy (BED 40 Gy_3). Dose-volume histogram curves reflect sparing effect on FLV-SPECT with V16 equal to 18% for FLV-SPECT (*blue line*) and 28% for LV-CT (*yellow line*).

To determine dose constraints of the liver which varies in size based on patient height, weight, and liver disease, a validated predicted functional liver volume (pFLV) is estimated from a formula used in hepatic transplantation (Urata et al. 1995) and 90Y radioembolization dosimetry (Kennedy et al. 2007):

$$pFLV = -794.41 + 1268.28 \times BSA$$

where BSA is body surface area in m^2 and pFLV is given in cm^3. In concordance with biologic equivalent dose of conventional liver tolerance (Russell et al. 1993; Leibel et al. 1987) and dose limits used in liver SBRT trials (Rusthoven et al. 2009; Goodman et al. 2010), we specify that 35% of the pFLV can receive no more than 16 Gy, 18 Gy, or 19 Gy, delivered in 4, 5, or 6 fractions, respectively. Functional treatment planning for patient with Child–Pugh B cirrhosis is illustrated in Fig. 3.

References

Andolino DL, Johnson CS, Maluccio M et al (2011) Stereotactic body radiotherapy for primary hepatocellular carcinoma. Int J Radiat Oncol Biol Phys 81:e447–e453

Bowen SR, Chapman TR, Borgman J et al (2016) Measuring total liver function on sulfur colloid SPECT/CT for improved risk stratification and outcome prediction of hepatocellular carcinoma patients. EJNMMI Res 6:57

Bujold A, Massey CA, Kim JJ et al (2013) Sequential phase I and II trials of stereotactic body radiotherapy for locally advanced hepatocellular carcinoma. J Clin Oncol 31:1631–1639

Cheng JC, Wu JK, Huang CM et al (2002) Radiation-induced liver disease after three-dimensional conformal radiotherapy for patients with hepatocellular carcinoma: dosimetric analysis and implication. Int J Radiat Oncol Biol Phys 54:156–162

Cheng JC, Wu JK, Lee PC et al (2004) Biologic susceptibility of hepatocellular carcinoma patients treated with radiotherapy to radiation-induced liver disease. Int J Radiat Oncol Biol Phys 60:1502–1509

Cheng JC, Chou CH, Kuo ML et al (2006) Radiation-enhanced hepatocellular carcinoma cell invasion with MMP-9 expression through PI3K/Akt/NF-kappaB signal transduction pathway. Oncogene 25:7009–7018

Cholongitas E, Papatheodoridis GV, Vangeli M et al (2005) Systematic review: the model for end-stage liver disease – should it replace Child-Pugh's classification for assessing prognosis in cirrhosis? Aliment Pharmacol Therapeut 22:1079–1089

Christiansen H, Saile B, Neubauer-Saile K et al (2004) Irradiation leads to susceptibility of hepatocytes to TNF-alpha mediated apoptosis. Radiother Oncol 72:291–296

Cucchetti A, Ercolani G, Vivarelli M et al (2006) Impact of model for end-stage liver disease (MELD) score on prognosis after hepatectomy for hepatocellular carcinoma on cirrhosis. Liver Transpl 12:966–971

Du SS, Qiang M, Zeng ZC et al (2010) Inactivation of kupffer cells by gadolinium chloride protects murine liver from radiation-induced apoptosis. Int J Radiat Oncol Biol Phys 76:1225–1234

El-Serag HB (2011) Hepatocellular carcinoma. NEJM 365:1118–1127

Everson GT, Shiffman ML, Hoefs JC et al (2012) Quantitative liver function tests improve the prediction of clinical outcomes in chronic hepatitis C: results from the Hepatitis C Antiviral Long-term Treatment Against Cirrhosis Trial. Hepatology 55:1019–1029

Fortune BE, Umman V, Gilliland T et al (2013) Liver transplantation for hepatocellular carcinoma: a surgical perspective. J Clin Gastroenterol 47(Suppl):S37–S42

Gayou O, Day E, Kirichenko A (2012) A method for registration of single photon emission computed tomography (SPECT) and computed tomography (CT) images for liver stereotactic radiotherapy (SRT). Med Phys 39:7398–7401.

Goodman KA, Wiegner EA, Maturen KE et al (2010) Dose-escalation study of single-fraction stereotactic body radiotherapy for liver malignancies. Int J Radiat Oncol Biol Phys 78:486–493

Guha C, Kavanagh BD (2011) Hepatic radiation toxicity: avoidance and amelioration. Semin Radiat Oncol 21:256–263

Hoefs JC, Wang F, Kanel G (1997) Functional measurement of nonfibrotic hepatic mass in cirrhotic patients. Am J Gastroenterol 92:2054–2058

Kamath PS, Kim WR (2007) Advanced Liver Disease Study G. The model for end-stage liver disease (MELD). Hepatology 45:797–805

Katz AW, Chawla S, Qu Z et al (2012) Stereotactic hypofractionated radiation therapy as a bridge to transplantation for hepatocellular carcinoma: clinical outcome and pathologic correlation. Int J Radiat Oncol Biol Phys 83:895–900

Kennedy A, Nag S, Salem R et al (2007) Recommendations for radioembolization of hepatic malignancies using yttrium-90 microsphere brachytherapy: a consensus panel report from the radioembolization brachytherapy oncology consortium. Int J Radiat Oncol Biol Phys 68:13–23

Kirichenko A, Gayou O, Parda D et al (2016) Stereotactic body radiotherapy (SBRT) with or without surgery for primary and metastatic liver tumors. HPB 18:88–97

Klein J, Dawson LA (2013) Hepatocellular carcinoma radiation therapy: review of evidence and future opportunities. Int J Radiat Oncol Biol Phys 87:22–32

Kudithipudi V, Day EE, Thai NV et al (2016) Hepatic failure progression is not hastened in intermediate-risk hepatocellular carcinoma after stereotactic radiation therapy (SRT) with functional treatment planning. Int J Radiat Oncol Biol Phys 96:E179–E180

Lasley FD, Mannina EM, Johnson CS et al (2015) Treatment variables related to liver toxicity in patients with hepatocellular carcinoma, Child-Pugh class A and B enrolled in a phase 1-2 trial of stereotactic body radiation therapy. Pract Radiat Oncol 5:e443–e449

Lawrence TS, Ten Haken RK, Kessler ML et al (1992) The use of 3-D dose volume analysis to predict radiation hepatitis. Int J Radiat Oncol Biol Phys 23:781–788

Leibel SA, Pajak TF, Massullo V et al (1987) A comparison of misonidazole sensitized radiation therapy to radiation therapy alone for the palliation of hepatic metastases: results of a Radiation Therapy Oncology Group randomized prospective trial. Int J Radiat Oncol Biol Phys 13:1057–1064

Liang SX, Zhu XD, Xu ZY et al (2006) Radiation-induced liver disease in three-dimensional conformal radiation therapy for primary liver carcinoma: the risk factors and hepatic radiation tolerance. Int J Radiat Oncol Biol Phys 65:426–434

Logan JK, Park PC, Wong FC et al (2016) Outcomes of patients with hepatocellular carcinoma and advanced cirrhosis after high-dose radiation therapy guided by functional liver imaging with Tc99m sulfur colloid liver SPECT-CT. Int J Radiat Oncol Biol Phys 96:E167–E168

Mendez-Romero A, Wunderink W, Hussain SM et al (2006) Stereotactic body radiation therapy for primary and metastatic liver tumors: a single institution phase i–ii study. Acta Oncol 45:831–837

Meng MB, Cui YL, Lu Y et al (2009) Transcatheter arterial chemoembolization in combination with radiotherapy for unresectable hepatocellular carcinoma: a systematic review and meta-analysis. Radiother Oncol 92:184–194

Russell AH, Clyde C, Wasserman TH et al (1993) Accelerated hyperfractionated hepatic irradiation in the management of patients with liver metastases: results of the RTOG dose escalating protocol. Int J Radiat Oncol Biol Phys 27:117–123

Rusthoven KE, Kavanagh BD, Cardenes H et al (2009) Multi-institutional phase I/II trial of stereotactic body radiation therapy for liver metastases. J Clin Oncol 27:1572–1578

Schneider PD (2004) Preoperative assessment of liver function. Surg Clin North Am 84:355–373

Seong J, Kim SH, Chung EJ et al (2000) Early alteration in TGF-beta mRNA expression in irradiated rat liver. Int J Radiat Oncol Biol Phys 46:639–643

Shirai S, Sato M, Suwa K et al (2010) Feasibility and efficacy of single photon emission computed tomography-based three-dimensional conformal radiotherapy for hepatocellular carcinoma 8 cm or more with portal vein tumor thrombus in combination with transcatheter arterial chemoembolization. Int J Radiat Oncol Biol Phys 76:1037–1044

Shirai S, Sato M, Noda Y et al (2014) Incorporating GSA-SPECT into CT-based dose-volume histograms for advanced hepatocellular carcinoma radiotherapy. World J Radiol 6:598–606

Teh SH, Christein J, Donohue J et al (2005) Hepatic resection of hepatocellular carcinoma in patients with cirrhosis: Model of End-Stage Liver Disease (MELD) score predicts perioperative mortality. J Gastrointest Surg 9:1207–1215. discussion 1215

Tello K, Christiansen H, Gurleyen H et al (2008) Irradiation leads to apoptosis of Kupffer cells by a Hsp27-dependant pathway followed by release of TNF-alpha. Radiat Environ Biophys 47:389–397

Tse RV, Hawkins M, Lockwood G et al (2008) Phase I study of individualized stereotactic body radiotherapy for hepatocellular carcinoma and intrahepatic cholangiocarcinoma. J Clin Oncol 26:657–664

Urata K, Kawasaki S, Matsunami H et al (1995) Calculation of child and adult standard liver volume for liver transplantation. Hepatology 21:1317–1321

Wiesner R, Edwards E, Freeman R et al (2003) Model for end-stage liver disease (MELD) and allocation of donor livers. Gastroenterology 124:91–96

Xu ZY, Liang SX, Zhu J et al (2006) Prediction of radiation-induced liver disease by Lyman normal-tissue complication probability model in three-dimensional conformal radiation therapy for primary liver carcinoma. Int J Radiat Oncol Biol Phys 65:189–195

Zuckerman E, Slobodin G, Sabo E et al (2003) Quantitative liver-spleen scan using single photon emission computerized tomography (SPECT) for assessment of hepatic function in cirrhotic patients. J Hepatol 39:326–332

Gastrointestinal Cancer: Pancreas

Linda Chen, Lauren M. Rosati,
and Joseph M. Herman

Contents

L. Chen • L.M. Rosati
Department of Radiation Oncology, Johns Hopkins
University School of Medicine, Baltimore, MD, USA

J.M. Herman (✉)
Department of Radiation Oncology,
University of Texas MD Anderson Cancer Center,
Houston, TX, USA
e-mail: jherma15@jhmi.edu

1   Introduction

Despite advances in surgical management and the use of multimodal therapy with chemotherapy and radiotherapy, pancreatic cancer continues to be an uncommon yet highly lethal malignancy. In the United States, the American Cancer Society estimated 53,070 new cases of pancreatic cancer and 41,780 deaths in 2016, making pancreatic cancer the 12th most common cancer and the 3rd leading cause of cancer-related death (American Cancer Society 2016). Thus, pancreatic cancer has a disproportionately high mortality rate with a 5-year overall survival of <6%. The term pancreatic cancer typically refers to pancreatic ductal adenocarcinoma, which is a disease of exocrine ductal glands that comprises 85% of pancreatic malignancies (Geer and Brennan 1993). Non-hereditary risk factors for development include cigarette smoking, high body mass index, and chronic inflammation in the setting of chronic pancreatitis

Med Radiol Radiat Oncol (2017)
DOI 10.1007/174_2017_97, © Springer International Publishing AG
Published Online: 27 July 2017

(Lowenfels and Maisonneuve 2006; Michaud et al. 2001; Stolzenberg-Solomon et al. 2008). The majority of neoplasms arise from the head of the pancreas, and common presenting symptoms include epigastric pain, jaundice secondary to obstruction, and weight loss in the setting of malabsorption and endocrine dysfunction (Porta et al. 2005). Following biopsy and histologic confirmation, staging is determined through dedicated thin-sliced computed tomography (CT) of the pancreas with triple-phase contrast enhancement to visualize disease extent and vessel involvement. The American Joint Committee on Cancer staging system is based on primary tumor (T), regional lymph node (N), and distant metastasis (M) staging; however, the National Comprehensive Cancer Network (NCCN) and a number of institutions frequently utilize a staging system which stratifies patients by resectability (American Cancer Society 2009; Tempero 2016). The NCCN staging reflects the extent of disease in terms of surgical resectability as resectable, borderline resectable, locally advanced (unresectable), and metastatic. This resectability-based staging is primarily determined by the presence of distant metastases, tumor involvement of adjacent structures, and tumor relation to arterial (the celiac axis, hepatic artery, and superior mesenteric artery) and venous (the superior mesenteric vein and portal vein) structures (Tempero 2016). While surgical resection remains the cornerstone of definitive therapy, 80% of patients present in more advanced, unresectable stages and, as a result, multidisciplinary care plays a critical role in determining both definitive and palliative treatment options.

2 Overview

2.1 Surgical and Chemotherapy Management

Surgery remains the mainstay of definitive treatment, and achieving resection with negative margins is currently the only potential curative option. Surgery for head-of-the-pancreas tumors consists of a classic pancreaticoduodenectomy (Whipple procedure), which involves resection of the head of the pancreas, a portion of the duodenum, proximal jejunum, common bile duct, gallbladder, and a partial gastrectomy. Modifications to the classic Whipple include the pylorus-preserving pancreaticoduodenectomy, and subtotal stomach-preserving pancreaticoduodenectomy. Body- and tail-of-pancreas neoplasms represent the minority of surgically eligible candidates, as few are detected prior to metastases. Surgical management for these cases consists of either a total pancreatectomy (some body lesions) or a distal subtotal pancreatectomy. Some of these cases are now being performed with a laparoscopic or robotic approach with decreased morbidity, thus allowing a more rapid initiation of adjuvant therapy (Wolfgang et al. 2013).

Even after surgery with complete tumor removal, the majority of pancreatic cancer patients ultimately succumb to disease and 5-year overall survival remains at 10–30% (Tempero 2016; Yeo et al. 1995; Cameron et al. 1993; Balcom et al. 2001; Kang et al. 2014). Long-term survival is achieved in a small subset of patients, and favorable prognostic factors include resection with negative margins, node-negative resection, small and well-differentiated tumors, and completion of the operation at high-volume pancreatic centers (Geer and Brennan 1993; Cameron et al. 2006; Yeo et al. 1997). However, the majority of pancreatic cancer patients present with advanced disease and are considered unresectable due to encasement of critical and non-reconstructable vasculature or due to metastatic disease. As such, a minority of patients are eligible for resection at diagnosis and multidisciplinary management is needed (Pawlik et al. 2008).

Chemotherapy plays a significant role in the management of pancreatic cancer, as the natural history is dominated by rapid progression to metastatic disease. Systemic therapy provides improved quality of life as well as prolonged survival, and key determinants in chemotherapy choices include goals of care, performance status, hepatic function, and renal function

(Tempero 2016). First-line therapy consists of single-agent gemcitabine as well as combination regimens such as gemcitabine and albumin-bound paclitaxel and FOLFIRINOX (leucovorin, infusional fluorouracil, oxaliplatin, irinotecan). While combination regimens have prospectively been shown to correlate with improved survival compared to gemcitabine alone in patients with metastatic disease, combination regimens are also associated with higher treatment-related morbidity that leads to intolerance in poor-performance-status patients (Ychou et al. 2007; Ueno et al. 2016; Poplin et al. 2016). Thus, goals of care, performance status, and patient preferences play a significant role in systemic therapy decision-making. Additionally, chemotherapy is used in the adjuvant setting to prevent local and distant recurrence in patients who undergo resection. Despite surgical resection with negative margins, even early-stage tumors have a propensity for developing metastatic disease in the lung, liver, and peritoneum as well as a local recurrence within the resection bed (Griffin et al. 1990; Tepper et al. 1976). In chemo-naïve patients who undergo surgical resection, there is category I evidence for adjuvant gemcitabine monotherapy based on the disease-free and overall survival benefit reported in the CONKO 001 trial (Oettle et al. 2013). A combination of 5-fluorouracil (5-FU)/leucovorin is another adjuvant category I option that has demonstrated similar survival outcomes to adjuvant gemcitabine in ESPAC-3 (Valle et al. 2014). The role of adjuvant chemoradiation therapy (CRT) remains controversial, but 5-FU or gemcitabine is commonly used in combination with radiation as a radiosensitizer (Regine et al. 2011; Neoptolemos et al. 2009). Finally, in borderline and locally advanced disease, there is an evolving role in utilizing neoadjuvant therapy to downstage disease with the goal of achieving a curative-intent resection. Clinical practice varies and regimens including FOLFIRINOX and gemcitabine + albumin-bound paclitaxel are typically recommended for 2–6 months prior to initiation of radiation therapy (Tempero 2016; Small et al. 2016; Jones et al. 2017; Coveler et al. 2016; Balaban et al. 2016).

2.2 Radiotherapy and Hypofractionated Radiation in Pancreatic Cancer

Radiation therapy is utilized for definitive and palliative management in pancreatic cancer and its clinical utility has been explored in all stages of disease. Radiotherapy is used to improve local control adjuvantly in resectable disease, neoadjuvantly in borderline resectable and non-metastatic locally advanced disease, definitively in unresectable locally advanced disease, and palliatively in select patients with metastatic disease. The benefit of adjuvant radiation following surgical resection is controversial and is being evaluated in the cooperative RTOG 0848 trial where patients are being randomized to chemotherapy alone or chemotherapy followed by CRT. Historically, radiation therapy in pancreatic cancer has been dominated by a conventionally fractionated CRT regimen of 45–54 Gy in 1.8–2 Gy fractions. However, conventionally fractionated regimens consisting of 5–6 weeks of daily therapy are associated with toxicity that often limits patients' ability to tolerate additional full-dose systemic therapy and offers limited effectiveness in both adjuvant and locally advanced disease.

Recently, there has been a rise in clinical trials investigating the role of hypofractionated therapy and stereotactic body radiation (SBRT), particularly in locally advanced pancreatic cancer patients. The critical importance of local control in pancreatic adenocarcinoma is seen in surgery, as complete surgical resection with negative margins is the only potential means of long-term survival. Given the poor survival outcomes in non-metastatic, unresectable disease despite chemotherapy and radiation, several trials have explored the use of SBRT to provide ablative biologic effective doses with curative intent. SBRT regimens involve highly conformal, high-dose-per-fraction radiation delivered in 1–5 fractions. SBRT is prescribed to lower isodose lines to allow for conformal treatments, promotes safety due to sharp dose fall-off near critical structures, and also provides dose heterogeneity within the planning target volume (PTV) (Myrehaug et al. 2016). SBRT in 3–5 fractions offers a number of clinical benefits including new data demonstrating local control, reduction of pain and improvement in quality of life, minimal toxicity, and reduced interruption of systemic regimens (Moningi et al. 2015a, b; Herman et al. 2015a). Moreover, recent exploration of neoadjuvant SBRT in borderline and locally advanced disease has been associated with increased rates of margin-negative resection for patients who are ultimately able to undergo resection (Moningi et al. 2015b).

However, pancreatic cancer, and head lesions in particular, is often in close proximity to a number of critical structures, namely the stomach, duodenum, and small bowel. As these are serial gastrointestinal structures, which result in significant toxicity or functional impairment when damaged, they represent significant dose-limiting organs at risk. Therefore, the ability to further escalate the dose of pancreas SBRT is likely reliant on radiation sensitizers to increase tumor response and/or radiation protectors to decrease treatment effect of the duodenum/stomach.

3   The Role of Radiotherapy in Locally Advanced Disease

While the natural history of locally advanced pancreatic cancer is dominated by metastatic disease, local progression significantly contributes to morbidity as well as mortality (Crane 2016). In an autopsy series, 30% of pancreatic patients died of locally destructive pancreatic cancer, and local failure has been reported as first site of failure in 58% of patients even with conventionally fractionated radiation (Iacobuzio-Donahue et al. 2009; Gastrointestinal Tumor Study Group 1985). Thus, while managing systemic disease is certainly critical in locally advanced pancreatic cancer, improving local control can offer symptom relief and improve quality of life, reduce local recurrence rates, and may prolong survival if coupled with effective systemic therapy.

After all, local control with surgery is potentially curative in a subset of patients, and the ultimate goal would be to optimize the use of radiotherapy to achieve long-term survival.

3.1   Conventionally Fractionated Chemoradiation in Locally Advanced Pancreatic Cancer

Historically, chemotherapy and consolidative radiation have been used in patients with non-metastatic, locally advanced pancreatic cancer (Moertel 1969; Moertel et al. 1981). However, due to the propensity for locally advanced pancreatic cancer to metastasize and considering evidence from several key randomized trials, the practice of routinely adding conventionally fractionated (CRT) to systemic therapy is in question (Gastrointestinal Tumor Study Group 1988; Chauffert et al. 2008; Loehrer et al. 2011; Klaassen et al. 1985; Hammel et al. 2016). Multiple prospective randomized trials sought to evaluate the benefit of the addition of radiation to systemic therapy with conflicting results (Gastrointestinal Tumor Study Group 1988; Chauffert et al. 2008; Loehrer et al. 2011; Klaassen et al. 1985; Hammel et al. 2016). The Eastern Cooperative Oncology Group (ECOG) 4201 compared gemcitabine alone vs. CRT using a standard RT dose of 50.4 Gy with concurrent gemcitabine (Loehrer et al. 2011). The CRT arm was associated with improved overall survival, but the cost of this survival benefit was increased grade 3–4 gastrointestinal toxicity. However, while there was a statistically significant improvement in survival, it is of note that the trial closed early due to poor accrual, decreasing statistical power. While ECOG 4201 favors a CRT approach, another recent trial, the FFCD-SFRO study, found a survival benefit in patients who received gemcitabine alone without CRT (Chauffert et al. 2008). Patients randomized to the CRT arm received 60 Gy in 30 fractions to a large radiation field coupled with an intensive chemotherapy regimen comprised of infusional 5-FU, intermittent cisplatin, and maintenance gemcitabine. Only 42% of patients in the CRT arm were able to complete the full treatment regimen due to intolerance of the intensive multi-agent chemotherapy regimen. Additionally, it is difficult to discern what clinical benefits or harms were due to the radiation given the significantly different chemotherapy regimens between the two arms. Finally, data from the largest and most recent prospective trial investigating CRT in locally advanced pancreatic cancer come from the LAP-07 trial (Hammel et al. 2016). Patients were initially randomized to 4 months of induction gemcitabine or gemcitabine plus erlotinib. This was followed by a second randomization to consolidative CRT (54 Gy, three-dimensional conformal radiation [3D-CRT] delivered concurrently with capecitabine) for patients who were free of systemic progression. Patients who received CRT had prolonged local progression-free survival, increased time between first-line and second-line chemotherapy, and no increase in grade 3–4 toxicity with the exception of nausea. However, there was no overall survival benefit for patients who were treated with CRT (10.1 months vs. 12.7 months from the second randomization) (Hammel et al. 2016). One factor which limits interpretation of the role of radiation in this trial is that only 37% of patients were treated with radiation per protocol, with 21% having major deviations and 50% having minor deviations in their radiation treatment plan. Thus, despite the historic use of consolidative radiation with chemotherapy in locally advanced pancreatic cancer, recent clinical trials have not resulted in a clear consensus. There were modest overall survival benefits associated with radiation in ECOG 4201 and a superior local progression-free survival in LAP-07. However, patients ultimately succumb to both progression and metastatic disease. It may be that the benefit of local control is not appreciable without improved systemic regimens, and published trials to date have not used more contemporary regimens such as FOLFIRINOX or nab-paclitaxel/gemcitabine. In spite of the conflicting evidence, it is clear that the prognosis for locally advanced pancreatic adenocarcinoma remains poor and requires further investigation.

3.2 SBRT in Locally Advanced Pancreatic Cancer

SBRT and hypofractionated radiation use higher doses per fraction to optimize the ablative tumor effect. A summary of clinical trials evaluating SBRT can be found in Table 1. The feasibility of using SBRT in LAPC was initially used in a dose escalation trial involving up to 25 Gy in one fraction reported by Koong et al. at Stanford University in 2004 (Koong et al. 2004). All patients enrolled on the trial had metastatic progression as the first site of progression, the primary objective of evaluating local control was achieved, and the trial was stopped early before any dose-limiting toxicity was observed. Not only did this trial demonstrate that SBRT could potentially be a well-tolerated and effective means of local control, but it also illustrated the importance of the use of systemic therapy. Integrating chemotherapy prior to SBRT not only allows for better control of micrometastatic disease, but its up-front use may be a means of screening out patients who will fail distantly and thus be less likely to benefit from SBRT. Moreover, given the small number of treatments involved in SBRT delivery, SBRT can easily be combined with chemotherapy, targeted therapies, and immunotherapy with minimal treatment delays. Groups including Schellenberg et al. (2008), Goyal et al. (2012), and Hoyer et al. (2005) have evaluated 25 Gy in one fraction and 45 Gy in three fractions in LAPC (Schellenberg et al. 2011; Goyal et al. 2012; Hoyer et al. 2005). However, the dose and fractionation regimen that best maximizes tumor ablation while maintaining tolerable dose to organs at risk remains under investigation.

Early SBRT studies (Koong et al. 2004; Hoyer et al. 2005) failed to incorporate clear dose constraints or establish methods for image-guided radiation therapy and therefore were associated

Table 1 Stereotactic radiation in locally advanced pancreatic cancer

Study	N	Treatment	BED10	Acute/late toxicity (≥Grade 3)	Median local PFS (months)	Median OS (months)
Koong et al. (2004)	15	15 Gy, 20 Gy, or 25 Gy in 1 fraction	37.5–87.5	0%/–	–	11
Hoyer et al. (2005)	22	45 Gy in 3 fractions	112.5	79%/–	4.8	5.7
Schellenberg et al. (2008)	16	Gemcitabine → 25 Gy in 1 fraction → Gemcitabine	87.5	6%/12%	8.4	11.4
Chang et al. (2009)	77	Gemcitabine → 25 Gy in 1 fraction (12% had prior pancreas radiation)	87.5	1%/10%	6.4	11.9
Polistina et al. (2010)	23	Gemcitabine → 30 Gy in 3 fractions	60	0%/0%	7.3	10.6
Rwigema et al. (2012)	71	18–25 Gy in 1 fraction	50.4–87.5	1%/0%	–	10
Schellenberg et al. (2011)	20	Gemcitabine → 25 Gy in 1 fraction → Gemcitabine	87.5	0%/5%	9.2	11.8
Mahadevan et al. (2011)	47	Gemcitabine → 24–36 Gy in 3 fractions → Gemcitabine	43.2–79.2	0%/9%	15	20
Goyal et al. (2012)	19	20–25 Gy in 1 fraction or 24–30 Gy in 3 fractions	43.2–87.5	–/16%	11.4	14.3
Gurka et al. (2013)	11	Gemcitabine + 25 Gy in 5 fractions	37.5	0%/0%	6.8	12.2
Tozzi et al. (2013)	21	45 Gy in 6 fractions	78.8	0%/0%	8	11
Herman et al. (2015a)	49	Gemcitabine + 33 Gy in 5 fractions	54	10%/6%	7.8	13.9

PFS progression free survival, *OS* overall survival

with high rates of acute and late gastrointestinal toxicity (Table 1) (Schellenberg et al. 2011, 2008; Goyal et al. 2012). Toxicities included duodenitis, gastritis, bleeding ulceration, and bowel perforation. These severe toxicities reinforce the need to prioritize gastric, duodenal, and small bowel constraints in close proximity to planning target volumes. Unlike SBRT to the lung and liver, which are surrounded by parallel structures, gastrointestinal organs at risk in pancreatic cancer are organized serially. In light of the gastrointestinal toxicity associated with pancreas SBRT, subsequent trials attempted to minimize toxicity by using modest fractionation, establish clear dose constraints for organs at risk, and incorporate image guidance at the time of treatment delivery. Thus far, studies incorporating 3–5 fractions appear to allow for some degree of normal tissue recovery (Chang et al. 2009). Additionally, the use of induction chemotherapy followed by restaging

to ensure the absence of metastases precludes administration of SBRT to patients who are unlikely to benefit (Mahadevan et al. 2011). Polistina et al. treated LAPC patients with sequential gemcitabine followed by 30 Gy in three fractions, with an 82.6% local response rate comprised of stable disease and partial tumor response (Polistina et al. 2010). Additionally, 9% of patients were found to have a complete response, and 8% were downstaged as resectable (Polistina et al. 2010). Furthermore, no grade ≥3 acute or late toxicity was noted. However, median local progression-free survival was 7.3 months and median overall survival from SBRT was 10.3 months. Thus, while the fractionated regimen was tolerable and provided local tumor response and pain control local control efficacy remained short-lived.

The optimal biologically effective dose (BED) for long-term local tumor control remains under investigation. Other recent groups such as

Mahadevan et al. investigated sequential gemcitabine and SBRT to a dose of 24–36 Gy in three fractions (Mahadevan et al. 2011). This regimen's BED closely approximated 25 Gy × 1, and favorable survival outcomes in locally advanced disease were reported, with a median progression-free survival of 15 months and median overall survival of 20 months after chemotherapy and SBRT (Table 1). However, while 0% of patients experienced severe acute toxicity, this radiation dose prescription resulted in 9% of patients with grade ≥3 long-term toxicity. As a result of these data, other groups investigated lower dose and five-fraction regimens. Gurka et al. evaluated gemcitabine and SBRT with 25 Gy in five fractions, with a BED10 of 37.5 Gy (Gurka et al. 2013). Although this regimen was tolerated very well with no grade ≥3 toxicity, local progression-free survival and overall survival from SBRT were only 6.8 months and 12.2 months, respectively. A recent prospective multi-institutional series was published in 2015 by Herman et al. that also examined a five-fraction regimen to a total dose of 33 Gy (Herman et al. 2015a). This phase II trial enrolled 49 patients who received the fractionated regimen coupled with three doses of induction gemcitabine followed by a 1-week break. Patients reported stable quality of life after SBRT from baseline, a significant improvement in pancreatic pain, and had a median overall survival of 13.9 months. Toxicity with this regimen was lesser compared to data from single-fraction trials; however, three (6%) grade 5 toxicities were noted that were related to *Clostridium difficile* infection, sepsis, and GI bleed as a result of direct tumor extension into the duodenum (Herman et al. 2015a).

Overall, there is no consensus with regard to a standard SBRT dose regimen, but the recent literature has peaked interest into further investigation of SBRT as a safe and effective regimen if careful consideration of normal tissue constraints is applied. Local control data are at minimum comparable to standard fractionation, and fractionated SBRT is a well-tolerated and convenient regimen that minimizes systemic treatment delays while improving patient quality of life. The incorporation of more aggressive, contemporary chemotherapy regimens as well as investigation of fractionation and optimal BED to provide tumor control on clinical trials are warranted.

3.3 Hypofractionated Radiotherapy in Locally Advanced Pancreatic Cancer

Conventional fractions of 1.8–2 Gy to 45–50.4 Gy have been ineffective in promoting long-term survival in locally advanced pancreatic cancer, even when using more conformal dose escalation with intensity-modulating radiation therapy (IMRT). Dose escalation to 70–72 Gy was evaluated by Ceha et al. in 2000 and again to 55 Gy by Ben-Josef et al. in 2004 (Ceha et al. 2000; Ben-Josef et al. 2004). Additionally, as discussed previously, trials using ablative BED of SBRT such as 45 Gy in three fractions by Hoyer et al. 2005 to a large field were associated with unacceptable severe treatment toxicity and poor survival outcomes (Hoyer et al. 2005). Thus, currently used SBRT regimens fractionate and prescribe to lower total doses in order to ensure patient safety. While such regimens have reported favorable tumor response rates, there are concerns that the reduced total dose limits the effectiveness of SBRT. Consequently, others have explored extended hypofractionated regimens to permit a total BED that is ablative to the tumor in a manner that allows for additional normal tissue recovery. In 2013, Tozzi et al. published a 45 Gy in six-fraction regimen with a BED10 of 78.8 Gy and Yang et al. have published a dosimetric evaluation of using integrated boost with pancreas SBRT (Tozzi et al. 2013; Yang et al. 2015). Crane et al. at MD Anderson have adopted a 15-fraction regimen to a dose of 67.5 Gy using a simultaneous integrated boost to the hypoxic tumor core in locally advanced pancreatic cancer (Crane 2016). The MD Anderson regimen was developed after extrapolating institutional pancreas and liver BED data, and provides an ablative BED10 of 97.8 Gy (Crane 2016). Institutional data suggest median local progression rates comparable to less advanced disease as well as surgical resection with a local progression-free survival of 15 months and 5-year survival rate of 18% compared to an expected

5-year survival rate of <6% (Crane 2016; Krishnan et al. 2016). Thus, dose escalation through simultaneous integrated boost delivering a definitive BED10 through 15 Gy in hypofractionated doses is a promising approach. However, these patients should be carefully selected because patients treated with this approach require at least a 1 cm separation between the tumor and bowel/stomach.

4 The Role of Adjuvant Radiotherapy in Resectable Disease

4.1 The Controversial Role of Adjuvant Chemoradiation

While there is category I evidence for adjuvant chemotherapy in pancreatic cancer, the role of conventionally fractionated adjuvant radiation remains controversial (Oettle et al. 2013; Evans et al. 2002). Even after curative-intent surgery with negative margins, 45–60% of patients experience local recurrence, with the majority of recurrences developing in close proximity to the celiac axis and superior mesenteric artery (Griffin et al. 1990; Dholakia et al. 2013a). Given this preponderance for local recurrence following surgical resection, several prospective and retrospective studies have examined the role of adjuvant local therapy with radiation. These adjuvant chemoradiation regimens consist of 40–54 Gy in 1.8 Gy fractions, using 3D-CRT or IMRT. While there may be a subset of patients who would benefit from adjuvant CRT, the literature suggests conflicting results with the majority of studies favoring adjuvant chemotherapy alone. As such, the role of adjuvant conventionally fractionated radiation remains unclear and controversial.

4.2 Surgery Alone vs. Adjuvant Chemoradiation

The Gastrointestinal Tumor Study Group (GITSG) (Kalser and Ellenberg 1985) and EORTC 40891 (Klinkenbijl et al. 1999) evaluated adjuvant CRT compared to surgery alone through randomized prospective trials which demonstrated a survival advantage with adjuvant CRT, though this trend was only statistically significant in the landmark GITSG trial (Kalser and Ellenberg 1985). The GITSG trial compared observation following resection to adjuvant CRT consisting of bolus 5-FU-based chemotherapy with a split course of external beam radiation of 40 Gy in 20 fractions followed by maintenance 5-FU (Kalser and Ellenberg 1985). This course of adjuvant CRT resulted in median overall of 20 months vs. 10 months in the control group; however, it was closed prematurely due to poor accrual and large survival differences between the study arms. Subsequently, in 1999, EORTC 40891 randomized patients to surgery alone vs. adjuvant CRT in ampullary and pancreatic cancers. Adjuvant chemotherapy consisted of continuous infusion of 5-FU without maintenance therapy and a similar split-course external beam radiation regimen of 40 Gy in 20 fractions was delivered. While adjuvant therapy demonstrated improved median overall survival (17.1 vs. 12.6 months), and 2-year overall survival (37% vs. 23%), these results were not statistically significant (Klinkenbijl et al. 1999). Another study, Radiation Therapy Oncology Group (RTOG) 9704, primarily explored the role of adjuvant chemotherapy; however, adjuvant radiation was incorporated into both trial arms. Patients were randomized to either gemcitabine or fluorouracil after resection, followed by concurrent 5-FU-based CRT to a radiation dose of 50.4 Gy. While both the adjuvant chemotherapy and radiation regimens differed and results cannot be directly compared to GITSG or EORTC 40891, the median overall survival of 20.6 and 16.4 in the gemcitabine and 5-FU arms, respectively, is similar to the median overall survival of pancreatic cancer patients who underwent resection and adjuvant chemotherapy in the aforementioned trials (Regine et al. 2011). Additionally, large retrospective series from the Johns Hopkins Hospital and Mayo Clinic have demonstrated an improved overall survival with adjuvant 5-FU-based CRT over observation (21.1 vs. 15.5 months) with a propensity score and matched-pair analysis (Herman et al. 2008; Corsini et al. 2008; Hsu et al. 2010).

4.3 Adjuvant Chemotherapy vs. Adjuvant Chemoradiation

Although there is some evidence to suggest that adjuvant therapy with CRT is beneficial compared to surgical resection alone, the bulk of prospective data favor adjuvant chemotherapy alone. Several large retrospective series including a National Cancer Database study and a large, multi-institutional pooled analysis have found a statistically significant benefit in median overall survival associated with adjuvant CRT compared to chemotherapy alone (Morganti et al. 2014; Kooby et al. 2013). Despite these large retrospective series, a meta-analysis of 9 prospective trials published in 2012 and another meta-analysis of 15 prospective trials with various chemotherapy regimens found that adjuvant chemotherapy was associated with improved patient outcomes but there was no statistically significant improvement in overall survival with adjuvant CRT (Ren et al. 2012; Liao et al. 2013). One particularly notable trial is the European Study Group for Pancreatic Cancer (ESPAC)-1, a multi-institution phase III trial with a 2 × 2 randomization of four patient groups: observation, adjuvant 5-FU-based chemotherapy, adjuvant concurrent CRT (using split-course radiation to 40 Gy and 5-FU-based chemotherapy), and adjuvant concurrent CRT followed by an additional six cycles of 5-FU/leucovorin. Survival outcomes favored adjuvant chemotherapy alone (21.6 months); however, the outcomes suggest that the addition of adjuvant radiation therapy to chemotherapy (19.9 months) was associated with improved survival outcomes than with observation alone (13.9 months) (Neoptolemos et al. 2009). Criticisms of this trial include the 2 × 2 randomization scheme, lack of radiation field guidelines or central review of radiation planning, and lack of restaging before adjuvant therapy (Herman et al. 2015b). The ongoing clinical trial RTOG 0848 will further clarify the role of adjuvant radiation therapy following surgical resection (Franke et al. 2015).

Other analyses have explored identification of select patients who may benefit from adjuvant CRT. In a meta-analysis of four randomized controlled trials, Butturini et al. found that chemoradiotherapy in patients with microscopically positive margins (R1) resulted in 28% reduction in the risk of death (HR 0.72, 95% CI 0.47–1.1) (Butturini et al. 2008). This was also demonstrated in another meta-analysis of five randomized controlled adjuvant CRT trials that demonstrated that CRT was more effective in patients with positive resection margins (Stocken et al. 2005). Finally, in a retrospective series from the Johns Hopkins Hospital of adjuvant CRT following resection in patients with distal disease, a subgroup of patients with node-positive disease who received adjuvant CRT correlated with a survival benefit (16.7 vs. 12.1 months) (Redmond et al. 2010). Therefore, there are conflicting data with regard to adjuvant CRT as a standard option, but there may be a subgroup of patients with pathologic features who may benefit.

4.4 Adjuvant Stereotactic Body Radiotherapy in Resectable Disease

Due to the conflicting evidence with regard to the therapeutic benefit of conventionally fractionated radiation, adjuvant chemotherapy alone is used in Europe and controversy surrounding routine adjuvant CRT after negative margins remains in the United States (Tempero 2016). Given the previously described adjuvant CRT data, some institutions reserve adjuvant CRT for patients with an R1 resection and node-positive disease (Tempero 2016). The role of adjuvant SBRT is exploratory, though some postulate that there is utility given that local recurrence is common after surgical resection and that use of SBRT in the margin-positive setting may be beneficial (Goodman 2016). One approach to adjuvant radiation therapy field design encompasses high-risk areas for local recurrence based on mapping of patterns of failure (Dholakia et al. 2013a). In 2012, Rwigema et al.

published a series of 24 patients who were treated with SBRT 20–24 Gy in one fraction adjuvantly after they were found to have close or positive margins (Rwigema et al. 2012). Retroperitoneal margins are the most common site of positive surgical margins, and 87.5% and 62.5% of patients with close and positive margins (respectively) achieved freedom from local progression following SBRT. Moreover, no patients experienced grade 3 or 4 toxicity and patients were able to receive adjuvant chemotherapy shortly afterwards following this short, well-tolerated treatment (Rwigema et al. 2012). However, data for SBRT are limited in the adjuvant setting and adjuvant SBRT remains an ongoing area of investigation.

4.5 Re-irradiation of Locally Recurrent Disease

The use of SBRT as an alternative or adjunct to conventional radiation has also been explored in the locally recurrent setting. The Stanford retrospective SBRT experience published in 2009 included 9 patients with locally recurrent disease who had received a prior course of radiation and 16 patients who received SBRT as a boost to fractionated external beam radiation to 45 Gy (Chang et al. 2009). This treatment was associated with significant toxicities with 25% of (1 of 4) acute toxicities and 33% of (3 of 10) late grade ≥2 toxicities occurring in patients who received external beam irradiation to the pancreas in addition to high-dose SBRT in a single fraction (Chang et al. 2009). Thus, in congruence with the locally advanced pancreatic cancer SBRT literature, single-fraction ablative SBRT regimens are associated with significant toxicities, and other series sought to determine the utility of fractionated regimens. A retrospective series from Georgetown University delivered a boost of SBRT (20–30 Gy in 3–5 fractions) to 28 patients with locally recurrent disease following a median conventional radiation dose of 50.4 Gy (Lominska et al. 2012). Salvage SBRT was well tolerated, though 7% of (2/28) patients experienced late grade 3 toxicity, and was associated with 85.7% freedom from local progression at 6 months

(Lominska et al. 2012). Other retrospective series have reported data on fractionated, lower BED SBRT regimens for re-irradiation of locally recurrent disease. Recently, a series reported by Dagoglu et al. report on 30 patients with locally recurrent or progressive disease following conventionally fractionated CRT to 50.4 in 28 fractions (Dagoglu et al. 2016). The SBRT dose of 24–36 Gy in five fractions was associated with a 78% 2-year local control rate, with 10% of patients experiencing grade III acute toxicity and 7% ($n = 2$) with a grade 3 late bowel obstruction (Dagoglu et al. 2016). Moreover, palliative BED prescriptions such as 25 Gy in five fractions have been shown to be well tolerated, associated with 0% acute grade 3 toxicity and a single case (6%) of grade 3 late toxicity in a series of 18 patients reported by the Johns Hopkins Hospital (Wild et al. 2013). Moreover 57% of patients reported palliation of back or abdominal pain, and local progression-free survival at 6 and 12 months was 78% and 62%, respectively (Wild et al. 2013). Therefore, these retrospective series provide evidence that fractionated SBRT may be a useful and tolerable treatment option for patients with local recurrence following prior conventional radiation.

4.6 Neoadjuvant Radiation in Borderline Resectable Disease

Borderline resectable pancreatic cancer (BRPC) is defined as a disease which contacts critical structures such as the superior mesenteric artery, but does not involve these structures to the extent that tumors are technically surgically unresectable (Tempero 2016; Bilimoria et al. 2007). This represents a distinct subset of patients, for which there is currently no standard treatment regimen. Primary management typically involves curative-intent surgery; however, due to the invasion of critical structures, there remains a concern that these patients are at increased risk for positive margins following resection. Currently, there is a lack of category I evidence for the use of neoadjuvant chemotherapy or radiation in borderline resectable patients. At a number of institutions, BRPC patients will undergo neoadjuvant gemcitabine-based or 5-FU-based chemotherapy (Tempero 2016; Rose et al. 2014). Frequently, neoadjuvant chemotherapy is followed by conventional CRT to a dose of 45–50.4 Gy in 1.8–2 Gy fractions (Katz et al. 2016); however, CRT has only been associated with a 12% RECIST criteria radiographic downstaging in a retrospective series (Katz et al. 2008, 2012; Dholakia et al. 2013b).

A meta-analysis of 111 studies compared neoadjuvant chemotherapy, neoadjuvant radiation, and neoadjuvant CRT in borderline resectable and unresectable pancreatic cancer (Gillen et al. 2010). In this study, while initially resectable patients did not benefit from neoadjuvant therapy, 33% of patients with borderline or unresectable disease were able to undergo surgery and had survival comparable to initially resectable tumor patients following surgery (Gillen et al. 2010). One potential concern for neoadjuvant CRT is that toxicities associated with treatment can potentially delay surgery (Breslin et al. 2001; Spitz et al. 2016). Delivery of fewer fractions of neoadjuvant therapy using hypofractionation has been investigated at MD Anderson, with reported outcomes of 132 patients who received either conventionally fractionated CRT to a dose of 45–50.4 Gy in 1.8 Gy fractions or 30 Gy in 3 Gy fractions (Breslin et al. 2001). The ten-fraction regimen was found to be less toxic although there was no statistically significant difference in survival outcomes. In an institutional review of 160 borderline resectable patients treated with neoadjuvant therapy, 82 patients were considered potentially operable after restaging following neoadjuvant CRT. The majority (80%) of patients were able to undergo surgical resection, with R0 and R1 resection rates of 94% and 6% (respectively), a median survival of 40 months, and a 5-year overall survival rate of 36% (Katz et al. 2008). The authors concluded that this neoadjuvant approach contributed to favorable survival outcomes and allowed for identification of patients who would benefit most from surgery (Katz et al. 2008).

SBRT prescriptions that further increase dose per fraction were also evaluated at Moffitt Cancer Center using gemcitabine-based chemotherapy followed by simultaneous integrated boost in 7–10 Gy in five fractions to the region of tumor-vessel abutment and 25–30 Gy in five fractions to the remainder of the tumor (Chuong et al. 2013). Of the 77 borderline resectable and locally advanced patients, 56% of the BRPC patients underwent surgical resection, with 16.3% of patients achieving a pathologic complete or near-complete response and an overall survival of 16 months. While locally advanced patients were not surgical candidates after neoadjuvant therapy, the authors reported favorable survival at 15 months following neoadjuvant chemotherapy and SBRT. Overall, the treatment regimen was tolerated well without high-grade acute toxicity, but 6% of patients had late grade 3 toxicities including bleeding and anorexia requiring feeding tube placement (Goodman 2016; Chuong et al. 2013). Additionally, data from Johns Hopkins in BRPC and LAPC patients who received neoadjuvant chemotherapy followed by SBRT 25–33 Gy in five fractions also suggest favorable resectability, pathologic outcome, and survival outcomes (Moningi et al. 2015b). Moningi et al. report their institutional experience with 74 LAPC and 14 BRPC patients, 19 (22%) of whom underwent surgery with an 84% margin-negative resection rate and minimal toxicity (Moningi et al. 2015b). Given the response rates, SBRT appears to be an attractive option due to efficacy, tolerability, and short treatment duration and the role of neoadjuvant SBRT in borderline resectable disease is the subject of the currently ongoing Alliance A021501 trial.

5 Stereotactic Body Radiation Treatment Delivery

5.1 Motion Management

The precise and highly conformal nature of SBRT requires effective patient immobilization and target localization in order to accurately target the tumor while allowing for a steep isodose gradient that spares organs at risk. Physiologic organ motion of the pancreas presents a unique challenge due to movement with breathing, gastric filling and emptying, as well as bowel displacement. CT simulation should be done with both intravenous and oral contrast. 4D imaging which tracks organ motion throughout the respiratory cycle is recommended as well as active breathing control (ABC) or an abdominal belt in order to minimize organ motion due to respiration. During ABC, an inspirational breath-hold technique is used such that treatment is only given during a breath hold to control for respiratory motion, while active respiratory tracking during treatment is also available at some institutions. If a patient is unable to tolerate ABC, an internal target volume (ITV) can be created from a 4D scan or an abdominal compression belt can be used to reduce full excursion of the tumor during the breathing cycle (Goodman 2016). Luminal organ motion is also minimized by encouraging patients to fast before simulation and before each treatment fraction. This allows for reduction in variability of gastric emptying and filling, and also decreases the amount of stomach in close proximity to the planning tumor volume.

5.2   SBRT Planning Volumes

A gross tumor volume (GTV) is defined by CT imaging. Fusion of a magnetic resonance imaging (MRI) scan or positron emission tomography (PET) can also be used to assist with identification of tumor extent. If there is direct tumor invasion of the duodenum and/or stomach on imaging and confirmed on endoscopy, SBRT should only be used if surgery is planned as these patients have a higher risk of bowel toxicity. In these cases, a more protracted regimen (15–30 fractions) is recommended. If ABC is not utilized during simulation, an ITV is created in order to encompass the tumor position when it is maximally displaced by the breathing cycle. An expansion from the GTV or ITV (if no ABC is used) to a planning target volume (PTV) of 1–5 mm is used, based on institutional and medical physics determination of margin required to account for daily setup error with SBRT. At the Johns Hopkins Hospital, the PTV is modified such that it does not overlap with the proximal stomach, duodenum, or bowel volumes more than 2 mm (Fig. 1).

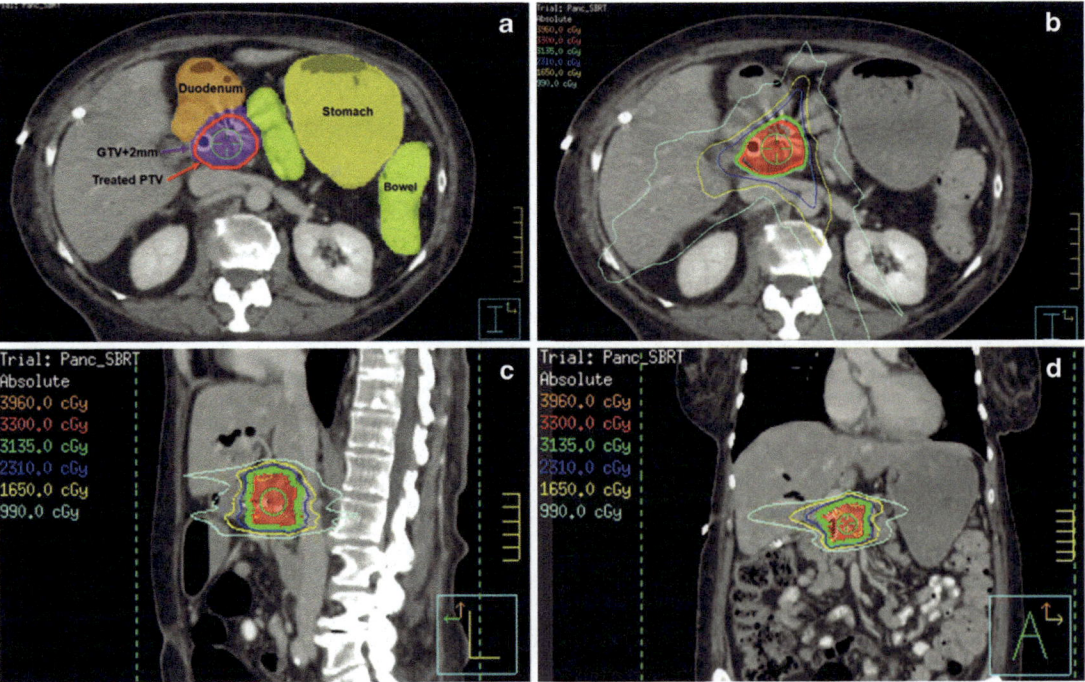

Fig. 1 Pancreas SBRT treatment planning. (**a**) Pancreas SBRT contours of proximal organs at risk and treated PTV. GTV+ 2 mm in *purple* is modified to the PTV used for treatment (*red*) such that there is a 2 mm space between proximal organs at risk and the PTV. (**b–d**) Axial, sagittal, and coronal dose distribution

This modification of PTV volume (modified PTV) is adapted based on the OARs plus a 2 mm (planning organ at risk volume, PRV) expansion. On some clinical trials, simultaneous integrated boost is utilized with 2 or more PTVs in order to boost tumor-vessel interface or the hypoxic tumor core while prescribing a lower dose to the entire PTV or any microscopic areas at risk (Crane 2016).

SBRT-associated duodenal toxicity in a cohort of 77 patients treated at Stanford (Murphy et al. 2010). They reported dose volume endpoints that were strongly correlated with toxicity. Specifically $V15 \geq 9.1$ cm^3 and $V20 > 3.3$ cm^3 were associated with 52% rate of duodenal toxicity compared to $V15 < 9.1$ cm^3 and $V20 < 3.3$ being associated with a 11% rate of toxicity (Murphy et al. 2010).

5.3 Treatment Planning and Dose Constraints

Dose is prescribed to the 60–90% isodose line, to allow for steep dose gradients to minimize dose to the stomach, duodenum, and bowel in close proximity to the PTV. Dose constraints in pancreas SBRT pose a unique challenge, as gastrointestinal organs are organized in serial subunits and proper function is affected by maximum doses. Additionally, the ablative doses of SBRT used in clinical trials exceed the maximum tolerated dose for these structures. The consequences of this were seen in early single-fraction series, which were associated with significant gastrointestinal toxicities. This has been addressed through fractionation, prescribing to lower BED, and modifying the PTV in a way that sacrifices coverage in order to adhere to dose constraints. Although there is currently no standard dose constraint, Murphy et al. published a dosimetric review of

5.4 Tumor Localization

Accurate delivery of SBRT requires confidence in tumor and normal structure location. Challenges to radiation delivery include inter- and intra-fraction tumor and critical organ motion. If SBRT is being utilized in the neoadjuvant or locally advanced setting, use of gold fiducials (ideally 3) placed under endoscopic guidance should be placed adjacent to or within the tumor for kV or MV image guidance. Cone beam CTs are fused with simulation imaging, and used to align patients based on bony anatomy as well as fiducial alignment for accurate target localization and to help evaluate patient setup (Fig. 2). Imaging must be taken immediately prior to delivery, and daily cone beam CTs allow for confirmation that the target volume and organ position are consistent and help to determine if replanning is necessary.

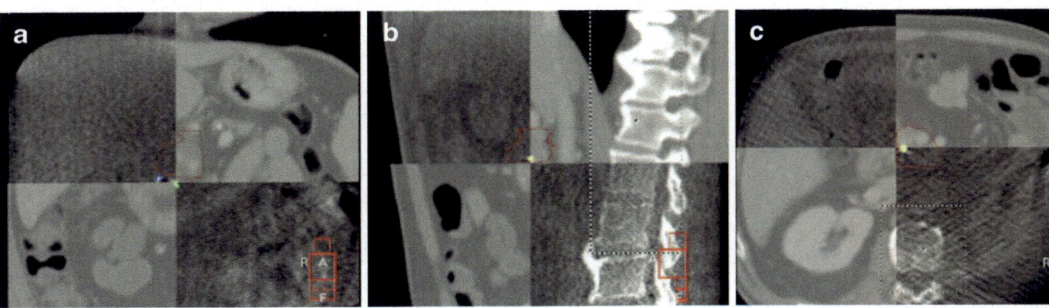

Fig. 2 Patient set-up is verified through daily cone beam CT (*top left*, *bottom right*) which is compared to the patient's reference simulation CT (*top right*, *bottom left*).

Patient is aligned to bone and fiducials (*blue*, *green*, and *yellow*) in (**a**) coronal, (**b**) sagittal, and (**c**) axial dimensions and the PTV (*red*) location is also referenced

Conclusion

SBRT in pancreatic cancer is an emerging therapy, which strives to provide local control with curative intent while limiting toxicity and delay in multi-agent chemotherapy administration. Much of the established literature involves locally advanced disease in which the importance of incorporating aggressive systemic therapy and the need to fractionate has been shown to be important in order to provide safe and effective therapy. However, the optimum dose and treatment approach require further investigation to maximize the therapeutic index with a short-course therapy that administers an ablative dose to the tumor while providing a well-tolerated therapy with minimal severe side effects. While the role of adjuvant radiation currently plays an uncertain role in management of disease with negative margins, use of adjuvant SBRT in the setting of positive margins needs further exploration. Moreover, palliatively dosed SBRT (5–6 Gy × 5) has been shown to be both feasible and effective for symptoms and local control in locally recurrent disease, even with re-irradiation. The utility of pancreas SBRT as neoadjuvant therapy for borderline resectable disease and downstaging locally advanced cancer is promising. With continued advancement, the use of pancreas SBRT in the multidisciplinary setting has the potential to provide substantial improvements in long-term survival. Finally, SBRT combinations with novel chemotherapy, targeted therapy, and immunotherapy should be evaluated in well-designed prospective clinical trials.

References

American Cancer Society (2009) Pancreas cancer staging, AJCC staging manual, 7th edn. p 1

American Cancer Society (2016) Cancer facts & figures 2016. pp 1–72

Balaban EP, Mangu PB, Khorana AA et al (2016) Locally advanced, unresectable pancreatic cancer: American Society of Clinical Oncology Clinical Practice Guideline. J Clin Oncol 34:2654–2668. doi:10.1200/JCO.2016.67.5561

Balcom JH, Rattner DW, Warshaw AL et al (2001) Ten-year experience with 733 pancreatic resections: changing indications, older patients, and decreasing length of hospitalization. Arch Surg 136:391–398

Ben-Josef E, Shields AF, Vaishampayan U et al (2004) Intensity-modulated radiotherapy (IMRT) and concurrent capecitabine for pancreatic cancer. Int J Radiat Oncol Biol Phys 59:454–459. doi:10.1016/j.ijrobp.2003.11.019

Bilimoria KY, Bentrem DJ, Ko CY et al (2007) Validation of the 6th edition AJCC pancreatic cancer staging system: report from the National Cancer Database. Cancer 110:738–744. doi:10.1002/cncr.22852

Breslin TM, Hess KR, Harbison DB et al (2001) Neoadjuvant chemoradiotherapy for adenocarcinoma of the pancreas: treatment variables and survival duration. Ann Surg Oncol 8:123–132. doi:10.1007/s10434-001-0123-4

Butturini G, Stocken DD, Wente MN et al (2008) Influence of resection margins and treatment on survival in patients with pancreatic cancer: meta-analysis of randomized controlled trials. Arch Surg 143:75–83. doi:10.1001/archsurg.2007.17

Cameron JL, Pitt HA, Yeo CJ et al (1993) One hundred and forty-five consecutive pancreaticoduodenectomies without mortality. Ann Surg 217:430–435. discussion 435–438

Cameron JL, Riall TS, Coleman J et al (2006) One thousand consecutive pancreaticoduodenectomies. Ann Surg 244:10–15. doi:10.1097/01.sla.0000217673.04165.ea

Ceha HM, van Tienhoven G, Gouma DJ et al (2000) Feasibility and efficacy of high dose conformal radiotherapy for patients with locally advanced pancreatic carcinoma. Cancer 89:2222–2229. doi:10.1002/1097-0142(20001201)89:11<2222::AID-CNCR10>3.0.CO;2-V

Chang DT, Schellenberg D, Shen J et al (2009) Stereotactic radiotherapy for unresectable adenocarcinoma of the pancreas. Cancer 115:665–672. doi:10.1002/cncr.24059

Chauffert B, Mornex F, Bonnetain F et al (2008) Phase III trial comparing intensive induction chemoradiotherapy (60 Gy, infusional 5-FU and intermittent cisplatin) followed by maintenance gemcitabine with gemcitabine alone for locally advanced unresectable pancreatic cancer. Definitive results of the 2000-01 FFCD/SFRO study. Ann Oncol 19:1592–1599. doi:10.1093/annonc/mdn281

Chuong MD, Springett GM, Freilich JM et al (2013) Stereotactic body radiation therapy for locally advanced and borderline resectable pancreatic cancer is effective and well tolerated. Int J Radiat Oncol Biol Phys 86:516–522. doi:10.1016/j.ijrobp.2013.02.022

Corsini MM, Miller RC, Haddock MG et al (2008) Adjuvant radiotherapy and chemotherapy for pancreatic carcinoma: the Mayo Clinic experience (1975–2005). J Clin Oncol 26(21):3511–3516. doi:10.1200/JCO.2007.15.8782;wgroup:string:Publication

Coveler AL, Herman JM, Simeone DM et al (2016) Localized pancreatic cancer: multidisciplinary management. Am Soc Clin Oncol Educ Book 35:e217–e226. doi:10.14694/EDBK_160827

Crane CH (2016) Hypofractionated ablative radiotherapy for locally advanced pancreatic cancer. J Radiat Res 57(Suppl 1):i53–i57. doi:10.1093/jrr/rrw016

Dagoglu N, Callery M, Moser J et al (2016) Stereotactic body radiotherapy (SBRT) reirradiation for recurrent pancreas cancer. J Cancer 7:283–288. doi:10.7150/jca.13295

Dholakia AS, Kumar R, Raman SP et al (2013a) Mapping patterns of local recurrence after pancreaticoduodenectomy for pancreatic adenocarcinoma: a new approach to adjuvant radiation field design. Int J Radiat Oncol Biol Phys 87:1007–1015. doi:10.1016/j.ijrobp.2013.09.005

Dholakia AS, Hacker-Prietz A, Wild AT et al (2013b) Resection of borderline resectable pancreatic cancer after neoadjuvant chemoradiation does not depend on improved radiographic appearance of tumor-vessel relationships. J Radiat Oncol 2:413–425. doi:10.1007/s13566-013-0115-6

Evans DB, Hess KR, Pisters P (2002) ESPAC-1 trial of adjuvant therapy for resectable adenocarcinoma of the pancreas. Ann Surg 236:694., author reply 694–696. doi:10.1097/01.SLA.0000037256.09376.FC

Franke AJ, Rosati LM, Pawlik TM et al (2015) The role of radiation therapy in pancreatic ductal adenocarcinoma in the neoadjuvant and adjuvant settings. Semin Oncol 42:144–162. doi:10.1053/j.seminoncol.2014.12.013

Gastrointestinal Tumor Study Group (1985) Radiation therapy combined with Adriamycin or 5-fluorouracil for the treatment of locally unresectable pancreatic carcinoma. Cancer 56:2563–2568. doi:10.1002/1097-0142(19851201)56:11<2563::AID-CNCR2820561104>3.0.CO;2-0

Gastrointestinal Tumor Study Group (1988) Treatment of locally unresectable carcinoma of the pancreas: comparison of combined-modality therapy (chemotherapy plus radiotherapy) to chemotherapy alone. JNCI 80:751–755. doi:10.1093/jnci/80.10.751

Geer RJ, Brennan MF (1993) Prognostic indicators for survival after resection of pancreatic adenocarcinoma. Am J Surg 165:68–72. discussion 72–73

Gillen S, Schuster T, zum Büschenfelde CM, et al Neoadjuvant therapy in pancreatic cancer: a systematic review and meta-analysis of response and resection percentages, PLoS Med 7 (2010) e1000267. doi:10.1371/journal.pmed.1000267.

Goodman KA (2016) Stereotactic body radiation therapy for pancreatic cancer. Cancer J 22:290–295. doi:10.1097/PPO.0000000000000206

Goyal K, Einstein D, Ibarra RA et al (2012) Stereotactic body radiation therapy for nonresectable tumors of the pancreas. J Surg Res 174:319–325. doi:10.1016/j.jss.2011.07.044

Griffin JF, Smalley SR, Jewell W et al (1990) Patterns of failure after curative resection of pancreatic carcinoma. Cancer 66:56–61. doi:10.1002/1097-0142(19900701)66:1<56::AID-CNCR2820660112>3.0.CO;2-6

Gurka M, Collins SP, Slack R et al (2013) Stereotactic body radiation therapy with concurrent full-dose gemcitabine for locally advanced pancreatic cancer: a pilot trial demonstrating safety. Radiat Oncol 8:44. doi:10.1186/1748-717X-8-44

Hammel P, Huguet F, van Laethem JL et al (2016) Effect of chemoradiotherapy vs chemotherapy on survival in patients with locally advanced pancreatic cancer controlled after 4 months of gemcitabine with or without erlotinib: The LAP07 Randomized Clinical Trial. JAMA 315:1844–1853. doi:10.1001/jama.2016.4324

Herman JM, Swartz MJ, Hsu CC et al (2008) Analysis of fluorouracil-based adjuvant chemotherapy and radiation after pancreaticoduodenectomy for ductal adenocarcinoma of the pancreas: results of a large, prospectively collected database at the Johns Hopkins Hospital. J Clin Oncol 26(21):3503–3510. doi:10.1200/JCO.2007.15.8469;page:string:Article/Chapter.

Herman JM, Chang DT, Goodman KA et al (2015a) Phase 2 multi-institutional trial evaluating gemcitabine and stereotactic body radiotherapy for patients with locally advanced unresectable pancreatic adenocarcinoma. Cancer 121:1128–1137. doi:10.1002/cncr.29161

Herman JM, Crane CH, Iacobuzio-Donahue C, Abrams RA (2015b). Pancreatic cancer. In: Gunderson LL, Tepper JE (eds) Clinical radiation oncology, 4th edn. Elsevier Health Sciences, pp 934–959

Hoyer M, Roed H, Sengelov L et al (2005) Phase-II study on stereotactic radiotherapy of locally advanced pancreatic carcinoma. Radiother Oncol 76:48–53. doi:10.1016/j.radonc.2004.12.022

Hsu CC, Herman JM, Corsini MM et al (2010) Adjuvant chemoradiation for pancreatic adenocarcinoma: the Johns Hopkins Hospital—Mayo Clinic Collaborative Study. Ann Surg Oncol 17:981–990. doi:10.1245/s10434-009-0743-7

Iacobuzio-Donahue CA, Fu B, Yachida S et al (2009) DPC4 gene status of the primary carcinoma correlates with patterns of failure in patients with pancreatic cancer. J Clin Oncol 27:1806–1813. doi:10.1200/JCO.2008.17.7188

Jones WE, Suh WW, Abdel-Wahab M et al (2017) ACR appropriateness criteria® resectable pancreatic cancer. Am J Clin Oncol 40:109–117. doi:10.1097/COC.0000000000000370

Kalser MH, Ellenberg SS (1985) Pancreatic cancer. Adjuvant combined radiation and chemotherapy following curative resection. Arch Surg 120:899–903

Kang MJ, Jang JY, Chang YR et al (2014) Revisiting the concept of lymph node metastases of pancreatic head cancer: number of metastatic lymph nodes and lymph node ratio according to N stage. Ann Surg Oncol 21:1545–1551. doi:10.1245/s10434-013-3473-9

Katz MH, Pisters P, Evans DB et al (2008) Borderline resectable pancreatic cancer: the importance of this emerging stage of disease. J Am Coll Surg 206:833–846. doi:10.1016/j.jamcollsurg.2007.12.020

Katz MH, Fleming JB, Bhosale P et al (2012) Response of borderline resectable pancreatic cancer to neoadjuvant therapy is not reflected by radiographic indicators. Cancer 118:5749–5756. doi:10.1002/cncr.27636

Katz MH, Shi Q, Ahmad SA et al (2016) Preoperative modified FOLFIRINOX treatment followed by capecitabine-based chemoradiation for borderline resectable pancreatic cancer: Alliance for Clinical Trials in Oncology Trial A021101. JAMA Surg 151:e161137. doi:10.1001/jamasurg.2016.1137

Klaassen DJ, MacIntyre JM, Catton GE et al (1985) Treatment of locally unresectable cancer of the stomach and pancreas: a randomized comparison of 5-fluorouracil alone with radiation plus concurrent and maintenance 5-fluorouracil—an Eastern Cooperative Oncology Group study. J Clin Oncol 3:373–378. doi:10.1200/JCO.1985.3.3.373

Klinkenbijl JH, Jeekel J, Sahmoud T et al (1999) Adjuvant radiotherapy and 5-fluorouracil after curative resection of cancer of the pancreas and periampullary region: phase III trial of the EORTC gastrointestinal tract cancer cooperative group. Ann Surg 230:776

Kooby DA, Gillespie TW, Liu Y et al (2013) Impact of adjuvant radiotherapy on survival after pancreatic cancer resection: an appraisal of data from the National Cancer Data Base. Ann Surg Oncol 20:3634–3642. doi:10.1245/s10434-013-3047-x

Koong AC, Le QT, Ho A et al (2004) Phase I study of stereotactic radiosurgery in patients with locally advanced pancreatic cancer. Int J Radiat Oncol Biol Phys 58:1017–1021. doi:10.1016/j.ijrobp.2003.11.004

Krishnan S, Chadha AS, Suh Y et al (2016) Focal radiotherapy dose escalation improves overall survival in locally advanced pancreatic cancer patients receiving induction chemotherapy and consolidative chemoradiation. Int J Radiat Oncol Biol Phys 94(4):755–765

Liao WC, Chien KL, Lin YL et al (2013) Adjuvant treatments for resected pancreatic adenocarcinoma: a systematic review and network meta-analysis. Lancet Oncol 14:1095–1103. doi:10.1016/S1470-2045(13)70388-7

Loehrer PJ, Feng Y, Cardenes H et al (2011) Gemcitabine alone versus gemcitabine plus radiotherapy in patients with locally advanced pancreatic cancer: an Eastern Cooperative Oncology Group trial. J Clin Oncol 29:4105–4112. doi:10.1200/JCO.2011.34.8904

Lominska CE, Unger K, Nasr NM et al (2012) Stereotactic body radiation therapy for reirradiation of localized adenocarcinoma of the pancreas. Radiat Oncol 7:74. doi:10.1186/1748-717X-7-74

Lowenfels AB, Maisonneuve P (2006) Epidemiology and risk factors for pancreatic cancer. Best Pract Res Clin Gastroenterol 20:197–209. doi:10.1016/j.bpg.2005.10.001s

Mahadevan A, Miksad R, Goldstein M et al (2011) Induction gemcitabine and stereotactic body radiotherapy for locally advanced nonmetastatic pancreas cancer. Int J Radiat Oncol Biol Phys 81:e615–e622. doi:10.1016/j.ijrobp.2011.04.045

Michaud DS, Giovannucci E, Willett WC et al (2001) Physical activity, obesity, height, and the risk of pancreatic cancer. JAMA 286:921–929

Moertel C (1969) Combined 5-flurouracil and supervoltage radiation therapy of locally unresectable gastrointestinal cancer. Lancet 294:865–867. doi:10.1016/S0140-6736(69)92326-5

Moertel C, Frytak S, Hahn RG et al (1981) Therapy of locally unresectable pancreatic carcinoma: a randomized comparison of high dose (6000 rads) radiation alone, moderate dose radiation (4000 rads + 5-fluorouracil), and high dose radiation + 5-fluorouracil. The Gastrointestinal Tumor Study Group. Cancer 48:1705–1710. doi:10.1002/1097-0142(19811015)48:8<1705::AID-CNCR2820480803>3.0.CO;2-4

Moningi S, Walker AJ, Hsu CC et al (2015a) Correlation of clinical stage and performance status with quality of life in patients seen in a pancreas multidisciplinary clinic. J Oncol Pract 11:e216–e221. doi:10.1200/JOP.2014.000976

Moningi S, Dholakia AS, Raman SP et al (2015b) The role of stereotactic body radiation therapy for pancreatic cancer: a single-institution experience. Ann Surg Oncol 22:2352–2358. doi:10.1245/s10434-014-4274-5

Morganti AG, Falconi M, van Stiphout RG et al (2014) Multi-institutional pooled analysis on adjuvant chemoradiation in pancreatic cancer. Int J Radiat Oncol Biol Phys 90:911–917. doi:10.1016/j.ijrobp.2014.07.024

Murphy JD, Christman-Skieller C, Kim J et al (2010) A dosimetric model of duodenal toxicity after stereotactic body radiotherapy for pancreatic cancer. Int J Radiat Oncol Biol Phys 78:1420–1426. doi:10.1016/j.ijrobp.2009.09.075

Myrehaug S, Sahgal A, Russo SM et al (2016) Stereotactic body radiotherapy for pancreatic cancer: recent progress and future directions. Expert Rev Anticancer Ther 16:523–530. doi:10.1586/14737140.2016.1168698

Neoptolemos JP, Stocken DD, Friess H et al (2009) A randomized trial of chemoradiotherapy and chemotherapy after resection of pancreatic cancer. N Engl J Med 350:1200–1210. doi:10.1056/NEJMoa032295

Oettle H, Neuhaus P, Hochhaus A et al (2013) Adjuvant chemotherapy with gemcitabine and long-term outcomes among patients with resected pancreatic cancer: The CONKO-001 Randomized Trial. JAMA 310:1473–1481. doi:10.1001/jama.2013.279201

Pawlik TM, Laheru D, Hruban RH et al (2008) Evaluating the impact of a single-day multidisciplinary clinic on the management of pancreatic cancer. Ann Surg Oncol 15:2081–2088. doi:10.1245/s10434-008-9929-7

Polistina F, Costantin G, Casamassima F et al (2010) Unresectable locally advanced pancreatic cancer: a multimodal treatment using neoadjuvant chemoradiotherapy (gemcitabine plus stereotactic radiosurgery) and subsequent surgical exploration. Ann Surg Oncol 17:2092–2101. doi:10.1245/s10434-010-1019-y

Poplin E, Feng Y, Berlin J et al (2016) Phase III, randomized study of gemcitabine and oxaliplatin versus gemcitabine (fixed-dose rate infusion) compared with gemcitabine (30-minute infusion) in patients with pancreatic carcinoma E6201: a trial of the Eastern Cooperative Oncology Group. J Clin Oncol 27(23):3778–3785. doi:10.1200/JCO.2008 .20.9007;subPage:string:Abstract;website:websit e:asco-site;issue:issue:10.1200/JCO.2009.24.27. issue-23;wgroup:string:Publication

Porta M, Fabregat X, Malats N et al (2005) Exocrine pancreatic cancer: symptoms at presentation and their relation to tumour site and stage. Clin Transl Oncol 7:189–197

Redmond KJ, Wolfgang CL, Sugar EA et al (2010) Adjuvant chemoradiation therapy for adenocarcinoma of the distal pancreas. Ann Surg Oncol 17:3112–3119. doi:10.1245/s10434-010-1200-3

Regine WF, Winter KW, Abrams R et al (2011) Fluorouracil-based chemoradiation with either gemcitabine or fluorouracil chemotherapy after resection of pancreatic adenocarcinoma: 5-year analysis of the U.S. Intergroup/RTOG 9704 phase III trial. Ann Surg Oncol 18:1319–1326. doi:10.1245/ s10434-011-1630-6

Ren F, YC X, Wang HX et al (2012) Adjuvant chemotherapy, with or without postoperative radiotherapy, for resectable advanced pancreatic adenocarcinoma: continue or stop? Pancreatology 12:162–169. doi:10.1016/j.pan.2012.02.002

Rose JB, Rocha FG, Alseidi A et al (2014) Extended neoadjuvant chemotherapy for borderline resectable pancreatic cancer demonstrates promising postoperative outcomes and survival. Ann Surg Oncol 21:1530–1537. doi:10.1245/s10434-014-3486-z

Rwigema JC, Heron DE, Parikh SD et al (2012) Adjuvant stereotactic body radiotherapy for resected pancreatic adenocarcinoma with close or positive margins. J Gastrointest Cancer 43:70–76. doi:10.1007/ s12029-010-9203-7

Schellenberg D, Goodman KA, Lee F et al (2008) Gemcitabine chemotherapy and single-fraction stereotactic body radiotherapy for locally advanced pancreatic cancer. Int J Radiat Oncol Biol Phys 72:678–686. doi:10.1016/j.ijrobp.2008.01.051

Schellenberg D, Kim J, Christman-Skieller C et al (2011) Single-fraction stereotactic body radiation therapy and sequential gemcitabine for the treatment of locally advanced pancreatic cancer. Int J Radiat Oncol Biol Phys 81:181–188. doi:10.1016/j.ijrobp.2010.05.006

Small W, Hayes JP, Suh WW et al (2016) Expert panel on radiation oncology-gastrointestinal, ACR appropriateness criteria® borderline and unresectable pancreas cancer. Oncology 30:619–624. 627–632

Spitz FR, Abbruzzese JL, Lee JE et al (2016) Preoperative and postoperative chemoradiation strategies in patients treated with pancreaticoduodenectomy for adenocarcinoma of the pancreas. J Clin Oncol. doi:10.1200/JCO .1997.15.3.928;issue:issue:10.1200/jco.1997.15.3.15. issue-3;page:string:Article/Chapter.

Stocken DD, Büchler MW, Dervenis C et al (2005) Meta-analysis of randomized adjuvant therapy trials for pancreatic cancer. Br J Cancer 92:1372–1381. doi:10.1038/sj.bjc.6602513

Stolzenberg-Solomon RZ, Adams K, Leitzmann KM et al (2008) Adiposity, physical activity, and pancreatic cancer in the National Institutes of Health-AARP Diet and Health Cohort. Am J Epidemiol 167:586–597. doi:10.1093/aje/kwm361

Tempero MA (2016) Pancreatic adenocarcinoma, The emperor of all pancreatic cancer maladies. J Oncol Pract 1:29–30. doi:10.1200/jop.2015.009753

Tepper J, Nardi G, Suit H (1976) Carcinoma of the pancreas: review of MGH experience from 1963 to 1973—analysis of surgical failure and implications for radiation therapy. Cancer 37:1519–1524. doi:10.1002/1097-0142(197603)37:3<1519::AID-CNCR2820370340>3.0.CO;2-O

Tozzi A, Comito T, FAlongi F et al (2013) SBRT in unresectable advanced pancreatic cancer: preliminary results of a mono-institutional experience. Radiat Oncol 8:148. doi:10.1186/1748-717X-8-148

Ueno H, Ioka T, Ikeda M et al (2016) Randomized phase III study of gemcitabine plus S-1, S-1 alone, or gemcitabine alone in patients with locally advanced and metastatic pancreatic cancer in Japan and Taiwan: GEST study. J Clin Oncol 31(13):1640–1648. doi:10.1200/JCO.2012.43.3680;page:string:Article/ Chapter

Valle JW, Palmer D, Jackson R et al (2014) Optimal duration and timing of adjuvant chemotherapy after definitive surgery for ductal adenocarcinoma of the pancreas: ongoing lessons from the ESPAC-3 study. J Clin Oncol 32:504–512. doi:10.1200/JCO.2013.50.7657

Wild AT, Hiniker SM, Chang DT et al (2013) Re-irradiation with stereotactic body radiation therapy as a novel treatment option for isolated local recurrence of pancreatic cancer after multimodality therapy: experience from two institutions. J Gastrointest Oncol 4:343–351

Wolfgang CL, Herman JM, Laheru DA et al (2013) Recent progress in pancreatic cancer. CA Cancer J Clin 63:318–348. doi:10.3322/caac.21190

Yang W, Reznik WR, Fraass BA et al (2015) Dosimetric evaluation of simultaneous integrated boost during stereotactic body radiation therapy for pancreatic cancer. Med Dosim 40:47–52. doi:10.1016/j. meddos.2014.09.001

Ychou M, Desseigne F, Guimbaud R (2007) Randomized phase II trial comparing folfirinox (5FU/leucovorin [LV], irinotecan [I] and oxaliplatin [O]) vs gemcitabine (G) as first-line treatment for metastatic pancreatic adenocarcinoma (MPA). First results of the ACCORD 11 trial. J Clin Oncol 25(18):4516

Yeo CJ, Cameron JL, Lillemoe KD et al (1995) Pancreaticoduodenectomy for cancer of the head of the pancreas. 201 patients. Ann Surg 221:721–731. discussion 731–733

Yeo CJ, Cameron JL, Sohn TA et al (1997) Six hundred fifty consecutive pancreaticoduodenectomies in the 1990s: pathology, complications, and outcomes. Ann Surg 226:248–257. discussion 257–260

Hypofractionation in Patients with Rectal Cancer

Te Vuong, Slobodan Devic, and Krzysztof Bujko

Contents

Abstract

Rectal cancers can be categorized into three clinical subgroups: early, intermediate, and those locally advanced. For the latter two cases, preoperative radiotherapy is recommended. An advanced type of cancer is diagnosed whenever a cT3 lesion threatens or invades mesorectal fascia or when a cT4 tumor overgrows into organs not readily resectable. For the intermediate-risk group, tumor shrinkage before surgery is not needed and preoperative radiotherapy is aimed at reducing the risk of local recurrence. There are two types of preoperative radiation treatment commonly accepted as standard for the intermediate risk group: (1) short-course (5 fractions of 5 Gy over 1 week) radiotherapy (RT) with surgery carried out within the next 5 days and (2) long-course chemoradiation (conventionally fractionated RT consisting of 25–28 fractions of 1.8 or 2 Gy over 5–5.5 weeks concomitantly used with 5-fluorouracil or capecitabine) with surgery carried out 6–8 weeks thereafter.

This chapter reports the experience of hypofractionation in patients with rectal cancer and includes two parts:

The first section is on the use of neoadjuvant short-course radiation with external beam radiation therapy followed by immediate surgery and supporting evidence of its efficacy and treatment-related toxicities in the literature. The second section introduces the innovative concept of the targeted volume at risk in the era of total mesorectal excision including quality magnetic resonance imaging in selected intermediate-risk patients.

The original version of this chapter was revised. The affiliations of the authors have been updated.

T. Vuong (✉) • S. Devic
Mcgill University, Montreal, QC, Canada
e-mail: tvuong@jgh.mcgill.ca

K. Bujko
The Maria Sklodowska-Curie Memorial Cancer Centre and Institute of Oncology, Warsaw, Poland

Med Radiol Radiat Oncol (2017)
DOI 10.1007/174_2017_36, © Springer International Publishing AG
Published Online: 13 April 2017

High-dose-rate endorectal brachytherapy was introduced in 1999 as a neoadjuvant modality for rectal cancer. The planning, technique, long-term oncological results, and most importantly the pattern of pelvic relapse are provided. This delivers highly conformal treatment to the target, but also provides dose distribution that more efficiently spares surrounding healthy tissue and in such a way paving the road for a better quality of life and avoidance of the well-documented normal tissue toxicities reported after external beam radiation therapy.

1 Introduction

1.1 External Beam Radiation Therapy

Presently, for rectal tumors, the two types of preoperative RT are used: either stereotactic radiotherapy (SRT) or long-course chemoradiation (Glimelius et al. 2013). The former schedule is preferred in Northern Europe but the latter schedule preferred in Southern Europe and the Americas. Currently, SRT-immediate (short course; usually five fractions in 1 week) is also gaining acceptance in the USA. The most recent version of the National Comprehensive Cancer Network (NCCN) guidelines recommends SRT-immediate as an option (National Comprehensive Cancer Network Guidelines 2016). However, is long-course chemoradiation or SRT-immediate preferable as preoperative radiotherapy in the intermediate-risk group?

1.1.1 Trials Exploring Preoperative SRT-Immediate, Surgery Alone, and Postoperative Long-Course RT

SRT-immediate was the most extensively tested radiotherapy regimen in randomized trials of rectal cancer, with approximately 6000 patients participating (Frykholm et al. 1993; Bujko et al. 2004; Ngan et al. 2012; Folkesson et al. 2005; Martling et al. 2001; Pettersson et al. 2010; Stockholm Colorectal Cancer Study Group

1990; Sebag-Montefiore et al. 2009). Four trials (all in Sweden) were performed with radiotherapy done before implementing total mesorectal excision (TME) and modern radiotherapy techniques. Thus, conclusions cannot be entirely generalized for currently treated patients. The Uppsala trial compared SRT-immediate against postoperative radiotherapy (60 Gy, 2 Gy per fraction) (Frykholm et al. 1993). No difference in overall survival was shown. At 5 years, the SRT-immediate group compared to the postoperative RT group had less local recurrences (13% vs. 22%, $p = 0.02$) and late small bowel obstructions (5% vs. 11%, $p < 0.01$). The Stockholm I (Stockholm Colorectal Cancer Study Group 1990), the Stockholm II (Martling et al. 2001), and the Swedish trial (Folkesson et al. 2005) compared SRT-immediate with surgery alone. The largest Swedish trial demonstrated improvement in overall survival at 13 years after preoperative radiotherapy compared to surgery alone, 38% vs. 30%, $p = 0.008$, and less local recurrences 9% vs. 26%, $p < 0.001$, respectively.

1.1.2 SRT-Immediate Versus Long-Course Chemoradiation in the Intermediate-Risk Group

There are two published randomized trials comparing SRT-immediate with neoadjuvant long-course chemoradiation: the Polish study of 312 patients (Bujko et al. 2004, 2006) and the Australian study of 326 patients (Ngan et al. 2012) (Table 1). The design of these two trials was similar. The Polish trial evaluated a hypothesized 15% or larger difference in the rate of sphincter-preserving surgery between the two treatment-assigned groups, and the Australian study evaluated a hypothesized 10% or larger difference in local recurrence rate. In the long-course chemoradiation groups, both trials used 50.4 Gy and 1.8 Gy per fraction. Fluorouracil and leucovorin in bolus were used concomitantly with radiation in the Polish trial and continuous infusion fluorouracil in the Australian study. The median follow-up was 4 years in the Polish study and 5.9 years in the Australian trial.

Table 1 The Polish (Bujko et al. 2004) and Australian (Ngan et al. 2012) randomized trials comparing neoadjuvant short-course radiation and neoadjuvant chemoradiation

	Polish study $N = 312$			Australian study $N = 326$		
	Short-course (%)	Long-course (%)	p-value	Short-course (%)	Long-course (%)	p-value
Overall acute toxicity	24	85	<0.001	72.3	99.4	<0.001
Grade III-IV acute toxicity	3	18	<0.001	1.9	27.1	<0.001
Deaths due to acute toxicity	0	1.3		0	1.2	
Acute neuropathic pain				5	4	
Adherence to the RT protocol	98	78		100	77	
Adherence to the RT + CT protocol	98	69				
Overall surgical complications	27	21	0.27	53.2	50.3	0.68
Postoperative deaths (30 days)	1.3	0.7		0	0	
Anastomotic leakage requiring re-operation	9	8	0.76			
All anastomotic leakage				7.1	3.5	0.26
Perineal wound complications	29	21	0.36	38.3	50	0.26
Permanent stoma rate	56.9	51.6	0.35	38	29.8	0.13
ypT0	1	16	<0.001[a]	1	15	<0.001[a]
ypN0	52	68	0.007	60	65	0.5
Positive circumferential margin	13	4	0.017	5	6	
Local recurrence	At 4 y. 10.6	15.6	0.21	At 3 y. 7.5	4.4	0.24
Distant metastases	Crude 31.4	34.6	0.54	At 5 y. 27	30	0.92
Disease-free survival	At 4 y. 58.4	55.6	0.82	At 5 y. 68	61	0.47
Overall survival	At 4 y. 67.2	66.2	0.96	At 5 y. 74	70	0.62
Overall late toxicity	28.3	27.0	0.81			
Grade III-IV late toxicity 53	10.1	7.1	0.36	5.8	8.2	0.
Late nerves damage	2.9	2.8				
QLQ-C30 global health status mean scores[b]	57	61	0.22	−9.9	8.2	0.44
Mean change from baseline[b]						
Poor anorectal function Defecation problems	59	64	0.52			0.47
Decline in sexual function male	80	69	0.56			NS
female	41	52	0.10			

Lack of data in the table confers that the data were unpublished
[a]This p-value compared ypT-downstaging (all ypT categories)
[b]The differences in the scores of all other scales of QLQ were also insignificant
QLQ quality of life questionnaire, *RT* radiotherapy, *CT* chemotherapy, *y* years, *NS* not significant

There are three advantages of SRT-immediate compared to long-course chemoradiation. Lower cost and better convenience: because five RT fractions are delivered over 1 week instead of 25–28 fractions over 5–5.5 weeks. The third advantage is lower acute toxicity. Grade III–IV acute toxicity was 3% in the SRT-immediate group and 18% in the long-course chemoradiation group, p <0.001 in the Polish trial (Table 1). The corresponding acute toxicity results in the Australian trial were 2% and 27%, respectively, p <0.001. In each of the two studies, two acute toxic deaths (1.2%) related to RT were reported in the long-course group and none in the SRT-immediate group.

Sacral pain was reported previously during SRT in 10% of patients in the Dutch TME trial (Marijnen et al. 2002). However, no difference in sacral pain was observed between randomized groups in the Australian trial. Lower early toxicity in the SRT groups translated into improved adherence to the protocol. The differences between randomized groups in all other clinical endpoints were insignificant (Table 1). The type, rates, and severity of postoperative complications were similar in the two randomized groups for both studies. There were also no differences in survival, local control, and permanent stoma rates (Table 1). When the two trials are evaluated together, any clear tendency in superior outcomes in either of the randomized groups cannot be distinguished. For example, in the Polish trial, the local recurrence rate was slightly lower in the SRT-immediate group than in the long-course group, 10.6% vs. 15.6%, $p = 0.21$, whereas the opposite tendency was seen in the Australian study at 7.5% vs. 4.4%, $p = 0.24$. The local efficacy of SRT-immediate or long-course chemoradiation was unrelated to the tumor location within the rectum (low-lying vs. high lesions) (Pietrzak et al. 2007). Additionally, no increase of late toxicity in the SRT-immediate groups was found when compared to the long-course chemoradiation groups (Table 1), although admittedly, in both trials, the follow-up was too short to draw definitive conclusions. Late neurotoxicity was observed in the early study with SRT. However, no difference in late neurotoxicity was reported

between the two randomized groups in the Polish trial (Table 1). In the two trials, no significant differences were observed between the randomized groups regarding quality of life, anorectal, and sexual dysfunction (Pietrzak et al. 2007) (Table 1).

It should be highlighted that despite more favorable postoperative pathology in the long-course groups (many more pathological complete responses and T- and N-downstaging) than in the SRT-immediate groups, the long-term oncological outcomes were similar (Table 1). This phenomenon can be explained by the strong dependence between manifestations of radiation-induced cancer cell damage and the interval duration between the beginning of radiation and surgery (Francois et al. 1999). In SRT-immediate, when surgery takes place within a few days following the start of radiation, nonviable cancer cells look morphologically intact microscopically. In long-course RT, such nonviable cells undergo lyses within the next few weeks that elapse between the beginning of radiation and surgery. This results in downstaging or in pathological complete response. The same explanation applies to the observation from the Polish study that rates of positive circumferential resection margin in patients treated with the SRT-immediate and long-course chemoradiation were, respectively, 13% and 4% ($p = 0.017$), while local recurrence rates were not different.

The management of patients with rectal cancer has dramatically changed with the introduction of quality surgery. Total mesorectal excision (TME) consists of complete excision of the rectum with an intact mesorectal fascia containing the immediate lymphatic drainage/perirectal nodes (MacFarlane et al. 1993; Martling et al. 2000). Two large randomized study groups, the Dutch TME trial and the MRC CR07 trial (Peeters et al. 2007; Quirke et al. 2009; Van Gijn et al. 2011), conducted randomized studies to examine the question of whether preoperative external beam radiation was still required. The Dutch trial compared TME alone to short-course external beam radiation therapy (EBRT) with 25 Gy in five fractions and TME surgery while the MRC CR07 trial (Sebag-Montefiore et al.

2009) compared SRT-immediate before TME vs. TME alone with the selective use of postoperative long-course radiochemotherapy for approximately 10% of patients who had a positive circumferential resection margin. Both trials showed a 50–60% relative reduction of local recurrence after SRT-immediate, although the absolute benefit was only 5–6%. Both trials showed no benefit in overall survival with SRT-immediate. In the MRC CR07 trial (Sebag-Montefiore et al. 2009) however, disease-free survival was significantly improved at 3 years in the SRT-immediate group. Nevertheless, these studies raised the question of the number of patients needed for treatment for the benefit of a small subset of patients. More than 15 years have passed since these studies were completed and long-term results show the persistent benefits of EBRT on local control (Van Gijn et al. 2011). However, there remains the issue of morbidity (Birgisson et al. 2007, 2008; Marijnen et al. 2005; Peeters et al. 2005; Bruheim et al. 2010; Wiltink et al. 2014) on normal tissues exposed to EBRT. The patients had worse bowel and sexual function (Birgisson et al. 2007, 2008; Marijnen et al. 2005; Peeters et al. 2005; Bruheim et al. 2010; Wiltink et al. 2014) and it was documented that the benefit of cancer-related survival (Van Gijn et al. 2011) was offset by noncancer-related mortality. The pattern of pelvic recurrence (Kusters et al. 2010) was reported in detail and, interestingly, showed that nodal contribution to local relapse was 2% actuarial rate at 5 years. In the meantime, quality pelvic imaging with magnetic resonance imaging (MRI) was introduced (Smith and Brown 2008). At the same time, there were also advancements in treatment planning and treatment delivery. Using a computerized software system coupled with an integrated imaging planning system now permitted highly targeted radiation delivery.

1.2   High-Dose-Rate Endorectal Brachytherapy: Rationale

In radiation oncology, brachytherapy (BT) is the most highly targeted radiation treatment. The inverse square law refers to the change of the dose rate inversely proportional to the square of the distance. The impact of the inverse square law allows brachytherapy to achieve higher levels of normal tissue sparing within the vicinity of the target volume. At McGill University in the early 1990s, high-dose-rate endorectal brachytherapy (HDREBT) was developed (Vuong et al. 2002, 2010) during the era of quality surgery with total mesorectal excision along with the introduction of magnetic resonance imaging (Smith and Brown 2008) in the staging of pelvic tumors. The HDREBT was tested as a neoadjuvant modality. Patients with nonobstructive tumors, large T4 tumors, or suspected extra-mesorectal or inguinal nodes were excluded. The rectal probe has a 2 cm diameter and measures 22 cm in length. It contains a distal opening to accommodate a guide wire that is useful to safely position the rectal applicator for middle third tumors that extend into the upper third rectum. Most patients having undergone a successful colonoscopy are eligible for HDRBT, but tumors with a thickness of more than 3 cm are not ideal for this treatment as there is a dose overspill that is not desirable within the context of delivering targeted RT treatment. Prior to treatment, radio-opaque clips are placed above and below the tumor as reference points. The patient takes daily enemas, and prior to each treatment, an exploratory view of the pelvis is obtained to ensure that there is no air interference. A rectoscopy (which now replaces the rectal digital exam) is done to ensure that there is no interference of stools/liquids at the interface of the tumor and the applicator prior to the positioning of the rectal probe. The rectal probe is positioned at the level of the proximal clips and then fixed on the treatment table. The target volume is identified using the diagnostic MRI and includes the tumor and its immediate intra-mesorectal extension. Nodes are not included unless they are adjacent to the tumor, or threatening the circumferential margin, as nodal contribution represents 2% of pelvic relapse, which was associated, in most of the cases, with systemic disease (Vuong et al. 2016).

The dose is customized to the patient and is prescribed at the deepest aspect of the tumor, slice

3D Conformal

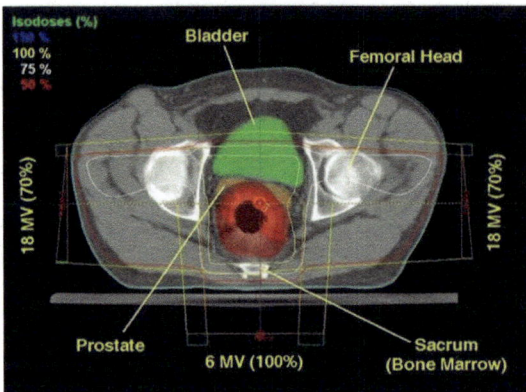

Brachytherapy

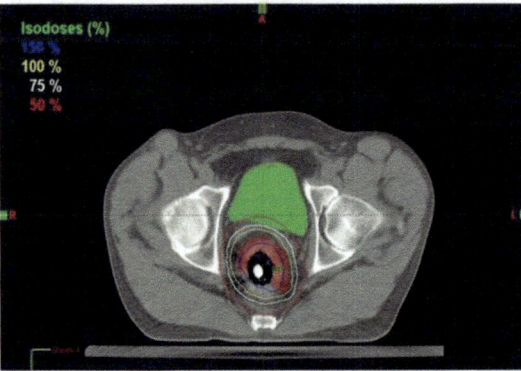

Fig. 1 Dose comparison for one rectal adenocarcinoma patient treated with high-dose-rate endorectal brachytherapy (*bottom*) to highly conformal external beam radiation therapy

by slice. At the level of dose distribution, a very high dose is observed close to the applicator based on the inverse square law as shown in Fig. 1. A total dose of 26 Gy in four daily fractions is delivered using a remote afterloader over various treatment times (10–30 min) depending on the tumor size and the actual isotope activity. This high dose mimics a boost within the tumor volume leading to the high sterilization rate of 27% (Vuong et al. 2010) observed in the pathological specimen compared to an expected 10% rate in the conventional long-course chemotherapy and EBRT. Indeed, the concern was that such a high dose might exceed mucosal tolerance but this was not a clinical issue as the treatment was delivered as a neoadjuvant modality and the tumor was resected within 4–8 weeks after treatment

completion. As a result, the clinical target volume (CTV) was relatively small when compared to EBRT and allowed for delivery of the entire treatment within 4 consecutive days. Over time, the technique evolved in conjunction with modern planning systems. The introduction of a CT simulator within the brachytherapy suite now allows for the adaptive treatment (Nout et al. 2016). On a daily basis, the CT is delineated and our experience shows that the CTV differs daily due to variation of the rectal applicator positioning, thus necessitating repeated daily treatment planning.

The accuracy of treatment delivery is possible as the applicator moves with the tumor, thereby eliminating the problem of intra-fractional organ motion encountered during EBRT and SBRT. There was no difference in the postoperative complication rate (Hesselager et al. 2013) when compared to those treated with EBRT. Patients treated with HDREBT are still being monitored for possible long-term normal tissue toxicity, but dosimetry data comparisons predict favorable outcomes with almost no dose to the small bowel and negligible dose to the bladder and, in particular, to the anal sphincter compared to EBRT for low tumors. For the patient, the convenience of having treatment completed within a week is appealing compared to the long course of 5 weeks of daily treatment with concurrent chemotherapy. This is an even more important consideration in North America where travelling long distances, at times in harsh weather conditions, is common in order to receive radiation treatments. EBRT poses a barrier to treatment acceptance in the elderly population, and is a burden to caregivers. However, the HDREBT is not without inconveniences to patients either. When compared to the short-course EBRT (25 Gy in five fractions), it is more invasive and requires daily placement of the intracavitary mold applicator and planning with an overall treatment time of 45–60 min. Patients expressed variable levels of anxiety (Néron et al. 2014) and reported different degrees of pain during treatment. Proctitis is the dominant and unique acute treatment-related toxicity, starting 7–10 days after treatment and lasting until the time of surgery. It is well managed with a prescription of steroid enemas, anti-inflammatory medication, and narcotics as needed.

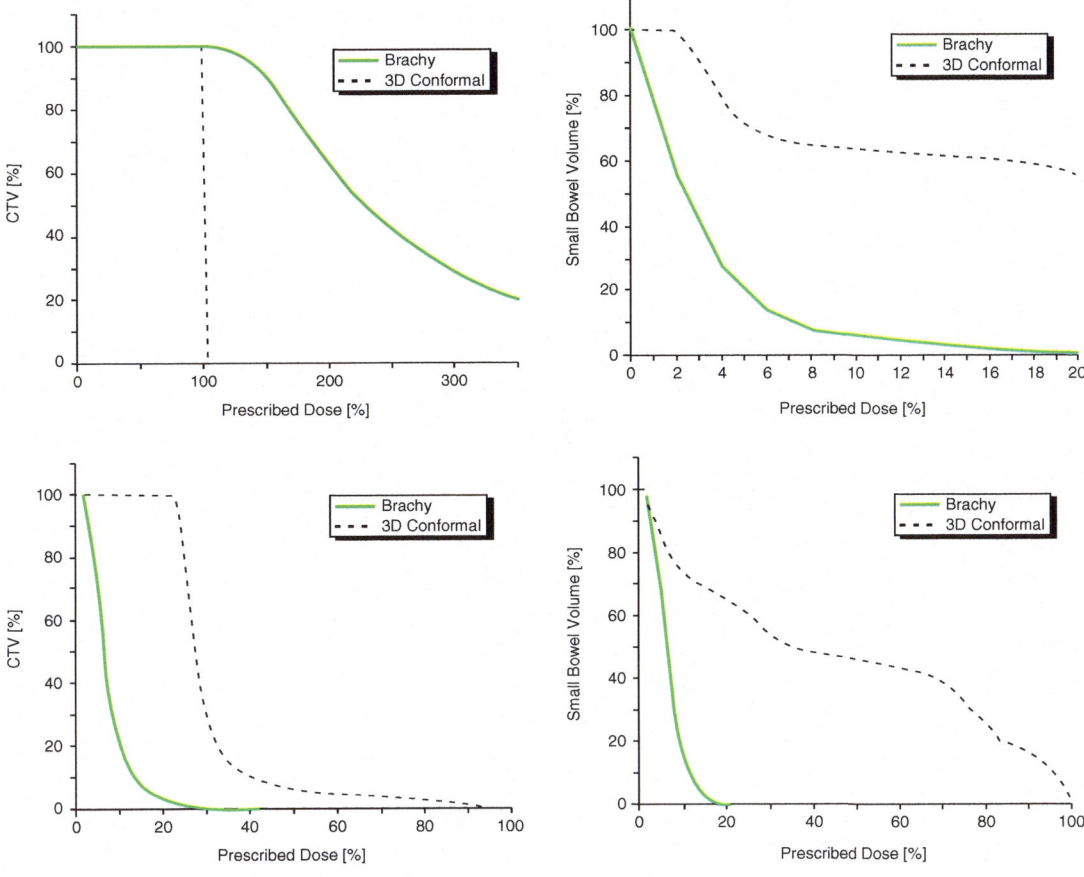

Fig. 2 DVH comparison between the three modalities (BT-brachytherapy, RA-Rapid Arc®, CK-Cyber Knife®) for CTV (*top*) and contralateral (to the target) rectal wall (*bottom*)

No treatment-related death has been observed and the 1% grade 3 toxicity rate was related to bleeding/tenesmus management requiring hospital admission which compared favorably to the 18–27% associated with EBRT (Bujko et al. 2004; Ngan et al. 2012; Sauer et al. 2004). Currently, there is no randomized study comparing EBRT to HDRBT. The major reason is related to the lack of expertise of GI radiation oncologists in brachytherapy and the long-time commitment associated with total treatment planning time (20–30 min for EBRT as compared to 3–4 h for HDRBT). On the other hand, the benefits not only to the patient but to society as well are easily predictable. Figure 2 shows the dose distribution demonstrating better avoidance of radiation exposure to the surrounding normal tissues. The tumor-specific benefits are yet to be shown in the absence of an RCT but

favorable tumor downstaging was observed in a matched pair study comparing HDRBT to EBRT (Breugom et al. 2015) during the same time period, with no statistically significant difference but with excellent tumor disease-free and overall survival rates.

2 Results and Discussion

From 1999 to 2015, 667 patients were treated, most of whom were diagnosed with T3 tumors (84%). The remainder presented with low T2 (13%) and early T4 (3%). Thirty-six percent of the patients had positive nodes on preoperative imaging. The pattern of pelvic relapse (Martling et al. 2000) was analyzed after 15 years from the time of its introduction.

Figure 1 illustrates a dosimetric difference between highly conformal EBRT (Cyber Knife™; Accuray, Inc., Sunnyvale California, USA and Rapid Arc™; Varian Inc., Palo Alto California, USA) and HDRBT for one patient in three different digitally reconstructed planes (axial, coronal, and sagittal). Brachytherapy plans were generated using the IPSA inverse planning module of MasterPlan® treatment planning system (Nucletron Inc.; Columbia Maryland, USA), which does not provide the impact of the midline shielding, used during HDRBT, while the CT data without applicator were used for planning on Cyber Knife™ and Rapid Arc™. Figure 2 shows a comparison between DVH curves for the same patient for CTV and the contralateral (to the target volume) rectal wall.

Figure 1 suggests that both EBT modalities provide very conformal dose distribution to the target. While EBT modalities provide generally better sparing of distal critical structures, the HDRBT shows a clear advantage in sparing the contralateral rectal wall (Fig. 2). Although all the EBT modalities use image-guided radiotherapy (IGRT) systems that allow repositioning of the patient (hence target) just before commencing the treatment fraction, it is difficult to ascertain the impact of daily intra-fractional rectal motility and gas interference on the CTV in this study. The higher dose within CTV (observed with HDRBT) is likely the most important factor for achieving complete tumor response.

The local failure rate in our patient population was 4.7% with a median follow-up time of 65 months for the 608 patients who were assessed after treatment completion (range 6–165 months) (Vuong et al. 2016). Twenty-eight patients developed pelvic recurrence, of which 25 were documented with MRI and 3 with CT scan. The imaging at the time of documented pelvic recurrence was reviewed by two radiologists. The locations of recurrence were identified as iliac or lateral nodes in 11 patients, anastomotic in 10 patients, inguinal nodes in 3 patients, anterior compartment in 4 patients, and presacral space in 1 patient (1 patient had more

than 2 sites). In the patients with pelvic nodal relapses, the relapse was isolated for three patients and in the other eight patients there were associated systemic relapses. These eight patients were asymptomatic and did not require pelvic irradiation while the former three patients underwent successful salvage radiation with intensity-modulated radiation therapy (IMRT) for one patient and stereotactic body radiation therapy (SBRT) for two patients. The other nine patients with anastomotic relapse without systemic recurrence received preoperative pelvic EBRT with salvage surgery. Pelvic nodal relapse actuarial rate was 2% and represented the most common site of recurrence. It is *associated in most of the cases with systemic relapse* and was *asymptomatic in the majority* of the patients. Interestingly, this 2% nodal relapse rate was similar to the observation arm reported in the Dutch TME trial (Kusters et al. 2010). In contrast, after EBRT, presacral recurrence was extremely low.

One can argue that short-course EBRT is more patient friendly than HDRBT. However, the avoidance of large-volume pelvic radiation is appealing in this time of highly effective chemotherapy regimens for patients with colorectal cancer. These systemic treatments are shown to be highly effective in metastatic stage cancer and there are numerous treatment regimens leading to long-term survival after the development of systemic disease. Therefore; sparing bone marrow reserves is important. Recent studies (Newman et al. 2016; Chan et al. 2012, 2016; Colaco et al. 2014; Yang et al. 2014) showed the impact of dose on bone marrow volume exposure to preoperative EBRT which has a strong impact on subsequent patient compliance and tolerance to adjuvant chemotherapy. In patients with nodal disease (stage III), the risks of systemic relapse are dominant (30–40%) when compared to the 2% of local relapse. Moreover, radiation technologies continue to evolve and SBRT is one among examples. In patients with lung cancer, SBRT was shown to be as effective as surgery in curing patients with limited treatment-related toxicity and offers practical hypofractionation. The SBRT modality is presently widely explored in clinical trials for patients with metastatic disease. In our center, we are currently exploring the treatment of patients with pelvic nodal relapse after HDRBT in a dose escalation study with the goal of offering a safe and efficient salvage radiation regimen with targeted treatment to the isolated nodes.

Conclusions

For patients with rectal cancer, there is evidence to support the use of hypofractionation with external beam radiation therapy as an effective neoadjuvant option compared to conventional long-course radiochemotherapy to improve the local tumor control.

In this era of high-quality tumor imaging, TME surgery, and highly targeted radiation treatment options, HDREBT is an appealing novel radiation modality for patients with rectal cancer allowing for highly efficient tumor downstaging and prevention of tumor recurrence in a selected patient population. It requires a dedicated team committed to delivering highly targeted treatment. This modality has a twofold practicality: it offers a 4-day treatment schedule, and, more significantly, spares the surrounding normal tissue from radiation exposure. It will be most useful in the future, to develop a randomized clinical trial to validate the McGill University experience and to record the long-term potential benefits of this highly targeted treatment over EBRT in order to avoid the well-documented long-term side effects of the latter treatment on normal tissues. Just as a similar experience for breast cancer patients documented lower toxicity in patients treated with targeted radiation such as intraoperative electronic brachytherapy or interstitial/intracavitary implant, the evaluation of cost-effectiveness and potential quality-of-life benefits for rectal cancer patients have become possible and are essential for patients, health care providers, and managers.

References

Birgisson H, Påhlman L, Gunnarsson U, Swedish Rectal Cancer Trial Group et al (2005) Adverse effects of preoperative radiation therapy for rectal cancer: long-term follow-up of the Swedish Rectal Cancer Trial. J Clin Oncol 23:8697–8705

Birgisson H, Påhlman L, Gunnarsson U et al (2007) Late adverse effects of radiation therapy for rectal cancer—a systematic overview. Acta Oncol 46:504–516

Birgisson H, Påhlman L, Gunnarsson U et al (2008) Late gastrointestinal disorders after rectal cancer surgery with and without preoperative radiation therapy. Br J Surg 95:206–213

Breugom AJ, Vermeer TA, van den Broek CBM et al (2015) Effect of preoperative treatment strategies on the outcome of patients with clinical T3, non-metastasized rectal cancer: a comparison between Dutch and Canadian expert centers. Eur J Surg Oncol 41(8):1039–1044

Bruheim K, Guren MG, Skovlund E et al (2010) Late side effects and quality of life after radiotherapy for rectal cancer. Int J Radiat Oncol Biol Phys 76:1005–1011

Bujko K (2013) Short-course preoperative radiotherapy for low rectal cancer. J Clin Oncol 31:1799

Bujko K, Nowacki MP, Nasierowska-Guttmejer A (2004) Sphincter preservation following preoperative radiotherapy for rectal cancer: report of a randomized trial comparing short-term radiotherapy vs. conventionally fractionated radiochemotherapy. Radiother Oncol 72:15–24

Bujko K, Nowacki MP, Nasierowska-Guttmejer A (2006) Long-term results of randomized trial comparing preoperative short-course radiotherapy with preoperative conventionally fractionated chemoradiation for rectal cancer. Br J Surg 93:1215–1223

Chan K, Vuong T, Kavan P, et al (2012) Does the compliance to adjuvant chemotherapy depend on neoadjuvant radiation therapy modality? In: 37th European Society for Medical Oncology (ESMO) Congress, September 28–October 2 2012, Vienna, Austria, Abstract #586P

Chen T, Newman N, Jabbour SK (2016) Normal tissue complication probability modeling of hematologic toxicity during postoperative chemotherapy in rectum cancer patients treated with preoperative chemoradiation therapy. 96(2):E219. doi:10.1016/j.ijrobp.2016.06.1141.

Colaco RJ, Nichols RC, Huh S et al (2014) Protons offer reduced bone marrow, small bowel, and urinary bladder exposure for patients receiving neoadjuvant radiotherapy for resectable rectal cancer. J Gastrointest Oncol 5(1):3–8

Folkesson J, Birgisson H, Pahlman L (2005) Swedish Rectal Cancer Trial: long lasting benefits from radiotherapy on survival and local recurrence rate. J Clin Oncol 23:5644–5650

Francois Y, Nemoz CJ, Bauliex J (1999) Influence of the interval between preoperative radiation therapy and surgery on downstaging and on the rate of sphincter-sparing surgery for rectal cancer: the Lyon R90-01 randomized trial. J Clin Oncol 17:2396–2402

Frykholm GJ, Glimelius B, Pahlman L et al (1993) Preoperative or postoperative irradiation in adenocarcinoma of the rectum: final treatment results of a randomized trial and evaluation of late secondary effects. Dis Colon Rectum 36:564–572

Glimelius B, Tiret E, Cervantes A et al (2013) Rectal cancer: ESMO Clinical Practice Guidelines for diagnosis, treatment and follow-up. Ann Oncol 24(Suppl 6):81–88

Hesselager C, Vuong T, Pahlman L et al (2013) Short term outcomes after neoadjuvant high dose rate endorectal brachytherapy versus short course external beam radiotherapy in resectable rectal cancer. Colorect Dis 15:662–666

Kusters M, Marijnen CA, Van De Velde CA et al (2010) Patterns of local recurrence in rectal cancer; a study of the Dutch TME trial. Eur J Surg Oncol 36(5):470–476

MacFarlane JK, Ryall RDH, Heald RJ (1993) Mesorectal excision for rectal cancer. Lancet 341:457–460

Marijnen CA, Kapiteijn E, van de Velde CJ et al (2002) Acute side effects and complications after short-term preoperative radiotherapy combined with total mesorectal excision in primary rectal cancer: report of a multicenter randomized trial. J Clin Oncol 20:817–825

Marijnen CA, van de Velde CJ, Putter H et al (2005) Impact of short-term preoperative radiotherapy on health-related quality of life and sexual functioning in primary rectal cancer: report of a multicenter randomized trial. J Clin Oncol 23:1847–1858

Martling AL, Holm T, Rutqvist LE et al (2000) Effect of a surgical training programme on outcome of rectal cancer in the County of Stockholm. Stockholm Colorectal Cancer Study Group, Basingstoke Bowel Cancer Research Project. Lancet 356(9224):93–96

Martling AL, Holm T, Johansson H et al (2001) The Stockholm II trial on preoperative radiotherapy in rectal carcinoma. Long-term follow-up of a population-based study. Cancer 92:896–902

National Comprehensive Cancer Network Guidelines. 2016 Rectal cancer version 2.1016, https://www.nccn.org/professionals/physician_gls/pdf/rectal.pdf. Accessed Nov 2016

Néron S, Perez S, Benc R et al (2014) The experience of pain and anxiety in rectal cancer patients during high-dose-rate brachytherapy. Curr Oncol 21(1):e89–e95

Newman NB, Sidhu MK, Baby R et al (2016) Long-term bone marrow suppression during postoperative chemotherapy in rectal cancer patients after preoperative chemoradiation therapy. Int J Radiat Oncol Biol Phys 94(5):1052–1060

Ngan SY, Burmeister B, Fisher RJ et al (2012) Randomized trial of short-course radiotherapy versus long-course chemoradiation comparing rates of local recurrence in patients with t3 rectal cancer:

Trans-Tasman Radiation Oncology Group Trial 01.04. J Clin Oncol 30:3827–3833

Nout RA, Devic S, Niazi T et al (2016) CT-based adaptive high-dose-rate endorectal brachytherapy in the preoperative treatment of locally advanced rectal cancer: technical and practical aspects. Brachytherapy 15(4):477–484

Peeters KC, van de Velde CJ, Leer JW et al (2005) Late side effect of short-course preoperative radiotherapy combined with total mesorectal excision for rectal cancer: increased bowel dysfunction in irradiated patients: a Dutch colorectal cancer group study. J Clin Oncol 23:6199–6206

Peeters KC, Marijnen CA, Nagtegaal ID, Dutch Colorectal Cancer Group et al (2007) The TME trial after a median follow-up of 6 years: increased local control but no survival benefit in irradiated patients with resectable rectal carcinoma. Ann Surg 246:693–701

Pettersson D, Cedermark B, Holm T et al (2010) Interim analysis of the Stockholm III trial of preoperative radiotherapy regimens for rectal cancer. Br J Surg 97:580–587

Pietrzak L, Bujko K, Nowacki MP (2007) Quality of life, anorectal and sexual functions after preoperative radiotherapy for rectal cancer: report of a randomized trial. Radiother Oncol 84:217–225

Quirke P, Steele R, Monson J et al (2009) Effect of the plane of surgery achieved on local recurrence in patients with operable rectal cancer: a prospective study using data from the MRC CR07 and NCIC-CTG CO16 randomized clinical trial. Lancet 373:821–828

Sauer R, Becker H, Hohenberger W et al (2004) Preoperative versus postoperative chemoradiotherapy for rectal cancer. N Engl J Med 351:1731–1740

Sebag-Montefiore D, Stephens RJ, Steele R et al (2009) Preoperative radiotherapy versus selective postoperative chemo-radiotherapy in patients with rectal cancer (MRC CR07 and NCIC-CTG C016): a multicentre, randomized trial. Lancet 373:811–820

Smith N, Brown G (2008) Preoperative staging of rectal cancer. Acta Oncol 47:20–31

Stockholm Colorectal Cancer Study Group (1990) Preoperative short-term radiation therapy in operable rectal carcinoma. A prospective randomized trial. Cancer 66:49–55

Van Gijn W, Marijnen CA, Nagtegaal ID et al (2011) Preoperative radiotherapy combined with total mesorectal excision for resectable rectal cancer: 12-year follow-up of the multicentre, randomized controlled TME trial. Lancet Oncol 12(6):575–582

Vuong T, Belliveau P, Michel R et al (2002) Conformal preoperative endorectal brachytherapy treatment for locally advanced rectal cancer: early results of a phase I/II study. Dis Colon Rectum 45:1486–1495

Vuong T, Richard C, Niazi T et al (2010) High dose rate endorectal brachytherapy for patients with curable rectal cancer. Semin Colon Rectal Surg 21(2):115–119

Vuong T, Desjardins F, Pelsser V, et al (2016) Patterns of relapse in rectal cancer patients following preoperative high dose rate brachytherapy. ESTRO 35. Turin, Italy. 30 Apr 2016. Oral presentation, abstract E35-0985

Wiltink LM, Chen T, Nout RA et al (2014) Health-related quality of life 14 years after preoperative short-term radiotherapy and total mesorectal excision for rectal cancer: report of a multicenter randomized trial. Eur J Cancer 50:2390–2398

Yang TJ, Oh JH, Apte A et al (2014) Clinical and dosimetric predictors of acute hematologic toxicity in rectal cancer patients undergoing chemoradiotherapy. Radiother Oncol 113(1):29–34

Hypofractionated Radiotherapy in Genitourinary Cancer: Better with Less

Ruud C. Wortel and Luca Incrocci

Contents

R.C. Wortel (✉) • L. Incrocci
Erasmus Medical Center, Rotterdam, The Netherlands
e-mail: r.wortel@erasmusmc.nl;
l.incrocci@erasmusmc.nl

Abstract

Over the years, most innovations in hypofractionated radiotherapy for malignancies of the genitourinary tract have involved treatment of prostate cancer, which will therefore be the main focus of this chapter. The rationale for hypofractionated radiotherapy, contemporary treatment techniques, and results of clinical trials of hypofractionated external beam radiation therapy (EBRT) or stereotactic body radiation therapy (SBRT) are discussed. Finally, the implications of clinical data on general practice and future directions of research are discussed.

1   Introduction

Prostate cancer is the second most common cancer in men worldwide, and the fifth leading cause of cancer-related death (Ferlay et al. 2015). Since the introduction of prostate-specific antigen (PSA) testing in the 1980s, the incidence of prostate cancer has doubled. More than one million men were estimated to have been diagnosed with prostate cancer in 2012 (http://www.cancerresearchuk.org/health-professional/cancer-statistics/statistics-by-cancer-type/prostate-cancer). Most patients are diagnosed with localized disease and are therefore candidates for curative treatment (http://www.cancerresearchuk.org/health-professional/cancer-statistics/statistics-by-cancer-type/prostate-cancer).

Med Radiol Radiat Oncol (2017)
DOI 10.1007/174_2017_37, © Springer International Publishing AG
Published Online: 26 Apr 2017

Patients with localized disease can be offered several treatment options including active surveillance, brachytherapy for selected patients, radical prostatectomy, and external beam radiation therapy (EBRT).

For several decades, EBRT has been delivered in conventional fractions of 1.8–2.2 Gy at 5 consecutive days per week. Clinical trials have demonstrated that dose-escalated EBRT for prostate cancer up to overall treatment doses of 74–78 Gy significantly improves local control as compared to previous schedules of 64–70 Gy (Peeters et al. 2006; Dearnaley et al. 2007; Pollack et al. 2002). These dose-escalated treatments are often associated with increased genitourinary and gastrointestinal toxicities (Peeters et al. 2006; Dearnaley et al. 2007; Pollack et al. 2002), which limit the options for further dose escalation using conventional 2 Gy fractions. Hypofractionated radiotherapy, in which fewer high-dose fractions are delivered, has the potential to increase the radiobiological dose to tumor.

In this chapter we discuss the rationale for hypofractionated radiotherapy in prostate cancer treatment and the technological improvements over the past two decades which have enabled delivery of high-dose conformal treatment plans with reduced dose to adjacent normal tissues. We also provide an overview of the clinical data on hypofractionated radiotherapy. For this purpose, we have reviewed randomized phase III trials of moderately hypofractionated (fraction doses of 2.4–3.5 Gy) EBRT and prospective clinical data from studies of stereotactic body radiation therapy (SBRT) to deliver extreme hypofractionation treatments (fraction doses of 5–10 Gy). Based on these results, we discuss the implications of hypofractionation in the general practice and future directions for clinical research.

2 Rationale for Hypofractionated Radiotherapy for the Treatment of Prostate Cancer

The α/β ratio is a radiobiological model used to express the sensitivity of tumor and normal tissues to changes in fractionation. After Brenner and Hall first suggested a uniquely low α/β ratio for prostate cancer of approximately 1.5, the interest in its radiobiology has considerably increased (Brenner and Hall 1999). Others have analyzed large clinical data sets and corroborated these earlier results (Dasu and Toma-Dasu 2012; Miralbell et al. 2012).

Tumors with low α/β ratios are generally resistant to low-fraction doses, and therefore require larger radiation doses per fraction to improve tumor control. Normal tissues surrounding the prostate are less sensitive to larger fraction doses due to suggested α/β ratios between 4 and 6 Gy (Brenner et al. 1998; Fowler 2005; Tucker et al. 2011). The proposed low α/β ratio of prostate cancer in relation to surrounding normal tissue demonstrates the potential benefit of hypofractionated radiotherapy as a means to improve clinical outcomes.

In general, two hypofractionation designs can be considered to exploit the hypothesized radiobiological advantages: (1) to achieve de-escalation of the normal tissue total dose while maintaining similar predicted tumor control, and (2) to achieve escalation of the radiobiological tumor dose while maintaining similar predicted late normal tissue effects (Ritter 2008). Hypofractionation schedules can be compared using the α/β ratio and the linear quadratic (LQ) model, in which the dose to tumor and normal tissue applied in each scheme are calculated in conventional 2 Gy fractions (Dale 1985). The LQ model is however subject to uncertainties, particularly with respect to the upper limit of fraction sizes for which it remains valid (Ritter 2008; Kirkpatrick et al. 2008).

3 Treatment Techniques

3.1 External Beam Radiation Therapy (EBRT)

The ability to deliver high-dose treatment fractions used for hypofractionated EBRT has greatly improved since the introduction of intensity-modulated radiotherapy (IMRT). This technique enables dose escalation to tumors with irregular shapes using beams of nonuniform radiation intensity with improved sparing of normal tissue (Wortel et al. 2015, 2016a).

More recently, image-guided radiotherapy (IGRT) techniques that include implanted intraprostatic fiducial markers have been developed. Daily imaging using two-dimensional portal images, three-dimensional cone-beam computed tomography (CBCT), or three-dimensional ultrasound localization allow for accurate prostate alignment before each fraction. IGRT techniques replaced previous protocols which were based on bony anatomy localization or skin marks matched to in-room lasers. As a result, the precision of radiotherapy has been further increased. Safety margins which are used to correct for variations in patient positioning, intrafractional prostate motion, and inaccurate dose delivery can be safely reduced from approximately 1 cm to a 5 mm margin using fiducials (Beltran et al. 2008). EBRT using IMRT and image guidance enables treatment planning with high conformity and steep dose gradients without compromising tumor coverage (Deutschmann et al. 2012; Nijkamp et al. 2008). Application of both techniques also significantly reduces the dose to adjacent organs at risk (OAR) and toxicity levels as compared to previous 3D-conformal radiotherapy (3D-CRT) techniques (Wortel et al. 2015, 2016a).

3.2 Stereotactic Body Radiation Therapy (SBRT)

According to the American Society for Radiation Oncology (ASTRO), SBRT is precise EBRT which is designed to deliver very high radiation doses, using a single dose or typically up to five fractions (Potters et al. 2010). Cross-firing beams of ionizing radiation and image guidance are used to achieve high levels of treatment conformality and rapid dose falloff.

In contrast to conventional EBRT, which is generally delivered via standard gantry-based linear accelerators (Linacs), SBRT can be delivered by several platforms (Table 1). Gantry-based Linacs can also deliver SBRT if daily image guidance is available. For example, the Calypso® system (Varian Medical Systems, Palo Alto, USA) is used for SBRT to enable real-time prostate monitoring via implanted transponders (Mantz 2014). In case of prostate motion beyond user-defined thresholds, typically between 3 and 5 mm, treatment is interrupted to enable patient repositioning.

Most prospective clinical data on SBRT are collected in studies using the CyberKnife® robotic radiosurgery system (Accuray, Sunnyvale, CA, USA). Cyberknife treatment is delivered via a linear accelerator which is mounted on a robotic arm (Kilby et al. 2010). Highly conformal dose distributions are delivered using multiple noncoplanar beams. Image guidance is based on implanted fiducial markers and orthogonal kV imaging with user-defined intervals during dose delivery (van de Water et al. 2014). Subsequent correction for intrafraction prostate motion occurs by adjusting the position and orientation of the robotic manipulator or treatment couch (van de Water et al. 2014).

Table 1 Treatment platforms

Platform	Treatment	Description	Image guidance	Correction
Gantry-based Linac	SBRT, EBRT (3D-CRT, IMRT, VMAT)	Linac on gantry with multileaf collimator	Intraprostatic fiducials, orthogonal X-rays, on-board CT	Prior to fraction
Calypso®	SBRT	Image guidance for gantry-based Linac	Intraprostatic transponders	Real-time, manual correction
CyberKnife®	SBRT	Noncoplanar beams delivered via Linac on robotic arm	Intraprostatic fiducials, orthogonal X-rays	Real-time, automated correction
Tomotherapy®	SBRT, EBRT	Linac with multileaf collimator in helical ring of CT scanner	On board CT	Prior to fraction

Abbreviations: *CT* computed tomography, *EBRT* external beam radiation therapy, *IMRT* intensity-modulated radiation therapy, *Linac* linear accelerator, *SBRT* stereotactic body radiation therapy, *VMAT* volumetric arc therapy

4   Hypofractionated External Beam Radiotherapy (EBRT)

4.1   Clinical Studies

The first hypofractionated EBRT treatments were mainly carried out to improve efficiency and patient convenience, and were generally well tolerated (Duncan et al. 1993; Read and Pointon 1989; Collins and Lloyd-Davies 1991). However, as these were nonrandomized studies mainly conducted before prostate-specific antigen (PSA) testing became routinely available, treatment efficacy was difficult to assess. The hypothesized high fraction sensitivity of prostate cancer has greatly increased clinical interest and ultimately led to the development of several randomized phase III clinical trials of moderate hypofractionation (2.4–3.4 Gy per fractions) (Table 2). In the following sections, clinical data, outcomes, and implications of the eight phase III trials using moderately hypofractionated EBRT that have been published are discussed.

4.2   Treatment Planning

Most of the recent studies applied IMRT and image guidance, whereas the earlier studies used 2D- or 3D-conformal techniques (Table 2). CT images were used for tumor delineation and normal tissue contouring in six of eight studies (Yeoh et al. 2011; Lukka et al. 2005; Arcangeli et al. 2010; Dearnaley et al. 2016; Hoffman et al. 2014; Lee et al. 2016), whereas magnetic resonance imaging (MRI)-based planning was introduced by Pollack and colleagues and Incrocci and colleagues (Incrocci et al. 2016; Pollack et al. 2013). Two studies reported that all patients received treatment of the prostate only (Lukka et al. 2005; Lee et al. 2016), whereas others also included the seminal vesicles in the target volumes. Expansion of the clinical target volume to yield the planning target volume was 10–15 mm in studies using 2D- or 3D-CRT techniques (Yeoh et al. 2011; Lukka et al. 2005; Arcangeli et al. 2010; Hoffman et al. 2014), and 5–10 mm in most studies using IMRT and image guidance

(Dearnaley et al. 2016; Lee et al. 2016; Incrocci et al. 2016; Pollack et al. 2013). In some studies, safety margins were reduced with 4–7 mm posteriorly to reduce the rectal dose (Lukka et al. 2005; Arcangeli et al. 2010; Hoffman et al. 2014; Pollack et al. 2013).

Conventional treatment fractions were always delivered on 5 consecutive days (e.g., Monday–Friday). Most studies also applied hypofractionation schedules with five fractions weekly (Table 2). In the HYPRO trial and the Arcangeli and colleagues study however, hypofractionated treatment was delivered at 3 and 4 days per week, respectively (Incrocci et al. 2016; Arcangeli et al. 2012). For acute toxicity, overall treatment time is an important factor and excessive acute effects can be avoided by prolonging the duration of treatment.

4.3   Treatment Efficacy

The first two trials published by Lukka and colleagues and Yeoh and colleagues were conducted before the era of dose escalation (Yeoh et al. 2011; Lukka et al. 2005) (Table 2). The prescribed treatment doses in both trials are well below current clinical doses, which might account for the low relapse-free survival (RFS) rates in both treatment arms. Two recently published randomized trials aimed to demonstrate superiority of a hypofractionated regimen compared to conventional with regard to RFS (Incrocci et al. 2016; Pollack et al. 2013). The Dutch HYPRO trial randomized 820 intermediate- to high-risk patients to 39 fractions of 2 Gy (5 weekly fractions) or 19 fractions of 3.4 Gy (3 weekly fractions). This study was designed to test whether an increased dose of 12.4 Gy in 2 Gy fractions using hypofractionated EBRT would achieve a significant increase in RFS of 10% as compared to conventional treatment (Incrocci et al. 2016). At a median follow-up of 60 months, no significant differences in RFS survival were achieved with RFS rates of 80 and 77% after hypofractionation and conventional fractionation (HR = 0.86, 95% CI 0·63–1·16); p = 0.36), respectively. In line with these results, Pollack

Table 2 Phase III studies of moderate hypofractionation for localized prostate cancer

Author	n	Patient population	Device and technique	Regimen	BED tumor ($\alpha/\beta = 1.5$)	BED OAR ($\alpha/\beta = 4$–6)	ADT (months)	FU (months)	RFS	Acute toxicity bladder	Acute toxicity bowel	Late toxicity bladder	Late toxicity bowel
Incrocci et al. (2016) and Aluwini et al. (2015, 2016) and HYPRO Trial The Netherlands	820	Intermediate-high-risk cT1b-T4 PSA < 60	Linac IMRT Fiducials	39 × 2 Gy (daily)	78 Gy	78 Gy	66% (6–36 m)	60	5-year bcRFS: 77%	RTOG-EORTC G2+ 58% 1× (<1%) G4	RTOG-EORTC G2+ 31%	RTOG-EORTC 3-year G2+ 39% 3× (<1%) G4	RTOG-EORTC 3-year G2+ 18%
				19 × 3.4 Gy (3 Fr/ weekly)	90.4 Gy	75.9–79.6 Gy			80% (NS)	61% (NS) 1× (<1%) G4	42% (p = 0.002)	41% (NS) 2× (<1%) G4	22% (NS)
Dearnaley et al. (2016) and CHHiP Trial United Kingdom	3216	Intermediate-high-risk cT1b-T3a PSA < 30	Linac IMRT 30% IGRT	37 × 2 Gy (daily)	74 Gy	74 Gy	97% (3–6 m)	62	5-year bcRFS 88%	RTOG G2+ 46%	RTOG G2+ 25%	RTOG 5-year G2+ 9%	RTOG 5-year G2+ 14%
				20 × 3 Gy (daily)	77.1 Gy	67.5–70 Gy			91% (NS)	49% (NS)	38% (p < 0.001)	12% (NS)	12% (NS)
				19 × 3 Gy (daily)	73.1 Gy	64.1–66.5 Gy			86% (NS)	46% (NS)	38% (p < 0.001)	7% (NS)	11% (NS)
Lee et al. (2016) and RTOG 0415 Trial USA	1115	Low-risk cT1b-T2c Gleason 2–6	Linac 3D-CRT/ IMRT Fiducials	41 × 1.8 Gy (daily)	73.8 Gy	73.8 Gy	0%	70	5-year bcRFS 85%	CTCAE G2+ 27%	CTCAE G2+10%	CTCAE G2+ 23% 1 × G4 (<1%)	CTCAE G2+ 14% 1 × G4 (<1%)
		PSA < 10		28 × 2.5 Gy (daily)	80 Gy	74.4–75.8 Gy			86% (NS)	27% (NS)	11% (NS)	30% (G2: p = 0.009)	22% (G2: p = 0.005)
Pollack et al. (2006, 2013) and Fox Chase USA	303	Intermediate-high-risk cT1–T3	Linac IMRT	38 × 2 Gy (daily)	76 Gy	76 Gy	47% (<4–24 m)	68	5-year bcRFS 79%	LENT/ RTOG G2+ 56%[a]	LENT/ RTOG G2+ 8%[a]	LENT/RTOG 5-year G2+ 13%	LENT/RTOG 5-year G2+ #9%
		PSA < 80		26 × 2.7 Gy (daily)	84.2 Gy	76.3–78.4 Gy	45% (<4–24 m)		77% (NS)	48% (NS)	18% (NS)	22% (NS)	#9% (NS)
Hoffman et al. (2014) and MD Anderson USA	203	Low-intermediate-risk cT1b-T3b	Linac IMRT	42 × 1.8 Gy (daily)	72.2 Gy	72.2 Gy	21% (4 m)	75	5-year bRFS 92%	Not reported	Not reported	RTOG 5-year G2+ 17%	RTOG 5-year G2+ 5%
		PSAS20	Fiducials	30 × 2.4 Gy (daily)	80.2 Gy	75.6–76.8 Gy			96% (NS)			16% (NS)	10% (NS)

(continued)

Table 2 (continued)

Author	n	Patient population	Device and technique	Regimen	BED tumor ($\alpha/\beta = 1.5$)	BED OAR ($\alpha/\beta = 4$–6)	ADT (months)	FU (months)	RFS	Acute toxicity bladder	Acute toxicity bowel	Late toxicity bladder	Late toxicity bowel
Arcangeli et al. (2010, 2011, 2012) and Italy	168	High-risk T1–T4 PSA≥100	Linac 3D-CRT No IGRT	40 × 2 Gy (daily)	80 Gy	80 Gy	100% (9 m)	70	5-year bRFS 79%	G2+ 40%	G2+ 21%	3-year G2+ 11%	3-year G2+ 14%
				20 × 3.1 Gy (4Fr/week)	81.5 Gy	70.5–73.4 Gy			85% (NS)	47% (NS)	35% (NS)	16% (NS) 1× (1%) G4	17% (NS)
Yeoh et al. (2011) and Australia	217	cT1–T2	Linac 2D/3D-CRT	32 × 2 Gy (daily)	64 Gy	64 Gy	0%	90	7.5-year bRFS 34%	Not reported	Not reported	LENT-SOMA (NS)	LENT-SOMA (NS)
			No IGRT	20 × 2.75 Gy (daily)	66.8 Gy	60.2–61.9 Gy			53% ($p < 0.05$)				
Lukka et al. (2005) and Canada	936	cT1–T2 PSA≤40	Linac 3D-CRT No IGRT	33 × 2 Gy (daily)	66 Gy	66 Gy	0%	68	5-year bcRFS 47%	NCIC G3+ 5%	NCIC G3+ 3%	NCIC G3+ 2%	NCIC G3+ 1%
				20 × 2.625 Gy (daily)	61.8 Gy	56.6–58.0 Gy			40%	9%	4%	2% (NS)	1% (NS)

Abbreviations: α/β alpha/beta ratio, *ADT* androgen deprivation therapy, *BED* biologically equivalent dose (in 2 Gy fractions), *CTCAE* common terminology criteria for adverse events, *EORTC* European Organization for Research and Treatment of Cancer, *Fr* fractions, *FU* follow-up, *G2+* grade 2 or worse, *G3+* grade 3 or worse, *G4* grade 4, *IGRT* image-guided radiotherapy, *IMRT* intensity-modulated radiotherapy, *NCIC* National Cancer Institute of Canada, *NS* not significant, *OAR* organs at risk, *PSA* prostate-specific antigen, *RFS* relapse-free survival, *SV* seminal vesicle, *3D-CRT* 3D-conformal radiotherapy

[a]Based on preliminary acute toxicity data (37), # estimated

and colleagues of the Fox Chase Cancer Center also could not demonstrate superiority of hypofractionation in 303 prostate cancer patients treated to 76 Gy in 2 Gy fractions or 26 fractions of 2.7 Gy (Pollack et al. 2013). It was hypothesized that the overall increase in treatment dose of 8.4 Gy in 2 Gy fractions using hypofractionation would result in 15% reduction of biochemical failure. At a median follow-up of 68 months, 5-year RFS was 77% for hypofractionation and 79% for conventional fractionation ($p = 0.75$). Both trials included a substantial proportion of patients receiving long-term androgen deprivation therapy (ADT) for at least 24 months, which might have had a substantial effect on RFS rates at follow-up. Additional follow-up could demonstrate whether the effects of androgen suppression on tumor recurrence have obscured the potential benefits of hypofractionated treatment.

The enormous advantages in terms of patient convenience and hospital logistics associated with hypofractionation justify noninferiority study designs, which in this case are a more prudent method to demonstrate clinical benefits of hypofractionated treatment. The CHHiP trial randomized 3216 patients with intermediate- or high-risk prostate cancer to conventional fractionation of 74 Gy in 37 fractions or two hypofractionation schedules: 57 Gy in 19 fractions or 60 Gy in 20 fractions (Dearnaley et al. 2016). Hypofractionated treatment using 60 Gy in 20 fractions was found noninferior to conventional treatment with 5-year RFS rates of 88 and 91% after conventional and hypofractionated treatment, respectively. The RTOG 0415 trial by Lee and colleagues also demonstrated noninferiority of hypofractionated EBRT of 70 Gy in 28 fractions versus 73.8 Gy in 41 fractions (Lee et al. 2016). This study included 1115 patients with low-risk prostate cancer only and as such complemented data from the CHHiP trial.

Whether low-risk patients are, in fact, the most clinically relevant study population with which to apply hypofractionation remains open to debate. Firstly, patients allocated hypofractionated EBRT in the RTOG 0415 trial received an increased radiobiological dose of 6.2 Gy in 2 Gy fractions (α/β ratio of 1.5) as compared to those allocated

conventional treatment (Lee et al. 2016). However, a previous Dutch dose-escalation trial (68 Gy vs. 78 Gy) demonstrated no effect of dose escalation on disease control in patients with low-risk features (Peeters et al. 2006). In addition, Arcangeli and colleagues randomized 168 patients to 80 Gy in 40 fractions or hypofractionated treatment of 62 Gy in 20 fractions over a period of 5 weeks (Arcangeli et al. 2010, 2011, 2012). Although no significant differences in RFS between both treatment arms were found, a benefit for hypofractionation (HR = 0.09, 95% CI 0.03–0.31) was suggested only in patients with aggressive tumors (e.g., Gleason $\geq 4 + 3$). Second and most important, many patients with low-risk features are candidates for active surveillance and may not need any curative treatment at all. Nonetheless, for those patients with low-risk prostate cancer who do prefer curative treatment, hypofractionation is a good option.

4.4 Radiation-Induced Toxicity

Toxicity was scored using the Radiation Therapy Oncology Group (RTOG) criteria, European Organization for Research and Treatment of Cancer (EORTC) criteria, the Common Terminology Criteria for Adverse Events (CTCAE), National Cancer Institute of Canada (NCIC) scoring criteria, or Late Effects of Normal Tissues/Subjective, Objective, Management, Analytic (LENT/SOMA) criteria (Table 2).

Normal tissues were estimated to receive a similar or lower biologically equivalent dose (BED) in 2 Gy fractions with hypofractionated treatments as compared to the conventional treatments. In practice however, reported grade 2 or worse acute bowel toxicities in several studies were substantially higher using hypofractionated regimens (Dearnaley et al. 2016; Pollack et al. 2006, 2013; Arcangeli et al. 2011; Aluwini et al. 2015). There was significantly more grade 2 or worse bowel toxicity in the CHHiP trial and the HYPRO trial (Dearnaley et al. 2016; Aluwini et al. 2015). In both trials however, the observed differences in bowel toxicity between arms had dissipated by 3–4 months after completion of treatment (Dearnaley et al. 2016; Aluwini et al. 2015). Interestingly, the CHHiP trial reported that acute toxicity peaked sooner in the hypofractionated schedules than in the control, at 4–5 weeks compared with 7–8 weeks (Dearnaley et al. 2016). In contrast to bowel toxicity, all trials reported comparable acute bladder toxicities between treatment schemes.

In terms of late toxicity, results of the RTOG 0415 trial demonstrated significantly increased grade 2 bowel (HR = 1.59, 95% CI 1.22–2.06) and bladder toxicity (HR = 1.31, 95% CI 1.07–1.61) in patients treated with hypofractionated EBRT (28 fractions of 2.5 Gy) as compared to conventional treatment (41 fractions of 1.8 Gy) (Lee et al. 2016). Results of the HYPRO trial could not demonstrate the postulated noninferiority of hypofractionation (Aluwini et al. 2016). In fact, a significantly increased cumulative incidence of grade 3 or worse bladder toxicity was found after hypofractionation (19% vs. 13%, respectively; $p = 0.021$). The risk of grade 3 nocturia (≥ 6/night) was significantly higher in patients allocated to hypofractionation (HR = 4.94, 95% CI 1.87–13.09) (Aluwini et al. 2016). Both the HYPRO trial and the Pollack and colleagues' study concluded that men with compromised urinary function at baseline were at risk of late bladder toxicity (Pollack et al. 2013; Aluwini et al. 2016). Specifically, Pollack and colleagues reported that patients with a baseline International Prostate Symptom Score (IPSS) >12 who receive hypofractionation were significantly associated with increased risk of late grade 2 or worse toxicity (Pollack et al. 2013).

4.5   Sexual Function

In contrast to radiation-induced bowel and bladder toxicity, sexual function has remained largely unaddressed in these trials. A substudy of the CHHiP trial of 2100 men addressed sexual function and quality-of-life domains assessed with the UCLA-Prostate Cancer Index (UCLA-PCI) and the Expanded Prostate cancer Index Composite (EPIC) questionnaires (Wilkins et al. 2015). Most patients used short-term ADT for 3–6 months. At 24 months, no significant differences were found between treatment arms. Dearnaley and colleagues also found no significant differences in sexual bother at a 5-year follow-up, and the proportion of LENT-SOM grade 2 or worse sexual toxicity was similar across treatment groups (Dearnaley et al. 2016). Results from the Dutch HYPRO trial showed no significant differences in erectile functioning between both treatment arms in patients who received no or short-term ADT (Wortel et al. 2016b).

4.6   Clinical Implications

We have sufficient evidence in the current literature supporting noninferiority of moderately hypofractionated EBRT as compared to conventional treatments. However, the HYPRO trial as well as the Pollack and colleagues' trial, that were both designed to demonstrate superiority of hypofractionation in terms of RFS, have failed to do so (Incrocci et al. 2016; Pollack et al. 2013). Based on these trials one might question the validity of the LQ model and the commonly suggested α/β ratio.

Figure 1 shows the calculated BED in 2 Gy fractions with corresponding control rates per treatment arm as reported by phase III studies applying overall treatment doses larger than 70 Gy. Treatment arms within each study are connected, demonstrating that the BED 2 Gy is higher in the hypofractionation arm of all studies. In four studies the BED 2 Gy was substantially increased with 6–12 Gy using hypofractionated treatment, with no substantial benefits in terms of RFS (Hoffman et al. 2014; Lee et al. 2016; Incrocci et al. 2016; Pollack et al. 2013; Kuban et al. 2010). Meta-analyses including all recently published data could establish whether the currently applied α/β ratio for prostate cancer of 1.5 might, in fact, be higher.

As most of the recent trials reported increased acute (Dearnaley et al. 2016; Aluwini et al. 2015) or late toxicities (Lee et al. 2016; Aluwini et al. 2016) with hypofractionation, it remains questionable whether hypofractionated regimens will become common clinical practice

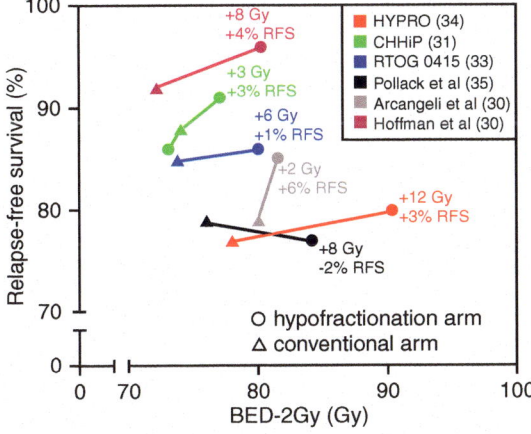

Fig. 1 Relapse-free survival rates per treatment arm in relation to biologically equivalent doses in 2 Gy fractions of phase III hypofractionation trials applying treatment doses >70 Gy. *Legend.* Conventional treatment arm (triangular shape) is connected with hypofractionation arm (round shape) within each study to demonstrate differences in biologically equivalent dose in 2 Gy fractions (BED-2 Gy) and relapse-free survival rates (RFS). The differences in BED-2 Gy and RFS between treatment arms are summarized for each study

given the absence of improved treatment efficacy. Dearnaley and colleagues of the CHHiP trial however concluded that their hypofractionated regimen of 60 Gy in 3 Gy fractions should be considered as new standard of care for EBRT of localized prostate cancer (Dearnaley et al. 2016). Incrocci and colleagues reported that the HYPRO treatment schedule of 19 fractions of 3.4 Gy can be offered to intermediate-high-risk patients with few bowel and bladder symptoms at baseline (Incrocci et al. 2016), whereas Lee and colleagues believe that the RTOG 0415 hypofractionation schedule of 70 Gy in 28 fractions can be prescribed in men with low-risk disease who opt for curative treatment, although an increase in late adverse events might be expected (Lee et al. 2016). In this setting, patient selection is paramount to safely deliver hypofractionated EBRT. The integration of hypofractionated treatment schemes in clinical practice together with prolonged follow-up of these phase III trials will help in clarifying the role of hypofractionation for prostate cancer in the near future.

5 Stereotactic Body Radiation Therapy (SBRT)

5.1 Clinical Studies

SBRT treatment schedules applying extreme fraction doses of 5–10 Gy have not been randomized and compared with other standard-of-care treatment modalities. At this point, prospectively collected data are only available from case series and single-arm phase I/II studies (Table 3).

5.2 Treatment Planning

In five studies, the CyberKnife® system was used to administer 35–51 Gy in 4–7 fractions, delivered either daily or on alternate days (Aluwini et al. 2013; Bolzicco et al. 2013; Fuller et al. 2014; Katz and Kang 2014a; King et al. 2012) (Table 3). Aluwini and colleagues treated 50 patients with the CyberKnife® up to 38 Gy in four daily fractions and applied an integrated boost to 11 Gy per fraction to the dominant lesion if visible on MRI (Aluwini et al. 2013).

Others used standard Linacs with daily image guidance for 5 weekly fractions of 7 Gy (Loblaw et al. 2013) or 9 weekly fractions of 5 Gy (Zimmermann et al. 2016). Mantz and colleagues used Varian Trilogy/Truebeam® (Varian, Palo Alto, CA, USA) Linacs with the Calypso® System for real-time tumor localization (Mantz 2014), whereas the Tomotherapy® (Accuray, Sunnyvale, CA, USA) ring gantry accelerator was used by Kim and colleagues (Kim et al. 2014).

Most of the studies (5 out of 9, 56%) used CT images fused with prostate MRI for accurate delineation (Aluwini et al. 2013; Bolzicco et al. 2013; Fuller et al. 2014; Katz and Kang 2014a; Kim et al. 2014), whereas others used CT imaging only. In two studies the clinical target volume consisted of the prostate with or without the seminal vesicles (Bolzicco et al. 2013; Fuller et al. 2014); the remaining studies treated the prostate only. Safety margins of 2–5 mm were added to the clinical target volume to yield the planning target volume. In the phase II study of Zimmerman and colleagues however, 3D-CRT was used and

Table 3 Prospective studies of extreme hypofractionation with at least 50 localized prostate cancer patients

Author	n	Patient population	Device and technique	Regimen	BED tumor ($\alpha/\beta = 1.5$)	BED OAR ($\alpha/\beta = 4$–6)	ADT (months)	FU (months)	RFS	Acute toxicity bladder	Acute toxicity bowel	Late toxicity bladder	Late toxicity bowel
Aluwini et al. (2013)	50	Low-intermediate-risk T1–T3a, PSA < 20 Gleason 6–7	Cyberknife fiducials	4 × 9.5 Gy (daily)	119 Gy	74–86 Gy	0%	23	2-year bcRFS 100%	RTOG-EORTC G2+ 23%	RTOG-EORTC G2+ 14%	RTOG-EORTC 2-year G2+ 16%	RTOG-EORTC 2-year G2+ 3%
Bolzicco et al. (2013)	100	Low-high-risk T1–T2c Gleason 4–10	Cyberknife fiducials	5 × 7 Gy	85 Gy	57–64 Gy	7% (3–36)	36	3-year bcRFS 94%	RTOG G2+ 12%	RTOG G2+ 18%	RTOG G2+ 4%	RTOG G2+ 1%
Fuller et al. (2014)	79	Low-intermediate-risk T1–T2 Gleason 5–7	Cyberknife fiducials	4 × 9.5 Gy (daily)	119 Gy	74–86 Gy	0%	NR	5-year bRFS 98% low risk 92% intermediate	CTCAE G2+ 10%	CTCAE G2+ 0%	CTCAE G2+ 15%	CTCAE G2+ 1%
Katz and Kang (2014a, b)	515	Low-high-risk T1a–T2a, PSA < 20 Gleason 6–9	Cyberknife fiducials	5 × 7/ 7.25 Gy (daily)	85–91 Gy	57–68 Gy	14%	72	7-year bRFS 96% Low risk 90% Intermediate 69% High	RTOG G2+ 4%	RTOG G2+ 4%	RTOG G2+ 9% (overall) 6% (5 × 7 Gy) 12% (5 × 7.25 Gy)	RTOG 2+ 4% (overall) 3% (5 × 7 Gy) 5% (5 × 7.25 Gy)
Kim et al. (2014)	91	Low-intermediate-risk T1–T2b Gleason 2–7, PSA < 20	IMRT/ Tomo fiducials/ Calypso	5 × 9/9.5/ 10 Gy (alternate days)	135–164 Gy	84–117 Gy	18%	25	NR	CTCAE G2+ 22%	CTCAE G2+ 21%	CTCAE G2+ 13%	CTCAE 2+ 29% 5% (5%) colostomy (G4)
King et al. (2012)	67	Low-risk T1c–T2b, PSA < 10 Gleason 6–7	Cyberknife fiducials	7 × 7.25 Gy (daily or alternate)	91 Gy	60–68 Gy	0%	32	4-year bRFS 94%	NR	NR	RTOG G2+ 8%	RTOG G2+ 2%
Loblaw et al. (2013)	84	Low-risk T1–T2b	IMRT fiducials	5 × 7 Gy (weekly)	85–91 Gy	57–68 Gy	0%	55	5 year bRFS 98%	CTCAE G2+ 20%	CTCAE G2+ 10%	RTOG G2+ 5%	RTOG G2+ 8% 1% (1%) fistula (G4)
Mantz (2014)	102	Low-risk T1c–T2a, PSA < 10, Gleason 6–7	Trilogy/ TrueBeam Calypso	5 × 8 Gy (alternate days)	109 Gy	70–80 Gy	0%	>60	5-year bRFS 100%	NR	NR	NR	NR
Zimmermann et al. (2016)	80	Low-risk T1a–T2a PSAS10, Gleason <6	3D-CRT Fiducials/ ultra-sound	9 × 5 Gy (weekly)	84 Gy	62–68 Gy	0%	83	5-year bRFS 96%	RTOG G2+ 36%	RTOG G2+ 14%	RTOG G2+ 31% 1% (1%) cystectomy (G4)	RTOG G2+ 30%

Abbreviations: α/β alpha/beta ratio, *ADT* androgen deprivation therapy, *BED* biologically equivalent dose (in 2 Gy fractions), *EORTC* European Organization for Research and Treatment of Cancer, *Fr* fractions, *FU* follow-up, *G2+* grade 2 or higher, *G3+* grade 3 or higher, *IGRT* image-guided radiotherapy, *IMRT* intensity-modulated radiotherapy, *NS* not significant, *OAR* organs at risk, *PSA* prostate-specific antigen, *RFS* relapse-free survival, *SV* seminal vesicle, *3D-CRT* 3D-conformal radiotherapy larger safety margins of 1–1.5 cm were applied in all directions except posteriorly (0.5–1.0 cm) (Zimmermann et al. 2016).

5.3 Treatment Efficacy

The BED in 2 Gy fractions of all treatment schedules exceeded 80 Gy, hypothetically offering a therapeutic benefit over most currently applied conventional treatment schemes. With follow-up ranging between 23 and 83 months, recurrence-free survival rates exceeded 90% in low- to intermediate-risk patients. It should be noted that only two studies included a small proportion of high-risk patients, ranging from 7% (Katz and Kang 2014a) to 17% (Bolzicco et al. 2013) of their respective patient populations. Benign PSA bounces with subsequent normalization occurred in 12–70% and after a median follow-up of 12–24 months (Mantz 2014; Aluwini et al. 2013; Bolzicco et al. 2013; Fuller et al. 2014; Loblaw et al. 2013; Zimmermann et al. 2016).

The currently available efficacy data are difficult to use comparatively; however the control rates are comparable to those reported in patients treated with high-dose conventional EBRT (Spratt et al. 2013).

5.4 Radiation-Induced Toxicity

The assessment of radiation-induced toxicities is a key factor in current reports on SBRT, as most patients had low- or intermediate-risk disease and can expect disease control regardless of treatment modality. Late grade 2 or worse bladder toxicity ranged between 4 and 31%, and bowel toxicity was reported in 1–30% of patients (Table 3). RTOG, CTCAE, and EORTC scoring criteria were used to report toxicity.

Of the studies using gantry-based Linacs for delivery, Kim and colleagues treated 91 patients up to 45–60 Gy in 5 fractions (Kim et al. 2014). With fraction sizes up to 10 Gy, they applied the most extreme hypofractionation schedule. Some patients were treated without intrafraction image guidance as they had implanted fiducial markers,

whereas others had Calypso®-based real-time monitoring. Five patients out of 91, all treated to 50 Gy (5%), required a diverting colostomy due to severe rectal toxicity or fistulation (Kim et al. 2014). A strong correlation between high-grade rectal toxicity and dose to rectal wall volume was found. Loblaw and colleagues treated 84 patients to 35 Gy in 5 weekly fractions with IMRT and fiducial based image guidance. After a median follow-up of 55 months, grade 2 or worse toxicity scores of 5% and 8% were found for bladder and bowel complaints, respectively. One patient developed a grade 4 fistula-in-ano requiring surgery. Somewhat higher toxicity scores were reported by Zimmermann and colleagues, who treated 80 patients with image-guided 3D-CRT (Zimmermann et al. 2016). Grade 2 or worse bowel and bladder toxicity ranged between 30 and 31%, and one patient developed hemorrhagic cystitis requiring cystectomy.

In studies applying CyberKnife® RRS, both acute and late toxicity were predominated by bladder complaints. Late grade 2 or worse toxicities ranged between 4 and 16% for bladder and between 2 and 5% for bowel (Aluwini et al. 2013; Bolzicco et al. 2013; Fuller et al. 2014; Katz and Kang 2014a; King et al. 2012). The largest series reported by Katz and colleagues consisted of 515 patients treated to 35 Gy in five fractions. After a median follow-up of 72 months, grade 2 or worse bladder and bowel toxicity was 9% and 4%, respectively (Katz and Kang 2014a). These toxicity scores are encouraging; however one should keep in mind that these data come from nonrandomized studies.

5.5 Sexual Function

Most studies reporting on sexual function used the EPIC questionnaire (Mantz 2014; Katz and Kang 2014a; Zimmermann et al. 2016), whereas others used the EORTC Quality-of-Life PR25 questionnaire (Aluwini et al. 2013) or the International Index of Erectile Function (IIEF) questionnaire (Fuller et al. 2014). Studies reporting on sexual function found a decrease in sexual function during the first 12 months posttreatment, with subsequent stabilization (Mantz 2014;

Aluwini et al. 2013; Fuller et al. 2014; Katz and Kang 2014a; Zimmermann et al. 2016). Fuller and colleagues and Katz and colleagues reported that 65–67% of the initially potent patients remained potent at last follow-up (Fuller et al. 2014; Katz and Kang 2014a).

5.6   Clinical Implications

Current clinical data provide excellent short-term control rates for SBRT; toxicity induced by extreme hypofractionation schedules does not appear to be substantially higher as compared to conventional treatments (Spratt et al. 2013; Michalski et al. 2013; Al-Mamgani et al. 2008, 2009). Severe toxicity (grade 4) might occur somewhat more frequently compared to conventional treatments, especially after dose delivery using gantry-based Linacs (Loblaw et al. 2013; Kim et al. 2014). We are eagerly awaiting long-term follow-up from current studies of extreme hypofractionation.

The ongoing phase III PACE trial (NCT01584258) addresses the need for randomized comparison with other treatment modalities and aims to randomly allocate more than 1700 hormone-naïve men with low- or intermediate-risk cancer between SBRT of 36.25 Gy in 5 fractions and laparoscopic prostatectomy (http://www.cancerresearchuk.org/about-cancer/find-a-clinical-trial/a-trial-comparing-surgery-conventional-radiotherapy-and-stereotactic-radiotherapy-for-localised-prostate-cancer-pace#undefined). If patients are unsuitable for or do not wish to undergo surgery, they are randomized between SBRT and conventional IMRT of 78 Gy in 39 fractions. Until comparative phase III studies have been completed, extremely hypofractionated SBRT can best be offered in the setting of prospective clinical studies.

6   Future Directions

6.1   Treatment Schedule

The concept of hypofractionated radiotherapy has such clear-cut advantages in terms of cost and time saving that future research activities will

continue to focus on novel and even more extreme SBRT treatment schemes. The optimal schedule has yet to be determined, since SBRT treatment fractions are now either delivered daily, on alternate days, or weekly (Table 3). The phase II PATRIOT trial (NCT01423474) aims to investigate the effects on bowel Quality-of-Life after SBRT to 40 Gy in five fractions delivered in 11 vs. 29 days. A similar phase II study from Switzerland (NCT01764646) randomizes patients between SBRT to 36.25 Gy in five fractions delivered either on alternate days or during weekly fractions. The primary endpoints are acute and late toxicity. These studies will help determine the safety of hypofractionation.

6.2   Hypofractionated Boost

The introduction of magnetic resonance imaging (MRI) for contouring has also provided new options for focal treatment of macroscopic tumor. The Dutch phase III FLAME trial (NCT01168479), which has completed accrual of 567 intermediate- or high-risk patients, randomized between conventional EBRT of 77 Gy in 35 fractions with or without a high-dose boost and 95 Gy in fractions of 2.7 Gy to the MRI-defined macroscopic tumor (Lips et al. 2011). The phase II hypo-FLAME study (NCT02853110) investigates whether SBRT of 35 Gy in 5 weekly fractions and an additional integrated focal boost of 50 Gy to the MRI-defined tumor volume is feasible and associated with acceptable toxicity (Clinicaltrials.gov 2016). Weekly MRIs will be performed as a preparation for MRI-guided treatments using novel MRI-Linacs. This technique can potentially better define soft-tissue changes as a result of rectum and bladder filling than currently available image guidance techniques, and could therefore play an important role in future hypofractionated treatments.

6.3   Treatment Technique

The reliance on imaging, position verification, and treatment technology will continue to increase if fraction doses are increased, and more patients with high-risk disease will be treated. The first experiences with fraction doses up to 10 Gy delivered by gantry-based Linacs demonstrated that severe grade 4 toxicities might occur in up to 5% (Kim et al. 2014). Novel dose-escalation studies might require CyberKnife® treatment, which has been shown to deliver treatment doses with submillimeter precision (Xie et al. 2008), and enables safety margins as low as 2 mm.

CyberKnife® dose-escalation studies will continue to occur in order to explore which treatment doses can safely be prescribed; however gantry-based Linacs are widely more available. Developing evidence using such techniques should be continued and might even impact clinical practice to a larger extent. The Swedish phase III HYPO-RT-PC trial (ISRCTN45905321) accrued 592 intermediate-risk prostate cancer patients between conventional treatment of 78 Gy in 39 fractions and 7 fractions of 6.1 Gy up to 42.7 Gy (http://www.cancerresearchuk.org/about-cancer/find-a-clinical-trial/a-trial-comparing-surgery-conventional-radiotherapy-and-stereotactic-radiotherapy-for-localised-prostate-cancer-pace#undefined; ISRCTN 2016). Both treatments are delivered using 3D-CRT or IMRT with daily fiducial-based image guidance. The primary endpoint is 5-year RFS.

6.4 Androgen Deprivation Therapy (ADT)

Randomized trials have demonstrated that addition of ADT significantly improves RFS or overall survival in intermediate- or high-risk prostate cancer patients treated by EBRT (Bolla et al. 2016; Jones et al. 2011; D'Amico et al. 2008). ADT is therefore generally added to EBRT in these patients. However, radiation treatment doses on which these results are based vary between 66 and 78 Gy (Bolla et al. 2016; Jones et al. 2011; D'Amico et al. 2008), and are therefore well below radiobiological doses as applied in some hypofractionated treatments. Further dose escalation using SBRT might obviate ADT in selected patient populations, reducing ADT-related severe side effects including

metabolic complications (Saylor and Smith 2009), erectile dysfunction (Kratzik et al. 2005), and increased risk of cardiovascular events (D'Amico et al. 2007). To date, only Katz and colleagues analyzed the impact of addition of ADT to SBRT on biochemical RFS among a subgroup of 97 high-risk patients included in their prospective trial (Katz and Kang 2014a). No significant benefit of ADT was found (Katz and Kang 2014b); however novel studies designed to specifically address these questions are warranted.

Conclusions

Sufficient evidence is available supporting the noninferiority of moderately hypofractionated EBRT for intermediate- to high-risk localized prostate cancer patients. However, these hypofractionated treatments are often associated with increased toxicities, but do offer logistic convenience and increase hospital capacity. Novel SBRT schedules, which should offer more therapeutic gain based on radiobiological models, yield excellent early control rates in low- to intermediate-risk groups. Long-term follow-up and results of comparative trials are needed before SBRT can be generally recommended in clinical practice. Future research will focus on identifying optimal treatment doses and schedules to improve disease control and reduce radiation-induced toxicity. Novel treatment techniques and imaging modalities will enable us to continue improving treatment delivery and conformality. Future research and improvements might also obviate the need for ADT in selected patients.

References

Al-Mamgani A, van Putten WL, Heemsbergen WD et al (2008) Update of Dutch multicenter dose-escalation trial of radiotherapy for localized prostate cancer. Int J Radiat Oncol Biol Phys 72:980–988

Al-Mamgani A, Heemsbergen WD, Peeters ST, Lebesque JV (2009) Role of intensity-modulated radiotherapy in reducing toxicity in dose escalation for localized prostate cancer. Int J Radiat Oncol Biol Phys 73:685–691

Aluwini S, van Rooij P, Hoogeman M et al (2013) Stereotactic body radiotherapy with a focal boost to the MRI-visible tumor as monotherapy for low- and intermediate-risk prostate cancer: early results. Radiat Oncol 8:84. doi:10.1186/1748-717X-8-84

Aluwini S, Pos F, Schimmel E et al (2015) Hypofractionated versus conventionally fractionated radiotherapy for patients with prostate cancer (HYPRO): acute toxicity results from a randomized non-inferiority phase 3 trial. Lancet Oncol 16:274–283

Aluwini S, Pos FJ, Schimmel E et al (2016) Hypofractionated versus conventionally fractionated radiotherapy for prostate cancer: late toxicity in the Dutch randomized phase III hypofractionation trial (HYPRO). Lancet Oncol 4:464–474

Arcangeli G, Saracino B, Gomellini S et al (2010) A prospective phase III randomized trial of hypofractionation versus conventional fractionation in patients with high-risk prostate cancer. Int J Radiat Oncol Biol Phys 78:11–18

Arcangeli G, Fowler J, Gomellini S et al (2011) Acute and late toxicity in a randomized trial of conventional versus hypofractionated three-dimensional conformal radiotherapy for prostate cancer. Int J Radiat Oncol Biol Phys 79:1013–1021

Arcangeli S, Strigari L, Gomellini S et al (2012) Updated results and patterns of failure in a randomized hypofractionation trial for high-risk prostate cancer. Int J Radiat Oncol Biol Phys 84:1172–1178

Beltran C, Herman MG, Davis BJ (2008) Planning target margin calculations for prostate radiotherapy based on intrafraction and interfraction motion using four localization methods. Int J Radiat Oncol Biol Phys 70:289–295

Bolla M, Maingon P, Carrie C et al (2016) Short androgen suppression and radiation dose escalation for intermediate- and high-risk localized prostate cancer: results of EORTC trial 22991. J Clin Oncol 34: 1748–1756

Bolzicco G, Favretto MS, Satariano N et al (2013) A single-center study of 100 consecutive patients with localized prostate cancer treated with stereotactic body radiotherapy. BMC Urol 13:49-2490-13-49

Brenner DJ, Hall EJ (1999) Fractionation and protraction for radiotherapy of prostate carcinoma. Int J Radiat Oncol Biol Phys 43:1095–1101

Brenner D, Armour E, Corry P, Hall E (1998) Sublethal damage repair times for a late-responding tissue relevant to brachytherapy (and external-beam radiotherapy): implications for new brachytherapy protocols. Int J Radiat Oncol Biol Phys 41:135–138

Cancer Research UK. http://www.cancerresearchuk.org/about-cancer/find-a-clinical-trial/a-trial-comparing-surgery-conventional-radiotherapy-and-stereotactic-radiotherapy-for-localised-prostate-cancer-pace#undefined, 2016a. Accessed 14 Oct 2016

Cancer Research UK. Prostate cancer statistics-key facts. http://www.cancerresearchuk.org/health-professional/cancer-statistics/statistics-by-cancer-type/prostate-cancer, 2016b. Accessed 6 Oct 2016

Clinicaltrials.gov. Hypofractionated focal lesion ablative microboost in prostatE cancer (Hypo-FLAME) (NCT02853110), 2016. Accessed 14 Oct 2016 2016

Collins CD, Lloyd-Davies RW, Swan AV (1991) Radical external beam radiotherapy for localized carcinoma of the prostate using a hypofractionation technique. Clin Oncol (R Coll Radiol) 3:127–132

D'Amico AV, Denham JW, Crook J et al (2007) Influence of androgen suppression therapy for prostate cancer on the frequency and timing of fatal myocardial infarctions. J Clin Oncol 25:2420–2425

D'Amico AV, Chen MH, Renshaw AA, Loffredo M, Kantoff PW (2008) Androgen suppression and radiation vs radiation alone for prostate cancer: a randomized trial. JAMA 299:289–295

Dale RG (1985) The application of the linear-quadratic dose-effect equation to fractionated and protracted radiotherapy. Br J Radiol 58:515–528

Dasu A, Toma-Dasu I (2012) Prostate alpha/beta revisited—an analysis of clinical results from 14,168 patients. Acta Oncol 51:963–974

Dearnaley DP, Sydes MR, Graham JD et al (2007) Escalated-dose versus standard-dose conformal radiotherapy in prostate cancer: first results from the MRC RT01 randomized controlled trial. Lancet Oncol 8:475–487

Dearnaley D, Syndikus I, Mossop H et al (2016) Conventional versus hypofractionated high-dose intensity-modulated radiotherapy for prostate cancer: 5-year outcomes of the randomized, non-inferiority, phase 3 CHHiP trial. Lancet Oncol 17:1047–1060

Deutschmann H, Kametriser G, Steininger P et al (2012) First clinical release of an online, adaptive, aperture-based image-guided radiotherapy strategy in intensity-modulated radiotherapy to correct for inter- and intrafractional rotations of the prostate. Int J Radiat Oncol Biol Phys 83:1624–1632

Duncan W, Warde P, Catton CN et al (1993) Carcinoma of the prostate: results of radical radiotherapy (1970–1985). Int J Radiat Oncol Biol Phys 26:203–210

Ferlay J, Soerjomataram I, Dikshit R et al (2015) Cancer incidences and mortality worldwide: sources, methods and major patterns in GLOBOCAN 2012. Int J Cancer 5:E359–E386

Fowler JF (2005) The radiobiology of prostate cancer including new aspects of fractionated radiotherapy. Acta Oncol 44:265–276

Fuller DB, Naitoh J, Mardirossian G (2014) Virtual HDR CyberKnife® SBRT for localized prostatic carcinoma: 5-year disease-free survival and toxicity observations. Front Oncol 4:321

Hoffman KE, Voong KR, Pugh TJ et al (2014) Risk of late toxicity in men receiving dose-escalated hypofractionated intensity modulated prostate radiation therapy: results from a randomized trial. Int J Radiat Oncol Biol Phys 88:1074–1084

Incrocci L, Wortel RC, Alemayehu WG et al (2016) Hypofractionated versus conventionally fractionated radiotherapy for patients with localized prostate cancer (HYPRO): final efficacy results from a randomized, multicentre, open-label, phase 3 trial. Lancet Oncol 8:1061–1069

ISRCTN Registry-Phase III study of HYPOfractionated radiotherapy of intermediate risk localized prostate cancer (ISRCTN45905321), 2016. Accessed 6 Oct 6 2016

Jones CU, Hunt D, McGowan DG et al (2011) Radiotherapy and short-term androgen deprivation for localized prostate cancer. N Engl J Med 365:107–118

Katz AJ, Kang J (2014a) Quality of life and toxicity after SBRT for organ-confined prostate cancer, a 7-year study. Front Oncol 4:301

Katz A, Kang J (2014b) Stereotactic body radiotherapy with or without external beam radiation as treatment for organ confined high-risk prostate carcinoma: a six year study. Radiat Oncol 9:1. doi:10.1186/1748-717X-9-1

Kilby W, Dooley JR, Kuduvalli G et al (2010) The CyberKnife® robotic radiosurgery system in 2010. Technol Cancer Res Treat 9:433–452

Kim DW, Cho LC, Straka C et al (2014) Predictors of rectal tolerance observed in a dose-escalated phase 1-2 trial of stereotactic body radiation therapy for prostate cancer. Int J Radiat Oncol Biol Phys 89:509–517

King CR, Brooks JD, Gill H et al (2012) Long-term outcomes from a prospective trial of stereotactic body radiotherapy for low-risk prostate cancer. Int J Radiat Oncol Biol Phys 82:877–882

Kirkpatrick JP, Meyer JJ, Marks LB (2008) The linear-quadratic model is inappropriate to model high dose per fraction effects in radiosurgery. Semin Radiat Oncol 18:240–243

Kratzik CW, Schatzl G, Lunglmayr G, Rucklinger E, Huber J (2005) The impact of age, body mass index and testosterone on erectile dysfunction. J Urol 174:240–243

Kuban DA, Nogueras-Gonzalez GM, Hamblin L et al (2010) Preliminary report of a randomized dose escalation trial for prostate cancer using hypofractionation. Int J Radiat Oncol Biol Phys 78:S58–S59

Lee WR, Dignam JJ, Amin MB et al (2016) Randomized phase III non-inferiority study comparing two radiotherapy fractionation schedules in patients with low-risk prostate cancer. J Clin Oncol 34:2325–2332

Lips IM, van der Heide UA, Haustermans K et al (2011) Single blind randomized phase III trial to investigate the benefit of a focal lesion ablative microboost in prostate cancer (FLAME-trial): study protocol for a randomized controlled trial. Trials 12:255-6215-12-255

Loblaw A, Cheung P, D'Alimonte L et al (2013) Prostate stereotactic ablative body radiotherapy using a standard linear accelerator: toxicity, biochemical, and pathological outcomes. Radiother Oncol 107:153–158

Lukka H, Hayter C, Julian JA et al (2005) Randomized trial comparing two fractionation schedules for patients with localized prostate cancer. J Clin Oncol 23:6132–6138

Mantz C (2014) A phase II trial of stereotactic ablative body radiotherapy for low-risk prostate cancer using a non-robotic linear accelerator and real-time target tracking: report of toxicity, quality of life, and disease control outcomes with 5-year minimum follow-up. Front Oncol 4:279

Michalski JM, Yan Y, Watkins-Bruner D et al (2013) Preliminary toxicity analysis of 3-dimensional conformal radiation therapy versus intensity modulated radiation therapy on the high-dose arm of the radiation therapy oncology group 0126 prostate cancer trial. Int J Radiat Oncol Biol Phys 87:932–938

Miralbell R, Roberts SA, Zubizarreta E, Hendry JH (2012) Dose-fractionation sensitivity of prostate cancer deduced from radiotherapy outcomes of 5,969 patients in seven international institutional datasets: alpha/beta = 1.4 (0.9–2.2) Gy. Int J Radiat Oncol Biol Phys 82:e17–e24

Nijkamp J, Pos FJ, Nuver TT et al (2008) Adaptive radiotherapy for prostate cancer using kilovoltage cone-beam computed tomography: first clinical results. Int J Radiat Oncol Biol Phys 70:75–82

Peeters ST, Heemsbergen WD, Koper PC et al (2006) Dose-response in radiotherapy for localized prostate cancer: results of the Dutch multicenter randomized phase III trial comparing 68 Gy of radiotherapy with 78 Gy. J Clin Oncol 24:1990–1996

Pollack A, Zagars GK, Starkschall G et al (2002) Prostate cancer radiation dose response: results of the M. D. Anderson phase III randomized trial. Int J Radiat Oncol Biol Phys 53:1097–1105

Pollack A, Hanlon AL, Horwitz EM et al (2006) Dosimetry and preliminary acute toxicity in the first 100 men treated for prostate cancer on a randomized hypofractionation dose escalation trial. Int J Radiat Oncol Biol Phys 64:518–526

Pollack A, Walker G, Horwitz EM et al (2013) Randomized trial of hypofractionated external-beam radiotherapy for prostate cancer. J Clin Oncol 31:3860–3868

Potters L, Gaspar LE, Kavanagh B et al (2010) American Society for Therapeutic Radiology and Oncology (ASTRO) and American College of Radiology (ACR) practice guidelines for image-guided radiation therapy (IGRT). Int J Radiat Oncol Biol Phys 76:319–325

Read G, Pointon RC (1989) Retrospective study of radiotherapy in early carcinoma of the prostate. Br J Urol 63:191–195

Ritter M (2008) Rationale, conduct, and outcome using hypofractionated radiotherapy in prostate cancer. Semin Radiat Oncol 18:249–256

Saylor PJ, Smith MR (2009) Metabolic complications of androgen deprivation therapy for prostate cancer. J Urol 181:1998–2006. discussion 2007–8

Spratt DE, Pei X, Yamada J et al (2013) Long-term survival and toxicity in patients treated with high-dose intensity modulated radiation therapy for localized prostate cancer. Int J Radiat Oncol Biol Phys 85:686–692

Tucker SL, Thames HD, Michalski JM et al (2011) Estimation of alpha/beta for late rectal toxicity based on RTOG 94-06. Int J Radiat Oncol Biol Phys 81:600–605

van de Water S, Valli L, Aluwini S et al (2014) Intrafraction prostate translations and rotations during hypofractionated robotic radiation surgery: dosimetric impact of correction strategies and margins. Int J Radiat Oncol Biol Phys 88:1154–1160

Wilkins A, Mossop H, Syndikus I et al (2015) Hypofractionated radiotherapy versus conventionally fractionated radiotherapy for patients with intermediate-risk localized prostate cancer: 2-year patient-reported outcomes of the randomized, non-inferiority, phase 3 CHHiP trial. Lancet Oncol 16:1606–1616

Wortel RC, Incrocci L, Pos FJ et al (2015) Acute toxicity after image-guided intensity modulated radiation therapy compared to 3D conformal radiation therapy in prostate cancer patients. Int J Radiat Oncol Biol Phys 91:737–744

Wortel RC, Incrocci L, Pos FJ et al (2016a) Late side effects after image guided intensity modulated radiation therapy compared to 3D-conformal radiation therapy for prostate cancer: results from 2 prospective cohorts. Int J Radiat Oncol Biol Phys 95:680–689

Wortel RC, Pos FJ, Heemsbergen WD, Incrocci L (2016b) Sexual function after hypofractionated versus conventionally fractionated radiotherapy for prostate cancer: results from the randomized phase III HYPRO trial. J Sex Med 11:1695–1703

Xie Y, Djajaputra D, King CR, Hossain S, Ma L, Xing L (2008) Intrafractional motion of the prostate during hypofractionated radiotherapy. Int J Radiat Oncol Biol Phys 72:236–246

Yeoh EE, Botten RJ, Butters J et al (2011) Hypofractionated versus conventionally fractionated radiotherapy for prostate carcinoma: final results of phase III randomized trial. Int J Radiat Oncol Biol Phys 81:1271–1278

Zimmermann M, Taussky D, Menkarios C et al (2016) Prospective phase II trial of once-weekly hypofractionated radiation therapy for low-risk adenocarcinoma of the prostate: late toxicities and outcomes. Clin Oncol (R Coll Radiol) 28:386–392

Fractionation Regimens
for Gynecologic Malignancies

Joanne Jang, Patrizia Guerrieri,
and Akila N. Viswanathan

Contents

The original version of this chapter was revised. The affiliations of the authors have been updated.

J. Jang
Beth Israel Deaconess Medical Center, Boston, MA, USA
e-mail: anv@jhu.edu

P. Guerrieri
Department of Radiation Oncology, Allegheny Health Network Cancer Institute, Pittsburgh, PA, USA
e-mail: anv@jhu.edu

A.N. Viswanathan (✉)
Sidney Kimmel Comprehensive Cancer Center, Johns-Hopkins University, Baltimore, MD, USA
e-mail: anv@jhu.edu

Abstract

Radiation therapy plays a large role in many gynecologic cancers. In cervical cancer, it can be used as curative treatment, often in the form of external beam radiation therapy (EBRT), followed by brachytherapy. For endometrial, vulvar, and vaginal cancers, often radiation can be used adjuvantly after surgery, but for patients with unresectable disease, or gross disease left in lymph nodes or elsewhere in the pelvis after surgery, it can also be used with definitive intent.

In many of these situations, radiation must be given to relatively high doses in order to eradicate the disease. Although brachytherapy can be used to deliver high doses to the cervix, vagina, vulva, or endometrium, if there is gross nodal disease in the pelvic, para-aortic, or inguinal nodes, EBRT must be used to deliver the high dose of radiation. In the era of 2D or 3D conformal radiation therapy, these doses often exceeded the tolerance of other organs at risk (OAR), especially the small bowel and femoral heads. The advent of intensity-modulated radiation therapy (IMRT) made the delivery of higher doses of radiation feasible, while still respecting normal tissue tolerances. Prior to the use of IMRT, patients with pelvic, para-aortic, or inguinal lymphadenopathy could not be treated adequately with EBRT, and so received only palliative doses of radiation or chemotherapy alone.

1   Radical Treatment of Gynecologic Malignancies

The first studies using IMRT for pelvic radiation in the management of gynecologic malignancies were reported starting in the early 2000s. Mundt et al. reported a retrospective series from the University of Chicago in which patients were treated with IMRT to the pelvis (Mundt et al. 2002, 2003). Although these patients only received a standard dose of 45 Gy to the pelvis, they showed that there was excellent coverage of target volumes, decreased dose to OAR, and decreased gastrointestinal and hematologic toxicities. Investigators reported the use of IMRT to deliver extended field radiation to the para-aortic lymph nodes (Salama et al. 2006; Beriwal et al. 2007), often giving higher doses to gross disease, with decreased doses to OAR and decreased toxicities (Poorvu et al. 2013).

These studies helped to define optimum doses for gross disease, as well as dose limits for OAR. Previously, older cervical cancer studies using predominantly or exclusively 3D conformal radiation suggested that doses of radiation above 50 or 54 Gy could improve nodal control (Niibe et al. 2006; Rash et al. 2013). With 3D conformal RT, doses in the range of 55–63 Gy resulted in nodal control rates of 60–70%, but resulted in high rates of toxicities (Rash et al. 2013; Small et al. 2007; Yoon et al. 2012). Multiple IMRT studies showed that 55–65 Gy of radiation can result in nodal control rates as high as 80–90%, with decreased toxicities (Ramlov et al. 2015; Vargo et al. 2014). One study of patients treated with IMRT for nodal recurrences in endometrial cancer showed that patients who received less than their median dose of 64.7 Gy to gross disease had higher rates of local failure than those who received 64.7 Gy or higher (Ho et al. 2015). The overall rate of toxicities in this study was relatively low. Another study reported on patients with endometrial cancer that had gross unresected nodes treated with dose-escalated IMRT (Townamchai et al. 2014). Gross nodes were treated to a range of 55–65 Gy (median total dose = 63 Gy) and a small bowel dose constraint of 5cc < 55 Gy recommended which resulted in a nodal control rate of 86%. Only one patient had acute grade 3 gastroin-testinal (GI) toxicity, and there were no grade 3 or higher genitourinary (GU) toxicities.

With the goal of treating extended fields or delivering high doses of radiation to gross disease using IMRT, often above 60 Gy, many investigations explored specific limits for OAR, with the most sensitive of these being the small bowel. Roeske et al. showed that limiting the amount of small bowel receiving 45 Gy (V45) to less than 195 cc minimized the risk of acute GI toxicity (Roeske et al. 2003). Another study showed that by using IMRT for extended field radiation to a median dose of 54 Gy and a maximum PTV dose of 65 Gy, only 6.5% of patients had acute or late GI toxicity greater than grade 3. There were no grade 4 or 5 GI toxicities, and there was no duodenal-specific toxicity (Poorvu et al. 2013). In this study the planning aim was a small bowel V55 < 5 cc. In another study of extended field radiation to the para-aortic nodes using IMRT to a median dose of 63 Gy, limiting the volume of duodenum receiving 55 Gy (V55) to less than 15 cc kept the risk of late duodenal toxicity including duodenal perforation to 7.4% (Verma et al. 2014; Xu et al. 2015). Similarly, Xu et al. found only a 3.9% risk of acute GI toxicity ≥ grade 3 by keeping the V55 to less than 15 cc (Xu et al. 2015). A series of 103 cervical cancer patients treated to the para-aortic nodes showed a 5 year DSS for 47%. Due to high toxicity rates with SIB, the authors recommend no more than 215 cGy per fraction to nodal volumes, with 50 Gy to the involved nodes while the clinical target volumes receive 45 Gy in 25 fractions, and the normal tissues do not receive more than 2 Gy per fraction. Patients with large nodes have a sequential boost. Mid-treatment replanning is required for large nodal volumes.

More recently, there have also been clinical outcomes reported regarding hematologic toxicities and the amount of bone marrow receiving radiation, which has become increasingly important with the use of concurrent and sequential chemotherapy. Researchers from the University of Chicago demonstrated that patients who had more than 90% of their pelvic bone marrow receiving at least 10 Gy had higher rates of grade 2 or higher leukopenia, and were more like to have their chemotherapy held (Mell et al. 2006). Similarly, Albuquerque et al. reported that there was a 4.5 times increased risk of grade 2 or higher hematologic toxicity if the amount of pelvic bone receiving 20 Gy was higher than 80% (Albuquerque et al. 2011).

Traditionally, higher doses of radiation are given as sequential boosts, with 45–50 Gy being given to the areas at risk for microscopic disease, such as the pelvic, para-aortic, or inguinal nodes, and an external beam boost given to nodal disease to escalate the total dose to over 60 Gy. In addition to an external beam boost, brachytherapy can be used during or after the course of external beam radiation therapy to deliver high doses of radiation to the primary tumor. Kavanagh et al. explored giving a second daily concomitant boost fraction with IMRT to deliver higher doses of radiation to positive lymph nodes (Kavanagh et al. 1997, 2001). Other institutions reported patients treated with hyperfractionated or accelerated hyperfractionated radiation (MacLeod et al. 1999; Faria and Ferrigno 1997). As part of the exploration of using altered fractionation schemes, several institutions started using simultaneous integrated boost (SIB).

With regard to the combination of external beam and brachytherapy, treatment times greater than 56 days have been associated with decreased local control. With multiple sequential EBRT boosts, the duration of external radiation needed to deliver greater than 60 Gy can already approach 7–8 weeks, requiring that physicians interdigitate the brachytherapy during the nodal boost. SIB with IMRT can deliver the first and boost courses of radiation therapy concurrently, using a smaller number of fractions and decreasing the overall treatment time. Shorter treatment duration also benefits the patient in terms of convenience and cost, but carries a higher risk of toxicity given the higher doses employed.

The boost volume, which usually encompasses targets with gross disease, often receives higher doses per fraction, increasing the biological equivalent dose (BED) compared to the same dose given with sequential EBRT boost. However, there are steeper dose gradients across the nodal target volume, resulting in relative dose inhomogeneity in the nodal tissue. In addition, tumor shrinkage over the course of treatment may result in the movement of normal tissues into the radiation field and when combined with the higher dose per fraction may increase the risk of acute toxicity (Dogan et al. 2003).

An early study from the Medical College of Wisconsin in 2005 proposed the use of SIB using IMRT, and used an example patient with bulky cervical disease that would not be adequately treated with a traditional tandem-based implant (Guerrero et al. 2005). They compared a variety of SIB IMRT plans to a conventional plan that used a sequential EBRT boost to the cervix, and also a plan with pelvic radiation followed by a high-dose-rate (HDR) brachytherapy boost. Their results suggest that an SIB IMRT plan can be equivalent in some cases to a plan using pelvic external radiation followed by a HDR boost. Even while controlling for the same BED for the cervical tumor, the SIB IMRT plan had improved sparing of normal tissues compared to the plan with sequential external beam boosts, and delivered treatment in a shorter amount of time overall. More recently, Feng et al. from the University of Chicago retrospectively designed a theoretical planning study with SIB plans for ten patients compared to sequential IMRT plans. They found that while target coverage was similar, hot spots were significantly decreased. There was better sparing of all contoured normal tissues, although only doses to the rectum and small bowel were significantly different statistically (Feng et al. 2016).

For vulvar cancer, definitive radiation doses can sometimes approach 70 Gy. In a study from McGill University, Bloemers et al. dosimetrically compared a variety of treatment plans for five patients getting definitive radiation for vulvar cancer, which included two SIB plans to 56 and 67.2 Gy, both given in 28 fractions (Bloemers et al. 2012). They found that all IMRT plans decreased doses to OAR compared to a 3D conformal plan. SIB IMRT plans for vulvar cancer had similar doses to OAR compared to IMRT plans with a sequential boost, but the authors note that SIB allows for a higher BED to both normal and target tissues.

Although SIB seems to have many dosimetric benefits, there are some concerns with its use as well. Since gross tumor volumes often receive higher doses per fraction, adjacent OAR also receive higher doses per fraction, particularly given the rapid shrinkage of gynecologic malignancies, increasing BED and potentially increasing both acute and late toxicities. Also, as with any IMRT plan, tumor shrinkage and motion and

OAR motion are significant concerns. Tumor volumes could potentially be under-dosed and OAR could potentially be overdosed, and the initial plans may not reflect the actual dose delivered. With the shortened treatment time and increased dose per fraction of SIB plans, this error can be amplified, potentially leading to worse tumor control and increased toxicity. In fact, one retrospective study of ten patients showed that treatment with SIB IMRT can cause lower doses to targets and higher doses to OAR than expected due to tumor regression and organ motion and recommended replanning during the course of treatment (Herrera et al. 2013).

However, there are now several series of patients treated with SIB that include toxicities and clinical outcomes. The first investigations looked into the feasibility and safety of SIB. Kavanagh et al. first reported a series of seven cervical cancer patients receiving SIB in 2002. Although the number of patients was small, they showed it was feasible and there were acceptable rates of GI and GU toxicities (Kavanagh et al. 2002). In a study by Gerszten et al., 22 patients with cervical cancer received extended field radiation using IMRT with concurrent cisplatin to 45 Gy in 25 fractions, with a simultaneous boost to 55 Gy to the involved nodes. There were no grade 3 or higher GI or GU toxicity, and two patients had chemotherapy held or had radiation treatment breaks due to hematologic toxicity, showing again that SIB was feasible and safe (Gerszten et al. 2006). SIB has also been shown to be feasible and safe in endometrial cancer, with investigators from Italy reporting 70 patients that were treated to the pelvis to 45 Gy in 25 fractions, with a simultaneous integrated boost to 55 Gy in one cohort, and to 60 Gy in the second cohort (Macchia et al. 2016a, b). Toxicities were deemed acceptable, with 24% and 20% having acute grade 2 or higher GI and GU toxicity, respectively. No patients experienced late grade 3 or higher GI or late grade 2 or higher GU toxicity.

As clinics became more comfortable with the technique and its feasibility and safety, the use of SIB became more widespread and investigators reported larger series. A group from Germany first reported their experience using SIB tomotherapy for 40 patients with cervical cancer, most of whom had laparoscopic staging before radiation (Marnitz et al. 2012). All patients received 50.4 Gy to the pelvic (±para-aortic) lymph nodes in 1.8-Gy fractions, and 59.36 Gy to the boost volume in 2.12-Gy fractions, all given in 28 fractions, with concurrent chemotherapy. Toxicities were relatively low, with no grade 4 or 5 acute toxicity, and only 2.5% acute grade 3 gastrointestinal (GI) toxicity, which was comparable to other series using IMRT. Mean doses to the small bowel were lower with SIB IMRT compared to other standard IMRT studies despite prescribing a higher dose to the target.

Researchers at Duke University retrospectively analyzed 39 patients with gynecologic cancers treated with a SIB technique, receiving 45 Gy in 1.8-Gy fractions to nodal regions at risk and 55 Gy in 2.2-Gy fractions to gross disease, all given in 25 fractions total (Boyle et al. 2014). Seven patients received an additional sequential boost. By the author's calculation, accounting for a shorter treatment time and higher dose per fraction, 55 Gy in 2.2-Gy fractions is equivalent to 64.8 Gy in 1.8-Gy fractions. This study similarly showed low rates of toxicities, with no grade 4 or 5 toxicity, 2.5% acute grade 3 GI toxicity, 25% acute grade 3 hematologic toxicity in those patients receiving concurrent chemotherapy only, and no grade 3 late toxicity. With 18 months of follow-up, local control was 77%, overall survival was 74%, and the rate of distant metastases was 30%.

Two other studies have evaluated SIB IMRT for the treatment of cervical cancer patients with positive lymph nodes in the PET/CT era (Vargo et al. 2014; Cihoric et al. 2014). Cihoric et al. describe ten patients with PET/CT-defined lymph node positive cervical cancer that received 50.4 Gy to the nodal volume and 55.8 Gy to the primary tumor in 1.8-Gy fractions, with a simultaneous boost to the gross nodal disease to 62 Gy in 2.0-Gy fractions, followed in most cases by brachytherapy. Only one patient developed grade 3 acute GU toxicity and one patient developed late grade 3 vaginal dryness. At 20 months of follow-up, seven patients were disease free. In the second study, investigators from the University of Pittsburgh describe 61 cervical cancer patients that received 45 Gy to the nodal regions at risk and 55 Gy to the positive pelvic or para-aortic nodes, as defined by PET/CT, all given in 25 fractions followed by brachytherapy. With an average 29 months of follow-up local control of the cervix was 76%, regional control of the lymph nodes was 94%, disease-free survival was 57%, overall survival was 69%, and distant control was 67%. Only one patient (4%) experienced grade 3 or higher late toxicity, which was a grade 4 rectovaginal fistula.

Finally, there are a handful of studies looking at other types of altered fractionation, including hyperfractionation, hypofractionation, or stereotactic body radiotherapy (SBRT). RTOG 92-10 described hyperfractionated RT 1.2 Gy per fraction, two fractions per day, 5 days per week for patients with cervical cancer (Grigsby et al. 2001). These patients received a total of 24–48 Gy to the pelvis, approximately 65 Gy to the parametria, 48 Gy to the para-aortic lymph nodes, and 54–58 Gy to the known involved lymph nodes with concurrent chemotherapy, in addition to a brachytherapy boost to the cervix. Unfortunately, there was an unacceptably high rate of toxicity, with 17% late grade 4 GI toxicity and one acute grade 5 toxicity, and no improvement in survival or tumor control. Viegas et al. enrolled stage IIIB cervical cancer patients on a phase I–II study in which they received 2.5 Gy per fraction given BID on 8 days spread out over 8 weeks with concurrent chemotherapy and a brachytherapy boost to the cervix (Viegas et al. 2004). Survival outcomes were comparable to contemporary studies using standard fractionation, and 12% and 3% of patients had late grade 3 or grade 4 toxicity, respectively.

Stereotactic body radiotherapy is a mechanism to deliver high doses of radiation to focal targets, typically using much higher doses per fraction than conventional fractionated radiation, and giving only 1–5 fractions in total. There have been reports of SBRT being used for gross pelvic or para-aortic lymphadenopathy, either in the primary or recurrent setting, as a substitute for brachytherapy, or for oligometastatic disease at other sites, such as the liver or the lung (Higginson et al. 2011). For gross lymphadenopathy and at oligometastatic sites, SBRT seems to result in local control rates ranging from 60–80% with acceptable toxicity (Hasan et al. 2016; Park et al.

2015; Seo et al. 2016). In terms of treating the primary site of disease, there is some evidence that although brachytherapy utilization may be decreasing and use of SBRT increasing, the use of IMRT/SBRT as a boost to the primary site may result in worse survival outcomes (Han et al. 2013). Although many consider SBRT to be technologically easier and more convenient, there is valid concern that compared to brachytherapy, SBRT may increase the volume of and dose to normal tissue, and that it does not account as well for target and organ motion. Nevertheless, SBRT may be an option for those patients that cannot tolerate brachytherapy, usually for medical or anatomical reasons. One group has published small series of patients with gynecologic cancers treated with an SBRT boost, suggesting that it may be feasible, well tolerated, and with acceptable survival outcomes in select patients (Molla et al. 2005; Jorcano et al. 2010). However, the use of SBRT needs to be validated with larger prospective and randomized studies.

Overall, these studies suggest that SIB IMRT may be safe when the per fraction dose is limited (@215cGy/fraction) and the lymph nodes are small, given the dose heterogeneity across a node in SIB regimens. However, many of these studies are retrospective, and may not have adequate follow-up to fully evaluate late toxicities, which could be affected by the higher than normal doses per fraction seen with SIB. A randomized trial would be needed to truly compare toxicities and outcomes between SIB IMRT and sequential IMRT boosts.

2 Palliative Treatment of Gynecological Malignancies

2.1 Rationale

In cases where the tumor has metastasized to multiple sites or the patient has too low a performance status that precludes radical intent, palliative radiation may be used to alleviate symptoms. In these instances a shorter course of radiation treatment with lower total dose is preferred to avoid the risk of grade 3 and above toxicity, while at the same time delivering a treatment that is clinically effective. Palliative radiation therapy can be applied therefore to different clinical scenarios and with diverse intents: for bleeding, pain, obstruction symptoms, or in case of re-irradiation.

For palliative intent cases, different fractionation schedules can be used and are present in the literature (Mohiuddin et al. 1990; Spanos et al. 1987, 1994; Rasool et al. 2011; Boulware et al. 1979; Fletcher 1980; Mishra et al. 2005; Van Lnkhuijzen and Thomas 2011; Onsrud et al. 2001; Rai et al. 2012; Patricio et al. 1987), but they usually gravitate around the concept of delivering a meaningful dose of radiation in a rather short period of time, that will not significantly interfere with other treatment modalities, like chemotherapy or other medical management and will allow for the patient to improve on her symptoms and obtain a better quality of life. Therefore palliative radiation is, in these instances, usually delivered using hypofractionation. Sometimes hypofractionation is required to deliver palliative doses of radiation in areas of the country, or of the world that have scarce access to radiation therapy machines.

In spite of the fact that palliative radiation in gynecological cancer is delivered to a significant percentage of the gynecological population, there are very few controlled multi-institutional or randomized studies and the data present in the literature are sparse. We will describe the clinical practice in terms of most and least used fractionation schedules and their results.

2.2 Clinical Aspects in a Palliative Setting

When facing a decision about palliative irradiation of a gynecological cancer patient, it is essential to evaluate the performance status and the presence of comorbidities. One must weigh the life expectancy and quality of life and assess the possible benefits of radiation treatment. Since a palliative treatment is not likely to increase life expectancy, we try to get an understanding of how long the patient can live with the tumor and what is the impact of treatment on quality of life.

How do we make a decision to administer palliative radiation in a gynecological cancer patient? There are two categories that we generally use for that: tumor status and the general health and strength of the patient.

Performance status alone has been shown to be an inadequate tool to predict toxicity in an elderly population (Tew 2016) while a more specific geriatric assessment (Repetto et al. 2002) and the advent of frailty ageing markers show some promise of usefulness (Dumas et al. 2016). Age alone is not a very useful parameter since chronological and physiological age can differ significantly and therefore the choice of a palliative treatment needs to take into account all of the variability already mentioned. Social and environmental assessment, financial support, spiritual resources, faith choices, and transportation issues all need to be part of the decision-making process (Gawande 2014).

For physicians the issues usually boil down to a simple question: do we have a reasonable expectation to get rid of the tumor or not? But we know too well that even such a simple question has today different answers in the developed and in the developing part of our world. Technology and medicine resources and access to the best technology and healthcare can affect life expectancy, although not lead to a better quality of life (Gawande 2014).

In everyday practice we are confronted with a variety of clinical situations that may or may not require active intervention. The most frequent situations that we are called to palliate in gynecological cancer can be summarized as follows: vaginal bleeding, pelvic or abdominal pain, vaginal discharge, bowel obstruction syndromes, urinary or colonic fistula formation, and palliation of metastatic sites. Palliation of metastatic sites is the topic of other chapters in this book; therefore we will focus on the abdomen and pelvis as geographic sites of irradiation for gynecologic cancer patients.

2.3 Palliation and the Radiobiologic Aspects of Altered Fractionation

Palliative treatment often involves the use of higher than conventional doses per fraction, which fall into the categories of moderately versus highly hypofractionated radiation schedules.

The main reason for this strategy is reducing overall treatment time and number of fractions, resulting in reduced treatment cost and less logistic burden for the patient and the family, while at the same time achieving good symptomatic control. These logistic advantages have exploited fundamental differences in radiobiology effects between low and high dose per fractions. Hypofractionation can be divided into two different categories with separate biological principles: schedules that use 3–6 Gy per fraction and schedules that use ≥8 Gy per fraction.

The former schedule can be approached using the "classical" linear quadratic model and be compared to standard fractionation by the use of biological effective dose (BED). They presumably follow the 4 Rs of radiation: repair, reassortment, re-oxygenation, and repopulation in a way similar to the standard fractionation of 1.8–2 Gy. The latter, better known as high-dose hypofractionation radiation therapy (HDHRT) is felt to cause four different radiobiological effects: intra-tumoral bystander and abscopal effects, where the high doses of radiation cause exposure of a massive amount of fractured tumoral antigens that can elicit unusual immunogenic reactions; tumor endothelial death; and targeting of tumor clones with different radiation sensitivity (Prasanna et al. 2014). An initial high dose per fraction could therefore potentially increase the tumor response to standard radiation therapy, but the problem is that a large dose per fraction can be safely administered only to rather small fields since toxicity, due to the presence of OARs, is the dose-limiting factor.

There are several mono-institutional and a few RTOG studies that employ schedules that belong to the abovementioned categories of moderately versus highly hypofractionated treatments (Spanos et al. 1987; Rasool et al. 2011). Results are sparse especially because evaluation points and metrics are very different and not always clearly defined.

The use of high dose per fraction to elicit biological effects like the bystander or abscopal effect or the radiation induced antigen presentation are possibilities in palliative pelvic radiation treatment even for large radiation fields by using an "old-new" technique: spatially fractionated radiation therapy. The concept derives historically from the use in the ortho-voltage or Cobalt-60 era of a grid with holes, to minimize superficial normal tissue dose while delivering tumoricidal doses in the depth (Mohiuddin et al. 1990). The concept is finding new flavor in the modern era, since it allows the irradiation of large fields using multiple nonconfluent pencil beams through a rather simple technique (a 2D grid or a 3D lattice). The irradiation of the target is nonuniform, but is spatially fractionated, so that part of the tumor can safely get the doses capable of triggering reactions in the tumor microenvironment such as vasculature effects and immunologic stimulation. Hypofractionation may be advantageous in overcoming the resistance of hypoxic cells especially when using a high dose per fraction, while, on the other hand, it might not take advantage of the in-between fraction re-oxygenation typical of the radiobiological concepts underlying standard fractionation (Hall and Giaccia 2012).

Looking at the fractionation schedules present in the literature we can use radiobiological models to compare them in terms of biological effectiveness. The most widely used is the linear quadratic model that classifies biological tissues into two broad categories (acute and late reacting); the model is presumably reliable for doses/fraction up to 6–7 Gy.

2.4 Fractionation Schedules and Techniques

Palliative treatment of gynecological malignancies can be carried out with external beam as well as intracavitary brachytherapy. Doses and indications vary according to institutional protocols and clinical presentations. There are different fractionation schedules reported in the literature that vary from daily fractions of 3–5 Gy to single fractions of 10–12 Gy repeated at 2–4 week intervals, as well as less used fractionation and techniques that will be summarized and grouped accordingly.

Table 1 lists examples of the most frequent choices in terms of radiation delivery for palliative treatments of gynecological malignancies.

Table 1 Fractionation schedules of palliative pelvic irradiation

Author	# patients	Dose/fraction	EQD2 α/β=3 Gy	EQD2 α/β=10 Gy	Timing/cycling	Technique
Rasool et al. (2011)	25	4 Gy × 5 5 Gy × 3	28 Gy 24 Gy	23.33 18.75	5 days[a] 5 days[a]	2D-RT (Co60)
Kim et al. (2013)	17	4 Gy × 5 5 Gy × 5	28 40	23.33 31.25	5 days[a]	3D-CRT
Spanos et al. (1987)	46	10 Gy × 1	26	16.67	Every 4 weeks up to 30 Gy total	2D-RT
Spanos et al. (1994)	290	3.7 Gy BID × 4	19.83	16.9	Every 2–4 weeks up to 3 times	
Patricio et al. (1987)	56 (43 stage III and IV)	6.5 Gy ×2[b] Repeated in 70% of stage III–IV)	24.7 49.6	17.88 35.75	48 h (interval time to second cycle not reported)	3D CRT
Cihoric et al. (2012)	62 (20 gyn)	EQD3 = 30 Gy$_3$[c]	Not known	30 Gy EQD3	Not known	3D CRT HDR BT
Rai et al. (2012)	72	8 Gy	17.6 Gy	12 Gy	Every 4 weeks up to 3 times	2D RT
Mishra et al. (2005)	100	10 Gy × 1 30 Gy LDR after second fx[d]	26 30	16.67 30	Every month up to 3 times	2D RT LDR-BT
Grigsby et al. (2002)	15	5 Gy × 2	16	12.5	At 1 week interval	HDR-BT (ring only)
Mohiuddin et al. (1990)	22	10–15 Gy × 1 (50–50 GRID)[e]	26–54	16.67–32.73	Repeated once at 4 weeks in some patients	Unopposed single field
Panek (2001)	55	18–62 Gy LDR 20–50 in 2 Gy/f	18–62 20–50	18–62 20–50	Standard fractionation	LDR 2D RT
Onsrud et al. (2001)	64	10 Gy × 1	26	16.67	Single fraction	2D RT 3DCRT

Key: *Co60* Cobalt 60, *BID* twice a day, *CRT* chemoradiation, *h* hours, *LDR* low dose rate radiation, *RT* radiation therapy, *HDR* high dose rate, *BT* brachytherapy, *fx* fraction, *Gy* Gray

[a]5 days: delivery over 5 consecutive working days
[b]All advanced cases received 6.5 Gy followed by a second dose of 6.5 Gy in 48 h; 70% received a second cycle of 6.5 × 2 in 48 h after an interval time that is not reported
[c]Different doses and fractionations were employed that were biologically equivalent to 30 Gy in 10 fractions by LQ model with α/β = 10; median doses 20 Gy (range 5–45 Gy)
[d]30 Gy LDR-BT after second fraction of 10 Gy in case of good response
[e]50% open, 50% 6.35 cm thick Cerrobend (5 HVL)
Note: The examples of EQD2 calculation must to be taken with caution since the LQ model does not apply in all cases, particularly with high dose/fraction and altered timing

Moderately hypofractionated regimens use doses/fraction from 3 to 6 Gy; they are generally administered in consecutive days. It seems safe to compare their biological effectiveness to standard fractionation using the linear quadratic model. As seen in Table 1, the biological effectiveness of the moderately hypofractionated regimens ranges from 16 to 54 Gy$_3$ (for an alpha/beta ratio = 3 Gy) and from 12.5 to 35.75 Gy$_{10}$ (for an alpha/beta ratio = 10 Gy) with a median of 28 Gy$_3$ and 23.33 Gy$_{10}$. Assessing late reacting tissue effect is critical, for in palliative treatment it is crucial not to harm the patient while delivering a reasonably effective palliative treatment.

Within the moderately hypofractionated regimen is the Quad-shot regimen described by Spanos et al. (1994) and derived from the randomized trial RTOG 8502. This trial prescribed 3.7 Gy BID for 2 consecutive days and the cycle was repeated up to three times with an interval of 2–4 weeks. The trial intent was to answer to the question about timing of the cycles, and no difference was found between the 2 versus 4 week interval. The trial was developed after the phase I-II RTOG 7905, where single doses of 10 Gy were administered up to three times with a 4 week interval, was closed due to toxicity. The biological equivalence of RTOG 8502 is 19.83 Gy$_3$ for late responding tissues and 16.9 Gy$_{10}$ for acute responding tissues like a squamous cell carcinoma of the cervix for every cycle. Interestingly, a 2 week interval is the average time it takes to the tumor to repopulate according to some radiobiologists, while for others the average time is about 3 weeks (Tarnawski et al. 2002; Huang et al. 2012). The trial shows no difference in terms of survival or side effects no matter the interval between cycles of radiotherapy (3–6 weeks in the pilot part or 2 versus 4 weeks in the randomized one), maybe due to the fact that it was not powered to show differences in such a variety of overall treatment times and/or to other factors playing a role in the final outcomes. The Quad-shot regimen is one of the few examples present in the literature of BID fractionation.

Several studies and institutions have adopted a single dose per fraction of 8–10 Gy administered at interval of 4 weeks up to a total of three times (Boulware et al. 1979; Fletcher 1980). The criteria for re-administration varied according to patient compliance, intervening death, or tumor response. If one were to evaluate the biological equivalence to standard fractionation of a single high dose fraction, the LQ model can be used as a guide (Brenner 2008), but it is probably not the best model to use when taking into account a large interval between fractions. One should be aware that the LQ model may reliably describe the shape of the survival curve only between 1 and 8 Gy (Brenner 2008).

For doses of 8 Gy and higher we should look at the straight part of the survival curve for late effects. According to some radiobiologists the survival curve at high doses per fraction becomes inverted between acute and late responding tissues compared to standard or moderately high doses/fraction. At high doses/fraction late responding tissues may be proportionally more resistant than acute responding. Others claim that the linear quadratic model can almost seamlessly fit the high dose per fraction models of SRT and SBRT, where advanced technology and imaging make possible the delivery of large doses to tumors with very small margins and high dose gradients outside the radiation target (Brenner 2008; Brown et al. 2014).

Should we apply the LQ formula to the HD-HRT regimens mentioned in the literature, they would have a biological equivalence to a standard fractionated dose of 17.6–26 Gy$_3$ for late effects and of 12–16.67 Gy$_{10}$ for tumor response, being in the same range of equivalence of the moderately hypofractionated regimens. There are several problems with this: (1) volumes of treatment are very different from the relatively small volume of SRT/SBRT; (2) timing and overall treatment times are based on split courses, rather than consecutive ones; (3) fractionation present in the palliative literature related to cervical cancer is often based more on empirical experience than on a choice guided by radiobiological models or by randomized trial results.

Since the widespread use of HDR brachytherapy, high dose per fraction has become quite common in the treatment of gynecological cancer. The linear quadratic model has been invaluable in guiding the choice of HDR dose/fraction schemes that summed with the pelvic external beam would allow for an overall biological effectiveness comparable to the 80–90 Gy of standard fractionation and LDR brachytherapy of the 2D-RT era. HDR brachytherapy can have a palliative role especially for bleeding, according to Grisby et al. who used a cervical ring to deliver a superficial treatment prescribed to 0.5 cm from the cervical ring in two fractions, 1 week apart, for hemostatic purposes prior to a more definitive type of treatment (Grigsby et al. 2002). A total of 30 brachytherapy treatments fashioned in this way delivered 10 Gy in two fractions to 15 patients. Computerized treatment planning calculated an average dose to the rectum of 1.75 Gy and average dose to the bladder of 1.65 Gy, while point A received an average dose of 0.85 Gy per patient. The patients then received definitive chemoradiation and brachytherapy according to standard of care. While the hemostatic cervical ring brachytherapy contribution to the total dose was not taken into account, it achieved complete bleeding palliation in 93% of patients (Grigsby et al. 2002).

Doses for GRID or 3D-Lattice radiation are usually prescribed in the nominal range of high dose per fraction and are usually delivered as split course, so that they could be assimilated to HD-HRT, but the fundamental difference is that only portions of the tumor get the prescribed dose, while the rest gets a gradient of low-intermediate doses in this "spatially fractionated" treatment. Mohiuddin et al. (Mohiuddin et al. 1990) report the experience on 22 patients with bulky symptomatic tumors (8 pelvic), who underwent single dose of 10–15 Gy through a 50:50 GRID. In eight patients the treatment was repeated after 4 weeks. Tolerance of the treatment was very good, with one patient developing an acute skin reaction, two developing mild diarrhea episodes, and one developing small bowel occlusion that was successfully relieved with surgery after receiving 60 Gy to the pelvis and 10 Gy GRID boost for a recurrent rectal cancer. Clinical response with palliation of symptoms and objective regression was observed in 91% of the patients and were seen primarily in patients treated with the GRID and an external beam irradiation of 50 or more Gy (Mohiuddin et al. 1990).

Intraoperative electrons have been used by Arians et al. for treatment of recurrent endometrial, vulvar, or cervical cancer after surgical excision, in Heidelberg (Arians et al. 2016). Twenty-six patients were treated with a median dose of 15 Gy and a median energy of 8 MeV after various degrees of surgical resection. Patients with recurrent cervical cancer had the worst outcome with 1 year overall survival (OS) of 44.5% and 5 years OS of 6.4%. Local progression-free survival (LPFS) was 0% at 2 years. Endometrial cancer patients fared the best LPFS with 61% of the patient be free of disease progression at 2 years and 40.6% at 5 years. In terms of toxicity, 50%, 61%, and 67% of endometrial, cervical, and vulvar cancer patients (respectively) developed complications. A total of 8.3% died of postoperative complications, 8.3% had femoral head toxicity, and neural affections occurred in 11.1% in spite of the dose being reduced to 10–12 Gy when major nerves were included in the treatment field. Postoperative disorders occurred in 22.2% of the cases and 8.3% and 5.6% developed lymphedema or lymphocele and thrombosis, respectively.

2.5 Primary Tumor Sites

All pelvic sites can be considered for palliative treatment with the technique and the doses described. Our focus here regards the gynecological sphere with tumor arising or recurrent from endometrium, cervix, vulva, ovary, or vagina, but the same modalities can be applied to other primary tumor sites like prostate, bladder, and urethra. As we have seen there could be differences in outcome for different primary sites, at least in part related to the type of primary treatment, and to the previous use of irradiation as well as to the extent of the tumor at presentation.

2.6 Palliative Intent

The most frequent symptoms requiring palliation in gynecological cancer arise from either a locally advanced cancer at presentation or a locally advanced recurrence. The lack of strong screening programs in the developing countries or underserved regions of the world make the use and availability of palliative tools extremely important in these situations.

Table 2 summarizes the most frequents signs and occurrence in the developed as well as in the developing countries in locally advanced primaries or recurrences of gynecological origin.

Overall, pelvic pain and vaginal bleeding are the most frequent symptoms for palliation, especially with radiation therapy. Other symptoms to palliate are vaginal discharge, frequently, foul smelling, leg lymphedema, and mass effect. There are really no substantial differences in terms of symptom frequency in the world geography of advanced pelvic diseases. Many authors are interested in reporting data regarding palliation of vaginal bleeding which usually represents an emergent situation especially when tumor originates in the uterine cervix. Therefore, there are reports focused exclusively on the role of radiation therapy or alternative tools in bleeding palliation.

Table 3 reports the efficacy of radiation therapy in controlling the most frequent signs of locally advanced disease in a palliative setting.

As already known for other tumor sites, radiation therapy is a highly effective hemostatic treatment with responses ranging between 83% and 100%. The degree of hemostatic effect is higher after higher doses of radiation, and it reached 100% after the third 10 Gy fraction in the highly hypofractionated regimens used in the RTOG 7905 phase I/II study. Misha et al. reported a 31% vaginal bleeding control rate after the first 10 Gy and 100% control after the third 10 Gy fraction (Spanos et al. 1994; Boulware et al. 1979; Mishra et al. 2005). Even the study published by Mohiuddin on the use of 10–15 Gy with the GRID device reports 100% vaginal bleeding control after just one treatment (Mohiuddin et al. 1990). Moderately hypofractionated treatments with dose/fractions between 2.5 and 6.5 Gy used by Rasool, Patricio, Kim, Cihoric, Macchia, and Grisby report vaginal bleeding control rates between 82% and 93.8% (Macchia et al. 2016b; Rasool et al. 2011; Patricio et al. 1987; Grigsby et al. 2002; Kim et al. 2013; Cihoric et al. 2012). Macchia evaluated the duration of response in a study of palliative radiation for nine elderly inoperable uterine cancer patients and found that 53.5% of them have a bleeding control at 2 years (Macchia et al. 2016a). Interestingly, if we look at the BED of the moderately hypofractionated regimens (MHRT) for which we can confidently use the linear quadratic model, they are in the range of 18–32 Gy_{10} with vaginal bleeding control rates ranging from 70% to 90% according to dose. It is more difficult to evaluate the highly hypofractionated regimens in terms of biological effectiveness since the dose per fraction is

Table 2 Most common signs of advanced pelvic cancer

Author	Country	# patients	Pain (%)	Vaginal discharge (%)	Foul discharge (%)	Vaginal bleeding (%)	Leg edema (%)	Mass effect (%)
Bates and Mijoya (2015)	Malawi	72	92	61	51	19		
Rasool et al. (2011)	India	25				100[b]		
Mishra et al. (2005)	India	100	48	69		67		
Kim et al. (2013)	Korea	19	47	10.5		84		
Panek (2001)	Poland	55	36.3	34.5		43.6	11	
Mohiuddin et al. (1990)	USA	22[a]	86.3			18	13.6	22.7
Cihoric et al. (2012)	Switzerland	62 (20 gyn)				100[b]		
Macchia et al. (2016a)	Italy	9				100[b]		
Grigsby et al. (2002)	USA	15				100[b]		
Patricio et al. (1987)	Portugal	56	25.6			69.8		

Note: [a]multiple types of pelvic malignancies; [b]only hemostatic treatments and patients treated with palliative therapies other than radiotherapy

Table 3 Symptom relief and grade 3–4 toxicity

Author	# patients	Pain (%)	Vaginal discharge (%)	Vaginal bleeding (%)	Edema (%)	Mass effect (%)	G3-4 toxicity Acute (%)	G3-4 toxicity Late (%)
Rasool et al. (2011)	25			88				
Patricio et al. (1987)	43	45.3		73				16.3
Mishra et al. (2005)	100	3, 41, 17 after first, second and third fx, respectively	20, 29, 14 after first, second and third fx, respectively	31 after first fx, 100 after third fx				10
Kim et al. (2013)	10	66.7		93.8			5	
Panek (2001)	55						15	2.7
Mohiuddin et al. (1990)	22	89 (CR + PR)		100	100	80		4.5
Choric et al. (2012)	62 (20 gyn)			82 (gr 0 and 1)				
Macchia et al. (2016a)	9			88.8, 2y actuarial rate 53.5				
Grigsby et al. (2002)	15			93				
Rai et al. (2012)	72	42 partial, 58 complete	66				6	
Boulware et al. (1979)	86	63		100				
Spanos et al. (1987)	46 (18 gyn)							24
Spanos et al. (1994)	290 (116 gyn)							6
Osrud et al. (2001)			39	90				6

Key: *fx* fraction, *y* year, *gyn* gynecologic cancer patients so high and the treatments are commonly 1 month apart. It is difficult also to understand the contribution of the palliative portion of the treatment to bleeding control in the experience reported by Grisby, Panek, and Mishra, since this was closely followed by a more definitive treatment in many of their patients (Mishra et al. 2005; Van Lnkhuijzen and Thomas 2011; Grigsby et al. 2002).

Unfortunately as delineated by van Lankhuijzen and Thomas (Van Lnkhuijzen and Thomas 2011), data are sparse and there are no real randomized studies for palliative radiation in gynecological cancers other than the RTOG 8502, but several mono-institutional experiences that do not report necessarily the same outcome in terms of results or toxicity. Nevertheless it is worth to look at the data and try to understand how the different palliative treatments can have an impact on the clinical history of diverse pelvic cancers. If we focus just on gynecological malignancies we see that another important symptom to consider is vaginal discharge, but the only studies that report results of control for this particular symptom used repeated doses of 10 Gy. Mishra reports 20, 29, and an additional 14% control after the first, second, and third fraction, while Osrud has 39% vaginal discharge control after just one fraction of 10 Gy. Rai reports a global 66% response after 1–3 fractions (Mishra et al. 2005; Onsrud et al. 2001; Rai et al. 2012).

Pelvic pain control is another parameter reported by the HDHRT users with 89% partial and complete control in Mohiuddin's GRID experience; 42% partial and 58% complete response for Rai and 63% overall response for the M.D. Anderson experience reported by Boulware in 1979 (Mohiuddin et al. 1990; Boulware et al. 1979; Rai et al. 2012). Mishra reports 3%, 41%, and 17% pelvic pain control after repeating single fractions

of 10 Gy one, two, or three times, respectively (Mishra et al. 2005).

Ten authors report grade 3 or more acute or late toxicities: from 6% to 16% in the MHRT and 6% to 24% in the HDHRT late toxicity rate, respectively, and 5–6% acute toxicity with either a MHRT or a HDHRT regimen (Rai et al. 2012; Kim et al. 2013). On the other end of the spectrum, Panek reports 15% acute and 2.7% late grade 3 or more toxicity in his re-irradiation experience with standard fractionation (Panek 2001).

One may hypothesize that:

1. It seems safe to use the LQ model and administer biologically equivalent doses up to 36 Gy_3 in a moderately hypofractionated fashion since these will carry a risk of grade 3 or more late toxicity of less than 5%.

2. With HDHRT one fraction of 10 Gy carries a risk of grade 3 toxicity close to 5%, whereas the use of two or three fractions of 10 Gy increases the risk of important and sometimes life-threatening toxicity as was shown in the RTOG 7905 study that reported a grade 3 or more toxicity in 25% of the treated patients and resulted in a switch to the Quad Shot regimen.

3. In the quad shot experience of 3.7 Gy BID ×4, a consistent risk of toxicity exists with repeat treatments for more than two times in patients that have a survival expectancy of more than 2–3 months, since the global biological equivalence of such a repeated treatment is close to 60 Gy_3.

In conclusion, higher dose fractionation regimens may be used in both curative and palliative management of patients with cervical cancer. These regimens must be used with caution given the potential for severe toxicity, and careful imaging in both planning and throughout treatment is necessary.

References

Albuquerque K, Giangreco D, Morrison C et al (2011) Radiation-related predictors of hematologic toxicity after concurrent chemoradiation for cervical cancer and implications for bone marrow-sparing pelvic IMRT. Int J Radiat Oncol Biol Phys 79(4):1043–1047

Arians N, Foerster R, Rom J et al (2016) Outcome of patients with local recurrent gynecologic malignancies after resection combined with intraoperative electron radiation therapy (IOERT). Radiat Oncol 11:44. doi:10.1186/s13014-016-0622-x

Beriwal S, Gan GN, Heron DE et al (2007) Early clinical outcome with concurrent chemotherapy and extended-field, intensity-modulated radiotherapy for cervical cancer. Int J Radiat Oncol Biol Phys 68(1):166–171

Bloemers MC, Portelance L, Ruo R et al (2012) A dosimetric evaluation of dose escalation for the radical treatment of locally advanced vulvar cancer by intensity-modulated radiation therapy. Med Dosim 37(3):310–313

Boulware RJ, Caderao JB, Delclos L et al (1979) Whole pelvis megavoltage irradiation with single doses of 1000 rad to palliate advanced gynecologic cancers. Int J Radiat Oncol Biol Phys 5(3):333–338

Boyle J, Craciunescu O, Steffey B et al (2014) Methods, safety, and early clinical outcomes of dose escalation using simultaneous integrated and sequential boosts in patients with locally advanced gynecologic malignancies. Gynecol Oncol 135(2):239–243

Brenner DJ (2008) The linear-quadratic model is an appropriate methodology for determining isoeffective doses at large doses per fraction. Semin Radiat Oncol 18(4):234–239

Brown JM, Carlson DJ, Brenner DJ (2014) The tumor radiobiology of SRS and SBRT: are more than the 5 Rs involved? Int J Radiat Oncol Biol Phys 88(2):254–262

Cihoric N, Crowe S, Eychmuller S et al (2012) Clinically significant bleeding in incurable cancer patients: effectiveness of hemostatic radiotherapy. Radiat Oncol 7:132. doi:10.1186/1748-717X-7-132

Cihoric N, Tapia C, Kruger K et al (2014) IMRT with [18]FDG-PET\CT based simultaneous integrated boost for treatment of nodal positive cervical cancer. Radiat Oncol 9:83. doi:10.1186/1748-717X-9-83

Dogan N, King S, Emami B et al (2003) Assessment of different IMRT boost delivery methods on target coverage and normal-tissue sparing. Int J Radiat Oncol Biol Phys 57(5):1480–1491

Dumas L, Ring A, Butler J et al (2016) Improving outcomes for older women with gynaecological malignancies. Cancer Treat Rev 50:99–108

Faria SL, Ferrigno R (1997) Hyperfractionated external radiation therapy in stage IIIB carcinoma of uterine cervix: a prospective pilot study. Int J Radiat Oncol Biol Phys 38(1):137–142

Feng CH, Hasan Y, Kopec M et al (2016) Simultaneously integrated boost (SIB) spares OAR and reduces treatment time in locally advanced cervical cancer. J Appl Clin Med Phys 17(5):6123

Fletcher G (1980) Textbook of radiotherapy, 3rd edn. Lea & Febiger, Philadelphia, pp 180–218. 103–179

Gawande A (2014) Being mortal, 1st edn. Macmillan, New York

Gerszten K, Colonello K, Heron DE et al (2006) Feasibility of concurrent cisplatin and extended field radiation therapy (EFRT) using intensity-modulated radiotherapy (IMRT) for carcinoma of the cervix. Gynecol Oncol 102(2):182–188

Grigsby PW, Heydon K, Mutch DG et al (2001) Long-term follow-up of RTOG 92-10: cervical cancer with positive para-aortic lymph nodes. Int J Radiat Oncol Biol Phys 51(4):982–987

Grigsby PW, Portelance L, Williamson JF (2002) High dose ratio (HDR) cervical ring applicator to control bleeding from cervical carcinoma. Int J Gynecol Cancer 12(1):18–21

Guerrero M, Li XA, Ma L et al (2005) Simultaneous integrated intensity-modulated radiotherapy boost for locally advanced gynecological cancer: radiobiological and dosimetric considerations. Int J Radiat Oncol Biol Phys 62(3):933–939

Hall EJ, Giaccia AJ (2012) Oxygen effect and reoxygenation. In: Radiobiology for the radiologist, 7th edn. Wolters Kluwer Health/Lippincott Williams & Wilkins, Philadelphia, PA, pp 86–103

Han K, Milosevic M, Fyles A et al (2013) Trends in the utilization of brachytherapy in cervical cancer in the United States. Int J Radiat Oncol Biol Phys 87(1):111–9

Hasan S, Ricco A, Jenkins K et al (2016) Survival and control prognosticators of recurrent gynecological malignancies of the pelvis and para-aortic region treated with stereotactic body radiation therapy. Front Oncol 6:249

Herrera FG, Callaway S, Delikgoz-Soykut E et al (2013) Retrospective feasibility study of simultaneous integrated boost in cervical cancer using tomotherapy: the impact of organ motion and tumor regression. Radiat Oncol 8:5. doi:10.1186/1748-717X-8-5

Higginson DS, Morris DE, Jones EL et al (2011) Stereotactic body radiotherapy (SBRT): technological innovation and application in gynecologic oncology. Gynecol Oncol 120(3):404–412

Ho JC, Allen PK, Jhingran A et al (2015) Management of nodal recurrences of endometrial cancer with IMRT. Gynecol Oncol 139(1):40–46

Huang Z, Mayr NA, Gao M et al (2012) Onset time of tumor repopulation for cervical cancer: first evidence from clinical data. Int J Radiat Oncol Biol Phys 84(2):478–484

Jorcano S, Molla M, Escude L et al (2010) Hypofractionated extracranial stereotactic radiotherapy boost for gynecologic tumors: a promising alternative to high-dose rate brachytherapy. Technol Cancer Res Treat 9(5):509–514

Kavanagh BD, Gieschen HL, Schmidt-Ullrich RK et al (1997) A pilot study of concomitant boost accelerated superfractionated radiotherapy for stage III cancer of the uterine cervix. Int J Radiat Oncol Biol Phys 38(3):561–568

Kavanagh BD, Segreti EM, Koo D et al (2001) Long-term local control and survival after concomitant boost accelerated radiotherapy for locally advanced cervix cancer. Am J Clin Oncol 24(2):113–119

Kavanagh BD, Schefter TE, Wu Q et al (2002) Clinical application of intensity-modulated radiotherapy for locally advanced cervical cancer. Semin Radiat Oncol 12(3):260–271

Kim DH, Lee JH, Ki YK et al (2013) Short-course palliative radiotherapy for uterine cervical cancer. Radiat Oncol J 31(4):216–221

Macchia G, Deodato F, Cilla S et al (2016a) Progestin-releasing intrauterine device insertion plus palliative radiotherapy in frail, elderly uterine cancer patients unfit for radical treatment. Oncol Lett 11(5):3446–3450

Macchia G, Cilla S, Deodato F et al (2016b) Simultaneous integrated boost volumetric modulated arc therapy in the postoperative treatment of high-risk to intermediate-risk endometrial cancer: results of ADA II phase 1–2 trial. Int J Radiat Oncol Biol Phys 96(3):606–613

MacLeod C, Bernshaw D, Leung S et al (1999) Accelerated hyperfractionated radiotherapy for locally advanced cervix cancer. Int J Radiat Oncol Biol Phys 44(3):519–524

Marnitz S, Kohler C, Burova E et al (2012) Helical tomotherapy with simultaneous integrated boost after laparoscopic staging in patients with cervical cancer: analysis of feasibility and early toxicity. Int J Radiat Oncol Biol Phys 82(2):e137–e143

Mell LK, Kochanski JD, Roeske JC et al (2006) Dosimetric predictors of acute hematologic toxicity in cervical cancer patients treated with concurrent cisplatin and intensity-modulated pelvic radiotherapy. Int J Radiat Oncol Biol Phys 66(5):1356–1365

Mishra SK, Laskar S, Muckaden MA et al (2005) Monthly palliative pelvic radiotherapy in advanced carcinoma of uterine cervix. J Cancer Res Ther 1(4):208–212

Mohiuddin M, Curtis DL, Grizos WT et al (1990) Palliative treatment of advanced cancer using multiple nonconfluent pencil beam radiation. A pilot study. Cancer 66(1):114–118

Molla M, Escude L, Nouet P et al (2005) Fractionated stereotactic radiotherapy boost for gynecologic tumors: an alternative to brachytherapy? Int J Radiat Oncol Biol Phys 62(1):118–124

Mundt AJ, Lujan AE, Rotmensch J et al (2002) Intensity-modulated whole pelvic radiotherapy in women with gynecologic malignancies. Int J Radiat Oncol Biol Phys 52(5):1330–1337

Mundt AJ, Mell LK, Roeske JC (2003) Preliminary analysis of chronic gastrointestinal toxicity in gynecology patients treated with intensity-modulated whole pelvic radiation therapy. Int J Radiat Oncol Biol Phys 56(5):1354–1360

Niibe Y, Kenjo M, Kazumoto T et al (2006) Multi-institutional study of radiation therapy for isolated para-aortic lymph node recurrence in uterine cervical carcinoma: 84 subjects of a population of more than 5,000. Int J Radiat Oncol Biol Phys 66(5):1366–1369

Onsrud M, Hagen B, Strickert T (2001) 10-gy single-fraction pelvic irradiation for palliation and life prolongation in patients with cancer of the cervix and corpus uteri. Gynecol Oncol 82(1):167–171

Osborne EM, Klopp AH, Jhingran A et al (2017) Impact of treatment year on survival and adverse effects in patients with cervical cancer and para-aortic lymph node metastases treated with definitive extended-field radiation therapy. Pract Radiat Oncol 7:3165–173

Panek G (2001) Reirradiation of late local recurrences of carcinoma of the cervix after primary radiotherapy. Nowotwory 51(5):502–505

Park HJ, Chang AR, Seo Y et al (2015) Stereotactic body radiotherapy for recurrent or oligometastatic uterine cervix cancer: a cooperative study of the Korean radiation oncology group (KROG 14-11). Anticancer Res 35(9):5103–5110

Patricio MB, Tavares MA, Guimaraes MF et al (1987) Haemostatic and antialgic effects of the 25 MV photon beam concentrated dose in the treatment of carcinoma of the cervix. J Surg Oncol 34(2):133–135

Poorvu PD, Sadow CA, Townamchai K et al (2013) Duodenal and other gastrointestinal toxicity in cervical and endometrial cancer treated with extended-field intensity modulated radiation therapy to paraaortic lymph nodes. Int J Radiat Oncol Biol Phys 85(5):1262–1268

Prasanna A, Amhed MM, Mohiuddin M et al (2014) Exposing sensitization windows of opportunity in hyper and hypofractionated radiation therapy. J Thorac Dis 6(4):287–302

Rai D, Khosla F, Patel M et al (2012) Palliative radiotherapy in advanced cancer of the cervix. Internet J Pain Symptom Control Palliat Care 9(1)

Ramlov A, Kroon PS, Jurgenliemk-Schulz IM et al (2015) Impact of radiation dose and standardized uptake value of (18)FDG PET on nodal control in locally advanced cervical cancer. Acta Oncol 54(9):1567–1573

Rash DL, Lee YC, Kashefi A et al (2013) Clinical response of pelvic and para-aortic lymphadenopathy to a radiation boost in the definitive management of locally advanced cervical cancer. Int J Radiat Oncol Biol Phys 87(2):317–322

Rasool MT, Manzoor NA, Mustafa SA et al (2011) Hypofractionated radiotherapy as local hemostatic agent in advanced cancer. Indian J Palliat Care 17(3):219–221

Repetto L, Fratino L, Audisio RA et al (2002) Comprehensive geriatric assessment adds information to eastern cooperative oncology group performance status in elderly cancer patients: an Italian group for geriatric oncology study. J Clin Oncol 20(2):494–502

Roeske JC, Bonta D, Mell LK et al (2003) A dosimetric analysis of acute gastrointestinal toxicity in women receiving intensity-modulated whole-pelvic radiation therapy. Radiother Oncol 69(2):201–207

Salama JK, Mundt AJ, Roeske J et al (2006) Preliminary outcome and toxicity report of extended-field, intensity-modulated radiation therapy for gynecologic malignancies. Int J Radiat Oncol Biol Phys 65(4):1170–1176

Seo Y, Kim MS, Yoo HJ et al (2016) Salvage stereotactic body radiotherapy for locally recurrent uterine cervix cancer at the pelvic sidewall: feasibility and complication. Asia Pac J Clin Oncol 12(2):e280–e288

Small W Jr, Winter K, Levenback C et al (2007) Extended-field irradiation and intracavitary brachytherapy combined with cisplatin chemotherapy for cervical cancer with positive para-aortic or high common iliac lymph nodes: results of ARM 1 of RTOG 0116. Int J Radiat Oncol Biol Phys 68(4):1081–1087

Spanos WJ Jr, Wasserman T, Meoz R et al (1987) Palliation of advanced pelvic malignant disease with large fraction pelvic radiation and misonidazole: final report of RTOG phase I/II study. Int J Radiat Oncol Biol Phys 13(10):1479–1482

Spanos WJ Jr, Clery M, Perez CA et al (1994) Late effect of multiple daily fraction palliation schedule for advanced pelvic malignancies (RTOG 8502). Int J Radiat Oncol Biol Phys 29(5):961–967

Tarnawski R, Fowler J, Skladowski K et al (2002) How fast is repopulation of tumor cells during the treatment gap? Int J Radiat Oncol Biol Phys 54(1):229–236

Tew WP (2016) Ovarian cancer in the older woman. J Geriatr Oncol 7(5):354–361

Townamchai K, Poorvu PD, Damato AL et al (2014) Radiation dose escalation using intensity modulated radiation therapy for gross unresected node-positive endometrial cancer. Pract Radiat Oncol 4(2):90–98

Van Lnkhuijzen L, Thomas G (2011) Palliative radiotherapy for cervical carcinoma, a systematic review. Radiother Oncol 98(2):287. 288–291

Vargo JA, Kim H, Choi S et al (2014) Extended field intensity modulated radiation therapy with concomitant boost for lymph node-positive cervical cancer: analysis of regional control and recurrence patterns in the positron emission tomography/computed tomography era. Int J Radiat Oncol Biol Phys 90(5):1091–1098

Verma J, Sulman EP, Jhingran A et al (2014) Dosimetric predictors of duodenal toxicity after intensity modulated radiation therapy for treatment of the para-aortic nodes in gynecologic cancer. Int J Radiat Oncol Biol Phys 88(2):357–362

Viegas CM, Araujo CM, Dantas MA et al (2004) Concurrent chemotherapy and hypofractionated twice-daily radiotherapy in cervical cancer patients with stage IIIB disease and bilateral parametrial involvement: a phase I–II study. Int J Radiat Oncol Biol Phys 60(4):1154–1159

Xu KM, Rajagopalan MS, Kim H, Beriwal S (2015) Extended field intensity modulated radiation therapy for gynecologic cancers: is the risk of duodenal toxicity high? Pract Radiat Oncol 5(4):e291–e297

Yoon MS, Ahn SJ, Nah BS et al (2012) Metabolic response of lymph nodes immediately after RT is related with survival outcome of patients with pelvic node-positive cervical cancer using consecutive [18F] fluorodeoxyglucose-positron emission tomography/computed tomography. Int J Radiat Oncol Biol Phys 84(4):e491–e497

Skin: The Case for Altered Fractionation in the Treatment of Both Malignant and Benign Conditions

James Fontanesi, Brian Kopitzki, and Richard Zekman

Contents

The original version of this chapter was revised. The affiliations of the authors have been updated.

J. Fontanesi, MD (✉)
William Beaumont Health Systems,
Farmington Hills, Cancer Center, Oakland University
School of Medicine, Rochester, MI, USA
e-mail: jfontanesi@comcast.net

R. Zekman, DO
Oakland Medical Oncology, Michigan Healthcare
Professionals, MI, USA

B. Kopitzki, DO
Clarkston Dermatology, Clarkston, MI, USA

Abstract

While most physicians recognize that skin is our largest organ, most lay people are unaware of this fact and the important role it plays not only in protection but also in temperature regulation and other activities that are essential to the overall general health of each individual. Despite the importance of this critical organ, we often subject it to various environmental, metabolic, and other stresses that cause changes, which can result in both malignant and benign conditions. Because of the obvious availability for visual inspection which can result in early detection, surgery often plays an initial and pivotal role in the primary diagnosis and treatment

Med Radiol Radiat Oncol (2017)
DOI 10.1007/174_2017_39, © Springer International Publishing AG
Published Online: 03 May 2017

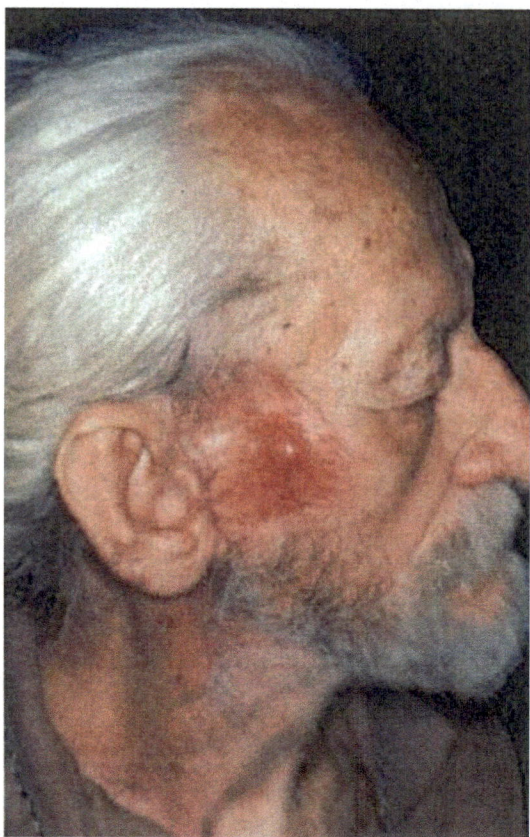

Picture 1 Advanced basal cell cancer of face

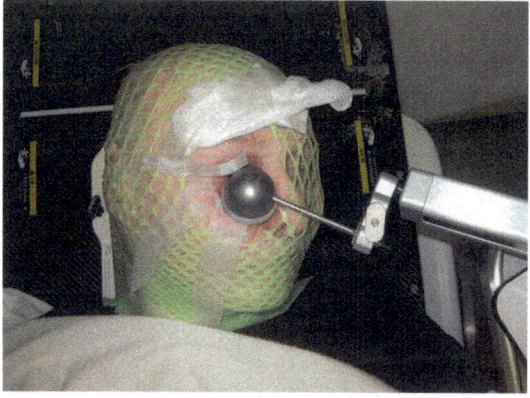

Picture 2 In treatment position for HDR brachytherapy of nasal skin

some cases involving unique locations such as the eyelid, or due to specific pathologic findings, radiation can be applied as a primary therapy or in the postoperative setting.

We must also be considerate of any past radiation exposures to any area which now manifest any skin malignancy, as these appear to have a more virulent course and are often found in unique sites especially when that radiation exposure was for benign conditions (Mizuno et al. J Craniofac Surg 17(2):360–362, 2006; McKeown et al. Br J Radiol 88(106):20150405, 2015).

1   Introduction

In this chapter our major focus will be on the use of external beam techniques, especially as they relate to "**altered**" fractionation but we will also endeavor to compare to limited conventional dose series and what we consider important brachytherapy series using "hypofractionated" techniques. We would be remiss if we did not also include important surgical series, especially randomized reports for comparisons.

We will not only look at the results but also review complication rates associated with various treatments and importantly look at issues related to second malignancies. These data are important because radiation has been utilized for many benign conditions such as acne, and that exposure has resulted in second malignant neoplasm (SMN) development. In addition, SMNs are increasingly being seen in irradiated areas in part due to improved cure rates for many pediatric and adult tumors. This knowledge is important when consulting patients and in obtaining informed consent regarding treatment. We will review nonmelanoma skin cancers (squamous and basal cell), melanoma, Merkel cell cancer, Kaposi sarcoma (all variants), and cutaneous lymphoma in this review.

2   Anatomy

The skin is comprised of three individual layers; they are:

1. The **epidermis**, which is the outermost layer. It provides a waterproof barrier and is responsible

in these conditions. It is often due to neglect or fear that patients will present with large lesions that have been years in the making.

Due to this ease with which we have access to our protective "coating" surgery is often the initial and only therapy needed. However in

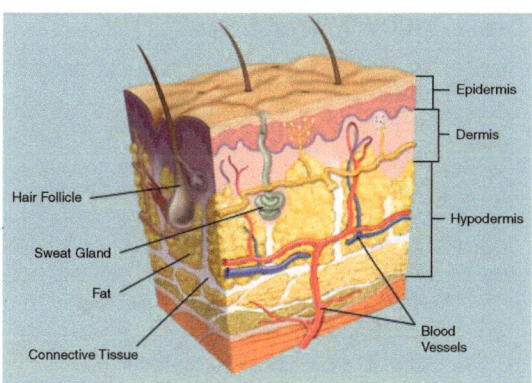

Fig. 1 Anatomy of skin

Table 1 Risk factors for development of NMSC

Sun exposure
Nordic ancestry
Older age
P-UVA in treatment psoriasis
Ionizing radiation
Arsenic exposure
Basal cell Nevis syndrome (Goblin's Disease)
Xeroderma Pigmentosum
Immunosuppression (medical/infectious)

for creating our skin tone. The epidermis is probably the single most abused organ in the human body on a daily basis.

2. The **dermis**, which lies below the epidermis. It contains connective tissue, hair follicles, and sweat glands.

3. The **hypodermis**, which is made up of fat and connective tissues. It also helps structurally and facilitates vascular supply (Fig. 1) (WebMD, LLC 2009).

2.1 Nonmelanoma Skin Cancer (NMSC)

The vast majority of nonmelanoma skin cancers are either basal cell or squamous cell carcinoma. It is estimated that approximately 80% of all NMSCs are basal cell carcinoma with the majority of the remaining being squamous cell carcinoma (American Cancer Society 2016). In the United States, it is estimated that about 3.3 million individuals will be diagnosed with NMSC in 2016 which represents an almost 300% increase since 1994 (Rogers et al. 2015). We must consider why we have seen such a dramatic rise in NMSC since the early 1990s. There are multiple factors, but clearly the single most important is UV (ultraviolet) radiation exposure, of which sun light exposure is the most important source. There is an excellent review discussing the various aspects of sunlight as it interacts with earth's atmosphere. Wavelengths shorter than those of visible light (400–700 nm)

are responsible for the development of the acute and chronic adverse effects seen in the skin (Hart et al. 2001). UVA accounts for 95% of the UV radiation reaching the earth. It is present with equal intensity throughout the year and during all daylight hours. It plays a major role in skin aging in addition to the development of skin cancer. Other risk factors such as past sunburn, being "fair" skinned, Nordic ancestry, and older age have been documented to enhance the development of NMSC (van Dam et al. 1999; Gallagher et al. 1995). More recently the explosive use of tanning beds has also been implicated in this increased incidence (Wehner et al. 2012) (Table 1).

Additional factors also include therapeutic exposures such as with use of P-UVA in the treatment of psoriasis (Stern et al. 1998) and the use of ionizing radiation in the treatment of both benign and malignant condition (Mizuno et al. 2006; McKeown et al. 2015; Turcotte et al. 2015). In fact, the use of therapeutic radiation (especially in children) must be followed carefully due to excess development of NMSC that have been reported often more than 10 years after initial therapy (Inskip et al. 2016).

However, no series has been able to link therapeutic intervention and casual sun exposure in terms of the additive effects they may have. It is also well known that chronic arsenic exposure is a factor for development of NMSC (Karagas et al. 1996), and certain genetic disorders such as Basal Cell Nevus syndrome (Gorlin's disease) (Bresler et al. 2016) and Xeroderma Pigmentosum (Black 2016) have a higher incidence of development of NMSC.

It is important to also note that immunosuppression for any reason, whether infectious (such as with HIV), or secondary to organ transplant, has been associated with increased incidence of NMSC (Song et al. 2016; Chen et al. 2015). Squamous cell carcinoma is by far the most common skin cancer in organ transplant patients occurring 65–250 times more often than basal cell carcinoma (Jensen et al. 1999).

3 Staging

Prior to any discussion regarding the use of external beam irradiation in the treatment of nonmelanoma skin cancers, it is important to review the staging system presently utilized. Although it is not frequently reported in peer-reviewed citations, nevertheless staging is important and we should take note that it should be utilized for each patient who is treated so one gets accurate information regarding the efficacy of therapy (Table 2).

Prior to reviewing altered fractionated external beam data, it would be beneficial to review some of the pathologic features found in NMSC which have been reported to affect local control.

3.1 Prognostic Factors Associated with Local Control for NMSCs

There have been various reports using univariate and multivariate analysis to determine which prognostic factors are associated with increased risk of local failure for NMSC. Most recently, perineural invasion has taken center stage in its importance and influence for local relapse. Its presence, either clinically or microscopically, has been shown to increase risk for local and regional failure (Panizza et al. 2014; Porceddu 2015). Others series have reported location (nasolabial fold) and lesional size (greater than 10 mm) having worse outcomes (Hernandez-Machin et al. 2007). Several series have also reported increased local failures related to the daily dose fractionation if less than 300 cGy (Locke et al. 2001; Lovett et al. 1990).

Table 2 AJCC skin cancer staging

Stage 0	**Tis**: Carcinoma in situ: the tumor is confined to the epidermis
	N0: The cancer has not spread to nearby lymph nodes
	M0: The cancer has not spread to distant organs
Stage I	**T1**: The tumor is 2 cm or smaller and has one or less high-risk feature
	N0: The cancer has not spread to nearby lymph nodes
	M0: The cancer has not spread to distant organs
Stage II	**T2**: The tumor is larger than 2 cm or is any size with two or more high-risk features
	N0: The cancer has not spread to lymph nodes
	M0: The cancer has not spread to distant organs
Stage III	**T3**: The tumor is larger than 4 cm
	N0: The cancer has not spread to lymph nodes
	M0: The cancer has not spread to distant organs
	T1 to T3, N1: The cancer has spread to ipsilateral lymph nodes which are 3 cm or less
	T1 to T3, M0: The cancer has not spread to distant organs
Stage IV	**T1 to T3, N2**: **N2a**: The cancer has spread to one ipsilateral lymph node which is larger than 3 cm but not larger than 6 cm
	N2b: The cancer has spread to more than one ipsilateral lymph node, none of which is larger than 6 cm
	N2c: The cancer has spread to contralateral lymph node(s), none of which are larger than 6 cm
	T1 to T3, M1: The cancer has spread to other parts of the body
	Any T, N3: The cancer has spread to any lymph node that is larger than 6 cm
	Any T4, M0: The cancer has not spread to other parts of the body
	T4, any N; N2a: The cancer has spread to one ipsilateral lymph node, larger than 3 cm, but not larger than 6 cm
	N2b: The cancer has spread to more than one ipsilateral lymph node, none of which is larger than 6 cm
	N2c: The cancer has spread to contralateral lymph node(s), none of which are larger than 6 cm

(continued)

Table 2 (continued)

	T4, MO: The cancer has not spread to other parts of the body
	Any T, any N; N2a: The cancer has spread to one ipsilateral lymph node, larger than 3 cm but not larger than 6 cm
	N2b: The cancer has spread to more than one ipsilateral lymph node, none of which is larger than 6 cm
	N2c: The cancer has spread to contralateral lymph node(s), none of which are larger than 6 cm
	Any T, any N, M1: The cancer has spread to other parts of the body

Table 3 Prognostic factors influencing local failure

Perineural invasion (clinical/or microscopic)
Location: nasolabial fold
Lesion size ≥ 10 mm
Daily fraction size (≤ 300 cGy)
Nuclear p53 immunoreactivity
Low BcL-2 expression
Subtype of cancer: sclerosing BCC
Treatment of locally failed lesions
T stage: T4 lesion
Positive N stage

Table 4 Summary of NCCN guidelines for squamous cell skin cancer (v 1.2016)

Tumor diameter	Dose schedules
<2 cm	64 Gy in 32 fractions
	55 Gy in 20 fractions
	50 Gy in 15 fractions
	35 Gy in 5 fractions
≥ 2 cm	66 Gy in 33 fractions
	55 Gy in 20 fractions
Postoperative adjuvant	50 Gy in 20 fractions
	60 Gy in 30 fractions

Regional disease: All doses at 2 Gy per fraction

• Post dissection (ECE = extracapsular extension)

Head and neck; (−) ECE	60–66 Gy over 6–6.6 weeks
Head and neck; (−) ECE	56 Gy over 5.6 weeks
Axilla/groin; (+) ECE	60 Gy over 6 weeks
Axilla/groin; (−) ECE	54 Gy over 5.4 weeks

• No dissection

At risk; clinically negative	50 Gy over 5 weeks
Clinically positive head and neck	66–70 Gy over 6.6–7 weeks
Clinically evident axilla, groin	66 Gy over 6.6 weeks

Nuclear p53 immunoreactivity and low BcL-2 expression have also been shown significantly correlated to the sclerosing subtype of basal cell carcinoma with a higher than projected failure rate when compared to non-sclerosing BCC (Zagrodnik et al. 2003). Treatment for locally failed, previously irradiated lesions, and advanced T stage have also been reported as negative factors for local control (Wilder et al. 1991). Some series have reported that the type of radiation used may also play a role in local failure (Lovett et al. 1990); however this is not universally accepted.

Regional nodal involvement, especially in squamous cell carcinoma, has also been reported to have inferior outcomes (Porceddu 2015; Stratigos et al. 2015; Moore et al. 2005; Hinerman et al. 2008). It is interesting to note that there seems to be increased controversy in terms of the importance of negative surgical margins as it relates to local control. Many reports do not correlate the surgical margins with other known prognostic factors including perineural involvement, size of the lesion, or other prognostic factors such as the p53/Bcl-2 which have been more recently investigated (Panizza et al. 2012) (Table 3).

There have been recommendations and guidelines that have been published by several international organizations for the treatment of various NMSC. These include the National Comprehensive Cancer Network, the Australian National Health Medical Research Council, and the French Dermatology Recommendations Association (Bonerandi et al. 2011).

The American College of Radiology has also published appropriateness criteria for "aggressive" NMSC of the Head and Neck (Koyfman et al. 2016) (Table 4).

The European Organization for Research in the Treatment of Cancer (EORTC) has also published its interdisciplinary guideline that includes various radiation options (Stratigos et al. 2015). It is interesting to note that EORTC uses various dose parameters that are often based on tumor diameter and whether or not treatment is applied in the postoperative setting. They do include various dose fractionation schemes that would be considered more traditional treatment regimens; however hypofractionated/altered fractionation recommendations are included.

3.2   Surgical Intervention in NMSCs

As initially discussed, due to the unique nature of our skin, surgical intervention is often the mainstay of treatment for NMSC. However, what is not clearly defined is which type of surgical procedure is best suited for which patient, which is often dependent on the primary site of lesion. For example, there is some debate as to whether or not Mohs micrographic surgery (MMS) or traditional surgical excision is best suited for the H-zone lesions of the face (Fig. 2).

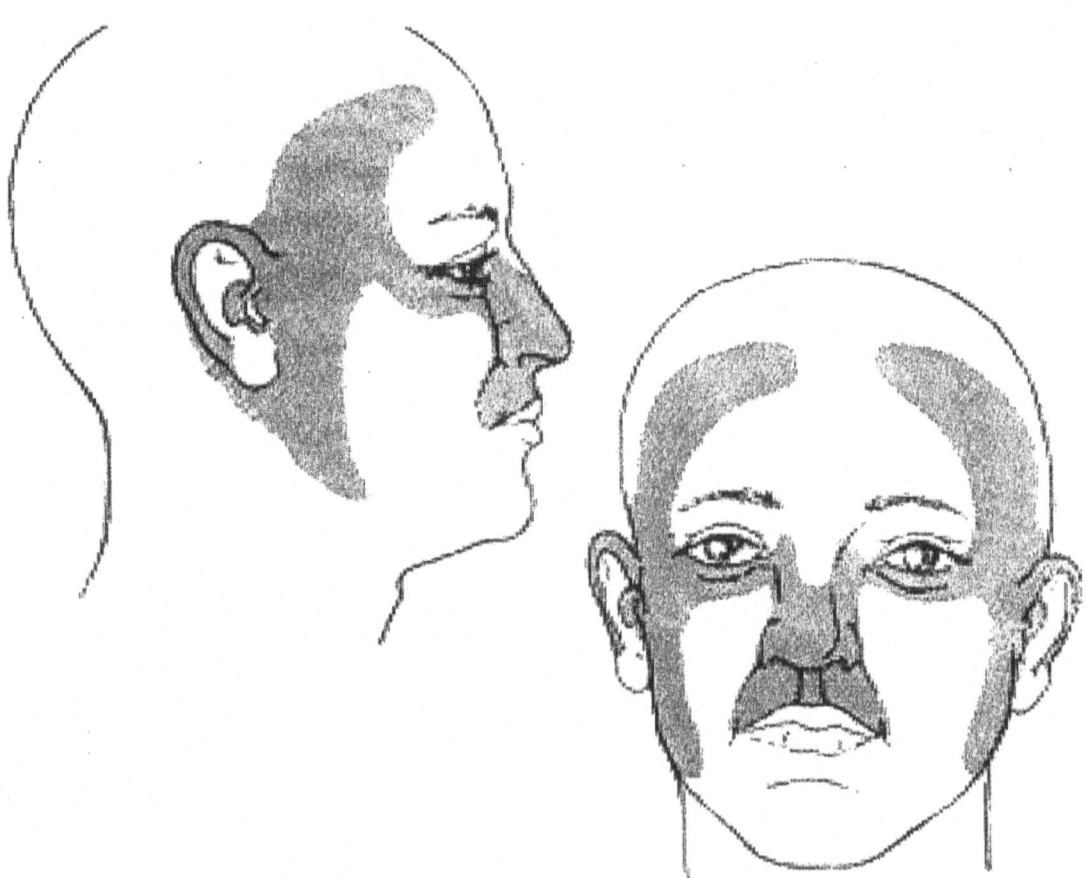

Fig. 2 H-Zone of face

Because of the importance of facial integrity and appearance which has been well documented in the literature (Andretto 2007; Biller and Kim 2009), there has been ongoing debate regarding preferential surgical treatment for this area.

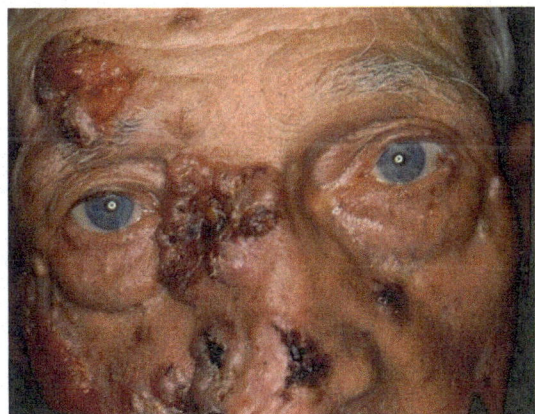

Picture 5   Advanced multifocal multicentric basal cell

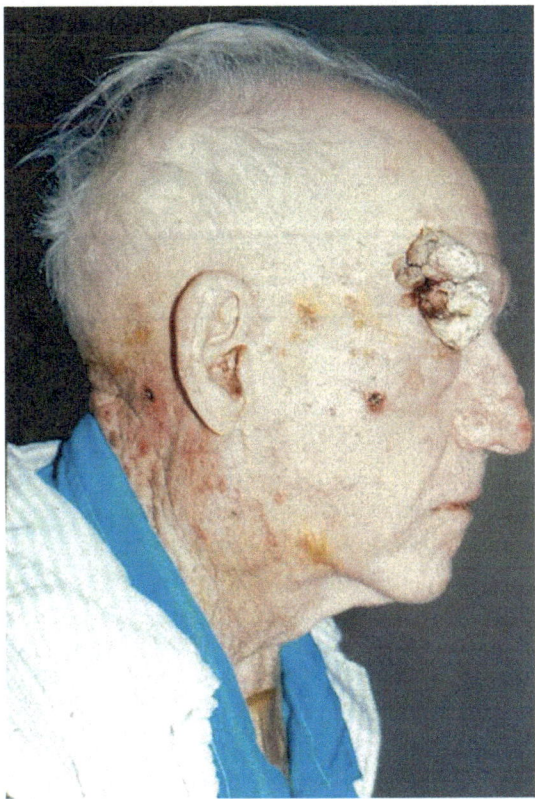

Picture 3   Advanced Squamous cell eye and cheek

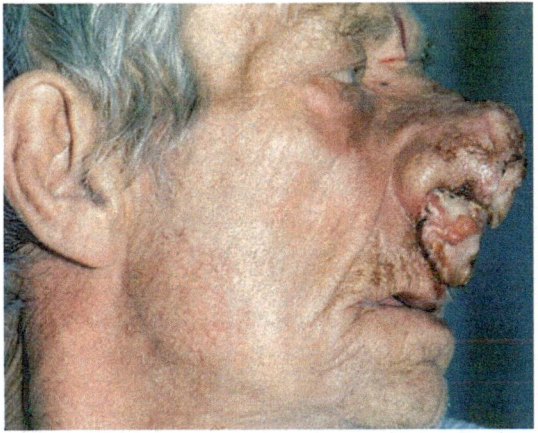

Picture 4   Advanced Squamous cell nasal

It would appear that in the H-zone, Mohs surgical procedures seem to have an improved cosmetic outcome which is desirable. Unfortunately there have been no randomized trials which have assessed the cosmetic outcomes related to the most common surgical interventions in the H-zone.

In non-H-zone lesions there have been reports evaluating various surgical techniques. Pereira et al. (2013) reported on 588 patients treated at the West Los Angeles Veterans Affairs Hospital of which 289 had non-H-zone extremity and truncal lesions. With a minimum follow-up of 3 years and noting that the traditional surgical excision (TSE) patients had larger lesions, the overall local recurrence rate was similar between the two groups. In their conclusions they felt that NMSC could be more effectively treated with TSE in "nonpremium" areas of the body.

Surgical excision is a highly effective treatment for NMSC. Complete surgical resection results in high cure rates especially for low risk, small lesions (Abide et al. 1984). However, there is continued discussion regarding what is considered an adequate surgical margin. Some reports suggest a minimum 3 mm peripheral margin; others report the need of up to 15 mm margins for histologically aggressive subtypes (Kimyai-Asadi et al. 2005). Moncrieff et al. (2015) did a retrospective audit of 253 cases of intraoperative frozen section analysis (IFSA). The combined rates of incomplete "very narrow"

(<1 mm) excisional margin rates were 28.7% for BCC and 27.5% for SCC. However, 94% of the errors were due to unrepresentative sampling of the excisional margins. Because of the large discrepancy, IFSA was abandoned at their institution. In one report on re-excision of incompletely resected NMSC, the presence of residual tumor was found in only 54% of cases, thus adding to the debate surrounding adequate margins and, more importantly, pathological assessment of surgical specimens (Wilson et al. 2004).

What becomes critical is the role that positive margins play in recurrence rates if no additional surgery or radiation is delivered. One report suggested that with negative margins, recurrence rates should be 2%. However with positive margins, recurrence rates of 30–40% should be anticipated (De Silva and Dellon 1985).

It is clear that when properly applied, surgical intervention is the mainstay of therapy for NMSC. With adequate margins, the local control rates should be in excess of 95% for most lesions less than 3 cm in size and without nodal involvement. The cure rate reported with Mohs surgery by most series is in the range of 97–100% for primary basal cell carcinoma (Mikhail and Mohs 1991).

3.3 Lymph Node Involvement in NMSC

As previously noted, lymph node involvement has been reported to result in poorer local regional control. This has led several groups to investigate whether sentinel lymph node biopsy (SLNB) may play a role in the management of NMSC. Unfortunately many published series report high sensitivity but have not demonstrated impact on survival, and have in general had small patient numbers (Wagner et al. 2004; Matthey-Gie et al. 2013). However in certain situations such as "high-risk" squamous cell cancers, identification of affected lymph nodes may help in the delineation of radiation fields. The information from SLNB may also be supplemented by the use of imaging studies. PET

scans have become more common in the workup of NMSC (Duncan et al. 2016; Ibrahim 2013; Siva et al. 2013).

To conclude, the use of imaging studies or SLNB may be instrumental in identifying lymph node involvement in "high-risk" NMSC. It remains that surgical intervention (when feasible) provides a high cure rate with excellent patient and physician perceived cosmetic acceptance. There are certain areas where different surgical techniques may be preferential (H-zone of face and Mohs) and certain sites where good postsurgical cosmesis is not feasible and/or the patient is not medically suitable for surgery. This is where radiation becomes an important intervention.

3.4 Systemic Therapy for NMSC

There have been various systemic agents that have been utilized for metastatic NMSC. Use of Smoothened (SMO) inhibitors, oral kinase inhibitors (which target epidermal growth factor receptors), and more traditional therapies such as 5-FU and capecitabine have all been looked at clinically with various reported response rates (Rudnick 2015).

The "Bolt" trial which utilized sonidegib, a Hedgehog signaling pathway inhibitor, in a randomized double blind phase 2 trial was recently published. The initial report on 230 patients determined that the best tolerated dose was 200 mg with only 14% experiencing severe side effects (Migden 2015). The **Erivance** BCC trial, which utilized a different Hedgehog pathway inhibitor, vismodegib, was also recently published. It was a non-randomized 2-cohort study for BCC patients with locally advanced or metastatic disease and NOT eligible for surgery or radiation. The dose used was 150 mg. With a median duration of exposure to vismodegib of about 14 months, the objective response rate was 33.3% for metastatic disease and 47.6% for locally advanced disease (Sekulic 2015).

Thus, while surgery or radiation plays critical roles in the initial management of NMSC, for those patients who, for various reasons, are not considered "curative" intent patients, there remain systemic therapies with known response rates and acceptable toxicity profiles.

4   Radiation Therapy for NMSC: Conventional External Beam

As noted, the number of newly diagnosed NMSC has exploded in the last 30 years. This has led to numerous reports on the use of radiation in their treatment. Many of these series have reported large numbers of patients that have been treated with quite different treatment regimens.

Due to technological issues, the earliest series were limited to orthovoltage irradiation. As equipment became more sophisticated, different radiation applications were utilized. Because many of these series that have been reported to span decades, there have also been various dose schedules reported. Our discussion about "conventional" irradiation will be limited to daily doses between 180 and 300 cGy per fraction delivered between three and five times per week.

However in the literature in which details are available, it appears that common themes arise. For example, one series compared weekly orthovoltage therapy to conventional daily orthovoltage treatment (Pampena et al. 2016). In that series, 436 tumors were retrospectively analyzed with no difference in outcomes or cosmesis between the treatment groups of once weekly 525 cGy × 7 fx vs. 15 × 300 cGy daily.

There are some series which have utilized conventional fractionation but report only on cosmetic results (Petit et al. 2010). In this series, Petit et al. utilized conventional orthovoltage radiation of 85–250 kV and fields were designed specifically for each case. Patients received up to 60 Gy. Twenty patients were treated with this technique and compared retrospectively in a nonrandomized fashion to irradiated patients. They routinely rated surgical intervention superior to radiotherapy between 6 and 48 months after treatment, but few observers were displeased with post-irradiation cosmesis.

Some series have focused on other factors. Zagrodnik et al. (2003) reported on recurrence based on histologic subtypes and expression of p53 and Bcl-2 in patients with lesions greater than 5 cm. Patients were treated with various conventional dose schedules. Patients typically received 26–30 fractions of 2 Gy per fraction with a margin of 10 mm. The overall 5-year recurrence rate for all regions was 15.8%. Unfortunately no data are given related to the doses that were delivered in patients who experienced local failure. It is important to note that the mean time to recurrence was 20 months with the 19 of 22 recurrences (86.4%) occurring within 3 years of treatment.

Washington University (Mallinckrodt) reported on 339 patients (Lovett et al. 1990). In that series, patients who received between 200 and 300 cGy experienced a relapse rate of approximately 11% while patients who received greater than 300 cGy per fraction had no local failures. This series was then updated by Locke et al. (2001) in which 531 lesions were analyzed (389 basal cell and 142 squamous cell). One hundred and sixty-seven patients of the total were treated at recurrence. With a median follow-up of 5.8 years, the overall local control was 89%. However when evaluating all patients, only those receiving ≤300 cGy/fx experienced local failure.

Princess Margaret Hospital (Tsao et al. 2002) reviewed 100 patients referred for radiotherapy between 1982 and 1993 for squamous cell carcinoma of the nasal skin. Lesions greater than 5 cm in size or lesions associated with bone or cartilage invasion were typically treated with more conventional radiation doses (50 Gy in 20 fx). The local relapse-free rate was 85% at 2 years. The univariate analysis could not identify any patient, tumor, or treatment factor that was a statistically significant prognosticator for local failure. Median follow-up was 2.9 years and there were ten total local failures of which five received doses between 2 and 3 Gy per fraction.

Table 5 Selected conventional external beam series

Author	Patients RT/or lesions	Median follow-up	Local fail	Cosmesis	Other
Petit	20			Favor surgery @ 48 months	
Zagrodnik	175	48 months	15.8% overall 7.8% nodular 16% superficial 21% sclerosing	–	Mean time to recur 20 months
Locke	531	5.8 years	Basal cell 9.3% if ≤300 cGy/fx 0% if >300 cGy/fx Squamous Cell 20% if < 300 cGy/fx 0% if > 300 cGy/fx	–	–
Tsao	96	2.9 years	10.6% (5/10 LF had ≤300 cGy/fx	–	–
Kahn	448	18.4 months	15.8% overall	–	Median time to fail 11.4 months Several univariate Multivariate factors for increased local failure
Mazeron	1676	24 months	6% overall 4.7% orthovoltage 19% mega voltage 3.3% brachytherapy	↓satisfaction when total dose ≥6200	–

The University of Toronto (Khan et al. 2014) reported on 448 patients where various fractionation schemes and modalities were used. The most commonly used dose schedules were either 50 Gy/20 fractions or 40 Gy/10 fractions. With a median follow-up of 18.4 months, overall local control was 84.2% with a median time to recurrence of 11.4 months. Multivariate factors found to lead to higher local failure rates included age, tumor size >2 cm, immunosuppression, and treatment modality.

Some series have reported only on recurrent lesions. The University of Arizona (Wilder et al. 1991) reported on 61 recurrent basal cell carcinomas. In that series, both orthovoltage and megavoltage irradiation were utilized and median follow-up was 57 months. Thirty-four of the patients were treated with orthovoltage irradiation (100 and 300 KVP) and 26 were treated using megavoltage irradiation. Unfortunately it is not delineated in the report which patients received conventional irradiation fractionation.

However 6 of the 61 lesions did fail, of which 5 of the 6 received between 2.5 and 3 Gy per fraction. In that report, only tumor size and stage had statistical significance on the ability to obtain complete remission and over half the patients had multiple recurrences prior to irradiation (Table 5).

5 Brachytherapy

One of the easiest ways in which to provide altered fractionation is with brachytherapy. There is a rich history of the utilization of brachytherapy in the treatment of NMSC. One French series (Gauden et al. 2013) reported on 236 lesions (median follow-up of 66 months) utilizing the Leipzig surface applicator. In this series, 36 Gy was delivered to a 3–4 mm depth using 3 Gy per fraction daily for 12 consecutive treatments. Local control was established at 98% with cosmetic results being considered excellent or good in over 88%.

Arenas et al. (2015) reported on 134 lesions (median follow-up of 33 months). Ninety-two were basal cell carcinomas and 42 were squamous cell. Those patients who were treated using the Leipzig applicator had a 95% local control rate at 5 years while patients with custom mold techniques had 88% local control. Cosmesis was rated as excellent or good in 82% of the patients. Local failure for basal cell was 6.5% and 4.8% for squamous cell carcinomas.

The European Curietherapy Group (GEC) reported on 570 nasal vestibule or nasal skin lesion (Mazeron et al. 1989). Various isotopes and dose schedules were reported. They reported a 3.3% overall failure rate with brachytherapy compared with 4.7% using orthovoltage energies and 19% with megavoltage treatment. Thus it is important to determine factors which would be beneficial in deciding whether external beam or brachytherapy techniques should be utilized. Perhaps the most important factors are the size of the lesion and the location. It would appear with larger lesions that are more deeply involved with the underlying tissues and that do not have any other adverse prognostic factors such as perineural invasion; external beam irradiation may be more beneficial to use. However, for small discrete lesions that are more superficial, it does appear that brachytherapy offers an attractive alternative to external beam irradiation.

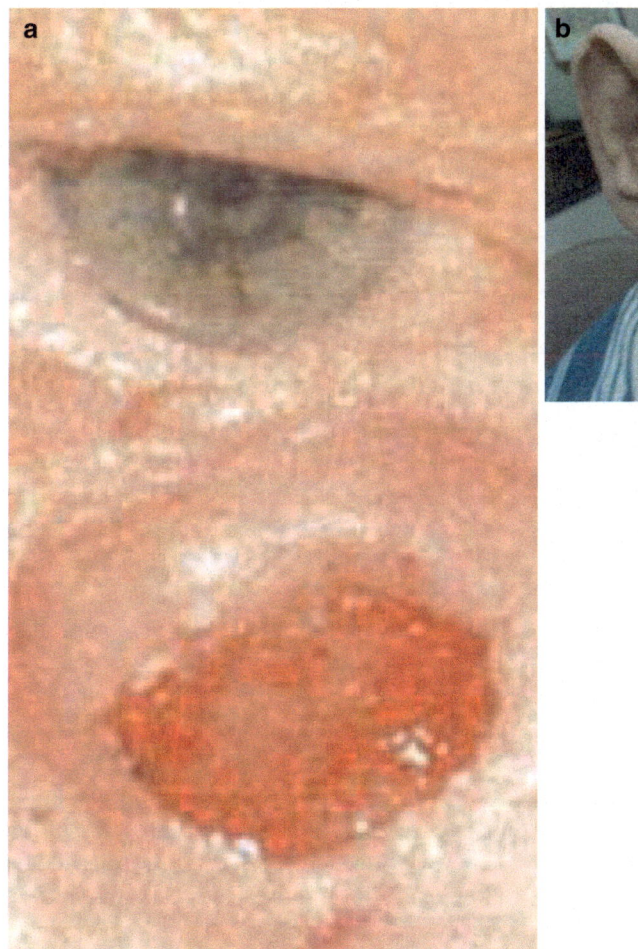
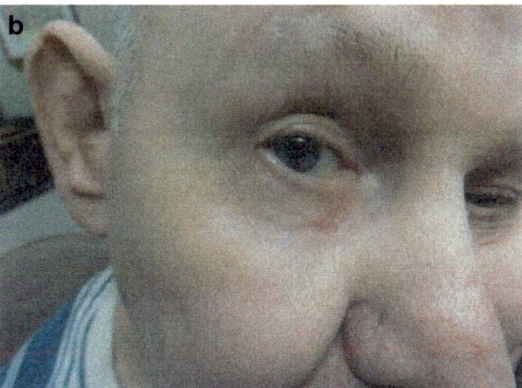

Picture 6 (a) Before contact application. (b) After contact application

6 Altered Fractionation with External Beam Irradiation

6.1 Orthovoltage

The utilization of external beam irradiation with altered fractionation/hypofractionation has a long-standing history. It began with orthovoltage series and has been extended into the modern era utilizing both electron beam and megavoltage irradiation. However it is important to look at the early series that utilized orthovoltage to help guide our travels through the decision-making process and how to treat using altered fractionation for NMSC.

Silverman et al. (1992) reported on 862 untreated basal cell carcinomas and 211 recurrent lesions. Utilizing a fractionation scheme of 5×680 cGy with a 100 KVP beam and a 0.9 mm HVL (Aluminum) over 9–12 days, they reported a 5-year recurrence rate of 7.4% in the untreated lesions and 9.5% in the recurrent lesions.

Buenaventura Hernandez-Machin (2007) reported on 710 lesions (604 basal cell, 106 squamous cell carcinomas) utilizing 4 Gy, three times a week, to a total dose of 45–55 Gy and then changed to a 9 Gy once a week regimen to a total dose of 36 Gy. This resulted in an overall 5-year relapse rate of 5.7%. What was also noted was a slight increased failure rate (7.3%) in lesions that were in the nasal labial fold or greater than 1 cm in size.

An Italian series (Ibrahim 2013) reviewed two different schedules using orthovoltage energies. Four hundred thirty-six lesions were treated with 525 cGy/once weekly/×7 (total 3675 cGy) or 15×300 cGy (total 4500 cGy) using 50–300 KVP. With a median follow-up of almost 32 months, 5.5% treated with the hypofractionated sequence relapsed compared to 3.7% with the more conventional regimen. Cosmesis was considered excellent or good in 85% with the hypofractionated sequence.

6.2 Megavoltage (Electron/ Photon)

In the modern era there is less usage of orthovoltage irradiation because of not only the lack of experience but also the lack of availability of these machines. As such, there has been an introduction of newer techniques utilizing electron beam and megavoltage irradiation. Recently, the utilization of what is considered "electronic brachytherapy" has also become popular. Bhatnagar (2013) reported on 171 lesions that received 5 Gy twice a week to a total dose of 40 Gy. With a mean follow-up of 10 months (range 1–28 months), there were no local failures. The shortcoming of this series is that the follow-up has not been long enough to establish a true efficacy rate. Doggett et al. recently reported on 524 lesions with a median follow-up of 12.5 months (Doggett et al. 2015). They used 8×500 cGy/4 weeks and reported only four local failures. However the main drawback is also the short follow-up of 12.5 months (1–16 months).

Leiden University Medical Center (van Hezewijk et al. 2010) reported on 434 lesions (332 basal cell, 102 squamous cell) treated with electron beam therapy utilizing 4–12 MeV electrons with a 1 cm margin. One hundred fifty-nine patients were treated with 18 fractions of 300 cGy while 275 of the patients received 4.4 Gy for 10 fractions. With a median follow-up of 42.8 months, the local failure rate for basal cell carcinoma was 2.4% for those patients receiving 54 Gy and 3.1% for those receiving 44 Gy. For squamous cell carcinoma it was 3% and 6.4%, respectively. The interesting part of this report was that the 44 Gy arm was established using an alpha-beta ratio of 3 to determine equivalent doses to 54 Gy.

Kouloulias (2012) reported on 42 patients that were treated using 3D conformal irradiation with five fractions of 600 cGy delivered once weekly. With a median follow-up of 15 months there were only local failures.

In a phase II trial, Ferro et al. reported on 31 patients who received 30 Gy in five fractions over 5 days (Ferro et al. 2015). Eligibility criteria were lesion size less than 3 cm without deep infiltration and patients greater than 70 years of age. There were three local failures (9.7%) at a median follow-up of 30 months. Cosmesis was noted as excellent or good in 96%.

Zagrodnik reported on patients who received 8 Gy delivered in five or six fractions over 7 days for lesions of up to 2 cm. For lesions between 2 and 5 cm, 10–13 Gy/fraction was delivered in four fractions (Zagrodnik et al. 2003). Unfortunately there were no data on the dose response but of the 175 basal cell carcinomas that were treated with this fractionation schedule (median follow-up of 48 months), the 5-year local recurrence rate was 16% and the median time to recurrence was 20 months, with 85% recurring within 3 years.

6.3   Conclusion

In the Wilder series, only a single patient received more than 3 Gy per fraction (Wilder et al. 1991). The Princess Margaret series utilized a fractionation sequence of 5 × 700 cGy for lesions less than or equal to 2 cm and ten fractions of 450 cGy for lesions between 2 and 5 cm in size. Local failure at 5 years was reported in ten patients of whom five received doses of greater than 300 cGy. It is of interest to note that six of ten were located on the bridge of the nose. Thus it would appear that based on these and other series, altered fractionation sequences that deliver greater than 300 cGy per fraction provide excellent local control and acceptable cosmetic results. It is interesting to note that, with various techniques, different margins, different type of radiation employed (orthovoltage, electrons, or megavoltage), and varying over all time to complete treatment did not seem to affect overall outcomes or cosmesis with the use of >300 cGy (Table 6).

Table 6 Altered fractionation outcomes

Author	Lesions treated	Median follow-up	Dose schedule	Technical data	Local fail	Cosmesis (excellent/ good)	Other
van Hezewijk	434	42.8 mos	18 × 300 (R = 159) or 10 × 440 (n = 275)	4–12 Electrons 1 cm margin	5/159 (3.1%) 10/275 (3.6%)	75% 100%	Used </3 = 3 for equivalent dose
Kouloulias	42	15 mos	5 × 600 cGy × 2/ week	3DC	2/42 (4.7%)	100%	–
Ferro	31	24 mos	5 × 600 cGy/daily	6-12 electrons Or 6mv photon 1.5-3.0 cm margin	3/31 (9.7%)	96%	PH II ≤ 3 cm > 70 Y.O. Used 0.5–1.0 cm bolus
Paravati	154	16.1 mos	8 × 500 cGy	Electrons	2/154 (1.3%)	97.5%	Electronic brachytherapy
Locke	531	5.8 mos	≤300 cGy/ Fx > 300 cGy/Fx	Orthovoltage electrons megavoltage	9.3% BCC 20% SCC 0% BCC 0% SCC	92%	No local failures with daily fraction ≥300 cGy
Zagrodnik	175	48 mos	40–54 Gy/5-6Fx (≤2 cm) or 40–54 Gy/4Fx (2–5 cm) 10 mm margin	20-50 KV	16%	N/A	Median time to recur 20 mos ↑ LF with sclerosing subtype and low Bcl-2 expression/p53 immunoreactivity
Tsao	79	2.9 years	700 cGy × 5 if ≤ 2 cm 450 cGy × 10 if 2–5 cm	75–250 kV 9–20 MV Electrons	10%	N/A	6/10 Local fail on bridge of nose
Pampena	383	31.8 mos	525 cGy × 7/i per week or 300 cGy × 15/ daily	50–300 kV	15/275 (5.5%) Or 6/161 (3.%)	85% or 95%	Hypofractionated excellent for elderly/travel impaired
Mazeron	1676	24 mos (66% >60 mos)	10.2 Gy × 3 5.2 Gy × 11 2.0 Gy × 35	Brachytherapy 100 kV Electrons Ext. Co6o	5.4%—ortho 22%—mega 3.3%—brachy	93% brachy therapy 83% ortho voltage 89% electron/co6o	↓ Local control with ↑ size

7 Altered Fractionation in Special Circumstance

7.1 Kaposi Sarcoma (KS)

Since first described by Morris Kaposi in 1872 (Kaposi 1872), this cutaneous sarcoma has been reported in multiple different clinical settings with unique epidemiology and prognosis. These include (1) classic Kaposi sarcoma (James 2005), (2) the endemic form, originally described in young Africans from the Sub-Saharan African region and of which there are two distinct forms (African lymphadenopathic and cutaneous variants), (3) that associated with immunosuppression, and (4)) the best known; HIV related KS (Cook-Mozaffari et al. 1998; Olsen et al. 1998; Luppi et al. 2000). In the United States, the AIDS-associated Kaposi sarcoma is most often referred for radiation management options. The KS lesions are not only found in the cutaneous regions of the body, but have also been found in mucosal and visceral sites.

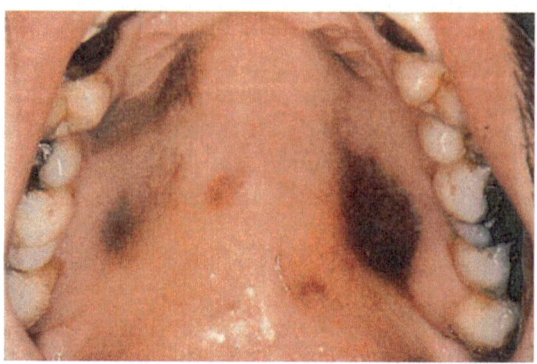

Picture 8 Kaposi sarcoma—oral Cavity

What is unique to all of these forms of Kaposi sarcoma is that they are associated with the Human Herpes Virus (HHV-8) (Ablashi 2002). Kaposi sarcoma has a unique "color" that presents because of spindle cells that form slit-like cavities which contain red blood cells. These highly vascular regions also contain irregular blood vessels that can leak red blood cells into surrounding tissue resulting in purplish color that is often the hallmark of KS (Weninger 1999).

The differential diagnosis can include arterio-venous malformation, venous malformation, pyogenic granuloma, or other vascular anomalies. The diagnosis can only be made by biopsy and detection of KSHV/HHV8 in the tumor cells. It had been noted that the cutaneous lesions associated with KS seem to enjoy a favorable response when treated with radiation; however it has also been noted that HIV-associated KS lesions often have enhanced and sometimes severe side effects from radiotherapy, especially in mucosal sites (Rodriguez et al. 1989).

While there have been numerous clinical reports on the use of radiation in the treatment of the different KS forms, the most recent series have dealt with the HIV-associated lesions. There have been two randomized prospective trials in the treatment of AIDS-associated Kaposi sarcoma. The first was from the University of Washington Medical Center (Stelzer and Griffin 1993). In that trial, patients were randomly selected to receive a single fraction of 8 Gy, 10 × 2 Gy, and 20 × 2 Gy to the area of the palpable tumor with a 2 cm margin. The more

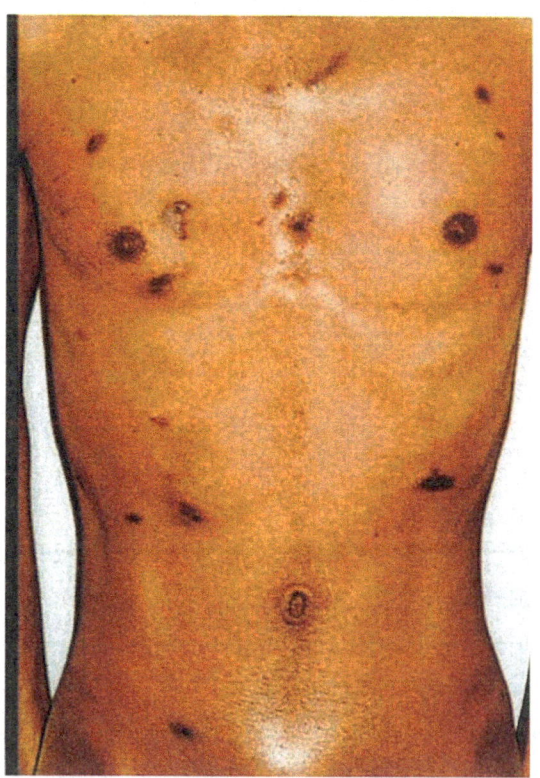

Picture 7 Kaposi sarcoma

protracted fractionated sequences provided improved local control and had less toxicity when compared with a single fraction of 8 Gy.

The second randomized trial was from South Africa. It also employed a hypofractionated radiation sequence. In this trial, patients were randomized to receive 24 Gy in 12 fractions or 20 Gy in 5 fractions. The two treatment arms produced equivalent results for treatment response, local recurrence-free survival, and toxicity (Singh et al. 2008). Other series have reported overall response rates of up to 92% with various dose schemes (Belembaogo et al. 1998; de Wit et al. 1990; Geara et al. 1991). Stein et al. reported on 56 patients that received 8–12 Gy in single fraction or 24–30 Gy fractionated over 1–3 weeks.

Symptomatic relief was noted in 80–100% regardless of schedule (Stein et al. 1993).

There were also several brachytherapy reports in the treatment of KS. Kasper et al. reported on 16 sites that received 24–35 Gy in 4–6 fractions over a 12-day period of time (Kasper et al. 2013). No lesion was greater than 2 cm and the median follow-up was a 41.4 months. They had no local failures.

Evans et al. reported on 120 lesions in 16 patients that were treated with iridium 192 surface applicators (Evans et al. 1997). Treatment ranged between 8 and 20 Gy (median dose 10 Gy) in a single fraction treatment and was well tolerated. However, those patients that received 20 Gy developed increased desquamation (Table 7).

Table 7 External radiation schemes for Kaposi sarcoma

Author	Ref	Year	PT#	Dose	F/U	CR/PR	Complications	Other
Stein	131	1993	28	8–10 Gy/x1 or 7–8 Gy × 3 or 4 week Total 14–24 Gy		76%		
Stelzer	132	1993	71	8 Gy × 1 2 Gy × 10 2 Gy × 20	37 wk 40 wk 40 wk	50% CR 79% CR 83% CR		≤50 reduction considered NR Med time to fail 8 Gy—13 wk 20 Gy—26 wk 40 Gy—43 wk
Chak	25	1988	24					
Piedbois	111	1994	453	Group A 2.5 Gy × 4/ wk → 10–20 Gy Group B 2Gy/day × 10 1 week break 2 Gy/ day × 5 → 30 Gy		87% 85%		71% recur @ 7.5 months
Singh	126	2008	60	12 × 2 Gy or 5 × 4 Gy	160 day for patients alive	21/30 CR 26/30 CR > No diff		Med time to recur 92 day
Belembaogo	12	1998	643	2.5 cGy × 4/wk total 20 Gy 1.9 cGy × 4/wk total 15.2 Gy For oral cavity		92% "Objective" response		23.4 GR III toxicity
deWit	33	1990	31	800 cGy × 1	86 % 34% objective response			2/3 Progressed @ 4 mos

PT patients, *F/U* follow up, *CR/PR* complete response, *NR* no response, *wk* Week

7.2 Conclusion

It appears that various radiation treatment schedules can be utilized in the treatment of the various forms of Kaposi sarcoma. However based on the two randomized trials, single fraction doses in excess of 8 Gy have not shown as durable a response when compared to more traditional dose schedules. However in certain circumstances, these single fraction treatments may be appropriate. If treated concurrently with chemotherapy or other systemic therapy, the radiation oncologist must consider the development of significant additive side effects into the radiation effects. In addition, the overall time frame for therapy and the location of the lesion (facial verses nonfacial sites) can have a tremendous role in decision making as it relates to therapy. However with improved antiviral therapy, the need for radiation for palliation of Kaposi sarcoma has become less frequent but it is good to know that is not found to be any less effective in those settings.

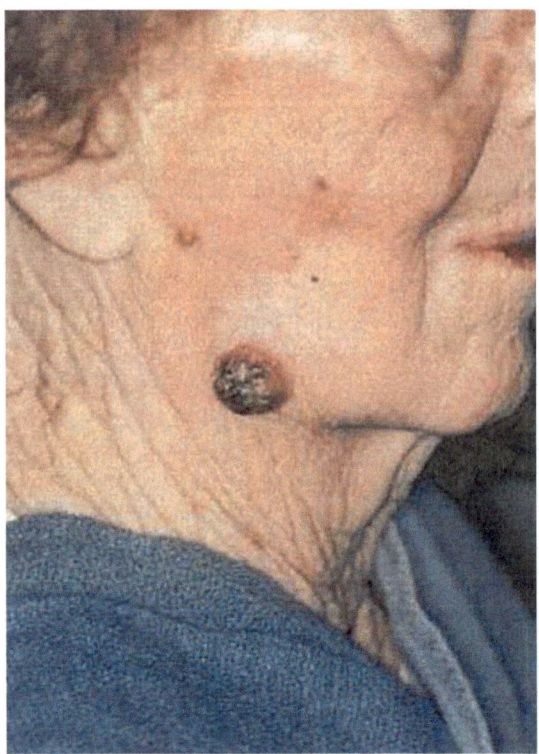

Picture 9 Merkel cell carcinoma

8 Merkel Cell Carcinoma (MCC)

Merkel cells were originally described in 1875 by J. Friedrich Meckel. They are unique tactile cells that are usually found within the basal layer of the epidermis (Han et al. 2012). It was not until 1972 when several cases of what was initially described as a "sweat gland" malignancy of the skin before being evaluated using electron microscopy for analysis, and then found to be originating from Merkel cells (Goessling et al. 2002; Toker 1972). Merkel cell carcinoma is a rare malignancy of the skin. It is estimated that about 1500 cases will be diagnosed in the United States in 2016 (American Cancer Society 2016). It has been reported that approximately 65% of cases present with local disease, 30% with nodal involvement, and up to 7% with distant metastases at diagnosis. Its incidence is 0.24/100,000 in the United States. It is more commonly found in men, Caucasians, in individuals older than 65, and in the head and neck region (Miller et al. 2009). Since being described, the instance of Merkel cell carcinoma has grown substantially in part because of the ability to identify Merkel cells.

There are various risk factors for the development of Merkel cell carcinoma which include exposure to high levels of UV light. Patients who are treated with oral Psoralen and UV-A phototherapy for psoriasis also have a greater chance of developing MCC. Additional risk factors include immunosuppression, immunodeficiency, fair skin, and infection with Merkel cell polyomavirus (Donepudi et al. 2012; Spurgeon and Lambert 2013). There is also geographic variation, with increased rates noted in Australia (Albores-Saavedra et al. 2010).

8.1 Staging and Work-Up

Prior to 2010 there were multiple competing staging systems. However in the eighth edition of the AJCC Staging System and based on a total of 9387 cases that were abstracted from the National Cancer Data base participant user file, a consensus staging system was developed (Harms et al. 2016) (Table 8).

Table 8 MCC staging system

	Clinical stage group (cTNM)[a]				Pathological stage groups (pTNM)[b]		
	T	N	M		T	N	M
0	T_{is}	N0	M0	0	T_{is}	N0	M0
I	T1	N0	M0	I	T1	N0	M0
IIA	T2−3	N0	M0	IIA	T2−3	N0	M0
IIB	T4	N0	M0	IIB	T4	N0	M0
III	T0−4	N1−3	M0	IIIA	T1−4	N1a(sn) or N1a	M0
					T0	N1b	M0
				IIIB	T1−4	N1b−3	M0
IV	T0−4	Any N	M1	IV	T0−4	Any N	M1
T		N		N			M
Tx, primary tumor cannot be assessed	cNx, regional lymph nodes cannot be clinically assessed (e.g., previously removed for another reason, body habitus)			pNx, regional lymph nodes cannot be assessed (e.g., previously removed for another reason) or not removed for pathological evaluation			M0, no distant metastasis
T0, no primary tumor							M1, distant metastasis
							M1a, metastasis to distant skin, distant subcutaneous tissue, or distant lymph nodes
T_{is}, in situ primary tumor	cN0, no regional lymph node metastasis by clinical or radiological evaluation			pN0, no regional lymph node metastasis detected on pathological evaluation			
T1, primary tumor ≤2 cm							
T2, primary tumor >2 cm but ≤5 cm	cN1, clinically detected regional nodal metastasis			pN1a(sn), clinically occult nodal metastasis identified only by sentinel lymph node biopsy			
T3, primary tumor >5 cm	cN2, in-transit metastasis without lymph node metastasis						M1b, lung
T4, primary tumor invades fascia, muscle cartilage, or bone				pN1a, clinically occult regional lymph node metastasis following lymph node dissection			M1c, all other distant sites
	cN3, in-transit metastasis with lymph node metastasis			pN1b, clinically or radiologically detected regional lymph node metastasis, pathologically confirmed			
				pN2, in-transit metastasis without lymph node metastasis			
				pN3, in-transit metastasis with lymph node metastasis			

[a]Clinical staging is defined by microstaging of the primary Merkel cell carcinoma (MCC) with clinical and/or radiological evaluation for metastasis

[b]Pathological staging is defined by microstaging of the primary MCC and pathological nodal evaluation of the regional lymph node basin with sentinel lymph node-biopsy or complete lymphadenectomy or pathological confirmation of distant metastasis

8.2   Work-Up and Staging

In addition to more traditional work-up of MCC patients that include a history and physical exam and more standard imaging evaluation such as plain films and other imaging modalities, there are multiple reports that support the use of 18F-FDG PET scans as part of the overall work-up of these patients.

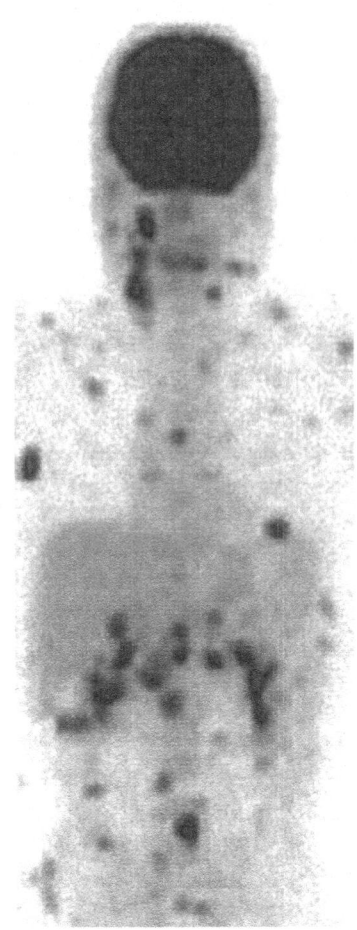

Picture 10 PET for MCC

8.3 Treatment

Patients who present with localized node negative disease generally undergo surgical intervention of the primary tumor followed by adjuvant
radiotherapy. It should be noted that there have
been no randomized trials to support any treatment sequence. There is controversy as to
whether or not clear margins are important since
adjuvant radiotherapy is often utilized. It has
been shown in a number of institutional reports
that adjuvant radiation does provide superior
local regional control when compared to surgery
alone. The issue regarding margins has been
borne out by the group from Brisbane,
Queensland, Australia, who reported on 112 consecutive patients diagnosed with MCC. In their
reports, surgical margins did not affect the local
relapse rate (Foote et al. 2010). This is also supported by the report evaluating 46 patients for
tumor size, depth of invasion, Clark's Level, and
margin status; there was no correlation between
tumor size or depth of invasion to survival or the
development of metastasis. However there was a
trend for increased local/regional failure with
increased size, depth, and positive margins
(Agelli and Clegg 2003). An excellent summary
article is also available for review that concluded
that microscopically positive margins were of no
consequence when postoperative radiotherapy
was used (Trombetta et al. 2011).

Siva et al. reported on 102 consecutive
cases in which PET had an impact on patient
management (Siva et al. 2013). Thirty-seven
percent were affected with 17% of patients
being upstaged while 5% were downstaged.
These results are paralleled by those reported
by other institutions (Duncan et al. 2016;
Ibrahim 2013).

There have also been several national and
international groups which have developed
consensus statements regarding treatment.
These include the European Consensus
Interdisciplinary Guideline (Lebbe and Becker
2015), in addition to those published by the
French Society of Otorhinolaryngology
(Durbec 2014) and the National Comprehensive
Cancer Network (NCCN) in the United States
(NCCN 2016).

8.4 Sentinel Lymph Node Biopsy Utilization

The use of SLNB in the staging and treatment of
MCC plays a critical part in overall management.
A meta-analysis in 2002 reported that 67% had
negative SLNB, and with a median follow-up of
over 7 months 97% remained disease free if they
were SLNB negative. Thirty-three percent had
positive findings and 1/3 of this cohort experienced local regional or distant relapse at 12
months. Those with positive SLNB who then
underwent completion lymph node dissection
(CLND) reported no local/regional recurrence.
Seventy-five percent of those who did not have
CLND had local/regional recurrence (Mehrany
et al. 2002). This is similar to multiple similar

reports including that from Servy et al. (2016). They retrospectively reviewed 87 patients and found that SLNB negativity was a strong predictor of longer OS ($p = 0.013$). The use of adjuvant radiation and negative SLNB were associated with improved disease-free survival ($p = 0.006$) and overall survival ($p = 0.014$).

A review by Fields et al. of 153 patients (median f/u 41 months) found that 45 patients (29%) had positive SLNB findings with localized disease (Fields et al. 2001). They reported that associated factors for positive findings on SLNB included primary tumor size (≥ 2cm) and presence of LVI. However, they could find no difference in recurrence or death rates between the two groups.

There is also a small group of patients who have primary tumors less than 2 cm and who have no evidence of lymphatic disease either by PET imaging or sentinel lymph nodes biopsy, clear surgical margins, and no adverse features such as lymph vascular involvement. These patients may be able to avoid radiotherapy in the adjuvant setting (Frohm et al. 2016).

8.5 Radiation Therapy in Management of MCC

The largest report to date regarding the use of radiation in the treatment of MCC is from Bhatia (Bhatia et al. 2016). A survival analysis was performed on 6908 cases from the National Cancer Data Base from 1996 through 2008. For Stage I ($n = 3369$) and II ($n = 1474$) patients who received surgery plus adjuvant radiation, a significant OS improvement when compared to surgery alone was noted ($p = <0.001$). However, no benefit was found with the addition of either adjuvant radiation or chemotherapy in Stage III ($n = 2065$) patients. Various radiation schedules were noted.

However, reports such as that from Moffitt Cancer Center (Strom et al. 2016) would suggest otherwise. In their report of 171 patients, wide excision included a 1–2 cm "clinical" margin. A total of 87.7% of patients underwent SLNB, of which approximately 35% were positive. Radiation daily doses ranged from 180 to 325 cGy although there was no mention of daily dose effect. They reported improved 3-year local

regional control, disease-free survival, and overall survival with postoperative irradiation. Disease-specific survival at 3 years was improved in node-positive patients but not node-negative patients.

This was similar to the report out of New South Wales in which 62 patients were treated with "radical" intent (Ashby et al. 1989). If radiation was given postoperatively there was statistical improvement in the 2-year local recurrence-free survival ($p < 0.001$). Immune status at time of diagnosis, if compromised, resulted in poorer outcomes. Radiation daily dose schedules were 200 cGy/day up to 60 Gy.

There has been a single trial in which 53 patients with high-risk MCC were treated with radiotherapy and 4 cycles of carboplatin and etoposide (Poulsen et al. 2003). Radiotherapy total doses were considered moderate at 30 Gy. (It should be noted that 62% of the patients presented with gross nodular disease.) The overall 3-year survival rates for local, regional, and distant control were 76%, 75%, and 76% respectively.

There have also been several reports which utilized external beam irradiation as monotherapy. The University of Washington reported on 50 patients (median F/U of 18 months), of which 26 had microscopic lymph node (LN) involvement and the remaining 24 had palpable LN involvement.

Unfortunately no specific radiation dose information is available. However, regional control was 100% in the microscopic LN group with a 2-year regional recurrence-free survival rate of 70–73% dependent on whether a CLND was done (Fong and Tanabe 2014).

Kitamura et al. reported on the Japanese experience with radiation monotherapy with a review of case reports cited over 20 years. Twenty-one out of 22 demonstrated a complete response (CR) to irradiation (Kitamura et al. 2015). A conventional daily dose was primarily used with total doses ranging from 30 to 70 Gy. Eventually, 7/22 had either loco-regional/or distant relapse. The total doses given to those who relapsed ranged from 30 to 70 Gy (med = 60 Gy). Similar local control rates are noted in other series; however patients included in these series are small (Ashby et al. 1989; Mortier et al. 2003; Pacella et al. 1988).

8.6 Conclusions

Thus it would appear that treatment recommendations should be as follows: Stages 1/11—Surgical resection with clear margins if possible followed by localized adjuvant radiation. There **does** not appear to be any advantage to "altered" daily dose scheduling. For Stage Ill with Microscopic nodal involvement, surgery followed by adjuvant radiation to the primary and nodal basin is recommended. There is no apparent advantage to altered daily fractionation other than shortening of the treatment time. For Stage III disease with clinically evident nodal disease, either surgery with lymphadenectomy followed by radiation or definitive radiation especially in the head and neck region is recommended.

9 Melanoma

Melanoma is a diagnosis that often strikes fear in the mind of patients. It conjures up fear of harsh treatment that is, in the layman's mind, ineffective and death due to the spread of the disease is inevitable. However, while this may be a more accurate assessment for individuals with locally advanced or metastatic disease at diagnosis; for the vast majority of patients, surgical resection can often provide a cure. The key is early detection and referral to a trained dermato-oncologist, experienced in diagnosis, work-up, and treatment because not all melanomas are the same and often have quite varied courses of disease even with an initial diagnosis of metastatic disease. In this section we will concentrate on cutaneous disease manifestation.

In 2016, it is estimated that over 76,000 individuals in the United States will be diagnosed with a melanoma, and worldwide this figure stands at somewhere in excess of 200,000 individuals (American Cancer Society 2016). It accounts for 1% of all skin cancers and 25% of all skin cancers that develop in individuals less than the age of 45. Cutaneous malignant melanomas are considered the most lethal form of skin cancer. They account for over 75% of all skin cancer deaths in the United States. It has also been noted that the incidence of melanoma has been increasing rapidly over the past 30 years.

Melanomas arise from melanocytes. Thus, any tissue in which melanocytes can be found can be a site for development of melanoma. These include not only cutaneous sites but also ocular and mucosal sites.

There are four distinct types of melanoma.

1. *Superficial spreading melanoma*—This is the most common and its hallmark is that of large melanocytes with mass formation along the dermal-epidermal junction. They often arise from precursor lesions such as dysplastic nevi (Forman et al. 2008).

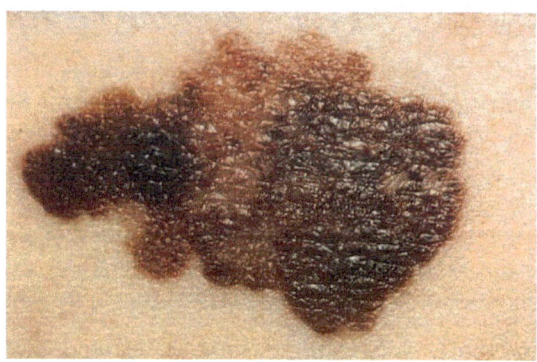

Picture 11 Superficial spreading melanoma

2. *Nodular melanoma*—These are considered the most aggressive of all the melanomas. It is thought that this is caused by the lack of a prodromal lesion and quick penetration into the underlying tissue planes (James 2005).

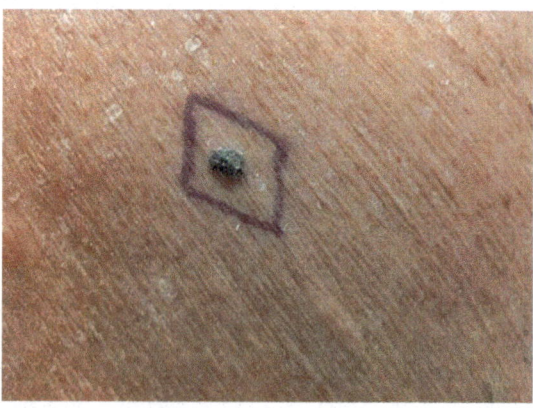

Picture 12 Nodular melanoma

3. *Acral melanoma*—These normally develop in nontraditional sites such as the palm, sole, and nails (Bradford et al. 2009).

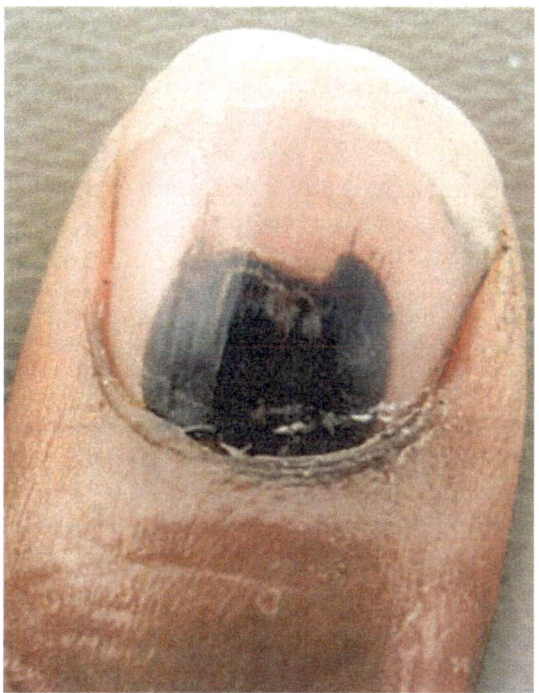

Picture 13   Acral melanoma

4. *Lentigo Maligna Melanoma*—These normally develop as a palpable mass or a nodule (Farshad et al. 2002).

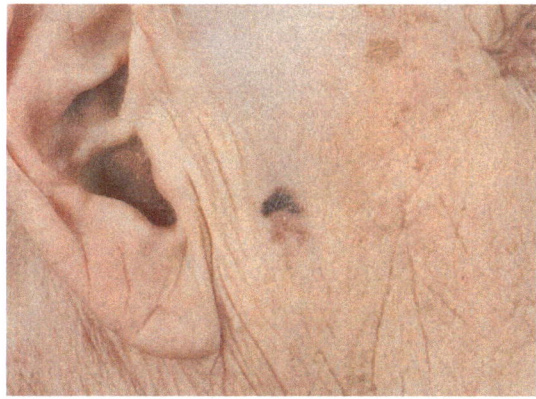

Picture 14   Lentigo Maligna melanoma

9.1   Risk Factors

It is well established that there are numerous factors that can increase the risk for development of melanoma. These include having large number of atypical nevi (also known as "moles"), being fair skinned, excessive use of tanning beds, high UV exposure, and severe sunburn at an early age. There appears also to be an increasing number of patients in increasing latitude regions which might be related to ozone depletion issues (Markovic et al. 2007).

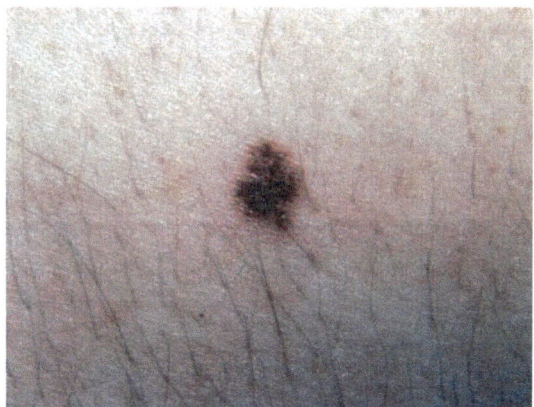

Picture 15   Atypical nevus

Family history also plays a role and there is a familial melanoma in which the specific genetic chains such CDKN2A, CDK4, and MITF have been implicated (Shi et al. 2016). In addition, other inherited conditions such as xeroderma pigmentosum, Li-Fraumeni syndrome, and Werners' syndrome also have an increased incidence of developing melanoma. A history of previous skin cancer, age above 40, and patients with weakened immune systems also increase the risk for development of malignant melanoma (Curiel-Lewandrowski et al. 2011; Lauper et al. 2013; Halkud et al. 2014).

Because of an early age at time of diagnosis for most cases there is also a significant economic cost associated with melanoma. In a report looking at 2000–2006 cost, the following was noted (Ekwueme et al. 2011):

(a) Death resulted in an average lifetime earning loss of about 413,000.00 dollars compared to 310,000 dollars for all other cancers
(b) On average, women lose 21.4 years of life and men 19 years
(c) Women have higher premature mortality
(d) Non-Hispanic whites have a higher health burden and economic cost associated with mortality

9.2 Staging

Until recently, two different "staging" systems for the evaluation of severity of melanoma were used: The Clark's Level and the Breslow System. However beginning in the seventh edition (2009) of American Joint Committee on Cancer, a unified staging system was created. It takes into consideration not only the depth of penetration but also ulceration and mitotic rates of lesions (Balch et al. 2009).

9.3 Risk Assessment Guidelines

Various organizations have created guidelines for staging and risk assessment for patients with melanoma (Dummer et al. 2016; Bichakjian et al. 2011; Coit et al. 2016). These guidelines include history and physical examination and certain laboratory assessments, especially as they relate to potential metastases in the liver. The imaging evaluation now often includes the use of PET scans which have been found to be quite useful in detecting metastatic and regional lymph nodal involvement. Other appropriate scans such as MRI of the brain will help identify CNS metastases prior to the development of symptomatology (Holder et al. 1998).

However when closely evaluated, there are distinct differences in the guidelines and they are usually based on the literature or expert panel consensus but often lack Level I consensus in critical recommendations (Fong and Tanabe 2014).

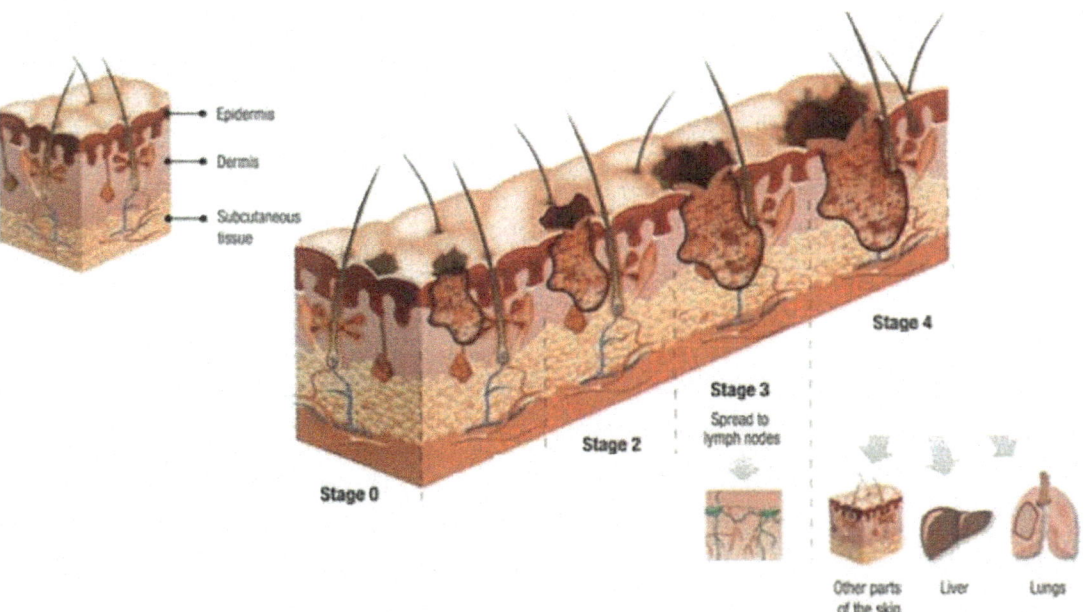

Picture 16 Melanoma staging cartoon

9.4   Diagnosis

As with all malignancies, histologic confirmation is desirable, if not imperative. Various recommendations have been made as to how to best determine, from a pathologic standpoint, a patient's disease severity. Recommendations from most organizations that have provided guidelines include wide local excision with various recommendations for margins. In addition, the use of SLNBs has been found to be quite useful in the identification of nonclinically apparent nodal disease, especially when paired with imaging techniques such as PET scans and followed by CLND, although controversy exists on these points (Morton et al. 2014; Jacques-Grob 2016).

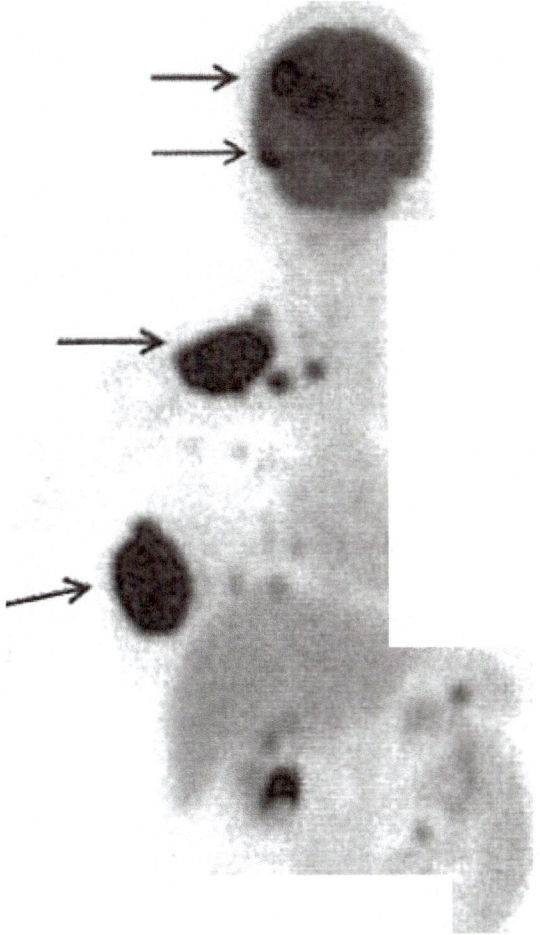

Picture 18 Melanoma PET

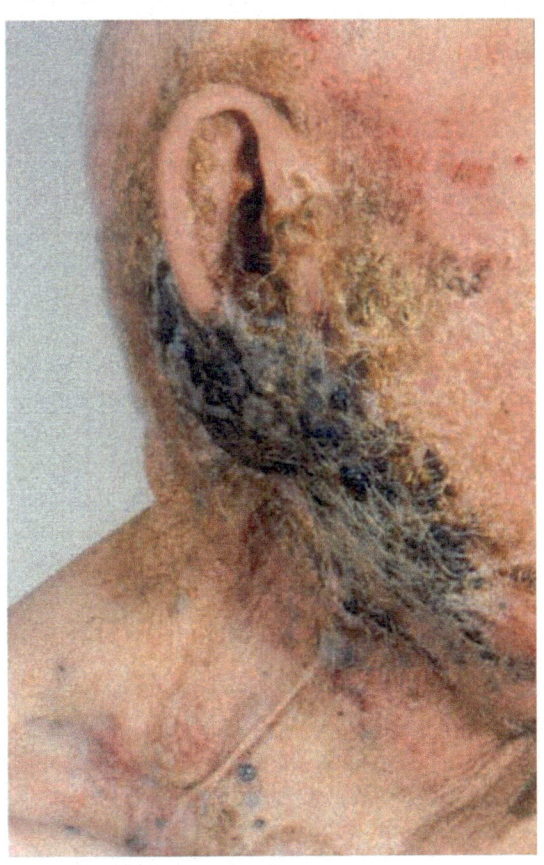

Picture 17 Melanoma clinical

9.5   Sentinel Lymph Node Biopsy/ Completion Lymph Node Dissection

There is further controversy as to whether or not CLND adds to overall survival or even disease-free survival in these patients when the SLNBs are found to be positive. As previously noted, identifying lymphatic metastatic disease is especially important in defining treatment options for patients with melanoma. When coupled with imaging studies such as PET scans, SLNBs help to identify patients who may benefit from local regional treatment such as radiotherapy and/or systemic therapies (Holder et al. 1998).

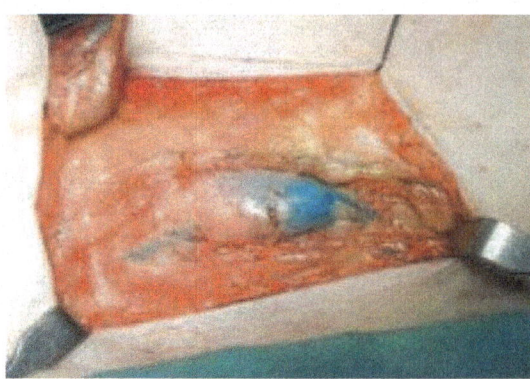

Picture 19 Sentinel lymph node biopsy

A multi-institution randomized trial, the Multicenter Selective Lymphadenectomy Trial (MSLT-1) study, sought to address the issue of SLNB/CLND and the role it plays in the treatment of patients with melanoma (Phan et al. 2009). This study randomized patients with intermediate thickness melanomas to SLNB and immediate CLND versus observation if the SLNB was positive. The initial report identified a 5-year survival rate of 72.3% in patients with positive sentinel lymph nodes verses 90.2% if they were negative ($p < 0.001$). There was no difference in overall survival; however there was a statistical improvement in the 5-year disease-free survival.

For those patients who had positive lymph nodes identified at the SLNB and who underwent immediate CLND, there was a noted improvement in the overall survival at 5 years when compared to those patients who had lymph node dissection only after they developed clinical disease. The conclusion from this initial article was that SLNB when performed on "acceptable" patients (Breslow depth ≥0.76 mm) was advantageous.

However, others had disputed this recommendation regarding the depth of the lesions. One series reviewed 1250 patients and found that only 5.2% of patients with lesions 1 mm or less in thickness were found to have lymph node metastases (Han et al. 2013). Another analysis which reviewed multiple databases concluded that "evidence is not sufficient to document a benefit of SLNB when compared to observation in individuals with primary localized cutaneous melanoma" (Kyrgidis et al. 2015).

However the final report from MSLT-1 in 2014 did report a mean 10-year disease-free survival benefit in the biopsy group with intermediate thickness (1.2–3.5 mm) and thick (>3.5 mm) lesions.

It concluded that SLNB-based management prolonged disease free for all patients and prolongs distant disease-free survival and melanoma-specific survival for patients with nodal metastases from intermediate thickness melanomas. However the question regarding thin and thick melanomas remains unresolved as to the impact of SLNB (Morton et al. 2014).

9.6 Radiation Therapy

Historically melanomas were thought to be radio-resistant malignancies. This was based on in vitro cell studies in which the radiation survival shoulder curves identified would suggest high capacity for melanoma cells to repair radiation damage (Bentzen et al. 1989; Fertil and Malaise 1985). From these data, further research tried to identify an alpha/beta ratio in which fractionation sequences could be developed. A report by Rofstad in 1994 suggested an alpha/beta ratio determined from ten different human melanoma xenograph lines that were measured in vivo and related to cellular radiation sensitivities that were measured in vitro using the Courtenay soft agar colony assay (Rofstad 1994). It showed that the alpha/beta ratio in vitro, when divided by an oxygen enhancement ratio of 2.8, resulted in estimates of 1 (±1 Gy) to 33 (±6.7 Gy). Seven of the ten lines that were investigated showed alpha/beta ratios similar to or higher than those of the acutely responding tissues.

This became known as Extrapolated Total Dose (ETD) which was initially suggested as a way to prescribe dose by Overgaard et al. in 1996 (Overgaard et al. 1985). In their initial report, they found that a 50% response for an ETD was 86 Gy. They identified a significant relationship between the dose per fraction and the response so that high doses per fraction yielded a significantly better response. As well, only 24% of patients treated with less than 4 Gy had a complete response, whereas 57% developed a CR for doses greater than or equal to 4 Gy per fraction ($p = 0.001$). They also noted a lack of influence of treatment time, thus allowing them to estimate an alpha-beta ratio of 2.5.

This same group also published a randomized study comparing two high dose rate per fraction schedules in recurrent or metastatic melanomas. Thirty-five tumors in 14 patients were treated with either 9 Gy × 3 fractions or 5 Gy × 8 fractions delivered twice weekly. The overall response rate was 97% and no difference was observed between the two treatment regimens (Overgaard et al. 1985).

Other groups have also looked at utilization of various dose sequences. To date however, there have been only two randomized trials looking at daily dose schedules. The first was conducted by the Radiation Therapy Oncology Group (RTOG 83-05) in which patients with measurable lesions were randomized to receive 4 fractions × 8 Gy in 21 days once weekly versus 20 fractions × 2.5 Gy in 26–28 days delivered 5 days a week (Sause et al. 1991). One hundred thirty-seven patients were randomized. The study was closed early when interim statistical analysis suggested that further accrual would not reveal a difference between the arms. There was no difference in CR/PR rates between the two arms; however it should be noted that the reported rates are less than seen in those series using the ETD calculation method.

Burmeister et al. published a randomized trial that included 123 patients that were randomly allocated to adjuvant radiotherapy compared to 127 who were allocated to observation after therapeutic lymphadenectomy (Burmeister et al. 2012). At a median follow-up of 40 months, they found that the risk for lymph node field relapse was significantly reduced in the adjuvant radiotherapy group compared to the observation group alone. The dose that was delivered was 48 Gy in 20 fractions. There was no difference in relapse-free survival or overall survival. They did note that the most common grade 3 and grade 4 adverse events were seroma and radiation dermatitis. This study noted that adjuvant radiotherapy improved lymph node field control in patients at high risk for in-field relapse. This series was recently updated in 2015 and the longer follow-up supported the previous findings (Henderson et al. 2015).

Two more recent series highlight variations of the radiation dose sequence saga. Georgetown University (Jahanshahi et al. 2012) published a series of 78 lesions, of which 21 were treated as "body" sites using dose calculations based on the ETD (vol) thresholds that were described by Overgaard (Overgaard et al. 1985). The 1-year local control rates were 72% at a follow-up ranging between 2 and 36 months (med = 9.2 months). Local control rates when treated above ETD (vol) thresholds of 100 Gy were 100% and 80% versus 74% and 59% below the threshold. Other institutional series have also evaluated various dose sequences. A German report reviewed 121 patients for palliative reason in advanced malignant melanoma (Seegenschmiedt et al. 1999). Seventy-seven received either 2 Gy × 5/week or 3.5 Gy × 3/week. The remaining 38 lesions were treated with 4–6 Gy delivered × 2 weeks with the majority (34/38) receiving 4 Gy (median dose = 48 Gy; range 20–66 Gy). At a very short follow-up of only 3 months, 64% achieved a CR and 100% had some form of response. Univariate analysis review of prognostic factors for complete response and long-term survival identified UICC stage, primary location of the head and neck, and total doses above 40 Gy as positive factors. Multivariate analysis revealed only UICC stage as a single independent prognostic factor ($p > 0.001$) (Table 9).

Table 9 Radiation altered fraction for melanoma

Author	Reference	Patients	Dose	Follow-up	Local control	Complications/other
Overgaard 1985	101	114 patients	≤4Gy		24%	No time effect
					($p =0.001$)	50% response rate
		204 lesions	>4 Gy		57%	For ETD(vol) = 86 Gy
Overgaard	102	14 patients	9 Gy × 3		97% response rate [no difference)	No difference in toxicity
		35 lesions	5 Gy × 8			
Sause	119	126	8 Gy × 40	N/A	20 LF in radiation group 34 LF in nonradiation group ($p = 0.041$)	No difference in acute toxicity
			2.5 Gy × 20			
Burmeister	23	123	Postsurgical 2.4 Gy × 20 vs No radiation	40	72% @ 1 year if ETD(vol) > 100 Gy 80% LC at 12 month <100 Gy 59% LC	Most common toxicity seroma/dermatitis
Jahanshahi	66	21 (body)	ETD (vol)	9.2	64% CR 100% CR/PR	(−)
Seegensehmieddt	120	121	All patients 3–6 Gy × 2 week total dose = 22–68 Gy 44 patients with 3.1–6 Gy total 24–56 Gy	3	Local control improved with total dose ≥50 Gy ($p < 0.01$)	RTOG toxicity GR I = 53% GR II = 17% 2 patients with soft tissue ulceration

vs versus, *LC* local control

9.7 Radiotherapy and Systemic Agents

Recently several articles have highlighted potential increased side effects when utilizing radiation with newer immunologic agents. Cornell reported on concurrent ipilimumab and non-CNS radiation in 29 patients for 33 treatment courses (Barker et al. 2013). Radiation was started either during induction or maintenance phase of ipilimumab. Daily dose was 2 Gy (EQD2) and median follow-up was 11 months for all patients. Median radiation dose was 30 Gy. Fifteen percent of patients experienced grade 3 adverse effects; one GR 4 event was noted.

A French report detailed increased skin reaction when pembrolizumab was used concomitantly with radiation (Sibaud et al. 2015). Radiosensitivity was also reported by the Germans when using vemurafenib (Forschner et al. 2014). Thus, one must be aware of potential increased side effects when both traditional and newer immunotherapies are utilized with external beam irradiation regardless of daily dose and total dose delivered.

It appears that the data that have been reported from the ETD (vol) dose analysis prescription series have resulted in excellent local control results and acceptable complication rates. In evaluating the RTOG study in CR/PR rates and despite the fact that the 4 × 8 Gy regimen would be considered an inadequate dose based on ETD (vol) evaluation, it would be reasonable to consider. Perhaps it is time to revisit this important topic, especially in light of the increasing number of patients being diagnosed.

10 Primary Cutaneous lymphoma (PCL)

Primary cutaneous lymphomas are skin associated but have the capacity like other non-Hodgkin's lymphoma to develop "metastatic" disease. They span the range of being localized to a single site in appearance, to that which involves the entire skin. Distinct types of cutaneous T-cell and B-cell lymphoma can be identified (Kim et al. 2007). The T-cell lymphomas comprise upwards of 80% of those found in the Americas and Europe with mycosis fungoides (MF) being the most common diagnosis. In Asia, non-MF T-cell lymphomas predominate.

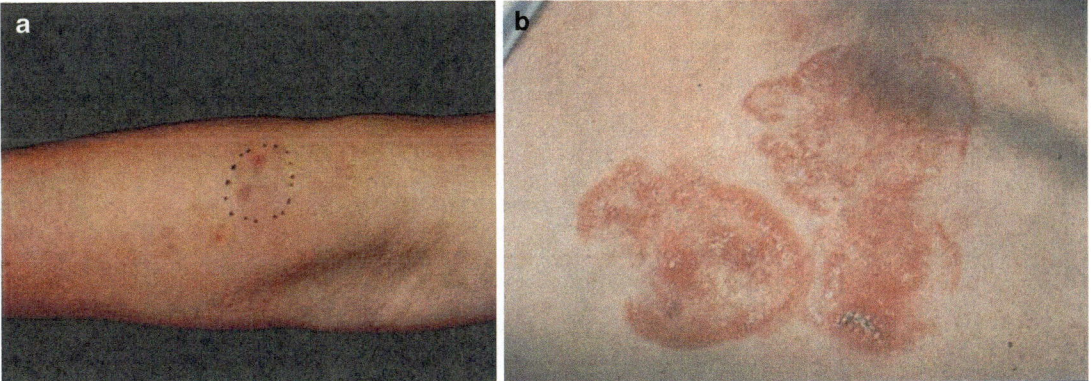

Picture 20 (**a**) Peripheral cutaneous lymphoma; (**b**) mycosis fungoides

10.1 Staging and Treatment

Staging for non-MF PCLs follows the guidelines developed through the International Society for Cutaneous Lymphomas and the EORTC (Willemze and Jaffe 2005). Recently the International Lymphoma Radiation Oncology Group has published Guidelines for field arrangement and doses. Based on their recommendations total doses range between 20 and 45 Gy and these conventional daily doses appear effective for local control (Specht et al. 2015).

Recently, with the improvement in genetics detection and sequencing, certain mutagens have been identified (UV radiation and recombination activating gene [RAG]), in addition to other potential treatment targets which include the NF-kB and the JAK-STAT pathways (Damsky and Choi 2016). While studies looking at these potential targets for systemic therapy are ongoing, radiation therapy remains an important tool in our treatment regimens. Most series have used conventional daily doses including those treating total skin electrons for MF patients. It should be noted that the most commonly utilized treatment technique for total skin electron is the Stanford technique utilizing six fields on alternating days (Hoppe 2003).

There have also been series which have looked at altered/hypo-fractioned irradiation for treatment of "localized" symptomatic lesions. One of the largest series reported was from Thomas et al. in which 58 patients (primarily MF) were treated with a single fraction to localized lesions (Thomas et al. 2013). Both electrons and photons

were utilized for the treatment of 270 lesions. The fraction size ranged from 4 to 9 Gy with only 3% receiving less than 7 Gy. Of the ten lesions rated as a PR, four were converted to CR with a second treatment. Complete responses were reported in 94.4% of the patients with a median follow-up of 41.3 months.

Neelis et al. reported on 18 patients with 44 treatment sites using an initial schedule of 4 Gy delivered in two fractions; however because of poor response to this fractionation, another group of 31 patients were treated utilizing 8 Gy in two fractions (Neelis et al. 2009). Complete response for cutaneous T cell lymphomas was noted to be 72%. However for mycosis fungoides patients, only 30% had a response to treatment with the 4 Gy regimen compared to 92% who received the 8 Gy regimen.

A case report from the Mayo Clinic documented a CR for a single patient treated for bulky cutaneous Tcell lymphoma of the head. That patient received four weekly fractions of 400 Gy (Ahmed 2016).

Conclusion

Despite the accessibility to visual exam, it is noted that both NMSC and melanoma are often found in more advanced stages which can lead to the need for combined modality treatment.

There are substantial data that altered/hypofractionated external beam irradiation >300 cGy/fraction can play an important role in establishing excellent local/regional control with acceptable cosmetic appearance in all of the cutaneous lesions.

As the population ages and more time is spent in the sun, combined with other known risk factors, the use of altered/hypofractionated therapy will play a more important role in management. Moreover, due to the financial constraints that our health care systems are experiencing and also considering the efficacy of this therapy and the convenience to the patient, physician-led groups are correctly redefining the long established paradigm.

References

Abide J, Nahai F, Bennett RG (1984) The meaning of surgical margins. Past Reconstr Surg 73:492–497

Ablashi DV (2002) Spectrum of Kaposi's sarcoma-associated herpesvirus, or human herpes virus 8, diseases. Clin Microbiol Rev 15:439–464

Agelli M, Clegg LX (2003) Epidemiology of primary Merkel cell carcinoma in the United States. J Am Acad Dermatol 49(5):831–841

Ahmed S (2016) Adaptation of Stanford technique for treatment of bulky cutaneous T-cell lymphoma of the head. Pract Radiat Oncol 6:183–186

Albores-Saavedra J, Batich K, Chable-Montero F et al (2010) Merkel cell carcinoma demographics, morphology, and survival based on 3870 cases: a population based study. J Cut Pathol 37((1)):20–27

American Cancer Society (2016). Cancer facts and figures. http://www.cancer.org/acs/groups/content/@research/documents/document/acspc-047079.pdf

Andretto A (2007) The central role of the nose in the face and the psyche: review of the nose and the psyche. Aesthetic Plast Surg 31:406–410

Arenas M, Arguis M, Diez-Presa L et al (2015) Hypo fractionated high-dose–rate plesiotherapy in nonmelanoma skin cancer treatment. Brachytherapy 14:859–865

Ashby MA, Jones DH, Tasker AD et al (1989) Primary cutaneous neuroendocrine (Merkel cell or trabecular carcinoma) tumour of the skin: a radioresponsive tumor. J Clin Radiol 40(1):85–87

Balch CM, Gershenwald JE, Soong SJ et al (2009) Final version of 2009 AJCC melanoma staging and classification. J Clin Oncol 279360:6199–6206. doi:10.1200/JCO.2009

Barker CA, Postow MA, Khan SA et al (2013) Concurrent radiotherapy and ipilimumab immunotherapy for patients with melanoma. Cancer Immunol Res. doi:10.1158/2326-6066.CIR-13-0082

Belembaogo E, Kirova Y, Frikha H et al (1998) Radiotherapy of epidemic Kaposi's sarcoma: the experience of the Henri-Mondor Hospital (643 patients). Cancer Radiother 2(1):49–52

Bentzen SM, Overgaard J, Thames HD et al (1989) Clinical radiobiology of malignant melanoma. Radiother Oncol. 16(3):196–182

Bhatia SJ, Storer BE, Iyer JG et al (2016) Adjuvant radiation therapy and chemotherapy in Merkel cell carcinoma: survival analyses of 6908 cases from the National Cancer Data Base. Natl. Cancer Inst 108(9). doi:10.1093/jnci/djw042. pii: djw042

Bhatnagar A (2013) Nonmelanoma skin cancer treated with electronic brachytherapy: results at 1 year. Brachytherapy 12:134–140

Bichakjian CK, Halpern AC, Johnson TM et al (2011) Guidelines of care for the management of primary cutaneous melanoma, American Academy of Dermatology. J Am Acad Dermatol 65(5):1032–1047. doi:10.1016/j.jaad.2011.04.031. Epub 2011 Aug 25

Biller K, Kim DW (2009) A contemporary assessment of facial aesthetic preferences. Arch Facial Plast Surg. 11(2):91–97. doi:10.1001/archfacial.2008.543

Black JO (2016) Xeroderma pigmentosum. Head Neck Pathol 10(2):139–144. [Epub ahead of print]

Bonerandi JJ, Beauvillain L, Caquant J et al (2011) Guidelines for the diagnosis and treatment of cutaneous squamous cell carcinoma and precursor lesions. For the French Dermatology Recommendations Association (aRED). J Eur Acad Dermatol Venereol 25(Suppl 5):1–51

Bradford P, Goldstein A, McMaster M (2009) Acral lentiginous melanoma: incidence and survival patterns in the United States, 1986-2005. JAMA Dermatol 145(4):427–434

Bresler SC, Padwa BL, Granter SR (2016) Nevoid basal cell carcinoma syndrome (Gorlin syndrome). Head Neck Pathol 10(2):119–124. [Epub ahead of print]

Burmeister BH, Henderson MA, Ainslie J et al (2012) Adjuvant radiotherapy versus observation alone for patients at risk of lymph-node field relapse after therapeutic lymphadenectomy for melanoma: a randomized trial. Lancet Oncol. 13:589–597

Chen C, Chung CY, Wang LH et al (2015) Risk of cancer among HIV-infected patients from a population-based nested case-control study: implications for cancer prevention. BMC Cance. 15:133. doi:10.1186/s12885-015-1099-y

Coit DG, Thompson JA, Algazi A et al (2016) NCCN Guidelines Insights: Melanoma, Version 3. J Natl Compr Canc Netw 14(8):945–958

Cook-Mozaffari P, Newton R, Burkitt DP (1998) The geographical distribution of Kaposi sarcomas and of lymphomas in Africa before the AIDS epidemic. Br J Cancer 78(11):1521–1528. doi:10.1038/bjc.1998.717. PMC: 2063225

Curiel-Lewandrowski C, Speetzen LS, Cranmer L et al (2011) Multiple primary cutaneous melanomas in Li-Fraumeni syndrome. J Arch Dermatol 147((2)):248–250. doi:10.1001/archdermatol.2010.428

van Dam RM, Huang Z, Rimm EB et al (1999) Risk factors for basal cell carcinoma of the skin in men: results from the health professionals follow-up study. Am J Epidemiol 150(5):459–468

Damsky WE, Choi J (2016) Genetics of cutaneous T-cell lymphoma: from bench to bedside. Curr Treat Options Oncol 17(7):33. doi:10.1007/s11864-016-0410-8

De Silva SP, Dellon AL (1985) Recurrence rate of positive margin basal cell carcinoma: results of a five-year prospective study. J Surg Oncol 28(1):72–74

Doggett S, Willoughby M, Willoughby C et al (2015) Incorporation of electronic brachytherapy for skin cancer into a community dermatology practice. J Clin Aesthet Dermatol 8(11):28–32

Donepudi S, DeConti R, Samlowski W (2012) Recent advances in the understanding of the genetics, etiology, and treatment of Merkel cell carcinoma. Semin Oncol 39:163–172

Dummer R, Siano M, Hunger RE et al (2016) The updated Swiss guidelines 2016 for the treatment and follow-up of cutaneous melanoma. Swiss Med Wkly. 146:w14279. doi:10.4414/smw.2016.14279. eCollection 2016

Duncan DJ, Carr D, Kaffenberger BH (2016) The utility of positron emission tomography with and without computed tomography in patients with nonmelanoma skin cancer. J Am Acad Dermatol 75(1):186–196. doi:10.1016/j.jaad.2016.01.045.   pii: S0190-9622(16)00125-0. [Epub ahead of print]

Durbec M (2014) Extension assessment and principles of resection in cutaneous head and neck tumors. Guidelines of the French Society of Otorhinolaryngology (SFORL), short version. Eur Ann Otorhinolaryngol Head Neck Dis 131(6):375–383

Ekwueme MS, Gery P, Li C et al (2011) The health burden and economic coasts of cutaneous melanoma mortality by race/ethnicity-United States, 2000 to 2006. J Am Acad Dermatol 65(5, Suppl 1):S133.e1–S133e12

Evans M, Yassa M, Podgorsak EB et al (1997) Surface applicators for high dose rate brachytherapy in AIDS-related Kaposi's sarcoma. Int J Radiati Oncol Biol Phys 39(3):769–774

Farshad A, Burg G, Panizzon R et al (2002) A retrospective study of 150 patients with lentigo maligna and lentigo maligna melanoma and the efficacy of radiotherapy using Grenz or soft x-rays. Br J Dermatol. 146(6):1042

Ferro M, Deodato F, Macchia G et al (2015) Short-course radiotherapy in elderly patients with early stage non-melanoma skin cancer: a phase II study cancer investigation. Cancer Invest 33(2):34–38. doi:10.3109/07357907.2014.998835

Fertil B, Malaise EP (1985) Intrinsic radiosensitivity of human cell lines is correlated with radioresponsiveness of human tumors: analysis of 101 published survival curves. Int J Radiat Oncol Biol Phys 11(9):1699–1707

Fields RC, Busam KJ, Chou JF et al (2001) Recurrence and survival in patients undergoing sentinel lymph node biopsy for Merkel cell carcinoma: analysis of 153 patients from a single institution. Ann Surg Oncol 18(9):2529–2537.   doi:10.1245/s10434-011-1662-y. Epub 2011

Fong ZV, Tanabe KK (2014) Comparison of melanoma guidelines in the U.S.A., Canada, Europe, Australia and New Zealand: a critical appraisal and comprehensive review. Br J Dermatol 170(1):20–30. doi:10.1111/bjd.12687

Foote M, Harvey J, Porceddu S et al (2010) Effect of radiotherapy dose and volume on relapse in Merkel cell cancer of the skin. Int J Radiat Oncol Biol Phys 77(3):677–684

Forman SB, Ferringer TC, Peckham SJ et al (2008) Is superficial spreading melanoma still the most common form of malignant melanoma? J Am Acad Dermatol 58(6):1013–1020. doi:10.1016/j.jaad.2007.10.650

Forschner A, Zips D, Schraml C et al (2014) Radiation recall dermatitis and radiation pneumonitis during treatment with vemurafenib. Melanoma Res 24(5):512–516. doi:10.1097/CMR.0000000000000078

Frohm ML, Griffith KA, Harms KL et al (2016) Recurrence and survival in patients with Merkel cell carcinoma undergoing surgery without adjuvant radiation therapy to the primary site. JAMA Dermatol. doi:10.1001/jamadermatol.2016.1428. [Epub ahead of print]

Gallagher RP, Hill GB, Bajdik CD et al (1995) Sunlight exposure, pigmentation factors, and risk of nonmelanocytic skin cancer. II. Squamous cell carcinoma. Arch Dermatol 131(2):164–169

Gauden R, Pracy M, Avery A-M et al (2013) HDR brachytherapy for superficial non-melanoma skin cancers. J Med Imag Radiat Oncol 57:212–217

Geara F, LeBourgeois JP, Piedbois P et al (1991) Radiotherapy in the management of cutaneous epidemic Kaposi's sarcoma. Int J Radiat Oncol Biol Phys 21(6):1517–1522

Goessling W, McKee P, Mayer R (2002) Merkel cell carcinoma. J Clin Oncol 20:588–598

Halkud R, Shenoym AM, Naik SM et al (2014) Indian Xeroderma pigmentosum: clinicopathological review of the multiple oculocutaneous malignancies and complications. J Surg Oncol 5(2):120–124. doi:10.1007/s13193-014-0307-6. Epub 2014 Apr 9

Han S, North J, Canavan T et al (2012) Merkel cell carcinoma. Hematol Oncol Clin N Am 26:1351–1374

Han D, Zager JS, Shyr Y et al (2013) Clinicopathologic predictors of sentinel lymph node metastasis in thin melanoma.   J   Clin   Oncol   31(35):4387–4393. doi:10.1200/JCO.2013.50.1114. Epub 2013 Nov

Harms K, Healy M, Nghiem P et al (2016) A analysis of prognostic factors from 9387 Merkel Cell carcinoma cases forms the basis for the new 8th edition AJCC staging system. Ann Surg Oncol. doi:10.1245/s10434-016-5266-4

Hart PH, Grimbaldeston M, Finlay-Jones JJ (2001) Sunlight, immunosuppression and skin cancer: role of histamine and mast cells. Clin Exper Pharmacol Physiol 28:1–8

Henderson MA, Burmeister BH, Ainslie J et al (2015) Adjuvant lymph-node field radiotherapy versus observation only in patients with melanoma at high risk of further lymph-node field relapse after lymphadenectomy (ANZMTG 01.02/TROG 02.01): 6-year follow-up of a phase 3 randomized controlled trial. Lancet Oncol 16(9):1049–1060. doi:10.1016/S1470-2045(15)00187-4. Epub 2015 Jul 20

Hernandez-Machin B, Borrego L, Gil-Garcia M et al (2007) Office-based radiation therapy for cutaneous carcinoma: evaluation of 710 treatments. Int J Dermatol 46:453–459

van Hezewijk M, Creutzberg C, Putter H et al (2010) Efficacy of a hypofractionated schedule in electron beam radiotherapy for epithelial skin cancer: analysis of 434 cases. Radio Oncol 95:245–249

Hinerman RW, Indelicato DJ, Amdur RJ et al (2008) Cutaneous squamous cell carcinoma metastatic to parotid-area lymph nodes. Laryngoscope 118(11):1989–1996. doi:10.1097/MLG.0b013e318180642b

Holder WD, White RL, Zuger JH et al (1998) Effectiveness of positron emission tomography for the detection of melanoma metastases. Ann Surg. 227(7):764–771

Hoppe RT (2003) Mycosis fungoides: radiation therapy. Dermatol Ther 16:347–354

Ibrahim SF (2013) 18F-fluorodeoxyglucose positron emission tomography-computed tomography imaging in the management of Merkel cell carcinoma: a single-institution retrospective study. Dermatol Surg. 39(9):1323–1333. doi:10.1111/dsu.12246. Epub 2013 Jun 18

Inskip PD, Sigurdson AJ, Veiga L et al (2016) Radiation-related new primary solid cancers in the childhood cancer survivor study: comparative radiation dose response and modification of treatment effects. Int J Radiat Oncol Biol Phys 94(4):800–807

Jacques-Grob J (2016) Personal communication. Skin Cancer Foundation

Jahanshahi P, Nasr N, Unger K et al (2012) Malignant melanoma and radiotherapy: past myths, excellent local control in 146 studied lesions at Georgetown University, and improving future management. Front Oncol 2:167. doi:10.3389/fonc.2012.00167. eCollection 2012

James W (2005) Andrews' diseases of the skin: clinical dermatology, 10th edn. Saunders, Philadelphia. ISBN: 0-7216-2921-0

Jensen P, Hansen S, Moller B et al (1999) Skin cancer in kidney and heart transplant recipients and different long-term immunosuppressive therapy regimens. J Am Acad Dermatol 40(2 Pt 1):177–186

Kaposi M (1872) Idiopathisches multiples Pigmentsarkom der Haut. Arch Dermatol Syphilis 4(2):265–273. doi:10.1007/BF01830024

Karagas MR, McDonald JA, Greenberg ER et al (1996) Risk of basal cell and squamous cell skin cancers after ionizing radiation therapy for the Skin Cancer Prevention Study Group. J Natl Cancer Inst 88(24):1848–1853

Kasper M, Richter S, Warren N et al (2013) Complete response of endemic Kaposi sarcoma lesions with

high-dose-rate brachytherapy: treatment method, results, and toxicity using skin surface applicators. Brachytherapy 12(5):495–499. doi:10.1016/j.brachy.2012.09.007. Epub 2013 Mar 1

Khan L, Breen D, Zhang L et al (2014) Predictors of recurrence after radiotherapy for non-melanoma skin cancer. Curr Oncol 21(2):e326–e329. doi:10.3747/co.21.1727

Kim YH, Wiiemze R, Pimpinelli N (2007) TNM classification system for system for primary cutaneous lymphomas other than mycosis fungoides and Sezary syndrome: a proposal of the International Society for Cutaneous Lymphomas (ISCL) and the Cutaneous Lymphoma Task Force of the European Organization of Research and Treatment of Cancer (EORTC). Blood 110:479–484

Kimyai-Asadi A, Goldberg LH, Peterson SR et al (2005) Efficacy of narrow-margin excision of well-demarcated primary facial basal cell carcinomas. Am Acad Dermatol 53:464–468

Kitamura N, Tomita R, Yamamoto M et al (2015) World J Surg Oncol. 13:152. doi:10.1186/s12957-0150564-2

Kouloulias V (2012) Efficacy, cosmesis and skin toxicity in a hypofractionated irradiation schedule for cutaneous basal cell carcinoma of the head and neck area. Head Neck Oncol 4(5):88

Koyfman S, Cooper JS, Beitler J et al (2016) ACR appropriateness criteria aggressive nonmelanomatous skin cancer of the head and neck. Head Neck 38(2):175–182. doi:10.1002/HED2016pp.175-82

Kyrgidis A et al (2015) Cochrane Database Syst Rev 16(5):CD 01037

Lauper JM, Krause A, Vaughan TL et al (2013) Spectrum and risk of neoplasia in Werner syndrome: a systematic review. PLoS One 8(4):e59709. doi:10.1371/journal.pone.0059709. Epub

Lebbe C, Becker JC, Grob JJ et al: Diagnosis and treatment of Merkel cell carcinoma. European consensus-based interdisciplinary guideline. European Dermatology Forum (EDF), the European Association of Dermato-Oncology (EADO) and the European Organization for Research and Treatment of Cancer (EORTC) 2015 Eur J Cancer; 51(16):2396-2403. doi: 10.1016/j.ejca.2015.06.131. Epub 2015 Aug 6.

Locke J, Karimpour S, Young G et al (2001) Radiotherapy for epithelial skin cancer. Int J Radiat Oncol Biol Phys 51:748–755

Lovett R, Perez C, Shapiro S (1990) External irradiation of epithelial skin cancer. Int J Radiat Oncol Biol Phys 19(2):235–242

Luppi M, Barozzi P, Schulz TF et al (2000) Bone marrow failure associated with human herpesvirus 8 infection after transplantation. N Engl J Med 343(19):1378–1385. doi:10.1056/NEJM200011093431905

Markovic SN, Erickson LA, Rao RD et al (2007) Malignant melanoma in the 21st century, part 1: epidemiology, risk factors, screening, prevention and diagnosis. Melanoma Study Group of the Mayo Clinic Cancer Center. Mayo Clin Proc 82(3):364–380

Matthey-Gie M-L, Boubaker A, Letovanec I et al (2013) Sentinel lymph node biopsy in nonmelanoma skin cancer patients. J Skin Cancer. doi:10.1155/2013/267474

Mazeron J, Chassagne D, Crook J et al (1989) Radiation therapy of carcinomas of the skin of nose and nasal vestibule: a report of 1676 cases by the Groupe Europeen de Curiethérapie. Radio Oncol 13:165–173

Mehrany K, Otley CC, Weenig RH et al (2002) A meta-analysis of the prognostic significance of sentinel lymph node status in Merkel cell carcinoma. Dermatol Surg 28(2):113–117

Migden MR (2015) Treatment with two different doses of sonidegib in patients with locally advanced or metastatic basal cell carcinoma (BOLT): a multicenter, randomized, double-blind phase 2 trial. Lancet Oncol 16(6):716–728. doi:10.1016/S1470-2045(15)70100-2. Epub 2015 May 14

Mikhail G, Mohs FE (1991) Mohs micrographic surgery. W. B. Saunders, Philadelphia, p 7. ISBN 978-0-7216-3415-9

Miller SJ, Alam M, Andersen J et al (2009) Merkel cell carcinoma. J Natl Compr Cancer Netw 7:322–332

Mizuno H, CagriUysal A, Koike S et al (2006) Squamous cell carcinoma of the auricle arising from keloid after radium needle therapy. J Craniofac Surg. 17(2):360–362

Moncrieff M, Shah AK, Igali L et al (2015) False-negative rate of intraoperative frozen section margin analysis for complex head and neck nonmelanoma skin cancer excisions. Clin Exp Dermatol 40(8):834–838. doi:10.1111/ced.12743. Epub 2015 Aug 19

Moore BA, Weber RS, Prieto V et al (2005) Lymph node metastases from cutaneous squamous cell carcinoma of the head and neck. Laryngoscope 115(9):1561–1567

Mortier L, Mirabel X, Fournier C et al (2003) Radiotherapy alone for primary Merkel cell carcinoma. Arch Dermatol 139(12):1587–1590

Morton DL, Thompson JF, Cochran AJ et al (2014) Final trial report of sentinel-node biopsy versus nodal observation in melanoma. N Engl J Med. 370:599–609

NCCN (2016) NCCN guidelines index, squamous cell skin cancer. NCCN guideline version 1. https://www.nccn.org/professionals/physician_gls/f_guidelines.asp

Neelis K, Schimmel E, Maaten H et al (2009) Low-dose palliative radiotherapy for cutaneous B-and T-cell lymphomas. Int J Radiat Oncol Biol Phys 74(1):154–158

Olsen SJ, Chang Y, Moore P et al (1998) Increasing Kaposi's sarcoma-associated herpesvirus seroprevalence with age in a highly Kaposi's sarcoma endemic region, Zambia in 1985. AIDS 12(14):1921–1925. doi:10.1097/00002030-1989

Overgaard J, von Der Maase H, Overgaaard M (1985) A randomized study comparing two high-dose per fraction radiation schedules in recurrent or metastatic malignant melanoma. Int J Radiat Oncol Biol Phys 11(10):1837–1839

Pacella J, Ashby M, Ainslie J et al (1988) The role of radiotherapy in the management of primary cutaneous neuroendocrine tumors (Merkel cell or trabecular carcinoma): experience at the Peter MacCallum Cancer Institute (Melbourne, Australia). Int J Radiat Oncol Biol Phys 14(6):1077–1084

Pampena R, Palmieri T, Kyrgidis K et al (2016) Orthovoltage radiotherapy for nonmelanoma skin cancer (NMSC): Comparison between 2 different schedules. Terracina, Reggio Emilia, and Naples, Italy. J Am Acad Dermatol 74(2):341–347

Panizza B, Solares CA, Redmond M et al (2012) Surgical resection for clinical perineural invasion from cutaneous squamous cell carcinoma of the head and neck. Head Neck 34(11):1622–1627. doi:10.1002/hed.21986. Epub 2011 Dec 23

Panizza B, Warren TA, Solares CA et al (2014) Histopathological features of clinical perineural invasion of cutaneous squamous cell carcinoma of the head and neck and the potential implications for treatment. Head Neck. 36(11):1611–1618. doi:10.1002/hed.23509. Epub 2013 Dec 18

Pereira C, Kruger EA, Sayer G et al (2013) Mohs versus surgical excision in nonmelanoma skin cancers: does location matter? Ann Plast Surg. 70(4):432–434. doi:10.1097/SAP.0b013e3182834b47

Petit JY, Avril MF, Margulis A et al (2010) Evaluation of cosmetic results of a randomized trial comparing surgery and radiotherapy in the treatment of basal cell carcinoma of the face. Plast Reconst Surg June 105(7):2544–2551

Phan GQ, Messina JL, Sondak VK et al (2009) Sentinel lymph node biopsy for melanoma: indications and rationale. Cancer Control. 16(3):234–239

Porceddu SV (2015) Prognostic factors and the role of adjuvant radiation therapy in non-melanoma skin cancer of the head and neck. Am Soc Clin Oncol Book: e513–e518. doi:10.14694/EdBook_AM.2015.35.e513

Poulsen M et al (2003) High risk Merkel cell carcinoma of the skin treated with synchronous carboplatin/etoposide and radiation: a Trans-Tasman Radiation Oncology Group Study, TROG 96:07. J Clin Oncol 21:4371–4376

Rodriguez R, Fontanesi J, Meyer JL et al (1989) Normal-tissue effects of irradiation for Kaposi's sarcoma/AIDS. Front Radiat Ther Oncol 23:150–159

Rofstad EK (1994) Fractionation sensitivity (alpha/beta ratio) of human melanoma xenografts. Radiother Oncol 33(2):133–138

Rogers HW, Weinstock MA, Feldman SR et al (2015) Incidence estimate of nonmelanoma skin cancer (keratinocyte carcinomas) in the U.S. population, 2012. JAMA Dermatol 151(10):1081–1086. doi:10.1001/jamadermatol.2015.1187

Rudnick EW (2015) Oral therapy for nonmelanoma skin cancer in patients with advanced disease and large tumor burden: a review of the literature with focus on a new generation of targeted therapies. Int J Dermatol. doi:10.1111/ijd.12961. [Epub ahead of print]

Sause WT, Cooper J, Rush S et al (1991) Fraction size in external beam radiation therapy in the treatment of melanoma. Int J Radiat Oncol Biol Phys 20(1):429–432

Seegenschmiedt MH, Keilholz L, Altendorf-Hofmann A et al (1999) Palliative radiotherapy for recurrent and metastatic malignant melanoma: prognostic factors for tumor response and long-term outcome: a 20-year experience. Int J Radiat Oncol Biol Phys 44(3):607–618

Sekulic A (2015) Pivotal ERIVANCE basal cell carcinoma (BCC) study: 12 month update of efficacy and safety of vismodegib in advanced BCC. J Am Acad Dermatol 72(6):1021–6.e8. doi:10.1016/j.jaad.2015.03.021

Servy A, Maubec E, Sugier PE et al (2016) Merkel cell carcinoma: value of sentinel lymph-node status and adjuvant radiation therapy. Ann Oncol 27(5):914–919. doi:10.1093/annonc/mdw035. Epub 2016 Jan 24

Shi J, Zhou W, Zhu B, et al (2016) Rare germline copy number variations and disease susceptibility in familial melanoma. J Invest Dermatol. doi:10.1016/j.jid.2016.07.023. pii: S0022-202X(16)32229-1. Epub ahead of Print

Sibaud V, David I, Lamant L et al (2015) Acute skin reaction suggestive of pembrolizumab induced radiosensitization. Melanoma Res. 25(6):555–558. doi:10.1097/CMR.0000000000000191

Silverman MK, Kopf A, Gladstein AH et al (1992) Recurrence rates of treated basal cell carcinomas. J Dermat Surg Oncol 18:549–554

Singh N, Lakier R, Donde B (2008) Hypofractionated radiation therapy in the treatment of epidemic Kaposi sarcoma. A prospective randomized trial. Radiother Oncol 88:211–216

Siva S, Byrne K, Seel M et al (2013) 18F-FDG PET provides high-impact and powerful prognostic stratification in the staging of Merkel cell carcinoma: a 15-year institutional experience. J Nucl Med. 54(8):1223–1229. doi:10.2967/jnumed.112.116814. Epub 2013 Jun 10

Song SS, Goldenberg A, Ortiz A et al (2016) Nonmelanoma skin cancer with aggressive subclinical extension in immunosuppressed patients. JAMA Dermatol. doi:10.1001/jamadermatol.2016.0192. [Epub ahead of print]

Specht L, Dabaja B, Illidge T et al (2015) Modern radiation therapy for primary cutaneous lymphomas: field and dose guidelines from the International Lymphoma Radiation Oncology Group. Int J Radiat Oncol Biol Phys 92(1):32–39

Spurgeon M, Lambert PF (2013) Merkel cell polyomavirus: a newly discovered human virus with oncogenic potential. Virol 435(1):118–130. doi:10.1016/j.virol.2012009.029

SR MK, Hatfield P, Prestwich R et al (2015) Radiotherapy for benign disease; assessing the risk of radiation-induced cancer following exposure to intermediate dose radiation. British J. Radiol 88(1056):20150405. doi:10.1259/bjr.20150405

Stein ME, Lakier R, Kuten A et al (1993) Radiation therapy in endemic (African) Kaposi's sarcoma. Int J Radiat Oncol Biol Phys 27(5):1181–1184

Stelzer K, Griffin T (1993) A randomized prospective trial of radiation therapy for aids-associated Kaposi's sarcoma. Int J Radiat Oncol Biol Phys 27(5):1057–1061

Stern RS, Liebman J, Vakeva L (1998) Oral psoralen and ultraviolet-A light (PUVA) treatment of psoriasis and persistent risk of nonmelanoma skin cancer. J Natl Cancer Inst 90(17):1278–1284

Stratigos A, Garbe C, Lebbe C et al (2015) Diagnosis and treatment of invasive squamous cell carcinoma of the skin: European consensus-based interdisciplinary guideline. European Organization for Research and Treatment of Cancer (EORTC); European Dermatology Forum (EDF); European Association of Dermato-Oncology (EADO). Eur J Cancer 51(14):1989–2007. doi:10.1016/j.ejca.2015.06.110. Epub 2015 Jul 25

Strom T, Carr M, Zager JS et al (2016) Radiation therapy is associated with improved outcomes in Merkel cell carcinoma. Ann Surg Oncol. doi:10.1245/s10434-016-5293-1

Thomas T, Agrawal P, Guitart J et al (2013) Outcome of Patients treated with a single-fraction dose of palliative radiation for cutaneous T-cell lymphoma. Int J Radiat Oncol Biol Phys 85(3):747–753

Toker C (1972) Trabecular carcinoma of the skin. Arch Dermatol 105:107–110

Trombetta M, Packard M, Velosa C et al (2011) Merkel cell tumor of the skin treated with localized radiotherapy: are widely negative margins required? Rare Tumors 3(1):e12. doi:10.4081/rt.2011.e12

Tsao MN, Tsang R, Liu F-F et al (2002) Radiotherapy management for squamous cell carcinoma of the nasal skin: the Princess Margaret Hospital experience. Int J Radiat Oncol Biol Phys 52(4):973–979

Turcotte LM, Whitton J, Friedman D et al (2015) Risk of subsequent neoplasms during the fifth and sixth decades of life in the childhood cancer survivor study cohort. J Clin Oncol 33(31):3568–3575

Wagner JD, Evdokimow D, Weisberger E et al (2004) Sentinel node biopsy for high-risk nonmelanoma cutaneous malignancy. Arch Dermatol. 140:75–79

WebMD, LLC (2009) Picture of skin, Anatomy of skin Fig. 1

Wehner MR, Shive ML, Chren MM et al (2012) Indoor tanning and non-melanoma skin cancer: systematic review and meta-analysis. BMJ 345:e5909. doi:10.1136/bmj.e5909

Weninger W (1999) Expression of vascular endothelial growth factor receptor-3 and podoplanin suggest a lymphatic endothelial origin of Kaposi's sarcoma tumor cells. Lab Invest 79:243–251

Wilder RB, Shimm D, John M, Kittelson J et al (1991) Recurrent basal cell carcinoma treated with radiation therapy. Arch Dermatol 127:1668–1672

Willemze R, Jaffe G (2005) WHO-EORTC classification for cutaneous lymphomas. Blood 105:3768–3785

Wilson AW, Howsam G, Santhanam V et al (2004) Surgical management of incompletely excised basal cell carcinoma of the head and neck. Br J Oral Maxillofac Surg 42:311–314

de Wit R, Smit W, Veenhof KH et al (1990) Palliative radiation therapy for AIDS-associated Kaposi's sarcoma by using a single fraction of 800 cGy. Radiother Oncol 19(2):131–136

Zagrodnik B, Kempf W, Seifert B et al (2003) Superficial radiotherapy for patients with basal cell carcinoma, recurrence rates, histologic subtypes, and expression of p53 and Bcl-2. Cancer 98(12):2708–2714

Radiotherapy for Primary and Metastatic Soft Tissue Sarcomas: Altered Fraction Regimens with External Beam and Brachytherapy

Sara Alcorn and Stephanie Terezakis

Contents

Abstract

This chapter describes altered fraction regimens used in the management of localized and metastatic soft tissue sarcomas. Rationale, disease outcomes, toxicity, and planning and delivery methodology are provided for stereotactic radiotherapy, interdigitated chemoradiation, intraoperative radiation therapy, and postoperative interstitial brachytherapy techniques.

1 Introduction

Soft tissue sarcomas are a relatively uncommon malignancy, accounting for 1% of adult cancers and resulting in 5000 deaths annually in the USA (Siegel et al. 2015). Arising from cells of mesenchymal origin, sarcomas are classified by the World Health Organization (WHO) into more than 100 histologic subtypes (Fletcher et al. 2013), demonstrating the high degree of heterogeneity within this disease entity. Primary location varies by histologic subtype and includes extremities (60%), trunk (30%), and head and neck (9%) sites (Lawrence et al. 1987). Staging and expected outcomes are based on tumor grade, size, deep versus superficial location, and presence of nodal and distant metastases (Edge et al. 2010).

Despite advances in both local and systemic management, 5-year overall survival from sarcoma remains at 50%. Approximately half of sarcomas are localized at diagnosis, corresponding to a 5-year overall survival of 83%, with survival declining to

S. Alcorn • S. Terezakis (✉)
The Johns Hopkins Hospital, Baltimore, MD, USA
e-mail: sterezak@jhmi.edu

Med Radiol Radiat Oncol (2017)
DOI 10.1007/174_2017_40, © Springer International Publishing AG
Published Online: 14 June 2017

54% and 16% for regional and distant disease involvement, respectively. However, there are few relapses among patients surviving past 5 years, suggesting that effective early local therapy can be curative (American Cancer Society 2016).

Historically, curative intent was achieved by aggressive primary surgery. Yet over time, surgical management evolved from extensive amputations to more conservative localized resections aimed at perseveration of function, with the addition of radiotherapy for enhanced local control (Tepper and Suit 1985; Lindberg et al. 1981). As such, current management for the majority of localized sarcoma is wide local excision with the addition of either external beam radiotherapy (EBRT) and/or brachytherapy (BT) (Holloway et al. 2013). The exception is superficial, low-grade tumors less than 5 cm that may be treated with surgery alone (Baldini et al. 1999; Pisters et al. 1996).

Radiotherapy may be administered in the preoperative, intraoperative, or postoperative setting. Data from the National Cancer Institute of Canada (NCIC) demonstrate no significant difference between preoperative EBRT to 50 Gy and postoperative EBRT to 66–70 Gy for 5-year local control (93% vs. 92%, respectively) and overall survival (73% vs. 67%, respectively) (O'Sullivan 2004). However, given high rates of fibrosis, edema, and joint stiffness in the postoperative setting, preoperative radiation is generally preferred despite the potential for increased wound complications (Davis et al. 2005). Intraoperative radiotherapy (IORT) has also been investigated and is reviewed in additional detail below.

Despite technologic advances in radiotherapy such as image guidance and intensity-modulated radiotherapy, the use of conventionally fractionated EBRT for sarcomas has its limitations. Primarily problematic are the relatively high doses needed to achieve local control as well as the relatively large margins used in both the pre- and postoperative setting for sarcoma. Preoperative EBRT is generally delivered to approximately 45–50 Gy and postoperative EBRT typically requires doses from 60 to 72 Gy, using GTV to CTV margins of approximately 1.5–2 cm radially and 3–3.5 cm in the longitudinal direction. Indeed, target size and dose may preclude the use of postoperative radiotherapy in the management of many retroperitoneal sarco-

mas due to side effects from nearby dose-limiting structures such as bowel (Ballo et al. 2007). Even in the postoperative setting, relatively high rates of complications including grade 2 fibrosis (31%) (Davis et al. 2005) may be amplified by the large volume used with EBRT. Moreover, both the preoperative and postoperative approaches require lengthy treatment courses ranging from 25 to 36 fractions.

As such, alternative approaches are being increasingly investigated, including the use of stereotactic radiotherapy (SRT) and interdigitated chemoradiation (ICR). These strategies allow for relative sparing of normal tissue through either reduction in the treatment volume or reduction of the total radiation dose, respectively, and provide novel means for addressing aggressive localized and metastatic sarcomas. Furthermore, although not a new technology, we also review the use of IORT and postoperative interstitial brachytherapy (IBT) as means for localized dose escalation. Each of these strategies not only offer the potential for an improved therapeutic index but also permit foreshortened treatment times—which may improve patient quality of life, lower health care costs, and reduce the time spent off systemic therapy when indicated.

2 Stereotactic Radiotherapy (SRT)

The use of SRT combines multiple noncoplanar beams with special immobilization procedures to deliver highly precise radiotherapy. Due to its characteristic rapid dose falloff and high conformality, high doses can be administered to the target with relative sparing to adjacent normal tissue. As such, SRT may avoid some of the pitfalls of traditional EBRT by delivering the high doses required to treat sarcomas while minimizing toxicity related to the large target volumes used in current practice. In addition, due to the direct cell kill afforded by high fractional doses of radiotherapy, SRT may also improve efficacy of treatment through the impact of vascular and stromal damage (Kirkpatrick et al. 2008). These additional means of cellular damage may be especially important in relatively radioresistant tumor types such as sarcoma. Although its use in a number of clinical settings is being investigated, SRT for sarcoma is best described in the management of localized sarcomas of the spine as well as in sites of metastatic involvement including the spine and lung. Lastly, SRT may have a specific role in the management of oligometastatic sarcomas.

2.1 Indications and Rationale

2.1.1 Primary Sarcomas of the Spinal Area

Primary sarcomas of the spinal area pose a unique management challenge. First, proximity to or involvement of the neuraxis may limit the extent of resection achievable, with one series showing that only 15% of patients with spinal sarcomas had tumors amenable to marginal or wide resection (Bilsky et al. 2001). Moreover, the doses needed to treat such sarcomas would often exceed the traditional dose tolerance of the spinal cord. Thus, it is unsurprising that one series by Merimsky et al. treating 19 patients with spinal cord compression from soft tissue sarcoma to a tolerable but palliative dose of 30 Gy in 8–10 fractions with conventional EBRT yielded modest outcomes, with a poor median survival of 5 months (Merimsky et al. 2004).

Conversely, delivery of SRT to primary spinal sarcomas using hypofractionated regimens shows significant promise. Chang et al. treated 32 spinal sarcomas including 10 primary tumors to doses ranging from 16 to 45 Gy in 1–3 fractions (Chang et al. 2012). SRT was the first line of therapy for 26 lesions and was the sole treatment modality for 17 of these lesions. The study reported a median overall survival of 29 months. Complications of treatment were not reported. Similarly, Levine et al. retrospectively evaluated 30 spinal sarcomas treated with SRT to a median dose of 30 Gy in 3 fractions (Levine et al. 2009). Seven patients were treated with definitive SRT, seven were treated with SRT following surgery with and without preoperative radiotherapy, and ten were treated for metastatic disease. Of those managed with definitive SRT for primary sarcomas of the spine, there were no deaths reported during the minimum follow-up interval of 12 months. Complications were uncommon, with two patients developing transient radiculopathy lasting <6 months. Table 1 summarizes these select studies regarding radiotherapy for spinal sarcomas. Such data support the role for SRT in this setting, particularly among patients who are not candidates for complete surgical resection.

2.1.2 Metastatic Sites

Although curative intent may not be possible, SRT appears to serve a vital role in the symptomatic management of metastatic sarcomas for sites

Table 1 Selected studies of radiotherapy for primary and metastatic spinal sarcomas

Study	Patient population	Radiotherapy delivered	Follow-up	Main outcomes
Merimsky et al. (2004)	23 spinal sarcomas causing spinal cord compression in 19 patients—17 metastatic and 2 primary tumors	30 Gy in 8–10 fractions using conventional radiotherapy with 1–2 fields	• Not specified	• 61% with improvement of neurological signs and/or Karnofsky performance status. • Median survival after diagnosis of spinal cord compression = 5 months
Levine et al. (2009)	30 spinal sarcomas in 24 patients—7 primary definitive, 7 primary postoperative, and 16 metastatic tumors	Median of 20–34 Gy in 1–5 fractions using SRT	• Mean 33 and 43 months for primary definitive and postoperative tumors, respectively. • Not specified for metastatic tumors	• 29% primary tumors treated recurred with no deaths for patients treated with definitive SRT • 50% complete, 44% partial, and 6% no pain response and mean survival of 11 months for metastatic tumors
Chang et al. (2012)	32 spinal sarcomas in 27 patients—10 primary and 22 metastatic tumors	16–45 Gy in 1–3 fractions using SRT	• Median 22 months	• 0.5-, 1-, and 2-year pain control = 89.3%, 68.2%, and 61.5%, respectively. • 0.5-, 1-, and 2-year radiologic local control = 96.7%, 78.3%, and 76.9%, respectively. • Median survival = 29 months

SRT stereotactic radiotherapy

including the brain, spine, and lung. Moreover, SRT may have a particularly efficacious role in the management of oligometastatic disease sites from sarcoma.

2.1.2.1 Brain Metastases

For management of brain metastases, there is evidence that hypofractionated SRT may improve efficacy of treatment vs. conventional EBRT. Whereas metastatic sarcoma is generally felt to be radioresistant to standard palliative whole-brain EBRT to 30 Gy in ten fractions, sarcoma brain metastases have been found to have local control rates that are equivalent or superior to those seen for radiosensitive histologies when treated with high-dose SRT (Boyd and Mehta 1999).

For example, Mehta et al. reported a complete response rate of 67% for sarcomas and melanomas after delivery of single-fraction SRT to a mean dose of 24 Gy. No significant acute toxicities were reported, with 10% of patients requiring long-term steroid use after treatment (Mehta et al. 1992). The incidence of symptomatic radionecrosis was not reported in the study, but a rate of 17% at 1 year has been reported for brain SRT treating to similar doses (Kohutek et al. 2015).

2.1.2.2 Spine Metastases

Similarly, improved outcomes have been seen for SRT delivered to spinal metastases from sarcoma. As noted, conventional EBRT with palliative doses of 30 Gy in 8–10 fractions has been delivered in the case of spinal cord compression, with small but measurable improvement in pain and performance status as reported by Merimsky et al. (2004). However, outcomes may be substantially improved through the delivery of SRT. The above studies by Chang and Levine also included patients with metastatic spinal sarcomas and showed substantially improved median survival and symptom control as compared to the 30 Gy regimen (Chang et al. 2012; Levine et al. 2009). See Table 1 for further details.

2.1.2.3 Lung Metastases

SRT for pulmonary metastases from sarcoma shows excellent local control rates and may be particularly useful in nonsurgical candidates. Navarria et al. treated 51 sarcoma lung lesions (not suitable for surgical resection) with SRT to doses including 30 Gy in one fraction, 60 Gy in three fractions, 60 Gy in eight fractions, and 48 Gy in four fractions (Navarria et al. 2015). Actuarial 5-year local control was 96%, with 5-year overall survival of 60.5%. Dhakal et al. similarly treated 74 pulmonary metastases from sarcoma to a preferred schedule of 50 Gy in 5 fractions over 2 weeks (Dhakal et al. 2012). Local control at 3 years was 82%, and medial survival was 2.1 years. Neither study reported any grade 3 or 4 toxicities.

2.1.2.4 Oligometastases

A subset of metastatic disease that may particularly benefit from SRT is oligometastatic disease. Oligometastasis refers to an intermediate disease state between localized disease and widespread metastasis, potentially associated with improved prognosis as compared to disseminated metastatic disease. Generally, this is defined as disease limited to 1–5 detectable metastases, although the specific number of metastatic sites varies by protocol (Milano et al. 2008; Salama et al. 2012). In such cases, aggressive local management including the use of SRT may be curative. Retrospective series evaluating the use of SRT to a limited number of extracranial metastases has shown local control rates of 67–95%, with 2- to 3-year survival of 30–64% (Corbin et al. 2013). These survival rates are comparable to those reported for surgical resection. Results from prospective protocols are similarly promising. Corbin et al. offer an excellent review of the use of SRT in oligometastatic disease including for patients with sarcoma (Corbin et al. 2013). Of note, sarcoma is one of the most frequently reported tumor histologies in surgical series of oligometastases, highlighting the role for treatment along a potentially curable paradigm for this disease entity.

2.2 SRT Procedure

2.2.1 Treatment Planning

Table 2 describes treatment planning and delivery methods commonly used for photon-based SRT in primary spine and metastatic sites. Proton therapy may also be utilized for highly conformal treatment of sarcoma but will not be described in the context of this review.

Table 2 Treatment planning techniques for stereotactic radiotherapy by disease site

Site	Primary planning modality	Image sets for fusion if indicated	Immobilization	Position	Respiratory motion management	Other considerations
Spine[a] (primary or metastatic)	CT or MRI	MRI, CT myelogram, PET	Thermoplastic mask or rigid frame for upper spine lesions, vacuum bag or alpha cradle for lower spine lesions	Supine, arms at sides for upper spine lesions, arms on chest for mid and lower spine lesions	–	Consider fiducial placement for target localization
Brain[a]	CT or MRI	MRI	Thermoplastic mask or rigid frame	Supine, arms at sides	–	–
Head and neck	CT	MRI, PET	Thermoplastic mask	Supine, arms at sides	–	–
Thorax	CT	MRI, PET	Vacuum bag or alpha cradle with wing board or U-frame	Supine, arms up	Consider 4-D CT, active breathing control, respiratory gating, or abdominal compression	Consider fiducial placement for target localization
Abdomen	CT	MRI, PET	Vacuum bag or alpha cradle	Supine, arms on chest	Consider 4-D CT, active breathing control, respiratory gating, or abdominal compression	Consider fiducial placement for target localization, consider NPO 1–3 h prior to treatment
Pelvis	CT	MRI, PET	Vacuum bag or alpha cradle	Supine, arms on chest	–	–
Extremity (metastatic)	CT	MRI, PET	Vacuum bag or alpha cradle	Supine or prone, in position that allows for greatest distance between the target and the trunk and/or contralateral extremity. Consider a neutral position for the limb to maintain reproducibility	–	–

NPO withhold food and fluids

[a]Spine and brain sites may be treated by either gantry- or robotic-based linear accelerator or Gamma Knife®. All other sites are generally treated by a gantry- or robotic-based linear accelerator

2.2.2 Target Volumes

2.2.2.1 Brain

The treatment target for brain metastases is typically the gross tumor volume identified on contrast-enhanced imaging (CT and/or T1-weighted MRI). Gamma Knife®-based (Elekta AB, Stockholm, Sweden) treatment is delivered without a margin, whereas gantry- and robotic-based linear accelerator treatments are delivered with a margin of 0–2 mm from gross tumor volume (GTV) to planning treatment volume (PTV). A clinical target volume (CTV) to account for subclinical disease spread is generally not included for brain SRT.

2.2.2.2 Spine

The International Spine Radiosurgery Consortium Consensus Guidelines (Cox et al. 2012) specify target volumes for spine SRT as follows:

- *GTV: Includes contrast-enhancing gross disease on CT, T1-weighted MRI, and/or CT myelogram. PET images may also assist in identification of the GTV.*
- *CTV: Includes the GTV plus areas of abnormal marrow signal on CT or T2-weighted MRI as well as adjacent normal-appearing bone felt to be at risk for subclinical disease involvement. The guidelines offer specific recommendations for the extent of adjacent bone that should be covered based on the site of gross involvement.*
- *PTV: Includes the CTV plus an expansion ≤3 mm.*

2.2.2.3 Lung

SRT for metastatic sarcoma generally follows guidelines for SRT management of primary lung lesions but may vary by protocol. However, a standard means for target delineation adapted from Radiation Therapy Oncology Group (RTOG) 0915 (RTOG Foundation 2014) is as follows:

- *GTV: Includes gross disease as defined on pulmonary CT windows. Although not specified by the protocol, PET and MRI images may also be fused to the primary CT image set to aid in target delineation.*
- *Internal target volume (ITV): A 4-dimensional CT (4-D CT) image can be performed to account for tumor motion with respiration. If performed, then an ITV can be defined to encompass maximal excursion of the GTV with respiratory motion.*
- *PTV without the use of 4-D CT: Includes GTV plus an expansion of 0.5 cm radially and 1 cm in the superior-inferior dimension.*
- *PTV with the use of 4-D CT: Includes GTV/ITV plus a uniform margin of 0.5 cm.*
- *PTV if additional measures are taken to account for respiratory motion such as active breathing control, respiratory gating, and abdominal compression: Includes GTV plus a uniform expansion of approximately 0.5 cm.*

2.2.2.4 Other Metastatic Sites Including Oligometastases

Target volume delineation of other metastatic disease is site dependent. Ahmed et al. offer a recent review including description of SRT trials of the spine, liver, lung, and other sites of oligometastases (Ahmed and Torres-Roca 2016).

2.2.3 Dose Prescriptions

2.2.3.1 Brain

Dose prescriptions for brain metastases vary by size of tumor and modality of delivery. RTOG 90–05 specifies maximum tolerable doses based on target size for single-fraction brain SRT as 24 Gy, 18 Gy, and 15 Gy for lesions ≤2 cm, 2–3 cm, and >3–4 cm, respectively (Shaw et al. 1996). The study was designed with treatment via Gamma Knife®, and doses were delivered to the 50–90% isodose line. Nieder et al. provide a review of single-fraction SRT for brain metastasis, including a range of doses utilized with and without whole-brain radiotherapy (Nieder et al. 2014).

Other hypofractionated stereotactic schemes are reported for lesions that are large in size, proximate to dose-limiting structures, or otherwise not amendable to single-fraction treatment. These include regimens to 21 Gy in three fractions, 24 Gy in four fractions, 40 Gy in four fractions, 30 Gy in five fractions, and 35 Gy in five fractions (Eaton et al. 2013; Fahrig et al. 2007).

2.2.3.2 Spine and Other Sites

Dose prescriptions for SRT of spine, lung, and other sites also vary widely by disease extent, location, and modality. For spine SRT, fractionation regimens reported include 16–24 Gy in one fraction, 24–27 Gy in three fractions, and 25–30 Gy in five fractions (Kumar et al. 2015). Extrapolating from primary lung cancer treatments, SRT to pulmonary sites can be delivered in regimens of 48–50 Gy in 4 fractions, 45–66 Gy in 3 fractions, 50–60 Gy in 5 fractions, and 60–70 Gy in 8–10 fractions, with single and three-fraction regimens preferred for small tumors (generally <2 cm) located >1 cm from the chest wall (Benedict et al. 2010; NCCN 2017). The RTOG recommends prescribing to the 60–90% isodose line, and dosimetric goals are listed for target coverage and avoidance of adjacent normal structures (RTOG Foundation 2014). A breadth of regimens have been described for the management of oligometastatic disease; as noted above, Ahmed et al. provided a recent review including fractionation regimens used and outcomes for spine, liver, lung, and other oligometastatic sites (Ahmed and Torres-Roca 2016). As an additional resource for management of a variety of sites with SRT, the American Association of Physicists in Medicine (AAPM) Task Group 101 includes a detailed description of dose prescriptions, beam selection, and normal tissue dose tolerances for SRT according to a number of fractionation regimens (Benedict et al. 2010).

2.2.4 Image Guidance

The majority of sites should be managed with daily pretreatment imaging using cone-beam CT, fluoroscopy, or kV/MV planar imaging modalities. Fiducials may be placed to assist with image guidance, particularly for lung, liver and other abdominal, and spine sites.

---

3 Interdigitated Chemoradiation (ICR)

3.1 Indications and Rationale

High histologic grade and large tumor size are predictive of poor outcome in sarcoma (Potter et al. 1985; Spiro et al. 1997). As a mean to address this particularly high-risk group, ICR regimens have been investigated. In this setting, ICR therapy is particularly attractive in that it both (1) shortens

the time spent without receiving systemic therapy for this group with high metastatic potential and (2) offers a means to preoperatively reduce large tumor bulk and improve resection rates. DeLaney et al. retrospectively reviewed treatment of 48 patients with high-grade extremity sarcomas ≥8 cm managed with ICR at a single institution (DeLaney et al. 2003). Patients received interdigitated mesna, adriamycin, ifosfamide, and dacarbazine (MAID) chemotherapy with EBRT to 44 Gy delivered as two courses of 22 Gy in 11 fractions. This was followed by surgical resection and a 16 Gy postoperative boost with EBRT for margin-positive disease, followed by three additional cycles of adjuvant MAID. Whereas the 5-year local control rate was comparable to that of historic controls (92% vs. 86%, respectively), overall survival rates were higher (87% vs. 58%) with the ICR regimen.

These data provided the basis for RTOG 9514, a phase II trial of a similar regimen of ICR administered to 64 patients with high-grade sarcomas of the extremities and torso measuring ≥8 cm (Kraybill et al. 2006). Results showed somewhat lower efficacy of therapy as compared to the DeLaney et al. report, with a 3-year local control rate of 82% and overall survival of 75%. This may have been in part due to a larger proportion of participants with grade 3 (as opposed to grade 2) sarcoma in the RTOG cohort. However, there was also significantly higher toxicity in the RTOG protocol group, with three treatment-related deaths (5%) and grade 4 toxicity (mostly hematologic) experienced by 83% of patients. This was felt to be attributable to the 25% increase in ifosfamide dose in the regimen administered by the RTOG. Of note, given low rates of local failure and favorable pathological response rates in both protocols, the radiotherapy dose delivered was felt to be appropriate for this high-risk group.

3.2 Procedure

Sequence of interdigitated therapy as per RTOG 9514 (Kraybill et al. 2006):

1. *First cycle of mesna, adriamycin, ifosfamide, and dacarbazine (MAID) chemotherapy*
2. *EBRT to 22 Gy in 11 fractions*

3. *A second cycle of MAID*
4. *An additional 22 Gy of EBRT*
5. *A third cycle of MAID*
6. *Surgical resection*
7. *A 16 Gy postoperative boost with EBRT for margin-positive disease*
8. *Three additional cycles of adjuvant MAID*

Neoadjuvant EBRT is prescribed to a total dose of 44 Gy in 22 fractions, delivered as a split course of 22 Gy in 11 fractions each over the course of 13–15 days. The first course of EBRT is delivered 3 days following the first cycle of MAID, and the second course is administered 3 days following the second cycle of MAID. Computed tomography and MR imaging are used to define the primary lesion and areas felt to be at risk for microscopic disease. Coverage of the entire compartment is not required. If the expansion extends beyond the compartment, the field can be reduced such that the volume encompasses the end of the compartment. Attempts should be made to not treat the full circumference of the extremity. Surgical resection is performed by day 80 following three cycles of MAID and 44 Gy of EBRT. This regimen is appropriate for patients in whom an R0 resection is felt to be achievable. Postoperative EBRT to 16 Gy in eight fractions is recommended for patients with margins positive for residual disease and should be delivered starting 14 days following surgery.

4 Intraoperative Radiation Therapy (IORT)

4.1 Indications and Rationale

IORT is delivered as a single fraction using electrons, low-energy photons, or BT techniques. Such approaches allow for delivery of high doses of radiation, with biological effectiveness of up to threefold higher than a similar total dose delivered with conventionally fractionated EBRT (Suit 1971). The therapeutic ratio is improved through protection of normal tissues by the use of lead shielding or exclusion from the treatment field via retraction. In general, electron- and photon-based IORT provides improved dose homogeneity throughout the depth of a target whereas BT-based IORT allows for concentration of dose at the surface of the target. While low-energy electrons are delivered with a rigid cone that may limit use in certain clinical situations, BT-based IORT uses flap applicators to enhance flexibility (Moningi et al. 2014; Calvo et al. 2006).

IORT is frequently used in combination with EBRT delivered before or after surgery (Pawlik et al. 2007). While specific clinical indications vary, IORT is likely most efficacious in settings where there is risk of residual microscopic disease and proximity to radiosensitive normal structures that may limit delivery of sufficient doses of conventionally fractionated EBRT. Patients with recurrent tumors at previously irradiated sites for which repeat EBRT is not feasible may also benefit from IORT.

4.1.1 Retroperitoneal Sarcomas

Although potentially beneficial in other clinical contexts, IORT has been best described in the setting of retroperitoneal sarcomas. As noted above, retroperitoneal location may limit the ability to deliver doses sufficient for tumor kill with conventionally fractionated EBRT due to proximity to radiosensitive normal structures such as the bowel. As such, IORT provides a means for dose escalation while limiting bowel toxicity.

A number of studies have evaluated the use of IORT alone and in combination with pre- or post-operative EBRT in this setting. Sindelar et al. completed the only randomized trial of IORT, with 35 patients randomized to treatment with 20 Gy electron-based IORT and postoperative EBRT to 35–40 Gy vs. postoperative EBRT to 50–55 Gy alone (Sindelar et al. 1993). Locoregional control was improved by the addition of IORT from 20% vs. 60%, although overall survival was similar between groups. Rates of enteritis were lower within the IORT arm than in the EBRT-alone arm (13% vs. 50%, respectively), but rates of peripheral neuropathy were higher (60% vs. 5%). Gieschen et al. retrospectively reviewed treatment of 37 patients with primary or recurrent retroperitoneal sarcomas managed with preoperative EBRT to 45 Gy followed by surgery, with or without electron-based IORT to 10–20 Gy (Gieschen et al.

2001). For the 29 patients with gross total resection, the 5-year local control was 83% vs. 61% and overall survival was 74% vs. 30% for those treated with vs. without IORT, respectively. The neuropathy rate among those who received IORT was 15%. Similar results are reported elsewhere (Ballo et al. 2007; Dziewirski et al. 2006; Schuck et al. 1997; Rachbauer et al. 2003; Krempien et al. 2006; Alektiar et al. 2000a) including with low-energy photon IORT (Dubois et al. 1995; Tran et al. 2008).

4.1.2 Extremity Sarcomas

Although its role is less well defined, literature exits regarding the use of IORT in combination with EBRT for extremity sarcomas as well. IORT in this setting may be particularly beneficial for recurrent disease limiting reirradiation with EBRT. Kretzler et al. treated 28 patients with localized recurrent, high grade, or incompletely resected sarcomas of the extremities with a median dose of 15 Gy using high dose rate (HDR) BT or linear accelerator-based IORT, with 90% of patients receiving postoperative EBRT to a mean dose of 50.6 Gy (Kretzler et al. 2004). Five-year local control and overall survival were 84% and 66%, respectively. Niewald et al. retrospectively reviewed treatment of 38 primary and recurrent sarcomas, 27 of whom had tumors located in the extremities (Niewald et al. 2009). All received HDR BT-based IORT to 8–15 Gy at 0.5 cm depth, followed by ERBT to doses of 23–56 Gy in 82% of patients. Five-year local control and overall survival were 63% and 57%, respectively. Late skin toxicity and wound healing complications occurred in 42% and 16% of patients, respectively, with no cases of neuropathy reported.

At least one study suggests that target volume-dependent fibrosis may limit the use of IORT in the extremities. Van Kampden et al. treated 53 patients with extremity sarcoma to 15 Gy using electron-based IORT followed by postoperative EBRT to a mean dose of 46 Gy (van Kampen et al. 2001). A target volume of 210 cm^3 was associated with a 5% risk (95% confidence interval 1–20%) of development of grade 3 or 4 fibrosis. This rate increased to 50% with IORT volumes >420 cm^3.

Other series reporting the use of electrons (Azinovic et al. 2003; Tran et al. 2006), low-energy photons (Dubois et al. 1995; Tran et al. 2008), and LDR (Llácer et al. 2006; Delannes et al. 2000) IORT for sarcoma of the extremities are available.

4.2 Procedure

Common to all IORT techniques, the operating physician and radiation oncology team must decide prior to surgery if IORT is potentially required. If so, treatment must occur in a space with sufficient shielding for a given IORT technique, either in the operating room or in the radiation oncology department. An exception is for self-shielding mobile electron devices, which may not require additional shielding (Beddar a et al. 2006). Staff specifically trained in interdisciplinary management of patients receiving IORT must be available, including anesthesiologists, medical physicists, and nursing (Moningi et al. 2014).

Once the tumor is maximally resected, surgical and radiation oncology staff collaborate to identify and measure the at-risk region of the surgical bed. Retraction of surrounding muscle and bowel should be optimized to isolate the target area and reduce dose to normal structures. Lead shielding (wrapped in wet gauze or wax to reduce backscatter) should be applied to sensitive structures that cannot be retracted such as the ureters. All IORT procedures should be performed with sterile methodology. Further IORT technique is then determined by the method of delivery, as described below. After completion of treatment, an appropriate radiation survey for exposure levels at controlled and uncontrolled areas must be performed.

4.2.1 Technique

4.2.1.1 HDR Brachytherapy

Flexible flap devices are most commonly used for HDR BT-based IORT, generally with an Ir-192 source. One such device is the Freiburg Flap (Nucletron, Elekta AB, Stockholm, Sweden), which utilizes a linear arrangement of silicone rubber balls connected in flexible sheets with predrilled holes through which 6-French afterloading catheters are threaded prior to treatment. Another similar device is the Harrison-Anderson-Mick (HAM) applicator (also a product of Nucletron, Elekta AB), which uses catheters that come preimbedded in a sheet of flexible plastic. The procedure is as follows:

- *The flap is cut to fit the target area of interest. In the case of the Freiburg applicator, catheters are inserted into the sheets and held in place with metal buttons.*
- *Labels are affixed to the catheters, generally with one numbered label at the proximal end of the catheter and with another label with the same number at the distal end of the catheter where it inserts into the flap. These numbers generally correspond to the channel number of the HDR afterloader.*
- *The flap is placed into the at-risk surgical bed and held in the desired location with packing material such as laparotomy sponges.*
- *An inactive dummy wire is threaded through the catheters to ensure safe passage and retraction of the active source.*
- *Because the intraoperative setting limits the time available for detailed dosimetric calculations, dwell times are determined according to an atlas corresponding to the size of the applicator and the curvature of the treatment field* (Thomadsen 1999).

Moningi et al. offer a useful safety checklist and flowchart for clinical decision making for IORT with the Freiburg flap (Moningi et al. 2014).

4.2.1.2 Electrons

Electron-based IORT generally utilizes either standard linear accelerators or mobile linear acceleration devices to generate electrons. Applicators are used to shape and confine the electron beam to the target volume of interest. Frequently used are cones of varying sizes and shapes (i.e., circular, rectangular) that can be affixed to the head of the electron-generating device. Cones with beveled edges may assist in

treatment sites such as the deep pelvis. The technique is as follows:

- *Once the operative bed is identified, the surgical and radiation oncology teams determine the appropriate applicator for the target.*
- *Electron energies are selected with the goal of covering the estimated thickness of the tumor bed target, using percent depth dose curves that account for the size and shape of the applicator used for a given delivery device* (Beddar a et al. 2006; Gunderson et al. 1982).
- *Beam modifiers such as bolus may be added to the end of the applicator or to the target surface if required to provide adequate superficial dose* (Beddar a et al. 2006).

4.2.1.3 Other

Description of less commonly used modalities including low-energy (e.g., orthovoltage) photon-based IORT (Dubois et al. 1995; Tran et al. 2008) and low dose rate (LDR) BT techniques (Llácer et al. 2006; Delannes et al. 2000). Specific review of these techniques is beyond the scope of this chapter.

4.2.2 Dose Prescriptions

Following neoadjuvant therapy, doses prescribed are generally 10–12 Gy for microscopic residual disease (R1 resections) and >12 Gy (up to 20 Gy) for macroscopic residual disease (R2 resections). In the setting of prior irradiation, doses of 15–20 Gy are administered, particularly if preoperative or postoperative EBRT to doses of 20–30 Gy can be administered. When IORT is used alone, doses to 25–30 Gy can be delivered if not limited by proximate normal structures (Moningi et al. 2014; Calvo et al. 2006; Gunderson et al. 1982).

For HDR BT-based IORT, doses are typically prescribed to a 0.5 cm depth. For electron-based IORT, dose is specified to the 90% isodose and the d_{max} is reported, per American Association of Physicists in Medicine (AAPM) Task Group No. 72 recommendations (Beddar a et al. 2006).

5 Postoperative Interstitial Brachytherapy

5.1 Indications and Rationale

Delivered in the postoperative setting, IBT also permits for the use of high radiation dose to the operative bed while minimizing dose to surrounding normal structures. The therapeutic advantage of IBT is due to the characteristic dose distribution afforded by the inverse square law, with exposure rate being inversely related to distance from the source. With the source inserted into the tumor bed, doses at the target are higher and fall off rapidly as distance from the target structure increases. Specific indications for IBRT include:

(a) *High-grade disease of the extremities and superficial trunk resected to negative margins*
(b) *Controversially, margin-positive disease in combination with EBRT*
(c) *Recurrent disease in combination with EBRT* (Holloway et al. 2013)
(d) *When there is a goal to limit or avoid EBRT due to specific toxicity (as in the case of radiation of pediatric extremity sarcomas near the growth plate)*

Use of IBT alone is limited by site, tumor grade, and extent to which catheters are able to adequately cover the operative bed. In the largest available series using postoperative IBT alone, Alektiar et al. retrospectively reviewed treatment of 202 patients with high-grade extremity sarcoma using postoperative IBT to a median dose of 45 Gy delivered over 5 days (Alektiar et al. 2002). Five-year local control and overall survival rates were 84% and 70%, respectively. Recurrence was significantly associated with upper extremity location and microscopically positive margins, suggesting that IBT alone may be most efficacious when applied in the setting of R0 resection to sites of the lower extremity. Toxicity rates included 12% wound complications requiring reoperation, 5% grade 3 or higher nerve damage, and 3% bone fracture. The benefit of IBT alone appears to be confined to high-grade

disease. Pisters et al. randomized patients with sarcoma of the extremity or trunk to either adjuvant IBT to 42–45 Gy over 5 days or no further treatment (Pisters et al. 1996). Five-year local control rates were significantly improved by IBT for high-grade lesions (82% vs. 69%), but there was no such benefit for IBT in low-grade lesions.

There have been no published randomized, controlled comparisons of IBT vs. EBRT in the management of sarcoma, and the role of combination IBT and EBRT is controversial. Alektiar et al. retrospectively reviewed treatment of 105 patients with primary or recurrent high-grade sarcoma of the extremity using postoperative IBT to 45 Gy over 5 days vs. combination IBT to 15–20 Gy and adjuvant EBRT to 45–50 Gy (Alekhteyar et al. 1996). While 2-year local control did not differ by management of IBT with and without EBRT (90% vs. 82%, respectively; *p*-value 0.32) across all patients, among patients with positive resection margins, there was a trend toward significant local control benefit for combination therapy (90% vs. 59%, respectively; *p*-value 0.08). Wound complication rates were similar across treatments. However, later work by the same group failed to show difference in control rates by radiotherapy type (Alektiar et al. 2000b). Regarding site of treatment, there may be increased toxicity when treating the lower extremity as opposed to the upper extremity with combination IBT and EBRT (Holloway et al. 2013; San Miguel et al. 2011). Per consensus recommendations of the American Brachytherapy Society (ABS), additional factors such as tumor grade and size and prior surgeries can further direct selection of EBRT and IBT. Moreover, combination IBT and EBRT is recommended when managing recurrent disease at sites that have not previously been irradiated (Holloway et al. 2013).

5.2 Procedure

5.2.1 Technique

IBT catheters are placed at the time of surgical excision under sterile procedure. Delivery is performed using LDR sources such as ribbons embedded with Ir-192 vs. HDR sources with a remote afterloader. A summary of ABR's consensus on technique (Holloway et al. 2013) is as follows:

- *The surgical and radiation oncology teams collaborate to define the tumor bed. They may potentially place radio-opaque clips to identify the tumor bed and dose-limiting structures for use in treatment planning. Spacers (e.g., gelfoam) can be used to create physical distance between the catheters and dose-limiting structures such as nerves.*
- *Catheters are spaced 1–1.5 cm apart and are inserted through the skin at least 1–2 cm from the surgical incision site. Catheter orientation is parallel or perpendicular to the incision, although dosimetry may be optimized by mixed arrangement with crossed ends.*
- *Catheters are sutured into the surgical bed and attached externally to the skin, usually with buttons. Care must be taken at wound closure to ensure that catheter placement and orientation are not disrupted.*
- *As with HDR BT-based IORT, catheters should be labeled at the proximal and distal ends with numbers that correspond to the numbered afterloader channels for HDR sources.*
- *CT-based simulation is performed for treatment planning.*
- *For LDR sources, treatment is delivered in the inpatient setting, with the patient restricted to an isolated room under radiation safety precautions for the duration of treatment. HDR delivered with an afterloader can be administered in the outpatient setting. Treatment generally begins at least 5 days after catheter placement to reduce toxicity (Alektiar et al. 2000c).*
- *Catheter removal should be conducted with attention to reducing the risk of infection.*

5.2.2 Target Volume

The target is comprised of the tumor bed and a margin, without dedicated coverage of drain paths or scars unless at high risk. Although determined by clinical scenario, margins of ≥2 cm in the superior-inferior and 1–2 cm radially are typically applied to the surgical bed, with smaller margins used for management of sites such as the hands and feet (Holloway et al. 2013).

5.2.3 Dose Prescriptions

As per ABR consensus recommendations, LDR-based IBT is delivered at a rate of 0.45–0.5 Gy per hour to 45–50 Gy over 4–6 days as monotherapy and to 15–25 Gy over 2–3 days in combination with 45–50 Gy of EBRT. HDR-based IBT is delivered at 2–4 Gy twice daily to 30–54 Gy over 4–7 days as monotherapy and to 12–20 Gy over 2–3 days in combination with 45–50 Gy of EBRT. Pulsed dose rate delivery is also described (Holloway et al. 2013).

6   Summary

Management of soft tissue sarcomas with conventionally fractionated external beam radiotherapy is limited by high doses and large treatment volumes required for adequate local control. Altered fractionation regimens including treatment with stereotactic radiotherapy, interdigitated chemoradiation, intraoperative radiation therapy, and postoperative interstitial brachytherapy are all associated with improved disease outcomes for specific sites of local and metastatic disease. Moreover, by shortening treatment time, these regimens may also improve quality of life, lower health care costs, and reduce delays until receipt of systemic therapy when indicated.

References

Ahmed KA, Torres-Roca JF (2016) Stereotactic body radiotherapy in the management of oligometastatic disease. Cancer Control 23(1):21–29. http://www.ncbi.nlm.nih.gov/pubmed/27009453

Alekhteyar KM, Leung DH, Brennan MF et al (1996) The effect of combined external beam radiotherapy and brachytherapy on local control and wound complications in patients with high-grade soft tissue sarcomas of the extremity with positive microscopic margin. Int J Radiat Oncol Biol Phys 36(2):321–324. http://www.ncbi.nlm.nih.gov/pubmed/8892454

Alektiar KM, Hu K, Anderson L et al (2000a) High-dose-rate intraoperative radiation therapy (HDR-IORT) for retroperitoneal sarcomas. Int J Radiat Oncol Biol Phys 47(1):157–163. http://www.ncbi.nlm.nih.gov/pubmed/10758318

Alektiar KM, Velasco J, Zelefsky MJ et al (2000b) Adjuvant radiotherapy for margin-positive high-grade soft tissue sarcoma of the extremity. Int J Radiat Oncol Biol Phys 48(4):1051–1058. http://www.ncbi.nlm.nih.gov/pubmed/11072162

Alektiar KM, Zelefsky MJ, Brennan MF (2000c) Morbidity of adjuvant brachytherapy in soft tissue sarcoma of the extremity and superficial trunk. Int J Radiat Oncol Biol Phys 47(5):1273–1279

Alektiar KM, Leung D, Zelefsky MJ et al (2002) Adjuvant brachytherapy for primary high-grade soft tissue sarcoma of the extremity. Ann Surg Oncol 9(1):48–56. http://www.ncbi.nlm.nih.gov/pubmed/11829430

American Cancer Society (2016) Sarcoma: adult soft tissue cancer. http://www.cancer.org/cancer/sarcoma-adultsofttissuecancer/detailedguide/sarcoma-adult-soft-tissue-cancer-survival-rates. Accessed 1 Jan 2016

Azinovic I, Martinez Monge R, Javier Aristu J et al (2003) Intraoperative radiotherapy electron boost followed by moderate doses of external beam radiotherapy in resected soft tissue sarcoma of the extremities. Radiother Oncol 67(3):331–337. http://www.ncbi.nlm.nih.gov/pubmed/12865183

Baldini EH, Goldberg J, Jenner C et al (1999) Long-term outcomes after function-sparing surgery without radiotherapy for soft tissue sarcoma of the extremities and trunk. J Clin Oncol 17(10):3252–3259. http://www.ncbi.nlm.nih.gov/pubmed/10506627

Ballo MT, Zagars GK, Pollock RE et al (2007) Retroperitoneal soft tissue sarcoma: an analysis of radiation and surgical treatment. Int J Radiat Oncol Biol Phys 67(1):158–163. doi:10.1016/j.ijrobp.2006.08.025

Beddar a S, Biggs PJ, Chang S et al (2006) Intraoperative radiation therapy using mobile electron linear accelerators: report of AAPM Radiation Therapy Committee Task Group No. 72. Med Phys 33(5):1476–1489. doi:10.1118/1.2194447

Benedict SH, Yenice KM, Followill D et al (2010) Stereotactic body radiation therapy: the report of AAPM Task Group 101. Med Phys 37(8):4078. doi:10.1118/1.3438081

Bilsky MH, Boland PJ, Panageas KS et al (2001) Intralesional resection of primary and metastatic sarcoma involving the spine: outcome analysis of 59 patients. Neurosurgery 49(6):1277–1286. http://www.ncbi.nlm.nih.gov/pubmed/11846926

Boyd TS, Mehta MP (1999) Stereotactic radiosurgery for brain metastases. Oncology (Williston Park) 13(10):1397–1409. 1409–10, 1413. http://www.ncbi.nlm.nih.gov/pubmed/10549566

Calvo FA, Meirino RM, Orecchia R (2006) Intraoperative radiation therapy first part: rationale and techniques. Crit Rev Oncol Hematol 59(2):106–115. doi:10.1016/j.critrevonc.2005.11.004

Chang UK, Cho WI, Lee DH et al (2012) Stereotactic radiosurgery for primary and metastatic sarcomas involving the spine. J Neuro-Oncol 107(3):551–557. doi:10.1007/s11060-011-0777-0

Corbin KS, Hellman S, Weichselbaum RR (2013) Extracranial oligometastases: a subset of metastases curable with stereotactic radiotherapy. J Clin Oncol 31(11):1384–1390. doi:10.1200/JCO.2012.45.9651

Cox BW, Spratt DE, Lovelock M et al (2012) International spine radiosurgery consortium consensus guidelines for target volume definition in spinal stereotactic radiosurgery. Int J Radiat Oncol Biol Phys 83(5):e597–e605. doi:10.1016/j.ijrobp.2012.03.009

Davis AM, O'Sullivan B, Turcotte R et al (2005) Late radiation morbidity following randomization to preoperative versus postoperative radiotherapy in extremity soft tissue sarcoma. Radiother Oncol 75(1):48–53. http://www.ncbi.nlm.nih.gov/pubmed/15948265

DeLaney TF, Spiro IJ, Suit HD et al (2003) Neoadjuvant chemotherapy and radiotherapy for large extremity soft tissue sarcomas. Int J Radiat Oncol Biol Phys 56(4):1117–1127. http://www.ncbi.nlm.nih.gov/pubmed/12829150

Delannes M, Thomas L, Martel P et al (2000) Low-dose-rate intraoperative brachytherapy combined with external beam irradiation in the conservative treatment of soft tissue sarcoma. Int J Radiat Oncol Biol Phys 47(1):165–169. http://www.ncbi.nlm.nih.gov/pubmed/10758319

Dhakal S, Corbin KS, Milano MT et al (2012) Stereotactic body radiotherapy for pulmonary metastases from soft tissue sarcomas: excellent local lesion control and improved patient survival. Int J Radiat Oncol Biol Phys 82(2):940–945. doi:10.1016/j.ijrobp.2010.11.052

Dubois JB, Debrigode C, Hay M et al (1995) Intra-operative radiotherapy in soft tissue sarcomas. Radiother Oncol 34(2):160–163. http://www.ncbi.nlm.nih.gov/pubmed/7597215

Dziewirski W, Rutkowski P, Nowecki ZI et al (2006) Surgery combined with intraoperative brachytherapy in the treatment of retroperitoneal sarcomas. Ann Surg Oncol 13(2):245–252. doi:10.1245/ASO.2006.03.026

Eaton BR, Gebhardt B, Prabhu R et al (2013) Hypofractionated radiosurgery for intact or resected brain metastases: defining the optimal dose and fractionation. Radiat Oncol 8:135. doi:10.1186/1748-717X-8-135

Edge SB, Byrd DR, Compton CC et al (eds) (2010) Soft tissue sarcomas. In: AJCC cancer staging manual, 7th edn. Springer, New York City. pp 291–296

Fahrig A, Ganslandt O, Lambrecht U et al (2007) Hypofractionated stereotactic radiotherapy for brain metastases--results from three different dose concepts. Strahlenther Onkol 183(11):625–630. doi:10.1007/s00066-007-1714-1

Fletcher CDM, Bridge JA, Hogendoorn PCW (2013) World Health Organization classification of tumours of soft tissue and bone, 4th edn. IARC, Lyon

Gieschen HL, Spiro IJ, Suit HD et al (2001) Long-term results of intraoperative electron beam radiotherapy for primary and recurrent retroperitoneal soft tissue sarcoma. Int J Radiat Oncol Biol Phys 50(1):127–131. http://www.ncbi.nlm.nih.gov/pubmed/11316555

Gunderson L, Shipley W, Suit H et al (1982) Intraoperative irradiation: a pilot study combining external beam photons with "boost" dose intraoperative electrons. Cancer 49:2259–2266

Holloway CL, DeLaney TF, Alektiar KM et al (2013) American Brachytherapy Society (ABS) consensus statement for sarcoma brachytherapy. Brachytherapy 12(3):179–190. doi:10.1016/j.brachy.2012.12.002

van Kampen M, Eble MJ, Lehnert T et al (2001) Correlation of intraoperatively irradiated volume and fibrosis in patients with soft tissue sarcoma of the extremities. Int J Radiat Oncol Biol Phys 51(1):94–99. http://www.ncbi.nlm.nih.gov/pubmed/11516857

Kirkpatrick JP, Meyer JJ, Marks LB (2008) The linear-quadratic model is inappropriate to model high dose per fraction effects in radiosurgery. Semin Radiat Oncol 18(4):240–243. doi:10.1016/j.semradonc.2008.04.005

Kohutek ZA, Yamada Y, Chan TA et al (2015) Long-term risk of radionecrosis and imaging changes after stereotactic radiosurgery for brain metastases. J Neuro-Oncol 125(1):149–156. doi:10.1007/s11060-015-1881-3

Kraybill WG, Harris J, Spiro IJ et al (2006) Phase II study of neoadjuvant chemotherapy and radiation therapy in the management of high-risk, high-grade, soft tissue sarcomas of the extremities and body wall: Radiation Therapy Oncology Group Trial 9514. J Clin Oncol 24(4):619–625. doi:10.1200/JCO.2005.02.5577

Krempien R, Roeder F, Oertel S et al (2006) Intraoperative electron-beam therapy for primary and recurrent retroperitoneal soft tissue sarcoma. Int J Radiat Oncol Biol Phys 65(3):773–779. doi:10.1016/j.ijrobp.2006.01.028

Kretzler A, Molls M, Gradinger R et al (2004) Intraoperative radiotherapy of soft tissue sarcoma of the extremity. Strahlenther Onkol 180(6):365–370. doi:10.1007/s00066-004-1191-8

Kumar R, Alcorn SR, Sahgal A et al (2015) Stereotactic radiation for spinal metastases. In: Fairchild A (ed) Palliative radiation therapy: utilization of advanced technologies. Nova Science, Edmontin, pp 227–244

Lawrence W, Donegan WL, Natarajan N et al (1987) Adult soft tissue sarcomas. A pattern of care survey of the American College of Surgeons. Ann Surg 205(4):349–359. http://www.ncbi.nlm.nih.gov/pubmed/3566372

Levine AM, Coleman C, Horasek S (2009) Stereotactic radiosurgery for the treatment of primary sarcomas and sarcoma metastases of the spine. Neurosurgery 64(2 Suppl):A54–A59. doi:10.1227/01.NEU.0000339131.28485.4A

Lindberg RD, Martin RG, Romsdahl MM et al (1981) Conservative surgery and postoperative radiotherapy in 300 adults with soft tissue sarcomas. Cancer 47(10):2391–2397. http://www.ncbi.nlm.nih.gov/pubmed/7272893

Llácer C, Delannes M, Minsat M et al (2006) Low-dose intraoperative brachytherapy in soft tissue sarcomas involving neurovascular structure. Radiother Oncol 78(1):10–16. doi:10.1016/j.radonc.2005.12.002

Mehta MP, Rozental JM, Levin AB et al (1992) Defining the role of radiosurgery in the management of brain metastases. Int J Radiat Oncol Biol Phys 24(4):619–625. http://www.ncbi.nlm.nih.gov/pubmed/1429083

Merimsky O, Kollender Y, Bokstein F et al (2004) Radiotherapy for spinal cord compression in patients with soft tissue sarcoma. Int J Radiat Oncol Biol Phys 58(5):1468–1473. doi:10.1016/j.ijrobp.2003.09.026

Milano MT, Katz AW, Muhs AG et al (2008) A prospective pilot study of curative-intent stereotactic body radiation therapy in patients with 5 or fewer oligometastatic lesions. Cancer 112(3):650–658. doi:10.1002/cncr.23209

Moningi S, Armour EP, Terezakis SA et al (2014) High-dose-rate intraoperative radiation therapy: the nuts and bolts of starting a program. J Contemp Brachytherapy 6(1):99–105. doi:10.5114/jcb.2014.42027

Navarria P, Ascolese AM, Cozzi L et al (2015) Stereotactic body radiation therapy for lung metastases from soft tissue sarcoma. Eur J Cancer 51(5):668–674. doi:10.1016/j.ejca.2015.01.061

NCCN (2017) Non-small cell lung cancer, version 1.2017. http://www.nccn.org/professionals/physician_gls/pdf/nscl.pdf. Accessed 10 Jan 2016

Nieder C, Grosu AL, Gaspar LE (2014) Stereotactic radiosurgery (SRS) for brain metastases: a systematic review. Radiat Oncol 9:155. doi:10.1186/1748-717X-9-155

Niewald M, Fleckenstein J, Licht N et al (2009) Intraoperative radiotherapy (IORT) combined with external beam radiotherapy (EBRT) for soft tissue sarcomas—a retrospective evaluation of the Homburg experience in the years 1995-2007. Radiat Oncol 4:32. doi:10.1186/1748-717X-4-32

O'Sullivan B (2004) Five-year results of a randomized phase III trial of pre-operative vs post-operative radiotherapy in extremity soft tissue sarcoma. J Clin Oncol 22(14S):2004

Pawlik TM, Ahuja N, Herman JM (2007) The role of radiation in retroperitoneal sarcomas: a surgical perspective. Curr Opin Oncol 19(4):359–366. doi:10.1097/CCO.0b013e328122d757

Pisters PW, Harrison LB, Leung DH et al (1996) Long-term results of a prospective randomized trial of adjuvant brachytherapy in soft tissue sarcoma. J Clin Oncol 14(3):859–868. doi:10.1200/jco.1996.14.3.859. http://www.ncbi.nlm.nih.gov/pubmed/8622034

Potter DA, Glenn J, Kinsella T et al (1985) Patterns of recurrence in patients with high-grade soft tissue sarcomas. J Clin Oncol 3(3):353–366. http://www.ncbi.nlm.nih.gov/pubmed/3973646

Rachbauer F, Sztankay A, Kreczy A et al (2003) High-dose-rate intraoperative brachytherapy (IOHDR) using flab technique in the treatment of soft tissue sarcomas. Strahlenther Onkol 179(7):480–485. doi:10.1007/s00066-003-1063-7

RTOG Foundation (2014) RTOG 0915 protocol information. https://www.rtog.org/ClinicalTrials/ProtocolTable/StudyDetails.aspx?study=0915. Accessed 10 Jan 2016

Salama JK, Hasselle MD, Chmura SJ et al (2012) Stereotactic body radiotherapy for multisite extracranial oligometastases: final report of a dose escalation trial in patients with 1 to 5 sites of metastatic disease. Cancer 118(11):2962–2970. doi:10.1002/cncr.26611

San Miguel I, San Julián M, Cambeiro M et al (2011) Determinants of toxicity, patterns of failure, and outcome among adult patients with soft tissue sarcomas of the extremity and superficial trunk treated with greater than conventional doses of perioperative high-dose-rate brachytherapy and external beam radiotherapy. Int J Radiat Oncol Biol Phys 81(4):e529–e539. doi:10.1016/j.ijrobp.2011.04.063

Schuck A, Willich N, Rübe C et al (1997) Intraoperative high-dose-rate brachytherapy after preoperative radiochemotherapy in the treatment of Ewing's sarcoma. Front Radiat Ther Oncol 31:153–156. http://www.ncbi.nlm.nih.gov/pubmed/9263811

Shaw E, Scott C, Souhami L et al (1996) Radiosurgery for the treatment of previously irradiated recurrent primary brain tumors and brain metastases: initial report of radiation therapy oncology group protocol (90-05). Int J Radiat Oncol Biol Phys 34(3):647–654. http://www.ncbi.nlm.nih.gov/pubmed/8621289

Siegel RL, Miller KD, Jemal A (2015) Cancer statistics, 2015. CA Cancer J Clin 65(1):5–29. doi:10.3322/caac.21254

Sindelar WF, Kinsella TJ, Chen PW et al (1993) Intraoperative radiotherapy in retroperitoneal sarcomas. Final results of a prospective, randomized, clinical trial. Arch Surg 128(4):402–410. http://www.ncbi.nlm.nih.gov/pubmed/8457152

Spiro IJ, Gebhardt MC, Jennings LC et al (1997) Prognostic factors for local control of sarcomas of the soft tissues managed by radiation and surgery. Semin Oncol 24(5):540–546. http://www.ncbi.nlm.nih.gov/pubmed/9344320

Suit H (1971) Radiation biology: a basis for radiotherapy. In: Fletcher G (ed) Textbook of radiotherapy, 2nd edn. Lea and Febiger, Philadelphia, pp 75–121

Tepper JE, Suit HD (1985) The role of radiation therapy in the treatment of sarcoma of soft tissue. Cancer Investig 3(6):587–592. http://www.ncbi.nlm.nih.gov/pubmed/3002565

Thomadsen B (1999) Achieving quality in brachytherapy. Institute of Physics, London

Tran QNH, Kim AC, Gottschalk AR et al (2006) Clinical outcomes of intraoperative radiation therapy for extremity sarcomas. Sarcoma 2006(1):91671. doi:10.1155/SRCM/2006/91671

Tran PT, Hara W, Su Z et al (2008) Intraoperative radiation therapy for locally advanced and recurrent soft tissue sarcomas in adults. Int J Radiat Oncol Biol Phys 72(4):1146–1153. doi:10.1016/j.ijrobp.2008.02.012

Stereotactic Body Radiotherapy

Gargi Kothari, Simon S. Lo, Matthew Foote,
Arjun Sahgal, Irene Karam, Michael Lock,
Gerrit J. Blom, Matthias Guckenberger,
Ben J. Slotman, and Shankar Siva

Contents

G. Kothari, MBBS, FRANZCR
Clinical Fellow, The Royal Marsden Hospital NHS
Foundation Trust, London, UK

S.S. Lo, MD, FACR (✉)
Professor and Vice Chair for Strategic Planning of
Radiation Oncology, Department of Radiation
Oncology, University of Washington School of
Medicine, Seattle, WA, USA
e-mail: simonsmlo@gmail.com

M. Foote, MBBS, FRANZCR
Co-Director Gamma Knife Centre of Queensland,
Staff Specialist, Radiation Oncology,
Princess Alexandra Hospital, Brisbane,
Queensland, Australia

Associate Professor, University of Queensland,
Brisbane, Queensland, Australia

A. Sahgal, MD, FRCPC
Professor, Department of Radiation Oncology,
University of Toronto, Sunnybrook Health Sciences
Centre, Toronto, Ontario, Canada

I. Karam, MD CM, FRCPC
Radiation Oncologist, Odette Cancer Centre,
Assistant Professor, Department of Radiation
Oncology, University of Toronto, Sunnybrook Health
Sciences Centre, Toronto, Ontario, Canada

M. Lock, MD, CCFP, FRCPC, FCFP
Chair, Division of Radiation Oncology, London
Health Science Centre, London, Ontario, Canada

Associate Professor, Department of Oncology, and
Department of Medical Biophysics, Western
University Radiation, London, Ontario, Canada

Associate Scientist, Lawson Health Research
Institute, London, Ontario, Canada

Staff Oncologist, London Regional Cancer Program,
London, Ontario, Canada

Associate Professor, Schulich School of Medicine
and Dentistry, University of Western Ontario,
London, Ontario, Canada

G.J. Blom, MD
Radiation Oncologist, Department of Radiation
Oncology, VU University Medical Center,
Amsterdam, The Netherlands

M. Guckenberger, MD
Professor and Chairman, Department of Radiation
Oncology, University Hospital Zurich (USZ),
Rämistrasse 100, CH-8091, Zurich

B.J. Slotman, MD, PhD
Professor and Chairman, Department of Radiation
Oncology, VU University Medical Centre,
Amsterdam, The Netherlands

S. Siva, MBBS, PhD, FRANZCR
Associate Professor, Radiation Oncologist, Division
of Radiation Oncology and Cancer Imaging, Peter
MacCallum Cancer Centre, Melbourne, Victoria,
Australia

Med Radiol Radiat Oncol (2017)
DOI 10.1007/174_2017_38, © Springer International Publishing AG
Published Online: 01 June 2017

Abstract

Stereotactic body radiation therapy (SBRT) consists of the delivery of precise, conformal, hypofractionated, and ablative therapy in a single or a small number of fractions to extracranial regions. Over the last decade, it is rapidly being integrated into mainstream radiation oncology practices. The indications for SBRT continue to grow, as does the technology associated with its delivery. This chapter presents a detailed overview of clinically relevant topics including patient selection and outcomes, and the technological aspects of planning and delivery of SBRT. The tumor streams covered in this chapter are lung, liver, spine, pancreas, renal cell carcinoma, adrenal, prostate, and head and neck. The chapter concludes by highlighting two novel areas, cardiac arrhythmias and pediatric oncology, in which the use of SBRT is emerging.

1   Introduction

Stereotactic ablative radiotherapy (SABR) or stereotactic body radiation therapy (SBRT) is the delivery of a single or a small number of high-dose-per-fraction ablative radiation treatments to extracranial sites. It is usually characterized by a very conformal isodose distribution with a rapid dose falloff, which allows for delivery of ablative doses to the target, while still protecting adjacent normal tissue from the late effects of this extreme form of hypofractionation.

The technique of SBRT is characterized by unique radiobiology compared to convention-ally fractionated radiotherapy. Most data regarding radiobiology were derived through the study of conventionally fractionated radiotherapy, from which the linear quadratic (LQ) model was established. At the ablative dose range, however, the LQ model likely overestimates the amount of cell kill that occurs (Park et al. 2008; Timmerman et al. 2007). This is relevant for both determining effective dose for tumour cell kill and respecting normal tissue constraints, and more prospective clinical data will help to guide us in the appropriate incorporation of such models into clinical practice.

Increasingly, research also highlights the importance of tumour microvasculature (Fuks and Kolesnick 2005). Animal studies suggest that the use of stereotactic radiotherapy results in a rapid wave of endothelial apoptosis at 1–6 h after irradiation followed by tumor cell death at 2–3 days. This is mediated via the acid sphingomyelinase pathway, which is not seen in conventionally fractionated radiotherapy (Garcia-Barros et al. 2003). Furthermore, animal studies have also suggested an immunomodulatory effect of stereotactic radiotherapy, with enhancement of T-cell priming in draining lymphoid tissue, followed by a reduction in primary and/or distant tumor in a CD8+ T-cell-dependent fashion (Lee et al. 2009a).

Stereotactic radiotherapy has developed over the last 20 years. However over the last decade, its use is increasing at an exponential rate, facilitated by a surge in the development and widespread incorporation of technology within radiation oncology practices. The development of SBRT followed on from the successes of intracranial stereotactic radiosurgery (SRS). The concept of SRS was developed in 1950s, pioneered by Lars Leksell, with the use of the GammaKnife® (Elekta AB, Stockholm, Sweden) and was proposed as a less risky alternative to open craniotomy. It was initially used to treat pain conditions, with targeting of intracranial metastases only becoming feasible after the development of contrast-enhanced CT and MRI scans in the mid-1970s. It was not until the early 1990s that groups began to investigate the use of stereotactic radiotherapy to extracranial sites including the spine and lungs through linear accelerator-based delivery methods, with the incorporation of rigid frame-based immobilization devices or body frames with inbuilt fiducial markers. Following the early successes of this treatment, the uptake and indications of SBRT continued to grow.

The landscape of SBRT today consists of a myriad of platforms for radiation delivery with numerous technological approaches. The key components, however, of any SBRT delivery system remain constant and include accurate immobilization, complex planning software capability, image guidance ability pre- (and often during) treatment, robust quality assurance, and motion management.

The CyberKnife® (Accuray, Inc., Sunnyvale, CA) is a purpose-built system conceived to bring stereotactic radiotherapy into the modern era and was used to treat its first patient in 1994. While initially developed to treat intracranial lesions, it is now widely used to also deliver SBRT. Today, it is composed of a compact linear accelerator with 12 circular collimators of varying sizes mounted upon a robotic arm, with six degrees of positional freedom, which allows for the delivery of numerous highly accurate noncoplanar beams. Radiation delivery is enhanced through the integration of a continuous real-time orthogonal X-ray and optic image guidance system through which tracking and correction based upon implanted fiducial markers and tracking of tumors that move with respiration and fiducial free spinal tracking can be performed. In this system, two orthogonal X-ray sources attached to the ceiling provide orthogonal images, which are continuously compared to the original digitally reconstructed radiographs (DRR) and adjusted near instantaneously. In addition, optimal markers may be attached to the patient's chest, and continuously monitored using three cameras, to adjust for respiratory motion during treatment. As a result a key feature of the CyberKnife® is that any positional changes of the patient or target are compensated for by adjustment of the robotic arm, rather than movement of the treatment couch, as is the case for conventional linear accelerators. CyberKnife® has developed a number of specialized tracking systems, including fiducial marker and spine tracking, Xsight® (Accuray, Inc.); Lung tracking, Synchrony® (Accuray, Inc.); respiratory motion tracking, Lung Optimized Treatment; and InTempo® (Accuray, Inc.) for prostate tracking. CyberKnife® uses the MultiPlan® (Accuray, Inc.) system to create an optimized treatment plan using forward or inverse-based planning. The planning process is based upon a set of predefined source positions called "nodes," with a set of these nodes called a "path." Depending upon the number of collimator sizes and on which optimization algorithm is applied, a plan is created, with the number of beams usually ranging from anywhere between 50 and 250.

Conventional linear accelerators can also be used to deliver SBRT, such as the Varian

Truebeam® (Varian Medical Systems, Palo Alto, CA) and Elekta Versa HD® (Elekta AB, Stockholm, Sweden) units which have integrated gantry-mounted kilovoltage (kV) cone beam CT to allow for repositioning immediately prior to treatment, as well as volumetric modulated arc therapy (VMAT) capability. The Novalis TX® (Varian Medical Systems, Palo Alto, CA, and BrainLAB, Munich) unit has kV cone beam CT as well as stereoscopic X-ray capabilities. The TomoTherapy HiArt System® (TomoTherapy, Madison, Wisconsin, USA) delivers intensity-modulated radiation therapy (IMRT) during continuous 360° rotations, and can obtain megavoltage (MV) CT images prior to treatment delivery. All of these systems have various advantages and disadvantages in their ability to deliver precise and accurate ablative therapy; however equally importantly they need to be complemented by knowledgeable support staff and a rigorous quality assurance program that will ensure the ongoing safety of patients and viability of any stereotactic radiotherapy center. The inherent advantage of conventional linear accelerator platforms is the versatility to function in a non-SBRT environment, which improves applicability in the resource-constrained environment that is typical in most clinical departments.

Although the use of stereotactic radiotherapy was founded on treatment of palliative conditions, increasingly its realm continues to widen. It now forms part of the armamentarium not only for palliation of patients with metastatic disease, but is being considered an alternative to both conventionally fractionated treatment and in some cases surgery for patients with localized disease. Its obvious attractions include reduced patient burden through provision of treatment in a single or few fractions, as well as its noninvasive yet ablative nature. In addition to this, there has been increasing data emerging regarding not only excellent local control (LC), but also reduced toxicities, improved quality of life (QOL), possible benefits in terms of cost-effectiveness, as well as its potential role in modulation of the immune system, in an era where systemic immunomodulatory agents are showing ever-promising results.

In addition to this, its role in a subset of patients with "oligometastatic" disease is an exciting and emerging field, in which the advantages of stereotactic radiotherapy seem to be so aptly suited. For decades, it was an accepted paradigm in oncology that patients with distant metastases from solid tumors are best served with palliative intent with treatments often involving the use of palliative radiotherapy and systemic chemotherapy, without expectation of long-term survival. This paradigm is increasingly being challenged, with the view that long-term survival may be achieved through aggressive treatment of metastases in selected cases (van Dongen and van Slooten 1978). In 1995 the term "oligometastasis" was introduced by Hellman and Weichselbaum as a consequence of the spectrum theory (Hellman and Weichselbaum 1995). This theory states that at the time of presentation, cancer represents a biological spectrum: some cancers remain a local disease and are not capable of metastasizing, and at the other end of the spectrum are cancers with widely metastatic disease at the onset of diagnosis. Most cancers behave somewhere in between these extremes and in some cases patients only develop a limited number of metastatic deposits without further progression. This intermediary oligometastatic state, variably defined as patients with up to three to five metastases, provides a therapeutic opportunity, in which the potential of long-term survival or even cure may exist. This forms a rationale, therefore, for the use of local therapies including SBRT, which may be used either in addition to systemic therapies or even to delay the use of systemic therapies, thereby allowing patients to minimize associated toxicities of treatment and perhaps improve QOL.

This chapter, therefore, aims to critically review the evidence for stereotactic radiotherapy in both the more established tumor streams and sites, including lung, liver, and spine lesions, as well as some of the emerging sites including renal cell carcinoma and head and neck cancers, and highlight issues relevant in clinical practice. This chapter also explores the role of SBRT in primary and oligometastatic disease as well as its role in palliation, patient selection, combining SBRT with systemic agents, and technical issues important in the delivery of safe and effective treatment.

We conclude the chapter by focusing on a couple of emerging and novel areas for SBRT.

2 Lung SBRT

Nonsmallcell lung cancer (NSCLC) contributes largely to cancer mortality worldwide (Ferlay et al. 2010). However, if diagnosed at an early stage, the 5-year overall survival (OS) is 50% (Rami-Porta et al. 2009). Historically surgery has been the standard treatment for stage I NSCLC. However, NSCLC is typically a disease of the elderly with one-third of newly diagnosed patients being greater than 75 years old (Edwards et al. 2002). Moreover, this group often has significant comorbidity with chronic obstructive pulmonary disease (COPD) diagnosed in 50–70% of patients (Loganathan et al. 2006). Therefore, a substantial proportion of these patients are not suitable for surgery due to their high risk of treatment-induced mortality and morbidity. As a consequence, this group may be less likely to receive active treatment leading to poor outcomes, with untreated early-stage NSCLC having a 5-year OS rate of less than 15% (Raz et al. 2007). There is, however, evidence to show that older patients who do receive active treatment have survival benefits that are similar to younger patients (Higton et al. 2010).

In the past, conventionally fractionated radiotherapy was used, leading to suboptimal outcomes (Rowell et al. 2003). Developments in image guidance, treatment planning, and delivery have led to the introduction of SBRT, and offer new opportunities to not only improve patient outcomes, but also allow for greater uptake of active treatment in patients that may otherwise have proved unable to undergo curative intent treatment (Haasbeek et al. 2012). This chapter section discusses the evidence in early-stage NSCLC for SBRT in medically inoperable patients, medically operable patients, patients with centrally based tumours, and patients without histopathological diagnosis; reviews the technical considerations for SBRT to the lung; follows up for SBRT; and concludes with a brief overview of the treatment of oligometastatic lung disease.

2.1 Inoperable Patients

The first experiences with SBRT as a treatment option for early-stage NSCLC were obtained in medically inoperable patients, in whom conventionally fractionated radiotherapy has been the standard of care. The Stereotactic Precision And Conventional radiotherapy Evaluation (SPACE) trial is the first randomized phase II trial that reported on the outcomes of SBRT to 66 Gy in three fractions vs. conventional radiotherapy to 70 Gy in 2 Gy per fraction in inoperable stage I NSCLC patients (Nyman et al. 2016). The results of this trial, which included 102 patients with a statistically significant greater number of patients with T2 tumors in the SBRT arm ($p = 0.02$), showed no difference in either progression-free survival (PFS) or overall survival (OS); however there were statistically significant lower rates of esophagitis, and improved health-related QOL measures for dyspnea, chest pain, and cough in the SBRT arm. Given the improved patient convenience and adverse effect profile with SBRT, this was recommended to be the standard of care for this group of patients. Two phase III randomized trials, Conformal Hypofractionated Image guided Stereotactic radiotherapy for inoperable Early stage Non-small cell Lung cancer (CHISEL, Clinical trials database: NCT01014130) and Stereotactic body radiotherapy vs. conventional radiotherapy in medically inoperable Non-small Lung cancer patients (LUSTRE, Clinical trials database, NCT01968941), are currently under way addressing the same question, and the results of these trials are eagerly awaited.

Several phase I and phase II trials have also investigated the use of SBRT. In a phase I trial, 37 medically inoperable patients with T1–2 N0 tumors were treated to different dose levels ranging from three fractions of 8 Gy to three fractions of 20 Gy (Timmerman et al. 2003). No dose-limiting toxicity was seen and patients receiving a dose per fraction of 18 Gy or higher had no local failure after a median follow-up of 15 months. Further dose escalation was investigated in a follow-up phase I study (McGarry et al. 2005).

Maximum tolerated dose was 66 Gy in three fractions for tumors larger than 5 cm. Severe grade 3–4 toxicity was observed in three out of five patients treated to 72 Gy in three fractions, including pneumonitis in two patients and tracheal necrosis in one patient. A Japanese study used a schedule of 48 Gy in four fractions and found no pulmonary complications greater than Common Terminology Criteria for Adverse Events (CTCAE) Grade 3 (Nagata et al. 2005). One of the largest phase II studies was reported by Nagata et al. for 164 patients receiving 48 Gy in four fractions (Nagata et al. 2015). Three-year LC was >85% with CTCAE grade 4 toxicity seen in two patients and no grade 5 toxicity. Shibamoto et al. reported on the 5-year outcome of lung SBRT for 180 patients receiving 44–52 Gy in four fractions, and found that for tumors greater than 3 cm LC was 73%, compared to 86% for smaller tumors (Shibamoto et al. 2015). Toxicity was also low, with only 13% grade 2 or higher toxicity and only 1% with grade 3 toxicity. Similarly a study of 70 patients delivering SBRT to 60–66 Gy in three fractions found a trend towards higher severe toxicity in centrally vs. peripherally based tumors (27.3% vs. 10.4%, respectively, p = 0.088) (Fakiris et al. 2009). Several other smaller phase II trials have shown good LC rates with low toxicity (Nagata et al. 2005; Baumann et al. 2009; Bral et al. 2011; Koto et al. 2007; Lindberg et al. 2015; Ricardi et al. 2010; Timmerman et al. 2010).

To compare clinical outcome after radiotherapy for different SBRT regimens and with conventionally fractionated radiotherapy, radiobiological modeling is necessary. The applicability of the linear-quadratic (LQ) model tumor control probability (TCP) was investigated using 395 patients from 13 centers treated with SBRT for early-stage lung cancer (Guckenberger et al. 2013a). A dose-response relationship was observed for fractionated SBRT; however for single-fraction radiosurgery local tumor control remained constant over a wide dose range. The traditional LQ concept was found to be an accurate model for local tumor control in this cohort, in which maximum dose at the isocenter correlated better with tumor control than dose at the planning target volume (PTV) periphery. A

strong dose-response relationship was also seen in a retrospective multi-institutional study evaluating TCP of SBRT for both primary lung cancer and lung metastases in 399 patients (Guckenberger et al. 2016). It was found that the tumor control dose (TCD) 90 (dose to achieve 90% TCP) was estimated to be 176 Gy (maximal dose) for primary lung cancer and 160 Gy for metastases (using BED_{10}). In another study prescription BED_{10} > 105 Gy and PTV_{mean} BED_{10} > 125 Gy demonstrated significantly higher LC rates than lower doses (Kestin et al. 2014). This suggests that sufficient dose for tumor control is lower than the maximum tolerated doses in the previously reported phase I studies.

Early experience on a larger scale with SBRT for early-stage NSCLC was obtained in Japan. A multi-institutional retrospective study reported on the outcomes of 257 patients treated between 1995 and 2004 at 14 institutions, of which the majority were medically inoperable (Onishi et al. 2007). This study showed promising 5-year OS of 35%. The local recurrence rates highly depended on the BED_{10}, being 8.4% if BED_{10} was 100 Gy or higher compared to 42.9% with lower biological doses. This study also showed limited adverse events with CTCAE grade 3 or higher toxicity seen in only 5% of patients. These results were further supported by a study from the Netherlands, in which 676 patients treated with SBRT were found to have a 5-year LC rate of approximately 90% (Senthi et al. 2012). The safety of SBRT for lung tumors was confirmed in a multi-institutional retrospective study (Guckenberger et al. 2013b). Of the 512 patients with toxicity data available, only 7.4% had grade 2 or higher pneumonitis with grade 5 pneumonitis documented for two patients. Similar results were seen in a report on a large, prospective database of 206 inoperable patients treated with SBRT in the Netherlands, with a very low local recurrence rate of 4% and severe late toxicity seen in only 3% of patients (Lagerwaard et al. 2008). Furthermore, in a propensity score-matched population-based analysis using the Surveillance, Epidemiology, and End Results (SEER) Medicare cohort, there was no difference seen in long-term survival between patients that underwent lobectomy and those that underwent SBRT, with short-term mortality <1% with SBRT and 4% with surgery (Shirvani et al. 2012).

Some groups also specifically addressed safety of SBRT in the elderly cohort, and found toxicity to be similarly low in this group, with SBRT associated with less than 10% late grade ≥3 toxicity (Haasbeek et al. 2010). This was further supported by a systematic review on lung SBRT in COPD patients, in which 196 patients with stage I NSCLC were treated with surgery or SBRT and the 1- and 3-year OS was found to be comparable, although SBRT was found to be much safer with 0% treatment-related mortality compared to 10% with surgery (Palma and Lagerwaard 2012).

2.2 Operable Patients

Although SBRT for early-stage lung cancer results in high LC rates and improved survival, historically surgery in the form of lobectomy and hilar/mediastinal lymph node dissection has been considered as the standard of care.

Initial data to support the role of SBRT in medically operable patients with early-stage disease was derived from retrospective data. A study of potentially operable patients with early-stage lung cancer who were treated with SBRT retrospectively identified patients from a prospective database of 706 patients (Lagerwaard et al. 2012). Of this group, 25% were eligible for surgery but refused or had a strong preference for SBRT. Median OS was 61.5 months, with a 3-year LC rate exceeding 90%. Predicted 30-day mortality with surgery using the Thoracoscore predictive model (Falcoz et al. 2007) would have been 2.6%, while no treatment-related mortality was seen with SBRT. The same group performed a propensity score-matched analysis between 64 patients receiving SBRT and 64 patients who underwent lobectomy (Verstegen et al. 2013). This revealed superior 3-year LC rates in favor of SBRT (93.3% vs. 82.6%, $p = 0.04$), although OS and distant recurrences were not significantly different.

Three randomized studies were also initiated to evaluate whether SBRT could be an alternative to surgery. The ROSEL and STARS trials compared SBRT to lobectomy, while the ACOSOG Z4099/RTOG 1021 study compared SBRT to sublobar resection in stage I operable patients. Unfortunately, all three trials ended prematurely due to slow accrual. Given the similar inclusion criteria of ROSEL and STARS, the data from both studies was combined in a pooled analysis of 58 patients (Chang et al. 2015). Median follow-up was 40.2 months for the SBRT group and 35.4 months for the surgical group. Notably, histological confirmation was not mandatory in the ROSEL trial and is often a major criticism of this study, although there is evidence to suggest that imaging-based diagnosis can be highly specific and sensitive (Herder et al. 2005; Verstegen et al. 2011). The results of the studies showed that pooled estimated OS at 3 years was significantly better in the SBRT arm (95% vs. 79%, $p = 0.037$). Recurrence-free survival also favored the SBRT arm, although the results were not significant (86% vs. 80%, $p = 0.54$). Freedom from local recurrence favored surgery, although the results were also not significant (96% vs. 100%, $p = 0.44$). Importantly, there were six deaths (one death directly related to a surgical complication) in the surgical arm, and only one death within the SBRT arm, suggesting that the poorer OS in the surgical arm may be related to worsening of preexisting comorbidities following surgery. Other toxicities seen included grade 3 toxicity in 10% of the SBRT patients (no grade 4), and grade 3–4 toxicity in 44% of the surgical patients. In addition, patient-reported outcomes have also been published for the 22 patients included in the ROSEL study (Louie et al. 2015). There was a significant difference found in European Organisation for Research and Treatment of Cancer (EORTC) global health status favoring SBRT (HR 0.19, $p = 0.038$). In addition, the Short Form Health and Labour Questionnaire (SF-HLQ) total productivity cost to society was lower for SBRT compared to surgery (95 vs. 3513, $p = 0.044$), as was the score for total degree of hindrance in paid and unpaid work (1.9 vs. 6.0, $p = 0.010$). While these results suggest that SBRT should be considered a viable alternative treatment option in operable patients, they should be interpreted with caution due to the lack of accrual to the individual studies and limited sample size. Perhaps these data provide the much-needed impetus needed to successfully conduct large randomized clinical trials to reveal the best evidence-based management strategy for this group of patients.

2.3 Central Lung Tumors

Earlier studies of SBRT to central lung tumors suggested higher rates of toxicity, and in general a cautious approach to these tumors is warranted. Timmerman et al. reported on the outcomes of SBRT in inoperable patients, including centrally located early NSCLC (Timmerman et al. 2006). In this phase II study, 70 patients were included with biopsy-confirmed T1–2 N0 NSCLC and treated to 60–66 Gy in three fractions. CTCAE grade 3–5 toxicity was seen in 20% of patients. Multivariate analysis showed that a strong predictor of toxicity was tumor location (hilar/pericentral vs. peripheral) and the authors concluded that this treatment should not be used for patients with tumors near the central airways because of poor LC and excessive toxicity. Another group also described their results of SBRT with comparable fractionation schedules for central lung tumors in 32 patients (Song et al. 2009). This study showed a 33% grade 3–5 toxicity rate. These initial publications initially led to the concept of a "no-fly zone," which is a region around the perihilar/central region reflecting the proximal bronchial tree around which SBRT should be avoided (Timmerman et al. 2006).

A more recent phase I/II study has explored further delivery of SBRT to early-stage central tumors, and aimed to determine the maximal tolerated dose and efficacy of SBRT (Bezjak et al. 2016). This study reported on 120 patients with positron emission tomography (PET) stage IA NSCLC that were within or touching the zone of the proximal bronchial tree or adjacent to mediastinal or pericardial pleura and who received escalated doses of between 10 and 12 Gy × 5 fractions. Dose-limiting toxicity was defined as any CTCAE grade 3 or worse toxic-

ity. The phase I part of the study found the maximum tolerated dose to be the highest dose used in the study, i.e., 12 Gy × 5 fractions. The phase II results reported on the long-term outcomes of the two cohorts which received the highest doses—11.5 Gy ($n = 38$) and 12 Gy ($n = 33$) × 5 fractions. The study showed 2-year LC to be 89.4% and 87.7%, and 2-year OS of 70.2% and 72.7%, respectively. Toxicity included two grade 5 toxicities in the 11.5 Gy group, and one grade 5 (pulmonary hemorrhage), one grade 4 (esophageal perforation), and three grade 3 late toxicities (one cardiac, two pulmonary) in the 12 Gy group.

In addition to the prospective data, there is a growing body of retrospective literature addressing the issue of SBRT to centrally based tumors. A systematic review on central lung tumors included 20 studies in which 563 central lesions (both primary tumors and metastases) were treated with SBRT (Senthi et al. 2013). Local tumor control rates were 85% or higher if a BED_{10} of at least 100 Gy was given and tumor location did not affect OS. Overall treatment-related mortality was 2.7 and 1% if normal tissue BED_3 was less than 210 Gy. Another study compared the outcomes of central vs. peripheral tumors of 613 patients sourced from German and Austrian databases (Schanne et al. 2015). Of the 613 patients, only 90 had central tumors, of which most were stage IB and received a lower median BED_{10} of 72Gy compared with peripheral tumors, of which the majority were stage IA and received a median BED_{10} of 84Gy. The outcomes, not unsurprisingly, revealed better outcomes for peripheral vs. central tumors with 3-year OS of 51% and 29%, and freedom from local progression of 84% and 52%, respectively. Toxicity for central tumors however was low, with no grade 3 or 4 toxicity, although there was one grade 5 toxicity at 60 days. The M.D. Anderson Cancer Center also reported on their long-term results of 100 patients treated for central lung tumors with a risk-adapted approach, and this showed high LC rates and no grade 4 or 5 toxicity after a median follow-up of 30 months (Chang et al. 2014a).

In conclusion, SBRT for central tumors may be able to provide high LC rates with acceptable toxicity when acceptable fractionation schedules are used. However, data from prospective studies particularly demonstrate that treatment-related deaths are concerning. The results of these studies should also be distinguished from situations where the PTV overlaps trachea or main bronchi, described by the term "ultra-central" tumors (Tekatli et al. 2016). For these tumors, generally more conventional schedules are suggested, because of the higher risk of fatal pulmonary hemorrhage, especially in cases of endobronchial tumor growth (Tekatli et al. 2016; Haseltine et al. 2016; Vansteenkiste et al. 2013).

2.4 Tumors without Pathology-Proven Disease

The introduction of SBRT led to an increased use of this therapy particularly in elderly unfit patients, many of whom were not only unfit for surgery, but also poor biopsy candidates (Haasbeek et al. 2012). Obtaining pathological diagnosis can be challenging as tumors are often outside the reach of endobronchial approaches and percutaneous biopsy is associated with a considerable risk of pneumothorax (Tomiyama et al. 2006). Therefore, in some institutions a substantial proportion of these patients are treated without pathological diagnosis (Lagerwaard et al. 2008). Other institutions require histopathological confirmation for all of their patients. Treatment without histopathology was performed based on the knowledge that in the Dutch population, in patients with new or growing FDG-PET-positive lesions, the risk of malignancy, estimated with a validated calculation model, is approximately 95% (Herder et al. 2005). This was further confirmed in an analysis by Verstegen et al., who evaluated outcomes in patients with and without confirmed pathological diagnosis (Verstegen et al. 2011). In this cohort of 591 patients, pathological diagnosis was obtained in only 35% of patients. At 3 years, there were no differences in LC (approximately 91% in both groups) and

OS. This suggests that it is unlikely that the survival benefits after the introduction of SBRT are biased by inclusion of a few patients without malignant disease. Nevertheless, these results should be interpreted with caution, as they are based on a population with a very low incidence of benign pulmonary FDG-PET avid disease, and this may vary widely depending on multiple factors including geographic location (Wahidi et al. 2007). The European Society of Medical Oncology (ESMO) guidelines now state that an attempt should be made to obtain a pathological diagnosis before SBRT, but when this is considered to be too hazardous, an 85% chance of malignancy is considered sufficient to initiate SBRT (Vansteenkiste et al. 2014).

2.5 Technical Considerations

The delivery of SBRT to lung lesions can present several challenges, including in particular management of tumor motion. Here, we briefly overview some of the most pertinent considerations with respect to patient setup, immobilization, motion management, contouring, planning, and treatment verification.

As with conventional treatment, patients are usually required to lie flat in the supine position with their arms over their heads. Immobilization can be achieved through a number of techniques including body frames or a vacuum immobilization mattress; however comparable results may be achieved without rigid immobilization (Dahele et al. 2012). Lung tumors can undergo significant motion in all directions with respiration, and this must be taken into account. Most commonly, this can be achieved by obtaining a four-dimensional computed tomography (4D–CT) during the simulation process, in which breathing phases are registered during acquisition of the imaging, using, for example, infrared markers or a belt system, followed by contouring an internal target volume (ITV). Other strategies depending upon local preference and expertise include the use of breath-hold techniques, which can be particularly useful in moving central tumors away from the mediastinum, abdominal compression, tumor tracking which may require the insertion of a fiducial marker with increased risk of pneumothorax, or respiratory gating, in which treatment is only delivered during a specific point in the patient's breathing cycle. Contouring an ITV using 4D-CT can be performed through various methods. PTV expansions will depend upon a number of factors, and should be modified according to department protocol, but will usually be in the order of 3–5 mm. Planning and dose prescription are also critical steps in the delivery of SBRT. Data suggests that a BED_{10} greater than 100 Gy results in improved 5-year local recurrence rates of 8.4% vs. 42.9% for less than 100 Gy (Onishi et al. 2007). This usually equates to 54–60Gy in three fractions, or 48–50 Gy in four fractions for peripheral tumors. Dose is usually prescribed to the 60–90% isodose, to allow for adequate peripheral tumor coverage, with some data suggesting that dose prescribed to the center of the tumor results in undercoverage at the tumor edge and resultant worsening in LC (Chang et al. 2011a). Organ-at-risk (OAR) dose constraints from the STARS and ROSEL trials are provided in Table 1.

There are multiple beam arrangement possibilities for lung SBRT, although they can usually be categorized into static coplanar, static noncoplanar, or arc. Noncoplanar beam arrangements usually have the advantage of being able to achieve greater conformality and steeper dose gradients compared to coplanar beam arrangements as well as reduced skin dose and complete sparing of the contralateral lung, however often resulting in greater volumes of lung receiving low dose, and longer treatment delivery times due to the need for couch and gantry rotations. Both forward-planned three-dimensional conformal radiotherapy (3DCRT) and IMRT are viable options when delivering SBRT. While IMRT may offer greater ability to sculpt dose around critical OAR, treatment times with IMRT are usually longer, and concerns regarding the interplay effect in the lung between tumor motion and collimator leaf movement should be taken into account, particularly when delivering large doses over only a single or a few fractions. The treatment planning algorithm used for SBRT is also of critical importance, particularly in the thorax, where there are sharp density gradients around the lung-air interface. In this situation, the Monte Carlo algorithm appears to outperform many other treatment planning algorithms, which have been shown to less accurately calculate dose resulting in reduction of tumor dose

Table 1 Organ at risk dose constraints

	ROSEL (54 Gy in 3 fractions)	STARS (50 Gy in 4 fractions)	ROSEL (60 Gy in 5 fractions)
Spinal cord	≤ 18 Gy	20Gy ≤ 1 cm³	< 25Gy
		15Gy ≤ 10 cm³	
Brachial plexus	≤ 24 Gy	Point ≤ 40 Gy	< 27 Gy
		35Gy ≤ 1 cm³	
		30Gy ≤ 10 cm³	
Lung	V20 < 5–10%	V20 ≤ 20%	V20 < 5–10%
		V10 ≤ 30%	
		V5 ≤ 50%	
Trachea	≤ 30 Gy	35Gy ≤ 1 cm³	< 32 Gy
		30Gy ≤ 10 cm³	
Bronchi	≤ 30 Gy	40Gy ≤ 1 cm³	< 32 Gy
		35Gy ≤ 10 cm³	
Esophagus	≤ 24 Gy	35Gy ≤ 1 cm³	< 27 Gy
		30Gy ≤ 10 cm³	
Heart	≤ 24 Gy	40Gy ≤ 1 cm³	< 27 Gy
		35Gy ≤ 10 cm³	

Gy **Gray,** *cc* **cubic centimeter**

coverage (Kry et al. 2013). Image guidance and treatment verification are obviously also crucial steps to deliver safe and accurate SBRT. Direct visualization of the lesion before and, if possible, during treatment delivery is recommended. Kilovoltage (kV) cone beam CT (CBCT) is the best method of soft-tissue delineation and target localization.

2.6 Follow-Up

Routine follow-up with CT scans every 6 months for 2–3 years is recommended for patients fit enough to undergo salvage treatment (Vansteenkiste et al. 2014). Although local recurrence is uncommon and usually occurs between 12 and 18 months (Senthi et al. 2012), CT changes can be seen in almost every patient at some point after treatment (Dahele et al. 2011). As changes on CT scans posttreatment can be diffuse or patchy, and may be mass-like, it can be difficult to distinguish recurrence from radiation-induced lung injury (RILI) such as fibrosis. A systematic review identified six high-risk features (HRF) on CT to better detect recurrence after SBRT: enlarging opacity at the primary site, sequential enlarging opacity, enlarging opacity at 12 months, bulging margin, loss of linear margin, and air bronchogram loss (Huang et al. 2012). These HRF were subsequently validated in a study that compared 12 patients with pathologically proven recurrence to a matched group of 24 patients without recurrence (Huang et al. 2013). All six HRF, and one additional HRF—cranio-caudal growth—were found to be significantly associated with local recurrence ($p < 0.01$). The two best individual predictors of recurrence were an enlarging opacity after 12 months (sensitivity 100%, specificity 83%), and cranio-caudal growth (sensitivity 92%, specificity 83%). In addition, the presence of three HRF was the best cumulative predictor of recurrence, with a sensitivity and specificity of 92%.

In case of a suspicion of recurrence, often a PET-CT is performed; however findings should be interpreted with caution. There is some evidence that high uptake values at 6 months are associated with high risk of local failure (Takeda et al. 2013); however hypermetabolic activity may persist 2 years after treatment without evidence of recurrence resulting in false-positive findings (Hoopes et al. 2007). Patients suitable for salvage treatment should therefore undergo a biopsy and routine use of PET-CT alone to detect disease recurrence is not recommended (Vansteenkiste et al. 2014).

Aside from detection of local recurrence, follow-up imaging is also useful for detection of new primary tumors, as the risk of developing a second primary lung cancer (SPLC) ranges from 3 to 6% per person per year (Lou et al. 2013). If selected properly, patients with SPLC can be offered radical treatment again with SBRT, leading to survival outcomes comparable to initial early-stage lung cancer (Griffioen et al. 2014).

2.7 Oligometastases

Lung parenchyma is a common site for metastatic spread of multiple cancer types, including colorectal cancer and sarcoma. The International Registry of Lung Metastases recorded 5206 cases of lung metastasectomy (Pastorino et al. 1997). Metastases were predominantly epithelial or sarcomatoid and the OS rates of completely resected cases at 5 and 15 years were 36% and 22%, respectively. Therefore, it seems feasible to treat lung metastases with local ablative therapy in selected cases.

If patients with lung metastases are unsuitable or refuse surgery, less invasive techniques such as SBRT are attractive. Typically, similar radiation schemes are used as for primary lung tumors. A systematic review performed in 2010 reported on the outcomes of hypofractionated lung SBRT for 564 lesions in 334 patients (Siva et al. 2010). The 2-year LC was 78% with a corresponding OS of 54%. Grade 3 or higher toxicity was seen in only 4%. Similar results were seen for single-fraction SBRT and the authors concluded that these outcomes were comparable with surgical alternatives with low rates of significant toxicity. Although promising, these results should be interpreted with caution as these data were not randomized and are prone to biases including patient selection. Therefore, the optimal choice of treatment cannot be made until results from randomized trials are available. Therefore, decisions should be made in the context of a multidisciplinary team.

Even more controversial is the existence of an oligometastatic stage in patients with lung cancer. While locally advanced and metastatic lung cancer has been approached with nihilism, increasingly there are data emerging that a group of patients who have truly oligometastatic disease may benefit from an aggressive approach. An individual patient meta-analysis of 757 NSCLC patients with oligometastatic disease (1–5 lesions), who had both the primary curatively treated and all sites of metastatic disease treated with ablative treatment, was analysed (Ashworth et al. 2014). Most patients received surgery (62.3%) while the remainder received conventional or stereotactic radiotherapy for their metastatic disease. The authors reported a higher than expected 5-year OS of 29.4%, with predictors of OS being synchronous vs. metachronous disease, N stage, and adenocarcinoma histology. A recursive partitioning analysis (RPA) was performed and found three risk groups: low-risk, metachronous metastases (5-year OS, 47.8%); intermediate-risk, synchronous metastases and N0 disease (5-year OS, 36.2%); and high-risk, synchronous metastases and N1/N2 disease (5-year OS, 13.8%). This suggests that we will increasingly be able to select a group of patients that may benefit from ablative treatment for oligometastatic disease. Additionally, a subset of patients with actionable mutations, including epidermal growth factor receptor (EGFR) and anaplastic lymphoma kinase (ALK) gene rearrangements, are now experiencing significantly improved survival, and small series are emerging of promising outcomes in patients treated with ablative therapies for oligoprogressive disease (Helena et al. 2013). The role of SBRT in this group of patients is also yet to be defined, including appropriate sequencing of SBRT with tyrosine kinase inhibitors (TKI), its potential in first-line or consolidation treatment for oligometastatic disease, and its role in oligoprogressive disease.

3 Liver SBRT

Liver cancer remains one of the most common and deadly cancers in the world (Ananthakrishnan et al. 2006). It continues to increase in incidence and is the fastest rising cause of cancer-related death in the USA (Mittal and El-Serag 2013). Based on the Continuous Update Project of the World Cancer Research Fund International (Ferlay et al. 2015), and the Surveillance Epidemiology, and End Results (SEER) statistics (Siegel et al. 2015), liver cancer is the sixth most common cancer with 83% of cancer diagnosed in less developed regions of the world. The function and anatomy of the liver also result in the liver being a significant site of metastases in as many as 40–50% of adult cancers (Ananthakrishnan et al. 2006; Lo et al. 2011).

The only local treatment considered curative is surgery: liver resection or transplant. Unfortunately, less than 30% of patients are eligible for surgery due to advanced disease, anatomical proximity to vascular structures limiting resectability, shortage of donor livers, or underlying comorbidity (Llovet et al. 2004). Given the suboptimal prognosis without surgery and expected increase in incidence, there has been active research investigating other local treatments such as transarterial chemoembolization (TACE), radiofrequency ablation (RFA), and radiotherapy. Initial data with TACE for hepatocellular carcinoma (HCC) suggested a significant improvement in 2-year survival, but subsequent meta-analysis by the Cochrane group has cast doubt on this initial data (Oliveri et al. 2011). Currently, the 5-year survival of patients undergoing transplant is 75% as compared to 10% with current local treatment options (TACE, RFA, and sorafenib) (Rose et al. 2013). Therefore, alternatives such as radiation are being investigated. Advances in our understanding of radiobiology and technical innovations have vastly improved our ability to treat liver cancer with radiation. Therefore, in this section we review both primary and secondary liver cancer radiotherapy with a focus on the rationale for the convergence of management options, particularly in patients where radiation plays an important role, technical issues, and future directions.

3.1   Radiobiology

The radiobiology of liver cancer has been well studied, principally in an effort to avoid a life-threatening radiation-induced liver disease (RILD) (Lawrence et al. 1995). Early data from Emami indicated that tolerance dose for whole-liver radiation was 30 Gy in conventional 2 Gy fractions (Emami et al. 1991). More recent data have suggested that whole-liver tolerance may be lower at 22–24 Gy in pretreated patients or those treated with high dose per fraction (Ruhl et al. 2010). As this is not a tumoricidal dose, partial liver irradiation with escalated dose has become the principal area of investigation. Liver has a large functional reserve and the radiobiologic tolerance increases with partial liver irradiation. Partial volume irradiation has shown promising results and is the current pathway of investigation (Lee et al. 2009b).

Initial investigations have focused on determining optimal treatment doses that balances sufficient dose for tumor control against the maximum dose tolerances of normal tissue. Greater understanding and new technology have spawned multiple trials using different dose regimens based on varied radiobiological assumptions (Hoyer et al. 2012; Klein et al. 2014). These wide-ranging studies have allowed us to access essential information on critical structure tolerances, dose-volume effects, impact of total dose on liver, and value of dose escalation.

Some of the earliest works using altered fractionation were performed by Dawson et al. (2002, 2006). Instead of standard dose escalation until a maximum tolerated dose was achieved, Dawson selected doses using radiobiological guidance. Data compiled from these studies provide parameters that allowed radiobiological prediction of normal tissue complication probability (NTCP) curves. Patients were provided individually selected doses specific to their cancer and anatomy, thus possibly treating them with the best therapeutic ratio. These dose escalation trials were mathematically based on the Lyman-Kutcher (LK) model for normal liver tissues (Ten Haken et al. 1993).

This evolution of dose regimen selection has brought the concept of V_{eff} (the effective liver volume defined as liver minus all gross tumor volume (GTV)) of the LK model to the fore-front of radiobiologically guided radiotherapy. V_{eff}, if irradiated uniformly to the treatment dose, would be associated with the same risk of liver toxicity as the nonuniform dose distribution delivered. This allows the nonuniformly irradiated liver dose distribution to be reduced to a single parameter that can be entered into the NTCP model (Dawson et al. 2006). Prescription doses are selected using an NTCP model (McGinn et al. 1998) and escalated based on three predefined liver V_{eff} strata. Using this NTCP model as a guide, 41 patients were treated with no cases of RILD seen and a median OS of 23 months for HCC (Tse et al. 2008). Doses ranged from 24 to 54 Gy in six fractions over 2 weeks.

3.2   Hepatocellular Carcinoma (HCC)

3.2.1   Rationale and Patient Selection

If surgery is not an option for HCC, other therapies remain limited to a small subgroup of patients or those with suboptimal outcomes. Options such as sorafenib and TACE have become standard and are included in several guideline recommendations including a merging of the European Association for the Study of the Liver and the European Organization for Research and Treatment of Cancer (EASL-EORTC), American Association for the Study of Liver Diseases (AASLD), and Japan Society of Hepatology (JSH) guidelines (Kudo 2015). Yet these options are commonly limited by the same restrictions (proximity to blood vessels and size of lesions) that precluded these patients from undergoing surgery in the first place. As lesions increase in size, the success of TACE and RFA drops precipitously (Shim et al. 2005). Radiation is not as limited by these restrictions, but has not been included in these guidelines. This is due to a lack of randomized controlled trials, no standardized liver radiotherapy management, and limited availability. Modern radiation for HCC has grown rapidly in the past decade with many critical questions converging on a few conclusions.

One of the primary questions is which patients should receive radiotherapy. This has been answered first by trials that have attempted to identify groups or parameters that predict for toxicity or poor outcome. Early surveys had suggested a wide range of indications, but based an accumulation of data from multiple trials (Klein et al. 2014), one subgroup has been identified that may benefit most from radiation. These patients are unresectable, have less than five lesions or a residual normal liver of over 700 cm^3, Child-Pugh (CP) class A-B7, and do not have extrahepatic metastases. There is no direct restriction on lesion size or vascular proximity. The Indiana group performed a series of trials in HCC (Cardenes et al. 2010). Patients received 36 Gy in three fractions escalating to 48 Gy in three fractions at a maximum of twice per week. The only grade 3 toxicities were in patients with CP greater than B7. Cardenes et al. also decreased the dose for CP B to 40 Gy in five fractions. For smaller isolated tumors, higher doses can be achieved with minimal toxicity and very good outcomes. For larger tumors, heavily pretreated or in close proximity to critical structures, higher dose may not be achievable and hypofractionation and dose escalation may not be necessary (Lausch et al. 2013; Vickress et al. 2017). Based on one of the larger published cohorts, Vickress et al. were also able to demonstrate that for patients with CP B, dose escalation did not impact on survival while there was a significant impact for CP A patients. With this information, a simple management approach based on size has come to be accepted for early-stage HCC and assists in coordinating care with other modalities (Barr et al. 2016). For lesions less than 2 cm, RFA has shown ability to achieve complete ablation. For intermediate lesions measuring 2–5 cm, SBRT may be preferred as benefits of RFA decline. Finally, larger lesions defined as greater than 5 cm are treated with TACE, SBRT, or a combination.

3.2.2 Patients with Special Indications

Radiation may be particularly useful for three specific subgroups: bridging to transplant, portal thrombosis, and palliative patients. Local treatments have been shown to be successful in downstaging or bridging to transplant with improvement in the ability to undergo transplant and perhaps survival (Pompili et al. 2013). Though based on a relatively small highly selected case series, radiation does seem to provide a comparable outcome to patients bridged with TACE. Post-TACE, complete responses range from 27 to 57% (Pompili et al. 2013) and 5-year survival rates as high as 90% (Lesurtel et al. 2006). Similar outcomes are found in radiation trials with similar levels of evidence though with significantly fewer trials. A summary of radiation pretransplant trials found five trials with outcomes as promising as 5-year 100% OS (Klein et al. 2014). Patients were highly selected and it is not clear how many patients would have failed transplant or progressed beyond transplant eligibility without radiation. The transplant rate achieved ranged from 38 to 100%. In addition, TACE failures may lead patients to fall off the transplant list and may be salvaged by radiation. Failure at the treatment periphery, where there is little penetration of doxorubicin or collateral vascular supply, can be encompassed by radiation in up to 100% of cases (Kelsey et al. 2005). In terms of treatment regimen, no standard has been demonstrated, but centers may rely on regimens such as the Andolino protocol (Andolino et al. 2011). This is the largest case series with 60 patients treated with 24–48 Gy (lower doses were given to CP B patients) over three fractions. About 40% went on to transplant with no local failures while on the transplant list. The patients had an actuarial 2-year survival rate of 96%.

Another group with few options are the patients found to have vascular thrombosis of the portal vein (PV) or inferior vena cava (IVC). Thrombosis is a poor prognostic factor and may play a role in the development of symptoms and fatal progression (Quirk et al. 2015). HCC patients with vascular thrombosis have an OS of 2–4 months compared to 10–24 months in those without it (Quirk et al. 2015; Lau et al. 2013). There is no level I evidence; only 13 case series were analyzed. The largest trial demonstrated a 43% 1-year OS with a median dose of 40 Gy in 2–5 fractions (Tanguturi et al. 2014; Yoon et al. 2012). In the only prospective case series, a subgroup of 56 patients with vascular thrombosis were treated using radiobiological guidance (Bujold et al. 2013). Doses ranged from 24 to 54 Gy in six fractions every other day. Thrombosis was the only patient parameter that significantly impacted on survival in multivariate analysis. The 1-year OS was 44% in patients with vascular thrombosis vs. 67% without it at baseline. Radiologic evidence of recanalization is seen in 71% of cases (Lin et al. 2006). Though survivals remain very poor in this group, these trials represent optimism for patients with limited options and should be investigated further.

The last subgroup that has a specific radiation indication relative to other treatments is that of the palliative patient. In this context, these patients are defined as those with very poor prognoses requiring treatment for symptom control. Liver cancer may cause capsular discomfort, fever, obstruction, anorexia, bleeding, and pain. In terms of radiosensitivity, a case series of HCC patients with metastases to sites such as bone derived a 73–83% relief from pain (Kaizu et al. 1989; Seong et al. 2005). Can whole-liver radiation result in a similar palliation rate? At least 18 publications have investigated whole-liver radiation with nine specifically addressing radiation alone (Hoyer et al. 2005). None investigated HCC alone and data were extrapolated from studies of liver metastases or combined data.

3.2.3 Results

A large body of work on radiotherapy for HCC comes from Asia where incidence rates are high (Siegel et al. 2015). One of the largest series and earliest publications retrospectively reviewed 398 patients from ten centers (Seong et al. 2009). This cohort had a 28% OS at 2 years and a median survival of 12 months. Most tumors were less than 5 cm, CP A, and

received greater than $53Gy_{10}$. These patients were treated during the conformal therapy era. With the advent of SBRT trials, outcomes may have improved. In the first SBRT trial of HCC alone, patients received doses of 25 Gy in five, 30 Gy in three, or 37.5 Gy in three fractions over 5–10 days (Mendez Romero et al. 2006). The study found a 40% 2-year survival. The literature now has over 20 trials using a wide range of SBRT regimens with a summary of the literature concluding that the 1-year OS rate is between 43 and 67% (Klein et al. 2014). Despite wide variation in dose regimens, LC rates are in the range of 80–90% and are dependent on factors such as the presence of thrombosis, size of lesion, and dose.

3.3 Liver Metastases

Liver metastases are common and often indicate an important change in prognosis (Ananthakrishnan et al. 2006). There is great interest in the use of radiotherapy for an oligometastatic state. Therefore, partial liver irradiation using high-dose-per-fraction radiotherapy has become well published with multiple phase I/II publications. A landmark paper entered 27 patients into a dose escalation protocol of 30 Gy in three, 50 Gy in five, and 60 Gy in five fractions (Rule et al. 2011). Actuarial LC for these three cohorts was 56%, 89%, and 100% at 2 years, respectively. There were no treatment toxicities greater than grade 1 with no dose-limiting toxicities. Patients were highly selected and conservative constraints were applied, such as ensuring that 700 mL of normal liver receives less than a 21 Gy cumulative dose. Only a small number of tumors were located near the hilum, which often reduces the ability to achieve this dose and further reduces generalizability. Therefore, if achievable, 60 Gy in five fractions appears to be a safe and very effective treatment. In the review of evidence by members representing the American Society of Radiation Oncology (ASTRO), the European Society for Therapeutic Radiology and Oncology (ESTRO), the Canadian Association of Radiation

Oncology (CARO), and the Trans-Tasman Radiation Oncology Group (TROG), there was a large variation found in patient selection and treatment (Hoyer et al. 2012). Ideal candidates for oligometastatic treatment were those with good hepatic function, no extrahepatic disease, and an uninvolved liver volume of 700 mL or greater. There is evidence of the benefit of dose escalation (Lausch et al. 2013), including a multicenter pooled analysis that indicated that a dose of 48–52 Gy in three fractions is required to achieve 90% control at 1 year (Chang et al. 2011b). Furthermore, there are data that suggest that there may be a threshold with 3-year LC rates dropping from 59–89% to 8% when dose dropped from over 54 Gy to less than 36 Gy (McCammon et al. 2009). As the 48 Gy in three-fraction regimen from the pooled analysis resulted in a relatively low risk of toxicity, this dose or biologically equivalent regimen has been recommended by the multi-society evidence-based review (Hoyer et al. 2012). Further research is required to better identify factors impacting on clinical outcomes including anatomical location, previous treatments, underlying liver function, dose, and concomitant treatments.

3.4   Technical Considerations

The implementation of a radiation program for liver lesions presents technical challenges. These technical challenges can be grouped into (1) localization and (2) motion management. At the time of simulation, standard immobilization techniques are employed, but localization with intravenous (IV) contrast is an important difference to other sites. Arterial phase and washout phase of IV contrast are often critical to identify and delineate HCC lesions. Portal venous phase is often helpful to identify metastatic lesions. These images can be obtained using time-based injection protocols or time-density assessments correlated to contrast entering the structures like the aorta (Beddar et al. 2008; Jensen et al. 2014). Active or patient-controlled breath holds are usually obtained in end expiration where motion is minimized for a longer period. MRI fused with the CT simulation is becoming more common due to the improved ability to localize the lesion and assist in contouring (Hussain and Semelka 2005). However, methods to control motion are required where extended acquisition times are necessary. During radiotherapy, localization can be difficult as lesions within the liver are often not well visualized on the treatment unit imaging technology. Localization using the diaphragm has been shown to be accurate with a superior-inferior 8 mm tumor margin sufficient to ensure that internal and systematic motions are covered (Vedam et al. 2003). Localization using other image-guided technology, including the use of internal markers, provides additional ability to reduce margins if the technology is available.

Motion management in liver is critical as the liver can move up to 2 cm (Keall et al. 2006) which results in problems with localization at contouring and at the time of treatment. Three major methods are employed to reduce the impact of motion. First, nongated strategies that rely on identifying the motion and encompassing the region of motion using margins, or physically minimizing the motion, need to be employed. For example, an encompassing technique is to simply assess the motion of the lesion via a surrogate marker or direct assessment, and then place a margin for treatment to sufficiently encompass this region of motion. Physical methods include abdominal compression where reduction in motion to 2–3 mm can be achieved (Eccles et al. 2011). Second, breath-hold strategies have been shown to reduce motion. Active breathing control (ABC) has been shown to reduce internal motion error to less than 5 mm (Brock 2011; Mageras and Yorke 2004). As with the first strategy, additional margins for setup error and inter- and intrafraction motion error are still required. Many patients are not able to tolerate these procedures. The third method is the use of surrogate markers to enable gating or tracking. Internal markers are the gold standard for motion management and advancement such as radio-transmitting markers can provide real-time continuous motion information. Markers visible on standard imaging such as gold seeds, surgical clips, lipiodol, or anatomical calcifications can be useful markers to track motion. Markers can be used to gate in a certain phase such as expiration, synchronize treatment via tracking, or as a surrogate of breath-hold techniques. Examples of the use of markers to synchronize delivery include delivering radiation when a marker is in a certain location, treat using a moving beam such as CyberKnife® (Winter et al. 2015), or move the treatment window using dynamic multi-leaf collimator (MLC) tracking (Vedam et al. 2001).

3.5 Toxicity

There is a wide range of selection criteria used for patient eligibility, dose regimen, technology, and safety constraints (Lock et al. 2012). This may explain some of the variation in the toxicity rate and grades reported in the literature. A comprehensive review of gastrointestinal SBRT toxicities found that grade 3 liver toxicity ranged from 0 to 35%, and that only one study reported a grade 4 toxicity (Thomas et al. 2014). Investigation of HCC has yielded data to identify patients that can undergo safe treatment and those that may undertake a greater risk. Two main approaches to determine this data have been the Toronto radiobiological approach described above (Tse et al. 2008) and the Indiana dose escalation program. Indiana conducted a series of standard dose escalation studies increasing from 36 Gy in three fractions using 2 Gy per fraction increments (Cardenes et al. 2010; Andolino et al. 2011). They found that CP A patients could escalate without dose-limiting toxicity to 48 Gy in three fractions, but two CP B patients developed grade ≥ 3 toxicities. Therefore, they have recommended these patients receive a maximum dose of 40 Gy in five fractions with dose to one-third of uninvolved liver to receive ≤ 18 Gy and 500 cm^3 < 12 Gy. This group cau-

Table 2 Dose constraints

Organ at risk	3 fraction	5 fraction
Normal liver	700 mL < 15 Gy	V10 < 70%
Esophagus	D1 mL < 21 Gy	D0.5 mL < 32 Gy
Stomach	D1 mL < 21 Gy	D0.5 mL < 30 Gy
Kidney	D35% < 15 Gy	Dmean < 10 Gy
Bowel and duodenum	D1 mL < 21 Gy	D0.5 mL < 30 Gy
Spinal Cord	Dmax < 18 Gy	D0.5 mL < 25 Gy
Heart	D1 mL < 30 Gy	D30 mL < 30 Gy

tions the use of SBRT for CP $\geq$ B7 patients. A list of constraints used in active multicenter clinical trials is given in Table 2. Within these constraints and parameters developed by the Indiana and Toronto groups, the risk of toxicity is likely insignificant.

What are the possible toxicities? RILD is a constellation of signs similar to Budd-Chiari syndrome. RILD has been formalized to include an elevation of transaminases or alkaline phosphatase of >2.5–5-fold and/or bilirubin >1.5–3-fold compared to the upper normal limit or pretreatment level, and/or nonmalignant ascites in the absence of disease progression within 3 months of SBRT (Jung et al. 2013). The pathologic appearance of central venous congestion and collagen deposition causing small vein obstruction without inflammation prompted the description of this entity to differentiate it from radiation-induced hepatitis (Lawrence et al. 1995). Only palliative therapies are available and include paracentesis, diuretics, use of enzyme changes to guide discontinuation of treatment, and vitamin K for coagulopathies.

Non-RILD hepatic complications may include gastrointestinal damage, chest wall pain, coagulopathies, reactivation of viral hepatitis, cardiac injury, and pneumonitis and may be a greater concern than RILD (Bae et al. 2012). This study consisted of a large retrospective series of 202 primary and secondary liver patients and was the first study to enumerate and provide predictive parameters for severe gastroduodenal toxicity. The Dmax of 38 Gy was associated with a 10% risk of severe toxicity with a clinical history of ulcers also being a strong predictor. In a prospective trial by the Toronto group, 7% of patients experienced grade 5 toxicity; specifically, one patient developed a fatal duodenal bleed and five developed liver failure (Tse et al. 2008). Use of antiulcer prophylaxis, monitoring of platelet count for increased bleed (particularly when combined with TACE), and biliary stenting have been recommended without strong evidence.

3.6 Future Directions

Management of primary and secondary liver cancer remains a priority for oncology given an increasing incidence, dire prognosis, and relative lack of effective treatments. Based on landmark work on radiobiological guidance, dose escalation studies, and pooled registries, we may be reaching a consensus on constraints and dose regimens. Three- and five-fraction regimens are now considered safe and effective (Tanguturi et al. 2014), thus allowing initiation of large multicenter randomized trials using consensus-based standards (Sahgal et al. 2012a). Treatments such as TACE and sorafenib alone have been investigated in randomized trials, and are included in standard guidelines. Many SBRT trials have shown that despite good LC, patients selected for treatment often have a failure rate beyond the region irradiated (Tse et al. 2008). Therefore, combination treatments may provide the best way to improve clinical outcomes. Two active examples are the RTOG 1112 (Dawson et al. 2013) and the Tata Memorial trial (Clinical trials database: NCT01014130). RTOG 1112 is assessing sorafenib plus a five-fraction radiobiologically guided regimen. The Tata Memorial trial is randomizing patients to SBRT in addition to TACE alone.

In addition to randomized trials, additional work to clarify other factors that can help categorize patients and provide prognostic information is needed. For example, identifying patients that have a high risk of extrahepatic failure, separation of the impact of lesion size vs. dose, and

sequence of treatment relative to other modalities will impact on patient selection and treatment. Work from Canada has shown that despite assessing a relatively large number of patients, there is significant residual statistical variation indicating that additional variables are yet to be identified (Vickress et al. 2017; Lock et al. 2014). To accomplish this, larger databases are required and will likely entail the need to combine data from many institutions. Lastly, better understanding of response assessment is required as the Response Evaluation Criteria in Solid Tumors (RECIST) alone is insufficient (Lock et al. 2016). We know that size alone does not accurately assess the impact of radiation, and even the inclusion of contrast can be misleading as radiation can cause increased contrast enhancement (Herfarth et al. 2003). New concepts such as assessment for lobulated enhancement in standard CT images may provide early and accurate information (Jarraya et al. 2015). Therefore, assessment of response using new technology, including possibly MRI, PET, immune markers, and circulating tumor cells, is needed to better provide predictive information for response based on primary clinical endpoints. If this move to randomized control trials and merging of databases can be accomplished, we may provide liver patients with truly personalized, guideline-based treatment and deliver better outcomes in the near future.

4 Spine SBRT

Although primary malignancy of the spine is rare, the spine is one of the most common sites of metastases, developing in more than 30% of patients during the course of their illness (Sciubba and Gokaslan 2006). Spinal metastases often result in pain and can potentially compromise neural structures such as the spinal cord and the cauda equina. Radiation therapy with or without surgical intervention is offered in most cases of spinal metastases to alleviate pain and to reverse or prevent neurologic complications (Lo et al. 2010).

A single fraction of conventional external beam palliative radiotherapy (EBRT) with 8 Gy has been recommended for patients with painful vertebral metastases (Bekelman et al. 2013; Chow et al. 2007; Lutz et al. 2011). However, this dose of radiation is associated with partial pain relief rates of up to approximately 60% and limited complete pain relief rates ranging from 0 to 20% within 3 months post-EBRT. Furthermore, EBRT is associated with retreatment rates of 10–20% due to pain progression or inadequate pain relief often within only 3 months following EBRT. The mean duration of response is approximately 6 months. This is clinically significant as the spine's cumulative dose exposure must be limited in order to respect spinal cord tolerance. Therefore, it can be argued that treatment impact should be maximized with the first course of radiation for spinal metastases, as opposed to allowing for retreatment in one in five patients treated with low-dose EBRT, such as 8 Gy in a single fraction, particularly in patients with an expected survival of greater than 3 months.

It is acknowledged, however, that a major challenge lies in predicting the spinal metastasis patient who will survive long enough to benefit from treatment, and validated scoring systems are emerging to enable selection of those subgroups that will survive beyond 3 months. For those patients with a reasonable prognosis, SBRT is a technique applied to the spine that provides a means to deliver an ablative dose of radiation to a spinal tumor while respecting safe OAR dose constraints in 1–5 fractions (Foote et al. 2011). Spine SBRT has been quickly adopted in the radiation therapy community as a viable treatment for selected patients (Pan et al. 2011); however, its broad clinical implementation is supported largely by retrospective single- and multi-institutional analyses (Guckenberger et al. 2014) and only a few prospective nonrandomized trials (Ryu et al. 2003; Wang et al. 2012). One of the areas of major growth for spine SBRT is in salvaging EBRT failures and this technique was initially developed for this indication; however, the application of spine SBRT for de novo spinal metastases is on the rise. It has particular utility in the management of the oligometastatic patient. Lastly, in the postoperative patient, the use of spine SBRT is increasing in awareness as a means of maximizing surgical outcomes.

4.1 Patient Selection

Common to SBRT in other sites, there are some general stipulations to be met for the patient to be eligible for spine SBRT. Although complete cure might be possible in a few patients with oligometastases, the aim of SBRT in general is to achieve LC and delay progression, and thereby postpone the need for further treatment. For this reason patient performance status and likely prognosis should be duly considered (Tree et al. 2013). Secondly, given the steep dose gradients and the risk of overdosing the critical neural structures resulting in myelopathy, the patient must be able to tolerate lying still in a near-rigid immobilization device for the duration of treatment (Lo et al. 2016).

Specifically for spine SBRT in the metastatic setting, given the wide variability in overall survival (OS) after treatment, an RPA has been developed to predict which patients may derive the greatest benefit (Chao et al. 2012). Factors predictive of an improved OS after spine SBRT include Karnofsky Performance Status (KPS) >70, age <70, and a longer time to progressive disease, which relates to disease-free interval. More recently a prognostic index for spinal metastases (PRISM) model based on patients from two prospective trials has been developed that predicts outcome in four groups (excellent prognosis–poor prognosis) based on several patient and treatment variables (Tang et al. 2015). Optimal inclusion criteria, relative contraindications, and major contraindications as outlined in Table 3 serve as a guide to assist in patient selection for spine SBRT (Jabbari et al. 2016).

Table 3 Inclusion, relative and major contraindications for spine SBRT

Optimal inclusion criteria for spine SBRT	Relative contraindication to spine SBRT	Major contraindications to spine SBRT*
Good to excellent performance status	Moderate performance status	Poor performance status (ECOG 3–4. KPS < 60)
Oligometastatic disease (5 sites extracranial metastases)	Oligoprogression in patients with widely metastatic and/or rapidly progressive disease	Widely metastatic and/or rapidly progression disease with limited life expectancy
Oligoprogression in a patient with oligometastatic disease		
No more than 3 spinal levels involved (contiguous or noncontiguous)	>3 spinal levels involved, but nondiffuse spine disease and no more than 3 continuous segments	>3 contiguous spinal levels involved, or diffuse spine disease
No or minimal spine instability (SINS 0–6)	Potential spine in-stability (SINS 7–12)	Spine in-stability (SINS 13–18)
No or minimal epidural disease (Bilsky 0–1)	Moderate-grade epidural disease (Bilsky 2)	High-grade epidural disease (Bilsky 3)
"Radioresistant" histology	"Radio-sensitive" histology	
No prior cEBRT to affected level, or prior cEBRT delivered 5 months prior to salvage spine SBRT	Prior cEBRT delivered 3–5 months prior to considered course of salvage spine SBRT	Prior cEBRT <3 months prior to considered course of salvage spine SBRT
Spine SBRT delivered 5 months of a considered second course of salvage SBRT	Spine SBRT delivered within 3 to 5 months of a considered second course of salvage SBRT	Spine SBRT delivered <3 of a considered second course of salvage SBRT
Robotic Linac or subcentimeter MLC based Linac delivery, CBCT and/or stereoscopic imaging IGRT, near-rigid body immobilization, fusion of thin-slice MRI sequences for target/CNS contouring and in selected post-op cases a treatment planning CT myelogram	If unable to have a MRI then a treatment planning CT myelogram for CNS structure contouring provided that the target is identifiable on CT alone with sufficient clinical detail as to paraspinal disease extension/epidural disease extension	Unable to tolerate near-rigid/supine immobilization. Unable to have a full spine MRI and/or CT myelogram

CNS in dicates central nervous system (spinal cord, thecal sac); ECOG, Eastern Cooperative Organization Group; IGRT, image-guided radiotherapy KPS, Karnofsky Performance Status; MLC, multi leaf collimator; mo, months
*Exceptions may exist based on Practitioner's Experience and Clinical Scenario

4.1.1 Up-Front Spine SBRT

A multi-institutional retrospective study has shown the safety and efficacy of using spine SBRT in patients with no previous radiation therapy at that spinal segment (Guckenberger et al. 2014). In this study, 387 spinal metastases were treated. The median follow-up was 11.8 months and LC at 2 years was 83.9%. On multivariate analysis, OS, male sex, performance status <90, presence of visceral, uncontrolled systemic disease, and >1 vertebra treated were correlated with worse outcomes. In one of the few prospective studies, spine SBRT was associated with significant reduction in pain scores with a 1-year progression-free survival of 80.5% (95% CI 72.9–86.1) and 72.4% (95% CI 63.1–79.7) at 2 years (Wang et al. 2012).

Spine SBRT is of particular interest in patients with oligometastases in an attempt to affect a cure. SBRT has been shown to be an effective, noninvasive alternative to surgery for treating oligometastases (Corbin et al. 2013) and given that en bloc resection with margin control in the spine is rarely achievable, spine SBRT has become a promising alternative for patients with oligometastatic disease to the spine. There is however scant literature on spine oligometastases. A retrospective review (Gill et al. 2012) showed that patients with spine-only oligometastases had a 2-year OS and freedom from local progression of 57% and 73%, respectively. Given that 35% of the treated patients had a sarcoma primary histology it is unlikely that these numbers are consistent with other institutions.

4.1.2 Retreatment Spine SBRT

Local failure following conventional palliative radiotherapy is a major problem as the traditional practice is to deliver a second course of palliative radiotherapy with a biologically effective dose lower than the first for fear of causing spinal cord damage. A trial in painful bone metastases has been reported showing poor efficacy of this treatment approach with only 30–50% of patients gaining any improvement in pain with second-course radiation therapy (Chow et al. 2014).

Early data suggested that spine SBRT is an effective salvage treatment for patients with recurrent metastases after previous radiotherapy (Sahgal et al. 2009) with 1- and 2-year progression-free probability of 85% and 69%, respectively. This has been replicated by others (Choi et al. 2010; Garg et al. 2011) which confirm that spine SBRT can be safely administered in patients who have previously had spine radiotherapy with good control rates and low rates of treatment-related complications. Furthermore, in a multi-institutional pooled analysis (Hashmi et al. 2016), the 6- and 12-month LC rates were 93% and 83%, respectively, with Karnofsky Performance Status (KPS) <70 being a significant prognostic factor for worse OS. There were no cases of radiation myelopathy and the vertebral compression fracture rate was 4.5% confirming the safety of this approach.

4.1.3 Postoperative Spine SBRT

Postoperative SBRT for metastatic spinal tumors is increasingly being performed in clinical practice and it is changing surgical paradigms away from large open (largely invasive and morbid) surgical procedures (Redmond et al. 2016). However, patients with high-grade malignant epidural spinal cord compression (MESCC) or those with a pathological fracture and clinical signs of mechanical instability will often benefit from spine surgery. This improves the chances for neurological recovery in patients with high-grade MESCC and can restore spinal stability; however, it may not provide durable LC (Sahgal et al. 2011). For patients receiving surgery and conventional adjuvant radiotherapy local recurrences of 57.9% at 6 months and 69.3% at 1 year have been reported (Klekamp and Samii 1998) which is unacceptably high for patients with a reasonable prognosis.

Based on these observations, spine SBRT has been utilized in the postoperative setting to optimize LC in an attempt to improve outcomes for these patients. Although technically more demanding, initial results suggest that utilizing spine SBRT in the postoperative setting is safe and effective (Redmond et al. 2016; Sahgal et al. 2011). Based on these findings investigators are exploring the role of limited surgery (thecal sac decompression and/or stabilization) followed by spine SBRT to reduce the morbidity associated with traditional spinal surgical approaches and attain durable tumor control and spinal stability.

4.1.4 Primary Spinal/Paraspinal Tumors

The most common malignant primary tumors of the spine include osteosarcoma, Ewing's sarcoma, chordoma, and chondrosarcoma. In general, outcomes are better with resection and clear margins; however, these are difficult to achieve and local recurrences are common (Yamada et al. 2013). Given the relative radioresistance of these tumors to conventional radiotherapy there has been an interest in exploring the role of spine SBRT to improve LC.

For chordoma of the sacrum and mobile spine, there is early data to suggest that spine SBRT is safe and effective in the recurrent and adjuvant setting using a range of dose fractionation regimens (Yamada et al. 2013; Chang et al. 2014b). Similarly, there are emerging data in the management of primary spine sarcomas with spine SBRT achieving high rates of LC at 2 years (Chang et al. 2012) with reasonable pain control and minimal toxicity (Miller et al. 2016). Although these preliminary results suggest a role of spine SBRT in the management of primary malignant spinal tumors, longer term prospective data are required before its routine use.

4.2 Technical Considerations

4.2.1 Modalities and Apparatus Dependence

Various apparatuses have been developed or modified to deliver spine SBRT. For example, a compact linear accelerator with a mobile robotic arm capable of six degrees of freedom (DOF) motion has been used (Chuang et al. 2007). The more widely available linear accelerators using subcentimeter multi-leaf collimators (MLC) for beam shaping and intensity modulation, and six DOF treatment couches to allow for submillimeter and subdegree patient positioning (Ryu et al. 2003; Hyde et al. 2012), are more commonly used. There are also data to support the use of various other devices including helical TomoTherapy® although these are more limited (Kim et al. 2013).

Fundamental to all modalities is the requirement for an image guidance system, patient immobilization, and a treatment planning system that is capable of computing the highly irregular-shaped plans with steep dose gradients at the spinal cord/thecal sac interface (Finnigan et al. 2016). Image guidance can be achieved using a stereoscopic X-ray system, a gantry-mounted cone beam computed tomography (CBCT), or both. The intent is to ensure that the patient is positioned within 1 mm and 1° of the planned position and maintains this positional accuracy despite long treatment times.

4.2.2 Volume Definition and Dosimetry

It is well accepted that consensus definitions are necessary to standardize the nomenclature and delivery of spinal radiosurgery. This enables comparison of results from different institutions, treatment platforms, and dose fraction schedules.

Early spine SBRT experience identified failures beyond the conformal targeted volume as the primary pattern of recurrence (Chang et al. 2007) highlighting the need for accuracy in target volume delineation.

The International Spine Radiosurgery Consortium developed consensus guidelines for volume definition in spinal stereotactic radiotherapy (Cox et al. 2012a). These guidelines largely focus on clinical target volume (CTV) definition in a range of common spine SBRT scenarios. Common to the various scenarios is that the CTV includes any abnormal marrow signal suspicious for microscopic invasion and an adjacent normal bony expansion to account for subclinical tumor spread in the marrow space. Furthermore, no epidural CTV expansion is recommended without epidural disease, and circumferential CTVs encircling the cord should be used only when the vertebral body, bilateral pedicles/lamina, and spinous process are all involved or there is extensive metastatic disease along the circumference of the epidural space.

For postoperative spine SBRT, the GTV should be outlined as any residual disease visualized on post-operative imaging. The CTV should follow similar concepts to those of the International Spine Radiosurgery Consortium guidelines but include areas of disease on preoperative imaging, disease found at the time of surgery (based on surgical notes), and any regions of concern based on personal communications with the surgeon. The surgical incision and any screws placed in areas of healthy tissue do not need to be covered in the CTV (Redmond et al. 2016).

Planning target volume contour recommendations are not proposed given the significant differences in inter- and intrafraction motion management techniques, treatment platforms, immobilization methods, and prescription dose fractionation schedules used. Generally, however, a PTV should include a uniform three-dimensional expansion around the CTV, keeping the CTV-to-PTV margin 3 mm or less (Cox et al. 2012a), but practice varies if the PTV overlaps with an OAR (Guckenberger et al. 2011). Figure 1 is an example of a spine SBRT plan.

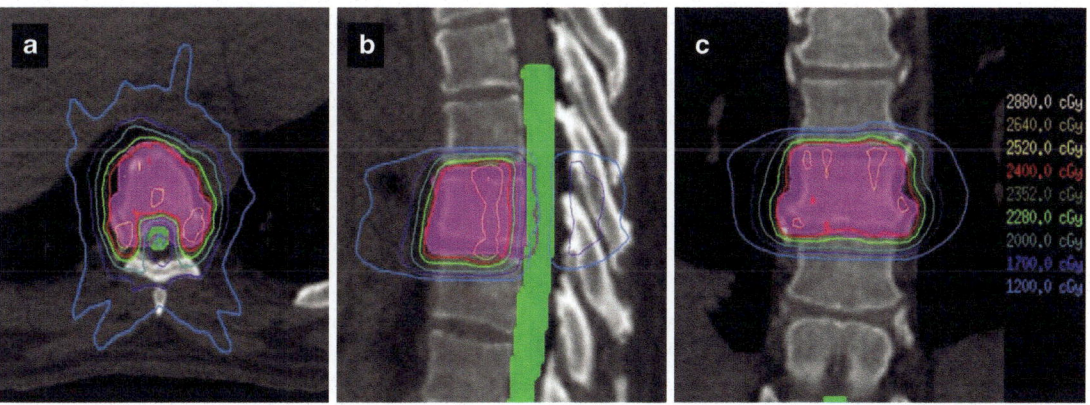

Fig. 1. Spine metastasis treated to 24 Gy in single fraction

4.2.3 Dose and Fractionation

At present, there are no prospective randomized studies comparing outcomes following single-fraction vs. multiple-fraction spine SBRT. As such a range of dose fractionation schedules are used ranging from a single dose of 18–24 Gy and various hypofractionated SBRT schedules of 18–30 Gy in 2–5 fractions (Lagerwaard et al. 2012; Pan et al. 2011; Guckenberger et al. 2011). Although open to debate, there is conflicting evidence that hypofractionated spine SBRT may provide superior longer term tumor control (Laufer et al. 2013; Heron et al. 2012). On the other hand, other groups have found single-fraction high-dose SBRT to be more effective for LC than hypofractionated approaches (Folkert et al. 2014). Hypofractionated spine SBRT schedules have a theoretical advantage in the postoperative spine SBRT settings (Hashmi et al. 2016). Irrespective, if strict dose constraints are used, toxicity appears similarly low with both single- and hypofractionated approaches.

4.2.4 Quality Assurance

Internationally, professional bodies have highlighted that SBRT is a specialized radiation therapy planning and delivery technique with defined roles as part of a multidisciplinary team (Sahgal et al. 2012a; Foote et al. 2015; Kirkbride and Cooper 2011; Potters et al. 2010). In general, it is recommended that specific protocols are used with emphasis on

maintenance of expertise, quality assurance, collection of data, and trial participation where applicable.

Specifically for spine SBRT, in a multinational report from high-volume centers, there was strong agreement that a formal or an informal credentialing process is an important component of a safe and effective spine radiosurgery program (Gerszten et al. 2013).

4.3 Local Outcomes

4.3.1 Local Failure

Patterns of failure have been described in an analysis of 285 consecutive patients with 332 spinal metastases treated with SBRT at the University of Texas MD Anderson Cancer Center (MDACC, Houston, Texas) (Bishop et al. 2015). Of the local recurrences, 48% were in-field and 52% were marginal. The marginal failures (typically at the thecal sac or spinal cord interface) tended to occur earlier (6 vs. 8 months) and, as expected, had more disease bulk at the interface. In attempting to identify dosimetric parameters accounting for local recurrence, GTV Dmin was the only factor of significance, which suggests that dose inhomogeneity may be an important factor (Bishop et al. 2015). The authors recommend maintaining a GTV Dmin above 14 Gy in one fraction and 21 Gy in three fractions, which may be difficult depending on the proximity of tumor to the critical neural structures and dose constraints used.

For postoperative spine SBRT, it has been reported that the most common site of failure is within the epidural space accounting for over 70% of failures. Patterns of epidural failure in the postoperative SBRT setting appear to be linked to the extent and location of preoperative epidural disease (Chan et al. 2016). In one study, grade 0 or 1 postoperative epidural disease (0, no epidural disease; 1, epidural disease that compresses dura only) predicted for LC (Al-Omair et al. 2013a). In that study, patients who had high-grade preoperative epidural disease downgraded surgically had superior LC suggesting that there is a theoretical biological advantage of debulking (potentially more aggressive) epidural disease.

4.3.2 Dependence upon Histology

There are some metastatic histologies that have been traditionally considered to be radioresistant, with poor response rates to conventional palliative radiotherapy. Included in these are sarcoma, renal cell cancer (RCC), and melanoma. There is conflicting data as to the impact of traditional "radioresistance" with spine SBRT. The International Spine Consortium suggested that LC was worse with primary histologies of NSCLC, RCC, and melanoma (Guckenberger et al. 2014). However, a report on 120 sarcoma metastases (88 patients) treated with SBRT spine reported a LC of 87.9% at 12 months with single-fraction treatment (Folkert et al. 2014). Others have reported similar outcomes for RCC metastases treated with spine SBRT with 12-month LC of 80–90% (Ghia et al. 2016; Thibault et al. 2014). Irrespectively, it appears that SBRT is challenging the notion of radioresistance where high doses per fraction seem very effective.

4.3.3 Toxicity After Spine SBRT

The risk of clinically significant pain flare has been reported in 68% of steroid-naïve patients treated with spine SBRT (Chiang et al. 2013). The initiation of rescue 4 mg dexamethasone was shown to significantly reduce the pain flare reaction over time. In a prospective observa-tional study, prophylactic 4–8 mg dexamethasone reduced the incidence of pain flare to 19% (Khan et al. 2015a) prompting the recommendation of routine use of prophylactic dexamethasone. Irrespectively, acute pain flare is a significant and common toxicity of spine SBRT that needs to be addressed in each individual patient.

When the practice of spine SBRT was initially introduced, radiation-induced myelopathy was the most feared complication. With accumulated data, the rates of radiation-induced myelopathy are considered acceptably low if appropriate tolerances are set on the critical neural structures. Given the high doses per fraction, steep dose gradients, and impact of small point maximum doses, traditional models to estimate spinal cord dose tolerance do not accurately predict tolerance in the setting of spine SBRT (Daly et al. 2012). In the up-front setting, based on known cases of spine SBRT-induced radiation myelopathy, a logistic regression analysis has established a guide to safe practice (Sahgal et al. 2013a). For a less than 5% risk of radiation myelopathy, it is recommended to limit the thecal sac (contoured surrogate for the spinal cord) Pmax volume dose to 12.4 Gy in a single fraction, 17.0 Gy in two fractions, 20.3 Gy in three fractions, 23.0 Gy in four fractions, and 25.3 Gy in five fractions. In the retreatment setting, guidelines on safe practices after EBRT have been published (Sahgal et al. 2012b). These guidelines are based on exposures to the spinal cord using the normalized BED (nBED), which is the 2 Gy equivalent BED using an alpha beta ratio of 2 and is essentially the same as the equivalent dose in 2 Gy per day fractions (EQD2). The guidelines are specific to a prior exposure of nBED ranging from 30 to 50 Gy2/2 and the rules for calculating the reirradiation thecal sac dose limit include the following:

1. *A thecal sac Pmax total nBED of no more than 70 Gy2/2*
2. *A SBRT thecal sac retreatment dose to the Pmax not exceeding 25 Gy2/2*
3. *A thecal sac SBRT Pmax nBED/total Pmax nBED ratio not exceeding 0.5*

4. *A minimum time interval to reirradiation of at least 5 months*

A detailed table of recommended dose limits in 1–5 fractions is reported in the publication. These guidelines represent a benchmark for safe practice. There is no doubt that some patients may tolerate even greater doses of radiation to the spinal cord. At this time there is no a priori method to determine which patients can tolerate higher doses. Furthermore, as the technology has improved over the past 5 years, the technical factors associated with myelopathy risk are diminished such that higher doses to the spinal cord may on occasion be reasonable.

The first report on SBRT-induced vertebral compression fracture (VCF) was by the Memorial Sloan-Kettering Cancer Center (MSKCC), which reported VCF in 27 (39%) of 71 sites treated with SBRT (Rose et al. 2009). This risk is prohibitive and further series including a comprehensive multi-institutional study clarified the risk of VCF (Sahgal et al. 2013b). In this study, Sahgal et al. reported a 1-year cumulative risk of 39% for VCF when the dose per fraction was 24 Gy or more; however, the risk was 19% when the dose per fraction ranged from 20 to 23 Gy and 10% when 19 Gy and less. Perhaps a more important and objective measure than the prescription dose per fraction is patient- and disease-specific factors which were identified as risk factors including lytic disease, baseline fracture, and spinal malalignment. More recently the Spinal Instability Neoplastic Score (SINS) was shown to predict for symptomatic VCF (Lee et al. 2016). In patients with high SINS (Hellman and Weichselbaum 1995; Ferlay et al. 2010; Rami-Porta et al. 2009; Edwards et al. 2002; Loganathan et al. 2006; Raz et al. 2007), 65.8% developed a VCF of which half were symptomatic. Patients with high SINS were more likely to experience symptomatic fractures (31.6%) than were patients with lower SINS (7.4%). With respect to the mechanism of radiation dose and VCF, clinicopathologic correlation analysis from biopsies of cases with post-SBRT VCF suggests that the underlying mechanism is radiation-induced osteoradionecrosis (Al-Omair et al. 2013b). It is highly recommended that the SINS be used as a tool to identify high-risk

patients for VCF and consultation with a spinal surgeon for patients who are frankly unstable. The safety of spine SBRT in these patients is unknown. Therefore, these patients may benefit from prophylactic stabilization to render them a candidate for SBRT; otherwise conventional radiation may be safer. Further research into the role of prophylactic stabilization is in progress especially in those with a potentially unstable spine.

Reported toxicities, other than those previously outlined, appear uncommon with spine SBRT. Potential esophageal toxicity should be considered when treating thoracic spinal/paraspinal lesions. In a study of 204 spinal or paraspinal metastases abutting the esophagus the rate of grade ≥ 3 acute or late esophageal toxicity was 6.8% when using single-fraction spine SBRT (Cox et al. 2012b). In a logistic regression model keeping the dose to the hottest 2.5 cm^3 of esophagus <14.5 Gy yields a grade ≥ 3 toxicity rate of <5% with a steep increase in toxicity after further increases in dose. Based on this, the authors recommend a V12Gy <3.78cm^3, V15Gy <1.87 cm^3, V20Gy <0.11 cm^3, and a point maximum of 22 Gy when using single-fraction SBRT. Chemotherapy appears to be a cofactor in high-grade esophageal toxicity with a median time to development of 4 months. Manipulation of the esophagus may also be contributory; thus endoscopy in the months after SBRT to the thoracic spine should only be undertaken if absolutely required. This highlights the need for conservative parameters to protect the esophagus when performing spine SBRT (Abelson et al. 2012).

4.4 Response Determination and Follow-Up Practice

There are a number of challenges in standardizing imaging-based assessment of LC and pain for spinal metastases. The SPine response assessment In Neuro-Oncology (SPINO) group is a committee of the Response Assessment in Neuro-Oncology working group comprised of a panel of international experts in spine SBRT tasked with reporting consensus criteria for tumor imaging, clinical assessment, and symptom-based response criteria in spine SBRT (Thibault et al. 2015).

Preliminary SPINO recommendations are as follows:

Imaging-based local tumor response

- *MRI preferred*
- *Images should be interpreted by a radiation oncologist and radiologist*
- *LC may be defined as the absence of progression within the treated area on serial imaging (two or three consecutive MRI scans 6–8 weeks apart)*
- *Local progression may be defined as:*
  - *Gross unequivocal increase in tumor volume or linear dimension*
  - *Any new or progressive tumor within the epidural space*
  - *Neurological deterioration attributable to preexisting epidural disease with equivocal increased epidural disease dimensions on MRI*
  - *Pseudo-progression and necrosis should be considered, with repeat imaging and biopsy to confirm when in doubt*

Pain response

- *Brief Pain Inventory (BPI) preferred, with assessment based on worst pain score*
- *International Consensus Pain Response Endpoints (ICPRE) guidelines should be adopted as standard for pain response*
- *Pain response should be assessed at 3 months after SBRT*

Imaging follow-up frequency

Spine MRI every 2–3 months after SBRT for the first 12–18 months, and every 3–6 months thereafter

4.5 Management of Spine SBRT Failure

Among patients with de novo, retreatment, and postoperative spine SBRT, 1-year LC rates of around 80% have been observed (Guckenberger et al. 2014; Sahgal et al. 2009; Redmond et al.

2016). However, this means that there are a significant number of spine SBRT failures and currently there are few data on how to effectively manage this scenario.

In a study of 56 metastatic spinal segments in 40 patients where salvage second SBRT course to the same level was delivered the 1-year LC rate was 81% and median time to local failure was 3.0 months (Thibault et al. 2015). No radiation myelopathy or VCF was observed with a median salvage second SBRT total dose and number of fractions of 30 Gy in 4 fractions (range 20–35 Gy in 2–5 fractions). These data suggest that second-course spine SBRT for spinal metastases that failed initial SBRT is a feasible and efficacious salvage treatment option; however the strength of any conclusions is limited by the paucity of quality data in this area.

4.6 Future Directions

The practice of spine SBRT will continue to evolve and become a standard of care for selected patients with spinal metastases internationally, in both oligometastatic patients and patients with widespread metastatic disease. Given the limitations of repeat fractionated treatment in the retreatment setting, spine SBRT will likely become a routine clinical practice to optimize pain and local tumor control in this group. In the up-front setting, clinical trials will further define the indications for spine SBRT. The role of postoperative spine SBRT appears promising to improve outcomes after surgery and the role of limited surgery with planned spine SBRT is a novel approach to improve oncologic outcomes as well as reduce treatment morbidity.

With the dissemination of immunotherapy in a wide range of patients with advanced disease, and the biological rationale of combining these treatments with ablative radiation (Gorayski et al. 2015) to enhance both local and systemic effects, it is likely that future developments in spine and other SBRT sites will be in the field of sequencing and combination with these systemic agents.

5 Kidney SBRT

The incidence of renal cell carcinoma (RCC) is rising due to multiple factors including an aging patient population and a greater number of incidental tumors found on imaging. In the USA, it is estimated that there will be almost 63,000 new cases in 2016, and just over 14,000 deaths (Siegel et al. 2016). The gold standard for management of localized disease is total or partial nephrectomy. There are, however, a number of situations in which surgery is not ideal, including cases of bilateral tumors, single kidney, preexisting chronic renal failure (CRF), and medically inoperable patients. In these cases, alternative strategies must be considered and include radiofrequency ablation (RFA), cryotherapy, microwave ablation, radiotherapy, and more recently SBRT. There are a number of advantages of SBRT that make it a particularly attractive option in primary RCC. We have found that SBRT is an ablative, yet noninvasive, outpatient procedure that shows promising LC rates accompanied by low rates of toxicity. In general, a broader range of patient and tumor locations can be approached than by alternative ablative treatments. This section reviews the radiobiology of RCC, treatment of primary RCC including patient selection, technical aspects of SBRT delivery, clinical outcomes, follow-up, and lastly metastatic RCC, including the role of SBRT, associated immunological effects, and role of systemic treatment options. Finally this section concludes by discussing future directions in this exciting field.

5.1 Radiobiology

Historically the role of radiotherapy in primary RCC has been limited due to the belief that RCC is inherently radioresistant. This notion followed studies using conventional radiotherapy doses of approximately 2 Gy per fraction. A review of preclinical studies on cell survival curves published in 1996 found RCC to be among the most radioresistant in vitro cell types to conventional radio-

therapy doses (Deschavanne and Fertil 1996). Clinical studies also appeared to corroborate these findings with two randomized studies on preoperative radiotherapy showing no survival benefit (Juusela et al. 1997; van der Werf-Messing 1973) and a more recent meta-analysis on postoperative radiotherapy showing similar results (Tunio et al. 2010). Although these studies had a significant negative impact upon clinician perspectives regarding the role of radiotherapy in RCC, they have a number of limitations, including the use of nonconformal radiation techniques, inadequate doses, and outdated technology in terms of image guidance and radiation delivery, that invalidate their applicability to modern clinical practice.

The advent of SBRT has assisted therefore in not only overcoming the technical hurdles of the past, but also gradually challenging and dispelling the concept of radioresistance in RCC. Experimental data studying the cell survival curves of two common human RCC cell lines (A498 and Caki-1) suggested that the α/β ratio of RCC is lower than seen in other cancers (2.6 and 6.9, respectively) and may therefore be more sensitive to higher dose per fraction (Ning et al. 1997). A preclinical study in which 12 nude mice with RCC (A498 cell line) were irradiated to 48 Gy in three fractions (once a week) and seven mice used as controls showed 30% tumor regression in the irradiated mice vs. tumor growth in the control mice at 7 weeks (Walsh et al. 2006). Furthermore, histological analysis revealed no active mitoses in the irradiated tissue as compared to 9–14 mitoses per high-powered field in the control mice. These preclinical studies are now supported by a growing body of clinical data showing excellent LC rates with the use of SBRT.

The differing outcomes seen with conventional radiotherapy vs. SBRT likely reflect the diverse pathways of cellular kill that are activated. Conventional radiotherapy results in oxygen-dependent DNA damage and P53-mediated programmed cell death. Unfortunately, this creates a state of hypoxia, in which proangiogenic factors accumulate, and protect the vascular endothelium, which is essential for the propagation of RCC. Ablative radiotherapy effects are partially mediated via novel apoptotic pathways, with translocation of ASMase, production of pro-apoptotic ceramide, and rapid endothelial cell death within 1 h of radiotherapy (Garcia-Barros et al. 2003; Li et al. 2010; Sathishkumar et al. 2005). This is particularly relevant in RCC in which survival is dependent upon an extensive vascular and angiogenic microenvironment. A comprehensive recent review of these mechanisms is provided by De Meerleer et al. (De Meerleer et al. 2014).

5.2 Primary Renal Cell Carcinoma

5.2.1 Patient Selection

While nephrectomy remains the standard of care in patients with localized disease, there are a number of patients in which nephrectomy may be inappropriate. SBRT may offer a more suitable alternative in medically unfit patients, patients with a single kidney, and patients with preexisting CRF. Svedman et al. reported the results of SBRT in patients with a single kidney and found that, in two out of seven patients, the posttreatment creatinine was moderately elevated at 160 µmol/L; however dialysis was not required. In the remaining five patients there was no worsening in kidney function (Svedman et al. 2008). Siva et al. reported on 21 patients, 9 of whom were assessed to be at high risk of requiring dialysis postoperatively, who were treated with SBRT to the primary tumor (Siva et al. 2016a). The mean baseline GFR was 52 mL/min and post-SBRT reduced to 43 mL/min. However once again, no patients required dialysis. The results of these studies suggest that SBRT may be a safe alternative to surgery in patients with a single kidney or deemed to be at high risk of dialysis postnephrectomy. However further studies with long-term data are required to better inform individual patients of their risk of nephron injury with SBRT.

Compared to other ablative techniques, SBRT has the advantage of being able to treat larger and fast-growing tumors, whereas RFA and cryotherapy are generally reserved for smaller

T1a tumors (Siva et al. 2016b; Swaminath and Chu 2015). SBRT is also an attractive choice when treating patients with centrally located tumors, or those adjacent to the collecting system and vessels. Patients with coagulopathies or frail patients should also be considered for SBRT as a noninvasive alternative that does not require anesthetic or sedation. Currently, no randomized data exist comparing any of these modalities to SBRT, although several retrospective studies and meta-analyses suggest comparable LC rates (Kunkle and Uzzo 2008).

Situations in which SBRT may not be appropriate include targets that are anteriorly placed close to bowel and very large tumors (Siva et al. 2016c), although the tumor size limit at which SBRT is no longer safe or effective is not well established. A recent retrospective study of large renal masses treated with SBRT included patients with tumors as large as 24 cm and reported relatively few associated side effects, although the patient with the largest tumor incurred grade 3 nausea as a toxicity (Correa et al. 2016).

5.2.2 Technical Considerations

Perhaps one of the most crucial aspects of SBRT delivery in RCC is motion management. The kidney moves with respiration; therefore methods for restricting and accounting for motion are vital. A review of studies investigating kidney motion revealed that mean kidney motion varied between 4.5 and 13.9 mm in free-breathing patients, between 4.6 and 18.1 mm through the use of the prone position or compression device, and between 10.1 and 41 mm through the use of deep breathing or breath-hold techniques (Pham et al. 2014a). Another study using a dual-vacuum stabilization device was shown to reduce kidney motion in six out of nine healthy volunteers, although motion was increased in one volunteer (Pham et al. 2015). These studies clearly highlight the complexities involved in accounting for respiratory-associated kidney motion and its management. Commonly therefore, individual tumor motion is also accounted for via the use of a thin-cut 4D-CT obtained during simulation and utilized to determine an appropriate ITV. Expansions of between 3 and 10 mm are usually added to produce a

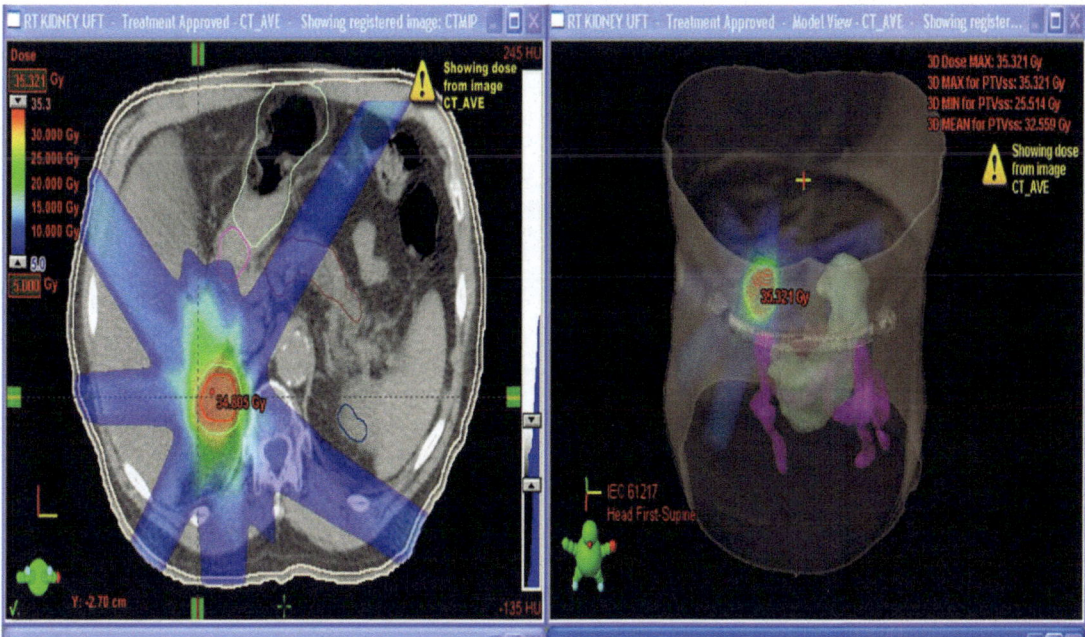

Fig. 2. SBRT plan for the right kidney

PTV (Siva et al. 2016c). Other strategies include respiratory gating and tumor tracking using implanted fiducial markers.

A range of stereotactic doses have been used in the literature to treat primary RCC which commonly varies between 30 and 45 Gy in 3–5 fractions, although more recent studies have also used single-fraction regimens of 25–26 Gy (Pham et al. 2014b; Staehler et al. 2015). The choice of fractionation depends upon multiple factors including tumor size and proximity to critical OAR, in particular the small bowel and contralateral kidney. A dose-response relationship may exist in RCC and two phase I dose escalation studies have already shown doses of 48 Gy in four fractions and 48 Gy in three fractions to be feasible and safe, with planning under way for further dose escalation to 60 Gy in three fractions, and we eagerly await the results of these trials (Ponsky et al. 2015).

Various planning techniques are used to treat RCC, and beam number and direction will therefore depend upon the technique used, tumor size, and position, and may be a combination of both coplanar and noncoplanar beams. A study by Pham et al. reported on 20 patients treated with 3DCRT and found that the median number of beams used varied depending upon the size of tumor (8 for PTV <100 cm^3 and 10 for PTV >100 cm^3) (Pham et al. 2014b). Furthermore, the intermediate dose spillage at 50% of the prescription dose (R50%) used as a measure of dose gradient was inversely proportional to the number of beams used. In general, all plans should aim to deliver adequate PTV coverage, usually prescribed to the 80 or 90% isodose, while achieving a steep dose gradient, and optimizing conformity, and thereby protecting adjacent OARs including small bowel, liver, and spinal cord. The authors highlighted that large bowel appears to be relatively robust to peak doses of SBRT. Ongoing studies will hopefully assist in creating guidelines and benchmarks for minimum PTV coverage and conformity indices, which will improve and standardize delivery of stereotactic radiotherapy in primary RCC. Figure 2 is an example of a SBRT plan for a right primary RCC.

5.2.3 Clinical Outcomes: Local Control and Toxicity

There are currently no randomized trials evaluating SBRT in primary RCC. The majority of reported studies are retrospective, with a few prospective trials emerging (see Table 4)

Table 4 Review of SABR literature for primary RCC

Author/year	N	Follow-up (median or mean)	Average marginal dose (Gy)	Outcome: crude local control	Estimated 2-year local control	Median overall survival	Toxicities
Chang et al. (2016)	16	19	30–40 Gy in 5 fractions	100%	NA	NA	Early: ×1 grade 2
							Late: ×2 grade 4
Gilson et al. (2006)	33	17	Median 40 Gy in 5 fractions	94%	92	NA	NA
Lo et al. (2014)	3	21.7	40 Gy in 5 fractions CyberKnife	100%	NA	NA	Early: 1× grade 1 nausea
							Late: nil
McBride et al. (2013) (abstract)	15	36.7	Median 33 Gy in 3 fractions	87% 1 failure at 30.7 months 1 failure at 31.2 months	NA	NA	1× grade 3 renal toxicity
							5× grade 1 fatigue
							2× grade 1 nausea
Nair et al. (2013)	3	13.3	39 Gy in 3 fractions	100%	NA	NA	Early: ×1 grade 1
							nausea
							Late: Nil
Nomiya et al. (2008)	10	57.5	Median 4.5 Gy × 16 fractions	100%	100	5-year OS 74%	10% grade 4 toxicity, no other toxicities > grade 1
Pham et al. (2014b)	20	6	26 Gy in 1 fraction 42 Gy in 3 fractions	NA	NA	NR	60% grade 1–2, nil else
Ponsky et al. (2015)	19	13.7	Max 48 Gy in 4 fractions	NA	NA	NA	5.2% grade 2
							15.8% grade 3–4
Qian et al. (2003)	20	12	40 Gy in 5 fractions	93%	86	NA	NA
Staehler et al. (2015)*	30[a]	28.1	25Gy in 1 fraction CyberKnife	98% (at 9 months)[b]	NA	Not attained after median 28.1 months[b]	13% grade 1–2, nil else
Svedman et al. (2006)	5	52	40 Gy in 4 or 5 fractions, 45 Gy in 3 fractions	80%	91	Median survival 32 months	89% grade 1–2
							4% grade 3
Svedman et al. (2008)	7	39	40 Gy in 4 fractions	86%	91	NA	58% grade 1–2, nil else
Teh et al. (2007)	2	9	24 Gy to 48Gy in 3– 6 fractions	100%	100	NA	NA
Wang et al. (2014)	9	38.3	36 to 51 Gy to 50% isodose line at 3– 5 Gy per fraction	5-year LC 43%	NA	5-year OS 35%	Early: 44% grade 1 (gastrointestinal, hematological) Late: 22% grade 2 (gastrointestinal)
Wersall et al. (2005)	8	37	40 Gy in 4 or 5 fractions, 45Gy in 3 fractions	100%	100	Median survival 58[b] months	20% grade 1–2
							19% grade 3
							nil grade 4[b]

[a]Report included an additional 15 patients with TCC
[b]Pooled results with patients treated for TCC

(Swaminath and Chu 2015). A systematic review was published in 2012 of ten studies on 126 patients treated with SBRT for inoperable RCC (Siva et al. 2012). Three studies were prospective and seven were retrospective. The weighted LC for all trials was 92.9% with a weighted rate of ≥grade 3 toxicity of 3.8%, although most trials had limited follow-up (median 2–3 years). More recent prospective studies also continue to report short- to medium-term high LC rates and low rates of toxicity as seen in previous studies (Pham et al. 2014b; Staehler et al. 2015; Ponsky et al. 2015; Chang et al. 2016). The main acute toxicities seen in the literature are self-limiting acute nausea and fatigue, followed by radiation dermatitis and enteritis. Severe toxicities reported include renal toxicity, duodenal ulcer, and skin toxicity, although the overall rates were low (Ponsky et al. 2015; Nomiya et al. 2008; McBride et al. 2013).

With respect to renal toxicity, despite the uncertainty regarding safe dose constraints, there are very few cases of dialysis seen post-SBRT, even with many patients being medically inoperable and some patients having single kidneys (Svedman et al. 2008; Siva et al. 2016a; Jackson et al. 2014). A recent prospective study of 21 patients using 51Cr-EDTA and 99mTc-DMSA SPECT/CT has suggested that there is a dose-response relationship, with regional kidney function being exponentially related to dose received, with minimal renal function deficit seen below 10 Gy, and plateauing above 100 Gy (BED_3) (Jackson et al. 2014). The R50% conformity index was also found to be correlated to GFR loss and the authors suggested that this could be used as a practical planning aid to minimize kidney damage. The authors also provided an equation derived from data using both single- (26 Gy) and three-fraction (3 × 14 Gy) treatment to estimate preserved local glomerular filtration rate as per DMSA SPECT, using an α/β ratio of 3, where a and b are the coefficients for the biexponential decline in local tracer uptake according to radiation dose and c is a parameter for residual perfusion to high-dose regions ($>100Gy_{BED}$):

$$GFR = a^* e^{-b*BED} + c$$

Renal atrophy has been demonstrated in the conventional radiotherapy setting, although there is limited data post-SBRT. A small study of 14 patients reported on a change in median irradiated kidney volume from 160.4 cm^3 to 137.1 cm^3 following SBRT for primary RCC in ten fractions (total doses 50–70 Gy) (Yamamoto et al. 2016). There was also a change in median creatinine levels from 1.1 mg/dL to a peak of 1.6 mg/dL, although no grade 2 renal toxicity or hemodialysis was reported. Renal atrophy was most strongly correlated with V20–V30 ($p < 0.01$), and patients with fiducial markers inserted were found to have a significantly lower ratio of renal atrophy.

5.2.4 Follow-Up

Following SBRT, determining the success of treatment can be particularly challenging. Follow-up is usually performed using CT or MRI. Various parameters may then be used to determine efficacy. The American Urological Association (AUA) defines recurrence after surgery as (1) a visually enlarging neoplasm; (2) a new nodularity in the same area of treatment, whether determined by enhancement of the neoplasm on post-treatment contrast imaging; (3) failure of regression in size of the treated lesion over time; (4) new satellite or port site soft-tissue nodules; and (5) biopsy-proven recurrence (Donat et al. 2013). By contrast, commonly in the context of radiotherapy, LC is measured using the RECIST system. Following RFA and cryotherapy, the absence of enhancement posttreatment is a defining criteria in determining therapeutic success (Iannuccilli et al. 2014). There are unfortunately multiple issues with these stipulations for SBRT. Size criteria can form a crude measurement, with many renal tumors displaying minimal reduction in size post-SBRT, occasionally even initial growth, with consequent evidence of reduced size only as a delayed effect (Nomiya et al. 2008). Furthermore, the presence of enhancement is expected following successful SBRT treatment and therefore proves an inadequate marker of treatment efficacy. Innovative strategies that may prove superior in SBRT assessment include use of diffusion-weighted MRI and dynamic contrast-enhanced MRI, which has been explored in a prospective setting in a small cohort of patients (Parameswaran et al. 2013), and has shown variable effectiveness in RCC diagnosis (Kang et al. 2015), and in the preclinical setting shown early changes post use of sorafenib (Jeon et al. 2015). Biopsy following treatment also poses its own difficulties, as shown by Ponsky et al. in which 64% of biopsies were positive following SBRT, despite lack of progression shown on subsequent follow-up imaging (Ponsky et al. 2015). The specific issue of biopsy timing is therefore being considered in a prospective study (Clinical trials database: NCT02141919). Novel methods of assessing posttreatment biopsy are required, and potentially mitotic index as investigated in preclinical data above (Walsh et al. 2006) may be one such parameter. Serum biomarkers provide another avenue for follow-up and may also prove useful in the future.

5.3   Oligometastases

Approximately one-third of patients diagnosed with RCC will present with metastatic disease and eventually over 50% of patients will develop metastatic disease (Motzer et al. 1996). While surgery in the form of cytoreductive nephrectomy (Flanigan et al. 2004) and metastasectomy (Daliani et al. 2009) combined with systemic therapy formed the backbone of treatment for metastatic RCC historically, its role in the era of targeted therapies is more uncertain, and the subject of ongoing trials (Clinical trials database: NCT02535351, NCT00930033, NCT01099423). The main goals of SBRT in the metastatic setting include LC and palliation of symptoms. Increasingly, SBRT is being considered as an alternative to metastasectomy in patients with oligometastatic or oligoprogressive disease, as a means of prolonging disease-free survival and potentially OS in certain patients, although evidence for this is still in its infancy stages.

5.3.1   Clinical Outcomes: Local Control and Toxicity

There is a rapidly growing body of literature supporting the use of SBRT in metastatic RCC, although it remains largely retrospective in nature (see Table 5) (Daliani et al. 2009). A systematic review on clinical outcomes associated with the use of SBRT in extracranial metastatic RCC found a total of 10 studies (2 of which were prospective) and included 389 patients with 730 targets (Kothari et al. 2015). The review found a weighted crude LC rate of 89%, and in the five studies that reported pain control, 69% of patients reported an improvement following SBRT. Grade 3–4 toxicities were low and ranged from 0 to 4%. There were only two treatment-related deaths, one due to electromechanical dissociation following 48 Gy in four fractions to a large metastatic lesion within the lung, and a second due to a fatal gastric hemorrhage 4 months after treatment for a metastasis within the pancreas. Several of the studies suggested that higher biological doses resulted in better LC. Zelefsky et al. reported that the 3-year local PFS (88%) with a high single dose (24Gy, $n = 45$) was greater than both a low single-dose (<24Gy, $n = 14$) or multiple-fraction regimens ($n = 46$) at 21% and 17%, respectively (Zelefsky et al. 2012). Multivariate analysis revealed that both a higher single dose compared with a lower dose and single-dose regimens compared with hypofractionation were significant predictors of improved PFS ($p < 0.01$). It is unclear whether the excellent control rates observed translate to improved OS in patients with oligometastatic disease. However, Ranck et al. reported on 18 patients, of whom 67% had oligometastatic disease and underwent SBRT to all known sites, and reported a high 2-year OS of 85% (Ranck et al. 2013). Wersall et al. compared median survival outcomes for patients with oligometastatic disease and found this to be higher than those with more widespread disease (37 vs. 19 months, respectively) (Wersall et al. 2005). Further research is required to see if it is possible to define a true state of oligometastatic disease in

Table 5 Extracranial SRS for metastatic RCC

Author, Date	N(n)	Locations	Average marginal dose (Gy)	Median follow-up (month)	Crude/1-year LC (%)	Median OS (month)	Toxicities (≥grade 3)
Gerszten et al. (2005) (Prospective)	48 (60)	Spine	Mean 16 Gy in a single fraction	37	88[a]/96	NA	0% radiation toxicity
Wersall et al. (2005)	50 (154)	117 lung, 6 adrenal gland, 12 kidney metastases, 5 thoracic wall, 4 bone, 3 mediastinum, 3 abdominal lymph gland, 2 liver, 1 spleen	Modal: 32 Gy in 4 fractions, 40 Gy in 4 fractions and 45 Gy in 3 fractions[b]	37[b]	98/99	NA	2% (1/58) mortality[b]
Svedman et al. (2006) (Prospective Phase II trial)	26 (77)	63 lung/ mediastinum, 5 kidney metastases, 5 adrenal, 4 thoracic wall, 3 abdominal glands, 3 liver, 1 pelvis, 1 spleen	40 Gy in 4 fractions[b]	52[b]	99/100	32[b]	4% (1/26) grade 5 toxicity
Teh et al. (2007)	47 (23)	Orbits, head and neck, lung, mediastinum, sternum, clavicle, scapula, humerus, rib, spine, abdominal wall	Modal 24 Gy in 3 fractions[b]	9[b]	86[a]/81	NA	None
Nguyen et al. (2010)	48 (55)	Spine	Modal 27Gy in 3 fractions	13	78/ 80	22	No grade 3 or 4 neurological toxicity (McCormick and associates scheme) 2% (1/48) grade 3 pain 2% (1/48) grade 3 anemia
Balagamwala et al. (2012)	57 (88)	Spine	Median 15 Gy in a single fraction unknown if marginal	5	77/ 50	12	2% (1/57) grade 3 nausea/ vomiting
							No grade 4 toxicity 8% (7/57) pain flare (not graded)
Jhaveri et al. (2012)	18 (24)	14 spine, 4 ribs/ clavicle, 6 pelvis	Modal 40 Gy in 5 fractions	10	NA/NA	NA	None
Zelefsky et al. (2012)	55[c] (Bujold et al. 2013)	59 spine, 22 pelvic bones, 14 other, 9 femur, 1 lymph node	Modal 24Gy in a single fraction	12	72[c]/72	NA	7% (4/55) fractures 2% (1/55) grade 4 erythema

(continued)

Table 5 (continued)

Author, Date	N(n)	Locations	Average marginal dose (Gy)	Median follow-up (month)	Crude/1-year LC (%)	Median OS (month)	Toxicities (≥grade 3)
Ranck et al. (2013)	18 (39)	11 bone, 10 abdominal lymph node, 7 mediastinum/hilum, 4 lung, 2 kidney metastases, 2 adrenal, 2 liver, 1 soft tissue	Modal 50Gy in 10 fractions, unknown if marginal dose	16	95/ 96	NA	None
Thibault et al. (2014)	116 (187)	187 osteolytic spine (15 cervical, 89 thoracic, 66 lumbar, 17 sacrum)	Median 16 Gy in 1 fraction	8.0	NA	11.0	34 (18%) vertebral compression fractures (not graded)
Altoos et al. (2015)	34 (36)	27 thorax, 3 skin and soft tissue, 6 abdomen	Modal 50 Gy in 5 fractions	16	NA/100	NA	Only 1 patient had ≥ grade 3 toxicity (1/31) 3%
Amini et al. (2015)	46 (50)	16 spine, 1 skull, 10 bony thorax, 15 bony pelvis, 3 bony upper extremity, 5 bony lower extremity	Modal 27Gy in 3 fractions	10	88/74	NA	Only 1 patient had grade 3 toxicity - dermatitis (1/46) 2%
							No grade 4 or 5 toxicity
Majewski et al. (2016)	34	Intracranial, Extracranial	NR	NR	70/NA	9.4[c] includes intracranial Patients	NA
Staehler et al. (2015)	55 (105)	Spine	Median 20 Gy in a single fraction	33	98/ 94	17	None
Tinkle et al. (2015) (abstract)	38[d]	Primary RCC, locally recurrent RCC; bone, soft-tissue metastases	Median BED_{10} 48 Gy	19.7	NA/88	1-year OS 82%	None
Ghia et al. (2016) (Prospective, non-randomized)	43 (47)	20 thoracic spine, 20 lumbar spine, 4 cervical spine, 3 thoracolumbar junction	Modal 24 Gy in 1 fraction	23	NA/82	22.8	Pain flare (13/40) – not graded posttreatment fracture (7/24) Grade 3 late radiculopathy/foot drop (1/43)
Hannan et al. (2016) (Prospective Phase II trial, abstract)	16	NR	Median 24.5 Gy for single fraction, 30 Gy for 3 fractions	9	95/NA	NA	None
Wang et al. (2016) (abstract)	91 (188)	75 bone, 28 lung, 18 liver, 22 lymph nodes, 45 other	8–60 Gy in 1–5 fractions	10.7	NA/91	1-year OS 76.5%	NA

N number of patients, *n* number of targets
[a]According to number of patients rather than targets
[b]Includes patients with metastatic and primary RCC
[c]Information obtained via personal correspondence
[d]Includes patients with primary/locally recurrent RCC

which durable LC may be able to achieve long-term survival in patients with RCC.

5.3.2 Renal SBRT and Systemic Therapy

Renal tumors are highly vascular and depend upon neo-angiogenesis for growth and survival. Multi-targeted TKI of vascular endothelial and platelet-derived growth factor receptors have been shown to be effective in improving OS in metastatic RCC (Motzer et al. 2009), although ultimately most patients will progress. At the cellular level, stereotactic radiotherapy is characterized by rapid endothelial cell apoptosis (Garcia-Barros et al. 2003); however VEGF and fibroblast-derived growth factor are believed to be involved in decreasing its effectiveness (Truman et al. 2010). Angiogenesis inhibitors may work by normalizing tumor vasculature and reducing intratumoral pressure, and improving oxygenation, or by increasing tumor apoptosis through inhibition of cell survival signals (Wong et al. 2014). There is a rationale therefore to combine the use of radiotherapy and targeted agents due to their complementary and synergistic effects. There are now a number of preclinical studies (Kleibeuker et al. 2015; Schueneman et al. 2003; Zhang et al. 2011) and phase I/II clinical studies (Kao et al. 2009; Kasibhatla et al. 2007; Staehler et al. 2011; Tong et al. 2012) that suggest increased efficacy and acceptable toxicity profiles with the combined use of these modalities. The largest of these clinical studies to consider metastatic RCC reported on 106 patients receiving concurrent stereotactic radiosurgery and antiangiogenic therapy in the form of sunitinib or sorafenib (Staehler et al. 2011). The authors of the study found that there was no skin toxicity, neurotoxicity, or myelopathy following SRS, and that SRS did not alter the side effect profile of systemic treatment. One patient died of a fatal cerebral bleed 3 months following SRS, and while on sunitinib, however, the death was not thought to be treatment related. The most common grade 3/4 toxicity IL-2 6 weeks of SRS was anemia in 11% of patients. Despite low toxicity rates reported in these studies, there are concerns regarding the rare but serious complications seen with combination therapy including bowel perforation and fatal hemorrhage (Inoue et al. 2012). There are also data from mixed and non-RCC tumor streams that suggest potential toxicities, including case reports of radiation recall effects (including pneumonitis and increased cerebral edema) (Wong et al. 2014), as well as a high rate (33%) of ≥grade 3 toxicities (Kao et al. 2014). Furthermore, issues raised in the preclinical setting regarding the optimal dose and scheduling of antiangiogenic agents with SRS still need to be addressed and validated in prospective clinical trials. NCT02019576 is a currently accruing phase II trial addressing the issue of SBRT for patients with oligoprogressive RCC on sunitinib and may help further elucidate some of these issues in the future.

5.3.3 Immunomodulation and the "Abscopal Effect" on RCC

The abscopal effect was first defined in 1953 as an effect which occurs "at a distance from the irradiated volume but within the same organism" (Mole 1953). The mechanism of action of the abscopal effect is poorly understood although there are a number of postulated mechanisms, most of which are believed to be immunologic phenomenona that can be instigated by therapies including stereotactic radiotherapy (Reynders et al. 2015; Siva et al. 2015). A recently published systematic review on abscopal effects found seven case reports in patients with RCC (Abuodeh et al. 2016). Therefore, the abscopal effect remains an intriguing but rare event, the potential of which remains yet to be translated to a clinical setting.

More recently there has also been increased interest in the use of immunomodulatory agents. Interleukin-2 IL-2 and more recently programmed cell death protein-1 (PD-1) inhibitors have been shown to be effective in metastatic RCC (Motzer et al. 2015a; Motzer et al. 2015b; Yang et al. 2003). It is hypothesized that radiation damage induces tumor antigen release and microenvironment changes that may enhance the effect of immunomodulatory agents. A phase I study looking at the combination of SBRT and IL-2 found it to be safe, and appeared to have increased activity over the use of IL-2 alone (Seung et al. 2012). A phase II study has since been performed considering this same combination in patients with RCC, and an interim report showed a 40% response rate, which is approximately twofold greater than historical controls (Hannan et al. 2016).

5.4 Future Directions

The emerging body of evidence demands that we shed historical concepts of radioresistance, and obliges us to continue to develop and report robust and scientifically sound studies that will allow for rational investigation of the therapeutic potential of SBRT in both primary and metastatic RCC. There is an urgent need for long-term data from prospective trials for both objective and patient-centric measures of SBRT in RCC. In addition, development of sophisticated follow-up measures, including laboratory and imaging modalities, to allow accurate response assessments and assessment of kidney function is needed. The abscopal effect requires further exploration to see if this is a phenomenon that may not only deepen our understanding of cancer, but may also be exploited for clinical benefit. Trials already under way considering many of these specific issues will hopefully continue to further inform physician decisions, and ultimately lead to improved patient care.

6 Adrenal SBRT

The adrenal gland is a common site for metastatic spread from many histologic tumor types and, in fact, ranks fourth worldwide after lung, liver, and bone metastases (Oshiro et al. 2011). While often clinically occult, it is being detected more commonly and earlier in the disease course, often when patients are still in an oligometastatic state (Kumar et al. 2004; Mitchell and Nwariaku 2007). The most common primary tumors associated with adrenal metastases are breast, lung, GI, and renal tumors (Abrams et al. 1950).

Historically, patients with adrenal metastases have been treated with palliative intent systemic therapy, with palliative conventional radiotherapy reserved for symptom control, which is effective in approximately 70–80% of patients (Soffen et al. 1990; Zeng et al. 2005). Increasingly however, metastasis-directed therapy is being employed for patients with oligometastatic disease, with the belief that this may result in prolonged disease-free survival. Particularly encouraging in the case of patients with adrenal oligometastases are reports of long-term survival following adrenalectomy, suggesting that a more aggressive and definitive intent treatment may improve survival and be appropriate in well-selected patients (Luketich and Burt 1996; Mittendorf et al. 2008; Muth et al. 2010; Tanvetyanon et al. 2008). Adrenalectomy can therefore be considered the gold standard in selected patients with oligometastatic disease; however not all patients are surgical candidates. In those who are, surgery is not without significant complication rates including a risk of perioperative death. An alternative option therefore listed by the National Comprehensive Cancer Network (NCCN) guidelines in 2013 is SBRT, which, in addition to being a noninvasive approach with potentially lower complication rates, also offers the advantage of better preservation of hormonal function (Katoh et al. 2008). This chapter section focuses on SBRT planning, delivery, LC, and toxicity for adrenal oligometastases. Treatment of primary adrenal tumors is not covered and is beyond the scope of this chapter.

6.1 Technical Considerations

As with SBRT to all abdominal sites, management of motion with respiration is critical to accurate delivery of treatment. A pilot study by Katoh et al. of nine patients in which fiducial markers were inserted near the adrenal gland revealed on average the markers moved 3.4, 5.4, and 9.9 mm in the left-right, anterior-posterior, and cranio-caudal directions, respectively (Katoh et al. 2008). There was no difference between patients treated in the supine and the prone position. A combination of patient immobilization, respiratory dampening using abdominal compression devices or breath-hold techniques, image guidance, and tumor tracking should be used with appropriate GTV to

PTV margins of 5–10 mm. The GTV is usually defined using either CT or MRI, although in some departments PET-CT may also be used.

There is limited evidence to guide us regarding the appropriate dose that should be used for adrenal metastases. There is a wide spectrum of dose used in the literature, which is largely retrospective in nature. There is some limited evidence to support a correlation between LC and BED (Desai et al. 2015). A number of OAR need to be considered including lung, stomach, duodenum, liver, kidneys, spinal cord, and small and large bowels. Dose constraints for these will depend upon the total dose and fractionation used. Planning techniques generally incorporate 3D-CRT or IMRT. A study by Scorsetti et al. (Scorsetti et al. 2011) compared different treatment plans with protons and photons for ten patients receiving a dose of 45 Gy in 7.5 Gy per fraction. Techniques assessed included RapidArc®, dynamic conformal arcs, 3D conformal static fields, IMRT, and intensity-modulated protons. The most conformal plans were achieved with IMRT and RapidArc®, while the lowest V10Gy and integral dose was achieved by protons.

6.2 Clinical Outcomes: Efficacy and Toxicity

A systematic review published in 2014 reviewed all studies that investigated the use of adrenalectomy, SBRT, and percutaneous catheter ablation (PCA) from 1990 to 2012 for adrenal oligometastases. In total nine studies (eight retrospective, one prospective) incorporating the use of SBRT were found, which included in total 178 patients, of which 68% had a lung cancer as their primary disease. The weighted 2-year LC for the SBRT group was 63% (range 27–100%) and 2-year OS was 19%, which compared unfavorably with the surgical group (84% and 46% respectively) (Gunjur et al. 2014). As seen in the range of LC reported however, some studies reported much higher rates of LC including the largest series of 48 patients that received a high median BED of 137.3 Gy and reported a 2-year LC of 90% (Casamassima et al. 2012), as well as the prospective series of 13 patients treated with a median BED of 85.5, in which no patients had local failure (Ahmed et al. 2013). A number of reasons

for the range in LC and OS outcomes between studies and between surgery and radiotherapy were discussed in the review, including the range of total doses and BED_{10} used (between 10 Gy and 60 Gy in 1 to 18 fractions; and 28 Gy and 110 Gy, respectively), as well as differences in the patient baseline characteristics between the surgical and SBRT groups, including the greater number of patients with isolated disease in the surgical group (75% vs. 48%) and the greater number of patients with lung cancer in the SBRT group (68% vs. 33%). Toxicities were noted in the review to have been inconsistently reported; however from the available information, there was no grade 3 or 4 acute toxicity reported. The commonest toxicity was grade 2 gastrointestinal toxicity, seen in up to 22% of patients ($n = 2$ out of 9) in one study (Guiou et al. 2012). There was also no grade 3–4 late toxicity seen, with studies reporting only grade 2 gastrointestinal toxicity, adrenal insufficiency, and fatigue. One study also looked at adrenal hormonal levels following SBRT and found no decline in function (Katoh et al. 2008). This suggests a low toxicity in patients treated with SBRT for adrenal metastases; however caution must still be applied, with one report of a fatal gastric ulcer with SBRT and concurrent vinorelbine in a patient treated with BED 185 Gy (Onishi et al. 2012).

More recent studies have shown similar LC and toxicity rates to those reported in the systematic review (Desai et al. 2015; Franzese et al. 2017; Jung et al. 2016), although prospective data continue to be lacking and future studies will hopefully provide higher level evidence to guide us to better understand the biology of adrenal oligometastatic disease, to allow for better patient selection, appropriate doses, and radiotherapy techniques, and allow us to translate this into better LC and survival outcomes in this growing field.

7 Prostate

Worldwide in 2012, there were more than one million new cases of prostate cancer and over 300,000 prostate cancer deaths, making it the second most commonly diagnosed cancer in men and the fifth leading cause of male cancer death (Torre et al. 2015). A number of established definitive treatment options exist for prostate cancer including radical prostatectomy, external beam radiotherapy, and brachytherapy. Hypofractionated and dose-escalated regimens using SBRT for prostate cancer may be more advantageous compared to conventional external beam radiotherapy. The relatively low α/β ratio of prostate cancer of 1.5–1.85 Gy may confer it sensitive to high dose per fraction (Brenner and Hall 1999; Dasu 2007). In addition, the α/β ratio of prostate cancer may be lower than surrounding OAR, including the rectum and bladder, thereby allowing hypofractionation to improve the therapeutic ratio and deliver similar rates of efficacy with the same or lower rates of complication compared to conventional fractionation (Dasu 2007). Randomized studies of slightly hypofractionated regimens of approximately 3 Gy per fraction, as well as dose escalation using conventional techniques, have been shown to be safe and effective (Arcangeli et al. 2012; Kupelian et al. 2007; Livsey et al. 2003; Lukka et al. 2005; Viani et al. 2009; Yeoh et al. 2011; Hodges et al. 2012; Yu et al. 2014). Apart from theoretical biological advantages, SBRT also has numerous practical advantages over both surgery and alternative radiotherapy options, including being noninvasive, time efficient, and cost effective (Hodges et al. 2012; Yu et al. 2014). This section outlines the specifics regarding planning and delivery of prostate SBRT and associated clinical outcomes, briefly reviews SBRT and oligometastatic prostate cancer, and outlines currently accruing studies and future directions in this field.

7.1 Technical Considerations

The majority of the literature published to date has incorporated the use of CyberKnife® to deliver SBRT, although more recent series have used gantry-based linacs with similar outcomes (Loblaw et al. 2013; Mantz et al. 2013). The main technical challenges in the delivery of SBRT to the prostate include management of inter- and intrafraction motion of the prostate gland, which is dependent on both rectal and bladder filling. Commonly real-time motion-tracking systems incorporating the use of three to four fiducial markers are used to minimize PTV margins, which are usually between 3 and 5 mm, with tighter constraints applied posteriorly to spare the rectum. Studies have also described vari-

ous techniques to control for bowel and bladder size, including prescription of a strict diet, bowel regimen and/or laxatives (Boike et al. 2011; Bolzicco et al. 2010; Katz and Santoro 2010; McBride et al. 2012), bladder catheterization (Bolzicco et al. 2010), or bladder emptying followed by a specified consistent intake of water (Boike et al. 2011). The rectum is of particular concern as not only an organ that contributes to target motion, but also as a critical OAR. Methods employed by some institutions to increase the distance between the prostate and the rectum include use of an endorectal balloon (Boike et al. 2011), and SpaceOAR® (Augmenix Inc., Waltham, Massachusetts, USA) hydrogel spacers (Alongi et al. 2013), although the use of these presents their own particular challenges.

Target delineation is critical in the use of SBRT, and the ongoing development and incorporation of imaging techniques are hoped to continue to improve our accuracy and confidence in this endeavor. Increasingly, image fusion of various MRI sequences as well as other modalities including ultrasound, and more recently PET, including prostate-specific membrane antigen (PSMA) PET, is being incorporated into practice, although ongoing research is required to better determine their applicability.

While a spectrum of total dose and fraction size is reported in the literature, most commonly doses in the order of 35 Gy in five fractions are employed based upon the iso-late-effects principle, which results in an EQD2 of 70 Gy for late effects ($\alpha/\beta = 3$Gy) and 85 Gy for tumor effects ($\alpha/\beta = 1.5$Gy). There is limited evidence for a dose-response effect beyond this (King et al. 2013a). Furthermore, concerns exist regarding toxicity with a prospective dose escalation study to 50 Gy in five fractions reporting a rarely seen late grade 4 rectal toxicity in the highest dose group (Boike et al. 2011). There is considerable variation applied to the scheduling of treatment within studies; however many choose not to treat on consecutive days. King et al. suggested that alternate-day treatment resulted in a favorable toxicity profile compared to daily treatment; however this is yet to be validated in a randomized setting (King et al. 2012). The ideal dosimetry for prostate plans is also still debated. In particular, it is unknown as to whether a homogenous distribution similar to external beam radiotherapy or a more heterogeneous distribution similar to that achieved using high-dose-rate brachytherapy is superior. Further research is required in this area.

Various dose constraints are applied for SBRT to rectum, bladder, penile bulb, urethra, and femoral head. Limited data exist for this, and are in part derived from our experience with conventional EBRT and also depend upon institutional preference.

7.2 Clinical Outcomes: Efficacy, Toxicity and Quality of Life

There are now multiple prospective trials investigating the use of SBRT, with the majority of patients included being low risk. The largest of the prospective series is a multi-institutional report on 1100 patients with clinically localized prostate cancer enrolled in separate phase II trials from eight institutions between 2003 and 2011 (King et al. 2013b). SBRT was delivered using CyberKnife® to a dose of between 35 and 40 Gy in 4 to 5 fractions. A majority of patients were at low risk (58%) with only 11% being high risk. Only 14% of patients received a short course of androgen deprivation therapy (ADT). The 5-year biochemical relapse-free survival (bRFS) rates defined as nadir +2 ng/mL were 95%, 84%, and 81% for low-, intermediate-, and high-risk patients, respectively. No correlation was shown with total dose used or ADT use. A subset of these patients ($n = 864$) also had complete quality of life (QOL) data collected (Bolzicco et al. 2010). Using the Expanded Prostate Cancer Index Composite (EPIC) the authors reported mean baseline urinary, bowel, and sexual domain scores of 89, 95, and 53, which worsened to 81.3, 83, and 47.9 at 3 months posttreatment. Patients subsequently showed recovery at 6 months in the urinary and bowel domains to 88.05 and 91.5 and subsequently to above baseline scores of 90.8 and 95.9, respectively, at 5 years. Sexual function continued to decline, initially likely reflecting posttreatment effect, and subsequently multifactorial effect in this elderly population with a median age of 69. The second largest series reported the results of 477 patients who received SBRT using CyberKnife® to be 35 Gy–36.25 Gy in five fractions for low- or intermediate-risk prostate cancer (Katz and Kang 2014a). Fifty-one patients also received ADT for 6 months. This study showed similar, if not slightly better, efficacy for low- and intermediate-risk patients, with a 7-year actuarial freedom from biochemical failure of 95.6% and 89.6%, respectively. Similar to the previous study, there was no difference seen between 35 Gy and 36.25 Gy. In 1.7% of patients, late grade 3–4 genitourinary toxicity was seen, comprising retention requiring surgery and bleeding requiring laser coagulation. All of these patients received 36.25 Gy. No severe late gastrointestinal toxicities were seen.

There are limited data on SBRT used as a boost in addition to pelvic radiotherapy; however there is evidence that pelvic radiotherapy does not improve efficacy in this setting and can worsen rectal toxicity (Katz and Kang 2014b).

The efficacy and toxicity outcomes in the above larger studies are similar to results published by other smaller series using CyberKnife®, as well as series using gantry-based linacs. In general, the results show excellent bDFS rates of 95% or greater for low-risk disease. The reported toxicities are also low, with late grade three genitourinary (GU) toxicities commonly under 2% and late severe gastrointestinal toxicities frequently negligible. Quality of life data also appear consistent across the literature with initial deterioration over the first few months in urinary and bowel domains, followed by subsequent recovery to baseline over the next 6–12 months (McBride et al. 2012; Meier 2015). Sexual function, however, usually declines post-SBRT without recovery (McBride et al. 2012; King et al. 2013b). The outcomes also appear to compare at least equally and perhaps favorably to conventional radiotherapy (Meier 2015), although the SBRT data are nonrandomized with relatively short median follow-up times. We await long-term results of randomized studies to validate the above findings.

7.3 Oligometastases

Most commonly patients that develop metastatic prostate cancer will develop multiple sites of bony metastatic disease, including spinal disease. The standard of care for first-line treatment of metastatic prostate cancer is ADT, with more recent data supporting the addition of docetaxel (James et al. 2016). In addition, radiotherapy has been found to be a safe and effective form of palliating patients with symptomatic bony metastases (Lutz et al. 2011). A detailed discussion on the use of SBRT to treat spinal metastases can be found earlier in this chapter.

There are limited data on the use of SBRT in oligometastatic prostate cancer, with the concept of oligometastases appearing to be somewhat more controversial in prostate cancer than other malignancies. Additionally, the conventional definition of oligometastatic disease of macroscopic metastases is confounded by the presence of a more sensitive diagnostic marker, the serum prostate-specific antigen (PSA), which usually detects disease recurrence earlier than currently available imaging techniques.

A systematic review published in 2014 on local treatments for oligometastatic (up to five lesions) prostate cancer found nine studies that included patients treated with SBRT (Yao et al. 2014). The endpoints used in these studies varied; however the LC rates were generally high (85–100%), although with a range of follow-up times varying from 6 to 43 months. Toxicities were also very low, with no grade 3 or 4 toxicities reported in patients treated for distant metastatic disease. Since this review, an individual patient data meta-analysis of treatment-naïve oligometastatic patients with one to three sites of metastases has also been published (Ost et al. 2016). This study included five studies within the above systematic review, and two newer studies. In total, there were 163 metastases in 119 patients. The median distant progression-free survival was 21 months. In addition, a higher BED was found to significantly correlate with better LC, with a 3-year LPFS of 79% for patients treated with a BED ≤100 Gy vs. 99% for patients treated with >100 Gy. Also, this group found that patterns of failure resulted in approximately a third of patients recurring in a limited "oligometastatic" pattern after SBRT and were suitable for further salvage SBRT. Fourteen percent of patients developed grade 1 toxicity, 3% developed grade 2 toxicity, and no patients developed grade ≥3 toxicity.

The results of these reviews suggest that the use of SBRT to treat metastatic prostate cancer presents a promising therapeutic option; however certainly more research is required prior to incorporating it into standard management for these patients.

7.4 Future Directions

The current scope of literature is promising for the future of SBRT in localized prostate cancer, and forms the basis of several currently accruing or maturing randomized studies that will hopefully provide answers to areas of uncertainty, including how the use of conventional radiotherapy compares to SBRT, and the optimal SBRT dose. Other interesting questions surround the use of SBRT and systemic therapies, and whether SBRT can either obviate the need for ADT in the localized setting or result in its delay in the oligometastatic setting which will provide areas for further research.

8 Pancreas

In spite of advances in therapies, pancreatic cancer remains the fourth leading cause of cancer death with a 5-year OS rate of 7% (Siegel et al. 2015). Its insidious onset has led to it commonly presenting at an advanced stage of disease at diagnosis. Controversies exist regarding the management of locally advanced pancreatic cancer. An Eastern Cooperative Oncology Group (ECOG) trial showed that the addition of conventional radiotherapy to gemcitabine chemotherapy improved both LC and OS (Loehrer et al. 2011). The proximity of the pancreas to critical structures such as the stomach and bowel limits the radiation dose that can be delivered safely to the region. Despite the development of highly conformal techniques of radiation delivery, significant short- and long-term side effects may develop due to radiation exposure to these organs. Given the shortcomings of conventional radiotherapy, SBRT is increasingly being used in the management of pancreatic cancer (Berber et al. 2013). Data on the use of SBRT for pancreatic cancer are emerging in the last 5 years, mainly in the locally advanced and, to a lesser extent, neoadjuvant and adjuvant settings.

8.1 Patient Selection

In most studies on SBRT for pancreatic cancer, only patients with nonmetastatic locally advanced pancreatic cancer were included (Berber et al. 2013). Inclusion criteria used in these studies include:

- *Biopsy-proven pancreatic adenocarcinoma*
- *Unresectable or borderline resectable disease*
- *Life expectancy of at least 12 weeks*
- *ECOG status of ≤2*
- *Tumor size less than 7.5 cm*
- *Absence of extensive vascular involvement, portal vein occlusion, and aorta or inferior vena cava invasion*

- *Leukocyte count of >3000/μL*
- *Absolute neutrophil count of >1500/μL*
- *Total bilirubin < x1.5 upper limit of normal*
- *Transaminases < x2.5 upper limit of normal*
- *Creatinine level within normal limits*

8.2 Technical Considerations

As in other disease sites, SBRT for pancreatic cancer requires proper target delineation, adequate respiratory motion control, meticulous treatment planning, and image guidance to facilitate accurate treatment delivery (refer to Fig. 3 as an example of a pancreatic SBRT plan).

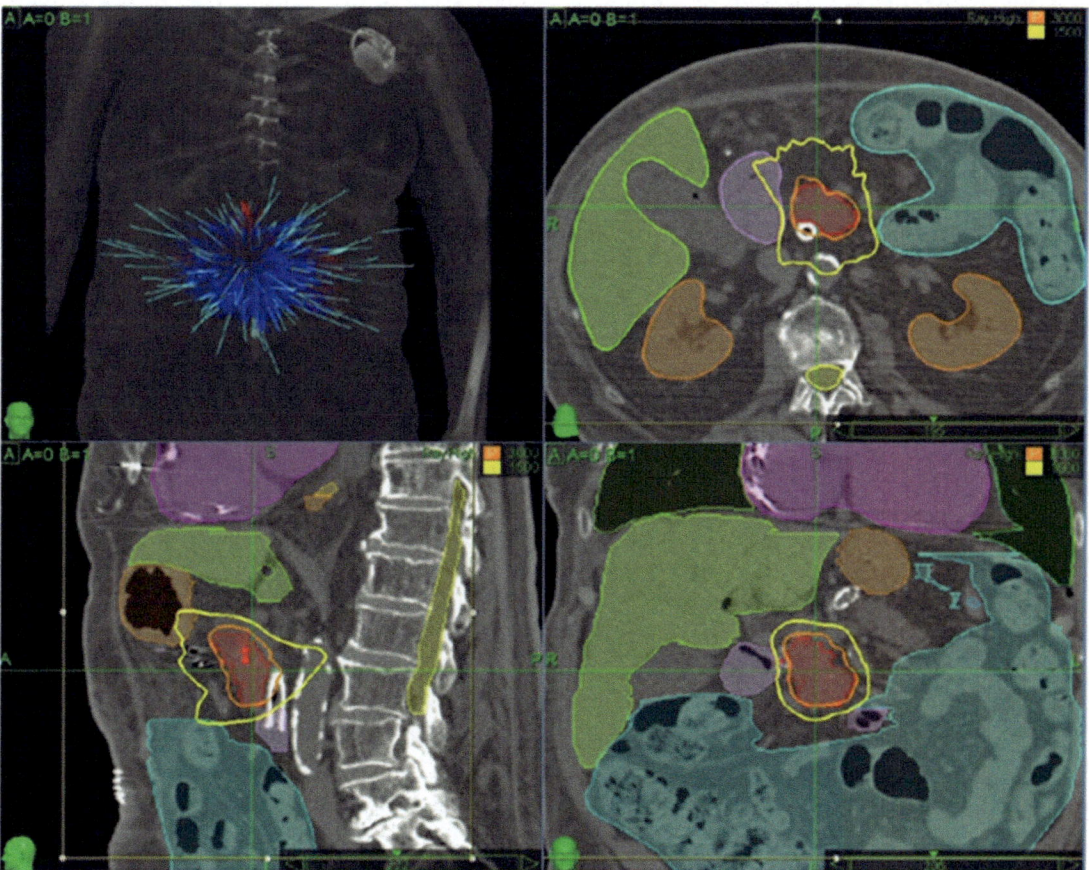

Fig. 3. Locally advanced pancreatic cancer treated with CyberKnife®-based SBRT to a dose of 30 Gy in three fractions. The orange line represents the prescribed isodose line (30 Gy at 70%) and the yellow line represents the 10 Gy line.

8.2.1 Target Delineation and Respiratory Motion Control

Challenges remain in the definition of the GTV. There is significant variability in the determination of optimal GTV for pancreatic SBRT. In general, a contrast-enhanced CT or MRI is used for the delineation of the GTV. A study from the Medical College of Wisconsin examined multiple imaging modalities (CT, PET, diffusion-weighted MRI, and dynamic contrast-enhanced MRI) for pancreatic cancer and discovered significant differences in GTV delineated using each modality (Dalah et al. 2014).

Given that the pancreas is an organ that moves with respiration, respiratory motion control is crucial to minimize margins and to avoid missing the tumor. An ITV or a PTV is created from a GTV based on the method of respiratory motion control used (Berber et al. 2013). Different strategies have been used, including the use of a 4D-CT alone, abdominal compression, breath hold, gating, and robotic tracking (only used in CyberKnife®) (Berber et al. 2013). A study from Stanford University found that 4D-CT may not be adequate in the assessment of pancreatic tumor motion during treatment with CyberKnife®. Tumor motion exceeded the predicted range by >10% in the majority of patients (Minn et al. 2009). Langen et al. showed that by using breath hold, the motion of the pancreas can be limited to 2.5 mm (Langen 2001). A study from Utrecht evaluated tumor motion with cine MRI, and found that average tumor motion observed was 15 mm in the craniocaudal dimension. By using gating at the end-expiration position, the target volume was reduced to 25% of the maximum craniocaudal breathing amplitude (Heerkens et al. 2014).

8.2.2 Treatment Planning, Image Guidance, and Treatment Delivery

Treatment planning technique depends upon the treatment device used. For linear accelerator-based systems, IMRT or VMAT treatment planning is typically used because

the pancreas is adjacent to various OAR including the duodenum, stomach, liver, and kidneys. Efforts must be made to limit the radiation exposure to these structures to avoid serious complications. If a CyberKnife® device is used, three to six cylindrical solid gold markers 3–5 mm in length are placed either endoscopically, laparoscopically, percutaneously under CT guidance, or via laparotomy within and around the tumor at a minimum mutual distance of 2 cm (Dalah et al. 2014). Usually, 5–7 days will be needed for the markers to stabilize in their positions.

To ensure accurate delivery of the radiation to the pancreatic tumor, pretreatment verification with image guidance is paramount. For linac-based systems, CBCT, mostly kV, is typically used. When Tomotherapy® is used, MV CBCT is used. CyberKnife® uses a pair of stereoscopic X-rays for pretreatment verification as well as intrafractional monitoring (Berber et al. 2013). Many centers obtain a midway CBCT to ascertain that there is no shifting of the patient's position during treatment.

Controversies exist with regard to the optimal method of tumor tracking during radiation delivery. Yang et al. found that image matching to skeletal anatomy was inadequate, and even when implanted fiducial markers were present, a PTV margin of at least 3 mm was deemed necessary (Yang et al. 2014). Huguet et al. evaluated the correlation of tumor motion with implanted fiducial marker or with biliary stent displacement and found that both stent and fiducial marker motion correlated well with tumor motion (Huguet et al. 2015). Other groups have quantitated pancreatic tumor motion and recommended that an asymmetric PTV expansion be utilized if a 4D-CT scan is not available to evaluate the tumor motion, even when biliary stents were present, as the mean +/− standard deviation superior-inferior stent excursion was found to be significantly greater than GTV motion (0.84 ± 0.32 cm vs. 0.55 ± 0.23 cm, respectively) (Goldstein et al. 2010). The need to exercise extra caution when using surrogates of tumor motion cannot be overemphasized.

8.2.3 Dose Selection

There has not been any phase III randomized trial comparing different doses and fractionation. An early trial from Scandinavia used 45 Gy in three fractions, resulting in prohibitive toxicities (Hoyer et al. 2005). The group from Stanford University started their phase I trials using a regimen of 24 Gy in one fraction and serious toxicities of the stomach and duodenum were observed (Schellenberg et al. 2011). They subsequently published their large experience of 167 patients treated with either single- or multi-fraction SBRT, showing no difference in LC or survival between the two treatment strategies, but significantly lower rates of grade ≥2 toxicity (Pollom et al. 2014).

In a recently published systematic review, outcome and toxicity of 16 trials (572 patients) of SBRT for pancreatic cancer were evaluated. All the prescribed doses were converted to EQD2 and BED. Pearson product-moment correlation coefficient, regression analysis, and Lyman-Kutcher-Burman modeling were used to correlate the EQD2 and BED to outcomes and toxicity in the multi-fraction group. Grade ≥2 late toxicity was highly correlated with EQD2/BED after linear and Lyman-Kutcher-Burman modeling with frequencies of 5% at 65 Gy and 80 Gy EQD2-$\alpha/\beta = 3$, respectively (Brunner et al. 2015). Although LC also correlated with dose, it appeared to be less dose dependent. The authors recommended a multi-fraction strategy with toxicity estimates according to EQD2/BED prescription doses, and dose constraints for the duodenum.

8.3 Clinical Outcomes: Local Control and Toxicity

There have been several retrospective studies and prospective trials on the use of SBRT for pancreatic cancer. Most of the studies pertain to locally advanced pancreatic cancer, either using SBRT as primary treatment or as a boost after conventional radiotherapy. Other studies examined the use of SBRT in the adjuvant or neoadjuvant setting.

8.3.1 Locally Advanced Pancreatic Cancer

Koong et al. from Stanford University reported the results of their first phase I trial of SBRT for locally advanced pancreatic cancer (Koong et al. 2004). Fifteen patients with an ECOG status of ≤2 received single-fraction SBRT to a dose of 15, 20, or 25 Gy to the primary pancreatic tumor. The GTV ranged from 19.2 to 71.9cm³ (mean 32.9cm³). The dose was prescribed to the 64 to 85% isodose lines and the 50% isodose line was only allowed to cover the proximal duodenal wall. No significant gastrointestinal toxicity was observed within 12 weeks of the treatment. Two and three patients developed grades 1 and 2 toxicities, respectively. For the 13 patients with follow-up CT, six developed metastatic disease at 4–6 weeks. The median survival was 11 months. For the six evaluable patients who received the highest dose of 25 Gy, the median OS was 8 months and the local tumor control was 100% until death or last follow-up. In a phase II trial study from Stanford University examining the use of single-fraction SBRT and sequential gemcitabine for patients with locally advanced pancreatic cancer, a single dose of 25 Gy in one fraction was delivered to an ITV with a 2–3 mm margin (Schellenberg et al. 2011). All patients were able to complete SBRT and a median of five cycles of gemcitabine-based chemotherapy. There was no acute grade 3 toxicity. However, four patients developed late toxicities: one patient developed late grade 4 duodenal perforation and three developed grade 2 duodenal ulcers. The median OS was 11.8 months and the 1- and 2-year survival rates were 50% and 20%, respectively. The 1-year freedom from local tumor progression rate based on CT was 94%. Hoyer et al. from Denmark reported the results of a phase II trial of SBRT for unresectable, locally advanced pancreatic carcinoma (Hoyer et al. 2005). A total of 22 patients were enrolled and 3 of them had a recurrence after a Whipple operation: 2 with primary recurrence and 1 with lymph node recurrence. A course of SBRT was administered within 5–10 days, delivering

45 Gy in three fractions. Two patients had a partial response, and six had local tumor recurrence. The actuarial local tumor control rate was 57% and the median time to local progression was 4.8 months. The 1-year progression-free survival and OS were 9% and 5%, respectively. Serious acute toxicities were observed with four patients developing severe mucositis or ulceration of the stomach or duodenum and one developing a nonfatal perforation of the stomach. The investigators concluded that SBRT was associated with a poor outcome, unacceptable toxicity, and questionable palliative effect.

Mahadevan et al. from Harvard University examined the use of CyberKnife®-based SBRT and gemcitabine in the treatment of locally advanced pancreatic cancer in 36 patients at Beth Israel Deaconess Hospital (Mahadevan et al. 2010). All patients had a follow-up of at least 12 months and the prescribed dose was 24–36 Gy in three fractions. The LC rate was 78% and median OS time was 14.3 months at a follow-up of 24 months. Distant metastases occurred in 78% of the patients and 17% were free of disease at last follow-up. Nine and five patients developed grade 2 and 3 toxicities related to SBRT, respectively. University Hospitals, Seidman Cancer Center, has also reported their experience with 20 patients treated with CyberKnife®-based SBRT for unresectable pancreatic cancer (Goyal et al. 2012). One patient received SBRT for a neuroendocrine tumor. The mean radiation dose was 25 Gy (range 22–30 Gy) in three fractions. Chemotherapy was administered in 68% of the patients. The mean total GTV reduction was 21% and 38% at 3 and 6 months after SBRT, respectively. At a median follow-up interval of 15 months, the freedom from local progression at 6 and 12 months was 88% and 65%, respectively. The 1-year OS was 56%. No complications related to placement of fiducial markers were observed. The SBRT-related complication rates were 11% for grade 1–2 toxicities and 16% for grade 3 toxicities. Chang et al. from Stanford University published the treatment outcomes of 77 patients with unresectable adenocarcinoma of the pancreas <7.5 cm treated with SBRT delivering 25 Gy in one fraction (Chang et al. 2009).

Seventy-two percent of the patients had locally advanced or medically inoperable disease, 19% had metastatic disease, and 8% had locally recurrent disease. Twenty-one percent of the patients also received conventionally fractionated radiotherapy and 96% received gemcitabine-based chemotherapy. The 1-year freedom from local disease progression was 84% at a median follow-up of 6 months for all patients (12 months for surviving patients). The local tumor control rate at 1 year was 95%. The overall progression-free survival at 1 year was 9% and the overall 1-year survival was 21%. Grade 2 or higher acute toxicities occurred in 5% of the patients; grades 2 and ≥3 late toxicities occurred in 4% and 9% of the patients, respectively. At 1 year, the rate of grade 2 or higher toxicity was 25%.

More recent studies typically use a five-fraction regimen combined with systemic chemotherapy. Herman et al. from Johns Hopkins University reported the results of a multi-institutional phase II study of SBRT followed by gemcitabine chemotherapy (Herman et al. 2015). The dose regimen used was 33 Gy in 5 fractions and a total of 49 patients were enrolled. The median OS was 13.9 months and the 1-year freedom from local progression rate was 78%. After SBRT, five patients (10%) were deemed to be resectable following treatment but one refused resection. The four remaining patients (8%) underwent successful margin- and lymph node-negative resections, with one showing pathologic complete response. One patient developed a grade ≥3 acute GI ulcer, and four developed grade ≥3 late fistula or ulceration. The overall rate of all grade ≥3 acute toxicities was 29%. Late toxicity was observed in 11% of patients. Quality of life evaluation was performed using the EORTC Quality of Life Questionnaire (EORTC QLQ-C30; version 3.0) and the pancreatic cancer-specific QLQ-PAN 26 questionnaire. Eighty-eight percent of the patients completed these questionnaires at baseline and 4 weeks after SBRT, and 51% completed questionnaires 4 months after treatment. Results from these assessments demonstrated favorable QOL after SBRT with stable QLQ-C30 global QOL scores from baseline to after SBRT, and significant improvement in pancreatic pain (25 at baseline, median change of −8, $P = .001$) 4 weeks after SBRT using the QLQ-PAN26 assessment. In a retrospective study of 88 patients with locally advanced or borderline resectable disease treated with five-fraction SBRT (25–33 Gy in five fractions), the median survival was 13.7 months and 1-year LC was 61% at a median follow-up of 14.5 and 10.3 months for locally advanced and borderline resectable disease, respectively (Moningi et al. 2015). The majority of the patients in the series had additional treatment with chemotherapy before and/or after SBRT (gemcitabine alone in 45 patients; gemcitabine-based regimens in 14 patients, and folinic acid/fluorouracil/irinotecan/oxaliplatin [FOLFIRINOX] in 18 patients). The toxicity profile was very favorable, with a grade ≥3 acute toxicity rate of 3.4% and a grade ≥2 late toxicity rate of 5.7%. Patients who received pre-SBRT chemotherapy had better survival compared to those who did not receive chemotherapy (median survival of 18.8 months vs. 9 months). There was no difference in survival between patients treated with gemcitabine-based chemotherapy or FOLFIRINOX. Chuong et al. from Moffitt Cancer Center reported the results of 73 patients treated with induction gemcitabine, docetaxel, and capecitabine (GTX-C) chemotherapy followed by SBRT (median dose delivered to the tumor was 25 Gy in five fractions and 35 Gy to the portion of tumor surrounding vasculature) for borderline resectable or locally advanced disease (Chuong et al. 2013). The corresponding median OS was 16.4 and 15.0 months, respectively. The 1-year LC was 81% with no acute grade 3 toxicity and 5.3% late grade ≥3 toxicity observed. A pilot study from Georgetown University reported on the use of concurrent gemcitabine (1000 mg/m²) with SBRT to 25 Gy in five fractions, followed by five more cycles of chemotherapy (Gurka et al. 2013). Eleven patients were enrolled. The median survival was 12.2 months, and no grade 3 radiation-related toxicities were observed.

There have been some studies evaluating the use of SBRT as a boost after conventional radiotherapy for pancreatic cancer for dose escalation. In a phase II trial from Stanford University, the efficacy of 45 Gy of conventional fractionated radiotherapy with concurrent fluorouracil, followed by a boost with SBRT of 25 Gy in 1 fraction to the primary pancreatic tumor in 16 patients, was tested (Koong et al. 2005). Two patients developed grade 3 toxicities and 15 of 16 patients achieved local tumor control until time of death. The median OS time was 8.3 months. In a retrospective study from South Korea, 30 patients with locally advanced pancreatic cancer were treated with external beam radiotherapy to a dose of 40 Gy in 20 fractions, followed by single-fraction SBRT to a dose of 14, 15, 16, or 17 Gy as a boost without a break (Seo et al. 2009). Chemotherapy was given to 21 patients. The 1-year survival and 1-year local progression-free survival were 60% and 70.2%, respectively. Grade 4 toxicity was observed in one patient (3%). Cancer antigen 19–9 response was found to be an independent prognostic factor predicting survival.

8.3.2 Neoadjuvant and Adjuvant SBRT

There have been a very limited number of studies evaluating the role of neoadjuvant or adjuvant SBRT in pancreatic cancer. In a retrospective study from University of Pittsburgh Medical Center, 12 patients who were deemed to be borderline resectable received neoadjuvant gemcitabine chemotherapy followed by SBRT (Rajagopalan et al. 2013). The R0 resection rate was 92% with complete response in 25% of the patients and <10% viable tumor cells seen in another 16.7%. Mellon et al. from Moffitt Cancer Center reported the treatment outcomes on a large series of 157 borderline resectable or locally advanced pancreatic cancer treated with neoadjuvant chemotherapy followed by SBRT (Mellon et al. 2015). In this cohort, 51% of patients initially deemed to be borderline resectable went on to surgical resection with an R0 rate of 96%. The toxicities of treatment were acceptable, with a grade 3 toxicity rate of only 7%. For those patients who were able to undergo surgical resection, the OS was much better at 34.2 months compared to 14.0 months for those without resection. Patients were usually taken to surgery between 1 and 2 months after SBRT. The results of this study underscore the importance of surgical resection on survival and the potential impact that aggressive systemic chemotherapy and SBRT may have in the neoadjuvant setting.

In the postoperative setting, the University of Pittsburgh Medical Center reported outcomes on 24 patients with postoperative close or positive resection margins treated with adjuvant SBRT to the tumor bed to a dose of either 20–24 Gy in one fraction ($n = 11$) or 30 Gy in three fractions ($n = 1$) (Rwigema et al. 2012). Postoperative SBRT was deemed to be safe and the acute treatment-related toxicities (12% grade ≤ 2) were acceptable. There were no late grade 3 toxicities observed. The median OS was 26.5 months, and the rates of freedom from local progression were 87.5% and 62.5% for patients with close or positive margins, respectively.

8.4 Future Directions

Despite reasonable LC with SBRT for pancreatic cancer, overall survival remains poor as there is a high risk for distant metastasis for patients with locally advanced pancreatic cancer. To improve survival, an individualized approach with refinement and integration of surgery, chemotherapy, and radiotherapy is necessary. Improvement in systemic therapy, including incorporation of targeted agents and/or immunotherapy, is necessary. To enhance the therapeutic index for SBRT, drugs that can decrease tumor hypoxia can be employed to potentially improve tumor reoxygenation with hypofractionation.

9 Head and Neck

According to the American Cancer Society, an estimated 48,330 new cases of head and neck cancers will be diagnosed in 2016 and 9570 deaths will occur (American Cancer Society 2016). Overall mortality rates have been decreasing over the past three decades, especially due to the cessation of smoking. However, from 2003 to 2012, rates have stabilized in men partly due to the increasing incidence of human papillomavirus (HPV)-related cancers, while they continued to decrease in Caucasian women. The standard treatment for head and neck cancers typically includes either surgery followed by postoperative radiation therapy or definitive radiation therapy, with concurrent chemotherapy reserved in locally advanced settings. In certain cases, when patients are not found to be suitable for radical treatment either due to medical comorbidities, poor performance status, unresectable recurrent locoregional disease, or metastatic disease, palliative doses of radiation therapy are considered. More recently, SBRT has become an attractive option for head and neck cancers due to its several advantages. SBRT allows delivery of an ablative dose while limiting toxicities due to its conformality around the target volumes and steep-dose gradients (Simpson et al. 2006). As an outpatient procedure, it provides a shorter nondaily treatment course with reduction of the overall treatment time to 1–2 weeks. In the most recent years, there have been an increasing number of institutions that reported their experiences on the use of SBRT for head and neck cancer patients with newly diagnosed or recurrent disease. This summary highlights the most recent findings in the diagnosis, treatment, and radiation planning and delivery of SBRT for head and neck cancers.

9.1 Primary Disease

9.1.1 Patient Selection

While the standard management of medically inoperable head and neck cancer patients remains definitive radiation therapy plus or minus chemotherapy delivered over 6–7 weeks, there are instances in which this treatment might not be suitable. When elderly patients present with multiple comorbidities and/or poor performance status, and require local treatment, a shorter course of radiation treatment might be more feasible. It is known that SBRT offers the advantages of limiting toxicities by offering conformal treatment plans with steep-dose gradients while delivering ablative doses over 1–5 fractions. Patients should be selected on a case-by-case basis at the discretion of a multidisciplinary head and neck tumor board, when it is felt that the patient might be unable to tolerate or is refusing a conventional treatment regime. Particular situations in which SBRT may be appropriate include well-lateralized lesions away from midline structures such as the larynx or hypopharynx due to concerns for toxicity (Vargo et al. 2014a). Furthermore, certain locally advanced head and neck cases might benefit from a specialized boost technique to maximize LC rates such as in cases of nasal cavity/ paranasal sinuses, or a nasopharyngeal carcinoma located near critical OAR such as brainstem or visual structures. Dose escalation is achieved via the use of a SBRT boost following a conventional course of external beam radiation therapy (Lee et al. 2012; Owen et al. 2015). This approach should be highly selective with limited volumes for the boost to minimize late complications.

9.1.2 Clinical Outcomes: Local Control and Toxicity

There are currently no randomized data summarizing SBRT for primary head and neck cancers. Some small retrospective series have been published, but most are subject to inherent biases including patient selection and short follow-up. These series are summarized in Table 6, and demonstrate LC rates in the range of 70–85% at 1 year with complete response rates of 40–85% (Karam et al. 2015). Data on toxicity are limited in these series, but a few studies describe grade 3 dysphagia, mucositis, osteoradionecrosis, brain necrosis, and cranial nerve palsies. Further validation from prospective trials is necessary to obtain longitudinal data specific to QOL measures and toxicity-related outcomes.

Dose escalation with SBRT/SRS boost is an interesting option in patients with locally advanced unfavorable disease. However, the risk of severe late toxicity is significant and should therefore be a highly selective option. Lee et al. reported on their experience using a hypofractionated SBRT boost for locally advanced head and neck cancer (Lee et al. 2012). The median SBRT dose was 21 Gy (range: 10–25 Gy) delivered in 2–5 fractions. The 2-year actuarial OS was 46% and the 2-year locoregional recurrence-free rate was 86%. The rate of severe late (grade ≥3) toxicity was relatively high as described in nine patients (34.6%), which included pontine necrosis, base of skull and soft-tissue necrosis, nasopharyngeal wall soft-tissue necrosis, temporal lobe

Table 6 Summary of data for primary SBRT

Author, date	N	Dose	Local control	Overall survival	Late toxicity ≥ grade 3
Siddiqui et al. (2009)	10	18–48 Gy in 1–8 fractions	1 year 83%	1 year 70%	Cataract (1)
					Pain (1)
Kodani et al. (2011)	13	19.5–42 Gy in 3–8 fractions	38% (complete response rate)	1 year 85%	None
Kawaguchi et al. (2012)	14	35–42 Gy in 3–5 fractions	71% crude	79% crude	Osteoradionecrosis (1)
Vargo et al. (2014a)	10	20–44 Gy in 1–5 fractions	1 year 69%	1 year 64%	Dysphagia (1)
					Mucositis (1)
Khan et al. (2015b)	17	35–48 Gy in 5–6 fractions	1 year 87%	1 year 60% (recurrent + de novo cases)	None
Owen et al. (2015)	63	14 Gy in 1 fractions 5%	1 year 41%	(recurrent + de novo cases)	Brain necrosis (15)
					Cranial neuropathy (11)
					Osteoradionecrosis (3)
					Stroke (1)

Table 7 Summary of Data for SBRT as a Boost in Nasopharyngeal Carcinoma

Author, date	N	Initial conventional dose	Boost dose	Local control	Overall survival	Late toxicity ≥ grade 3
Tate et al. (1999)	23	64.8–70 Gy	7–15 Gy in 1 fraction	3 year 100%	Not available	None
Le et al. (2003)	45	64.8–70 Gy	7–15 Gy in 1 fraction	3 year 100%	3 year 75%	Retinopathy (1)
						Temporal lobe necrosis (3)
						Transient cranial nerve weakness (4)
Chen et al. (2006)	64	64.8–68.4 Gy	12–15 Gy in 3 fraction	3 year 93.1%	3 year 84.9%	None
Hara et al. (2008)	82	64.8–70 Gy	7–15 Gy in 1 fraction	5 year 98%	5 year 69%	Retinopathy (3)
						Carotid aneurysm (1)
						Temporal lobe necrosis (10)

necrosis, mucosal ulcer/necrosis, radiation retinopathy, and optic neuropathy. Two SBRT-related deaths were reported from massive oral bleeding and pontine necrosis. The authors demonstrated that SBRT boost volume was a significant parameter predicting severe late complication. Therefore, when considering a hypofractionated SBRT boost in locally advanced head and neck cancers, one should be careful of the treatment volume especially if located near critical structures.

A retrospective series by Owen et al. demonstrated that treatment of skull base disease with stereotactic radiosurgery is a viable option (Owen et al. 2015). They reported on long-term outcomes of 215 cases treated with GammaKnife®, of which 109 received a stereotactic radiosurgery (SRS) boost mainly for base-of-skull disease. Other intents were for palliative SRS alone (n = 63), or salvage SRS alone with curative intent (n = 43). One-year locoregional control and OS rates at a median follow-up of 17.4 months were 82% and 40%. They reported on 14 (7.5%) grade ≥3 toxicities, including radiation necrosis of the brain and cranial nerve palsies, being the most common ones. The authors noted that although most complications occurred within the first 5 years after GammaKnife® SRS treatment, the risk of grade 3 and above late effects increased significantly beyond 5 years, thus showing the impor-

tance of long-term follow-up in this patient population.

The role of a stereotactic boost in the treatment of locally advanced nasopharyngeal carcinoma has been extensively studied after radical external beam delivery with boost doses ranging from 7 to 15 Gy delivered in 1–3 fractions with concurrent chemotherapy (Chen et al. 2006; Hara et al. 2008; Le et al. 2003; Tate et al. 1999). Reported 3-year LC rates have been excellent ranging from 90 to 100% at 3 years (Table 7). Minimal late grade 3 toxicities were noted, but follow-up was relatively short. The largest institutional experience was reported by the Stanford group, describing 82 nasopharyngeal cancer patients treated with a stereotactic boost with late toxicities including radiation-related retinopathy in three patients, carotid aneurysm in one patient, and radiographic temporal lobe necrosis in ten patients, of which two were symptomatic (Hara et al. 2008).

9.2 Recurrent Disease

9.2.1 Patient Selection

Despite improvements with radiation delivery, use of concurrent systemic therapy or molecularly targeted agents, locoregional failure remains the most common cause of death in patients with head and neck cancers, estimated in the range of 20–50% (Farrag et al. 2010; McDonald et al. 2011; O'Sullivan et al. 2013). When patients present with unresectable recurrent disease, or if they are medically unfit or decline radical surgery, reirradiation remains the only potential curative option. A course of IMRT, when used either in the definitive setting or after salvage surgery, is a feasible option with acceptable 2-year LC rates of 59% and OS rates of 51% (Takiar et al. 2016). However, it has been shown to be associated with significant treatment-related toxicity (2-year grade ≥3 toxicity rate of 32% and 5-year rate of 48%), especially when treatment volumes are >50 cm^3 or if concurrent chemotherapy is being used. Hyperfractionation can be employed with the goal of reducing late toxicity, but this type of treatment can be time intensive for some patients who might be unable to attend treatments twice daily. It is speculated that recurrent tumors are morphologically distinct from primary disease and thus might benefit from ablative radiation doses with rapid dose falloff outside tumor volumes near critical structures, allowing for increased conformity and smaller treatment volumes (Takiar et al. 2016). However, this type of technique is limited by the size of treatment volume, as toxicity has been demonstrated to increase with >25cm^3 treatment volumes (Vargo et al. 2014b). Therefore, careful patient selection remains of significant importance when considering retreatment options for patients with recurrent disease in the SBRT setting.

9.2.2 Clinical Outcomes: Local Control and Toxicity

Recent institutional published data for recurrent head and neck cancers treated with SBRT are summarized in Table 8. The reported that 1- to 2-year LC rates are broad ranging from 30 to 80% with OS rates from 20 to 60% (Karam et al. 2015). Even though SBRT for recurrent head and neck cancers is a viable option, serious acute and late complications in the range of 1–20% have been reported due to the high cumulative doses used (Karam et al. 2015).

Notably, the Pittsburgh group recently published on their 10-year institutional experience on reirradiation with SBRT (Ling et al. 2016). A total of 291 patients were treated with SBRT for recurrent head and neck cancer with a 5-year actuarial OS rate of 17%. The median dose delivered was 44 Gy. Eleven percent of their patients experienced grade ≥3 acute toxicity and 19% experienced grade ≥3 late toxicity. Half of their patients treated for a laryngeal/hypopharyngeal recurrence experienced severe late toxicity compared to 6–20% for other sites, demonstrating that location is a significant predictor of late toxicity. Grade 5 late toxicities included carotid blowout syndrome (CBOS) in the absence of recurrent disease in three patients, dysphagia in two patients, laryngeal edema in one patient, and mucosal bleeding in one patient.

The risk of CBOS in the recurrent setting remains of significant concern when considering SBRT and has been documented in several institutional experiences (Ling et al. 2016; Cengiz et al. 2011; Ozyigit et al. 2011; Unger et al. 2010; Yamazaki et al. 2015). Some authors have described predisposing disease factors that increase the risk of CBOS, including patients with carotid invasion >180°, skin ulceration, or location of nodal irradiation (Cengiz et al. 2011; Yamazaki et al. 2015). Cengiz et al. reported that the risk of blowout is unrelated to tumor volume, response to treatment, or time elapsed between SBRT and previous radiation (Cengiz et al. 2011). Therefore, careful patient selection is important when considering patients for retreatment with SBRT, and use of alternate-day treatment schedules, avoidance of hot spots in the carotid artery, assigning a dose constraint to the carotid artery <34 Gy in five fractions, or using an alternate fractionation schedule such as hyperfractionation are all strategies reported in order to decrease the rates of late complications such as CBOS (Cengiz et al. 2011; McDonald et al. 2012; Thariat et al. 2011; Yazici et al. 2013).

Table 8 Summary of data for reirradiation with SBRT

Author, date	N	Reirradiation dose	Time to reirradiation (median)	Margins	Local control	Overall survival	Late toxicity ≥ grade 3
Voynov et al. (2006)	22	10–36 Gy in 1–8 fractions	Not applicable	PTV = GTV	2 year 26%	2 year 22%	None
Roh et al. (2009)	36	18–40 Gy in 3–5 fractions	24 months	PTV = GTV + 2 -3 mm	2 year 52%	2 year 31%	Bone necrosis (1) Soft tissue necrosis (2) Trismus (2) Chronic ulcer (2) Death (1)
Heron et al. (2009)	25	25–44 Gy in 5 fractions	13 months	PTV = GTV	17.4% (response rate)	Median 6 months	None
Siddiqui et al. (2009)	21	18–48 Gy in 1–8 fractions	19 months	PTV = GTV/C TV	2 year 40.4%	2 year 14.3%	Dysphagia (1) Fistula (3) Mandibular necrosis (1) Ulceration (1)
Unger et al. (2010)	65	21–35 Gy in 2–5 fractions	26 months	PTV = CTV = GTV + 2–10 mm	2 year 30%	2 year 41%	Arterial bleeding (2) Dysphagia (2) Soft tissue necrosis (1) Fistula formation (1) Death (1)
Rwigema et al. (2011)	96	15–50 Gy in 5 fractions	19.4 months	PTV = GTV	2 year 30.7%	2 year 28.4%	Dysphagia (2) Fibrosis (1)
Kodani et al. (2011)	21	19.5–42 Gy in 3–8 fraction	Not applicable	PTV = GTV/ITV	29% (complete response rate)	2 year 58.3%	Pharynx hemorrhage (2) Severe mucositis (2) Dysphagia (2) Skin necrosis (1) Death (2)

(continued)

Table 8 (continued)

Author, date	N	Reirradiation dose	Time to reirradiation (median)	Margins	Local control	Overall survival	Late toxicity ≥ grade 3
Cengiz et al. (2011)	46	18–35 Gy in 1–5 fraction	38 months	PTV = GTV	1 year 84%	1 year 47%	Soft tissue necrosis (1) Mandibular necrosis (1) Dysphagia (3) Carotid blowout (8) Deaths (7)
Ozyigit et al. (2011)	24	30 Gy in 5 fractions	38 months	PTV = GTV	2 year 82%	2 year 64% (CSS)	Cranial neuropathy (1) Carotid blowout (4) Brain necrosis (1)
Vargo et al. (2012)	34	30–44 Gy in 5 fractions	53 months	PTV = GTV	1 year 59%	1 year 59%	Osteoradionecrosis (1) Pain (1)
Lartigau et al. (2013)	60	36 Gy in 6 fractions + cetuximab	38 months	PTV = CTV +1 mm CTV = GTV + 5 mm	3 months 91.7%	1 year 47.5%	Fibrosis (1) Xerostomia (2) Fistula (1) Death (1)
Khan et al. (2015b)	7	35–48 Gy in 5–6 fractions	Not available	PTV = GTV + 2 – 3 mm	1 year 50%	1 year 60%	None
Vargo et al. (2015)	50	40–44 Gy in 5 fractions + cetuximab	18 months	PTV = GTV + 3 – 5 mm	1 year 60%	1 year 40%	Dysphagia (1) Fistula (1)

9.2.3 SBRT and Systemic Therapy

Various strategies to improve outcomes of patients with unresectable locally recurrent previously irradiated head and neck cancers have been explored in the past years, including the addition of concurrent cetuximab with SBRT delivery. The Pittsburgh group recently reported on their prospective experience with SBRT and concurrent cetuximab in 50 patients with recurrent head and neck malignancies treated to a median dose of 40–44 Gy in five fractions (Vargo et al. 2015). The 1-year local progression-free survival rate was 60% and OS rate was 40%. The treatment was relatively safe with 6% of patients experiencing grade 3 acute and late toxicity. Late toxicities included dysphagia requiring feeding tube dependence, moist desquamation, tracheoesophageal fistula, and leakage extending into neopharynx requiring a feeding tube. There was no grade 4 toxicity reported.

Similar to the Pittsburgh group, the French group also reported on a phase II trial that enrolled 60 patients treated to a slightly lower dose of 36 Gy in six fractions with concurrent and adjuvant cetuximab and SBRT (Lartigau et al. 2013). The 1-year OS rate was similar to the above study at 47.5% and 18 (30%) patients presented with grade 3 toxicity including mucositis, dysphagia, and fibrosis. Interestingly, neither group reported rates of CBOS, partly due to delivery of radiation on alternate days and exclusion of patients with disease wrapping around carotid vessels by the French group. In summary, the benefits of this approach allow patients to complete treatment over a short period while optimizing LC rates.

Moreover, it is well known that SBRT can elicit antitumor immunity through the upregulation of different immunomodulators and release of cytokines, inflammatory mediators, or necrosis factors leading to activation of tumor-specific T cells (Karam et al. 2015; Song et al. 2014). The ability of SBRT to enhance antitumor immunity can be improved with the use of immunotherapy, with possible enhancement of the abscopal effect in visceral lesions (Karam et al. 2015; Formenti 2015; Sharabi et al. 2015). As a result, the use of PD-1 antibodies such as pembrolizumab, or CTLA-4 antibodies, such as ipilimumab, delivered concurrently with SBRT might lead to optimization of LC rates. This will be further explored through an RTOG trial on SBRT delivered concurrently with pembrolizumab in the recurrent/metastatic setting.

9.3 Technical Considerations

There is significant heterogeneity in the treatment techniques reported for head and neck SBRT among treating institutions. Treatment delivery systems may include a linear accelerator with CBCT, robotic SBRT, Co-60 SRS, and proton systems (Owen et al. 2015; Cengiz et al. 2011; Unger et al. 2010; McDonald et al. 2012; Lartigau et al. 2013; Heron et al. 2009; Khan et al. 2015b; Kodani et al. 2011; Roh et al. 2009; Rwigema et al. 2011; Siddiqui et al. 2009; Vargo et al. 2012, 2015; Voynov et al. 2006). CBCT, robotic tracking, optical based surface alignment, or CT-on-rail can be used as part of pretreatment imaging verification and intrafractional monitoring.

The use of margin expansions for target volumes, including the use of margins to account for microscopic disease, varies among institutions (Table 8). The Pittsburgh group (Wang et al. 2013, 2016) assessed the impact of adding margins to the GTV in patients after SBRT recurrences. Based on their results, they recommended a 3–5 mm PTV expansion on the GTV in order to prevent recurrences. Our institution uses a 3 mm PTV expansion on the GTV and does not include a margin for microscopic disease.

A range of SBRT doses have been published to treat primary and recurrent head and neck cancers and vary between 14–22 Gy in one fraction and 30–50 Gy in five or six fractions (Table 6 and Table 8). Heron et al. published a phase I dose escalation trial of 25 patients treated in five dose tiers up to 44 Gy delivered in five fractions. There were no grade 3/4 or dose-limiting toxicities reported and therefore SBRT delivered up to 44 Gy was felt to be relatively safe and well tolerated by patients in the acute setting (Heron et al. 2009).

9.4 Future Directions

The use of SBRT for primary and recurrent head and neck disease will likely increase in popularity due to its potential advantages. However, there remains a lack of standardization in SBRT planning and delivery and randomized trials with objective measures and patient-reported outcomes are lacking. In addition, the benefit of concurrent potential cancer biological agents is unknown and requires further exploration. Interinstitutional prospective trials are necessary to allow standardization of approaches in the implementation of head and neck SBRT.

10 Novel Applications for SBRT

10.1 Cardiac Arrhythmias

Atrial fibrillation (AF) is the most common form of cardiac arrhythmia (Camm 2005). Currently four million people have AF in America (Naderi et al. 2014). Seventy percent of these people are between 65 and 85 years old (Karamichalakis et al. 2015). Symptomatic AF can significantly affect QOL, as well as increase the risk of stroke, thromboembolism, and even death (Naderi et al. 2014). Treatment options for AF can be divided into rate control and rhythm control. Rate control is usually combined with the use of antithrombotic drugs, which carry a risk of major bleeding events. Rhythm control includes the use of antiarrhythmic drugs and catheter ablation. The most common antiarrhythmic drugs are amiodarone and sotalol, and are limited by their proarrhythmic and noncardiovascular toxicities and their modest antiarrhythmic efficacy (Zimetbaum 2012). The most effective established treatment option for AF is catheter ablation (Bhatt et al. 2016), although it is invasive and technically challenging, and usually requires the use of con-

current anticoagulation. Catheter ablation is usually performed using radiofrequency energy; however other modalities such as cryoablation, ultrasound, and laser have also been used. In the case of AF, the catheter is directed to the junction between the pulmonary veins and left atrium. In the less common case of atrial flutter, the catheter is directed towards the cavotricuspid isthmus of the right atrium. The success rate of catheter ablation is approximately 60% after 5 years and often requires repeat procedures (Takigawa et al. 2014). It is also associated with procedural complications at a rate of approximately 6%, including bleeding, stroke, myocardial infarction, infection, thromboembolism, and death, although the rate can be significantly higher in certain groups including the elderly (9.37%), diabetics (17.83%), patients with COPD (23.25%), and patients with renal failure (23.25%), which is partly related to atypical or diseased vascular anatomy (Calkins et al. 2012; Deshmukh et al. 2013). Cardiac tamponade, the most life-threatening complication, occurs in 1.5–6% of patients (Deshmukh et al. 2013). Ventricular tachycardia (VT) is a reentrant rhythm that can also cause significant mortality and morbidity (Moss et al. 2004). In addition to implantable cardioverter defibrillators (ICD), catheter ablation may be used to treat VT. In cases where this is not successful, cardiac surgery is an option; however it can be associated with serious complications, and is only suitable in patients with minimal comorbidities who are fit for surgery.

In recent times, there is increasing interest in the use of SBRT as a noninvasive option for AF, based on the theory that radiation, like radiofrequency energy, may be able to create localized scar tissue that can block the aberrant signals which cause cardiac arrhythmias. It may also allow for treatment in an increased patient population, particularly in patients that have failed or are not candidates for established treatment options such as catheter ablation and cardiac surgery, as well as result in improved safety and clinical outcomes. Although the heart is usually not a target but rather an OAR to be avoided given the known radiation-related cardiac toxicities including pericarditis and coronary artery disease (Darby et al. 2010), SBRT allows for greater precision in radiotherapy delivery and avoidance of critical structures such as the coronary arteries and apex of the heart, which may allow minimization of cardiac toxicities in these patients. It has also been shown to be a feasible option in the treatment of tumors in or adjacent to the heart (Soltys et al. 2008).

There are, however, several challenges that cardiac SBRT for arrhythmia present. Firstly, the structures of the heart are difficult to identify on CT without contrast, as is the actual target. Secondly, motion management in the heart is complicated and has two facets: cardiac motion that occurs with respiration and deformation and motion that occurs during cardiac contraction/relaxation. In addition, the amount of movement depends upon the location within the heart, with the apex moving the most, and the posterior structures moving the least (Gardner et al. 2012). While systems have been developed to allow for tracking of motion with respiration, often using fiducials, the authors are not aware of any commercial systems available currently to track the contractile motion of the heart for the purposes of radiotherapy delivery. Lastly, there are critical organs adjacent to the target which need to be avoided. The pulmonary veins straddle the esophagus and the left atrium is immediately anterior. This means that not only are steep-dose gradients required to both treat the pulmonary vein ostia and avoid the esophagus, but also that the dose distribution must be extremely accurately delivered, even through the complexities of cardiac motion.

Despite these hurdles, a few animal studies have now shown that SBRT for AF is feasible (Gardner et al. 2012; Blanck et al. 2014; Bode et al. 2016; Maguire et al. 2011; Sharma et al. 2010). Sharma et al. reported on the results of 16 Hanford-Sinclair mini-swine that received SBRT to the cavotricuspid isthmus, AV node, pulmonary vein-left atrial junction, or left atrial appendage (Sharma et al. 2010). Target localization for treatment of AF can be particularly challenging due to complex respiratory

and cardiac motion. In this study, a gated cardiac CT was used to define the anatomic targets and an ITV created. Some animals additionally underwent real-time tracking to compensate for respiratory and cardiac motion. A surgically implanted or catheter tip fiducial marker at the target site was used to assist with both registration and tracking. The results of this study showed that at least 25 Gy was required to cause electrophysiological effects at the cavotricuspid isthmus, usually in 30–90 days. The authors noted a significant reduction in voltage to less than 0.05 mV at the pulmonary vein-left atrial junction and left appendage after treatment, which is comparable to that attained by an invasive catheter ablation procedure. In addition, there were no spontaneous arrhythmias following treatment and pathology specimens showed no radiation damage to areas outside the PTV at 6 months. This is promising, although it is noted that cardiac toxicity from radiotherapy often manifests many years following the initial treatment. Blanck et al. reported on a dose escalation study in nine mini-pigs. Animals were randomized to either 0 or 17.5–35 Gy in 2.5 Gy steps to the right superior pulmonary vein atrium (Blanck et al. 2014). The MRI and electrophysiology studies occurred prior to and 6 months after treatment. Transmural scarring was noted to occur at doses of ≥ 32.5 Gy, although complete circumferential scarring was not seen. The extent and intensity of fibrosis significantly increased with dose, with the 50% effective dose for intense fibrosis being 31.3 Gy. Heart function and adjacent structures were not adversely affected as verified by MRI/electrocardiogram and pathology, respectively. Another dose escalation and feasibility study by the same group looked at eight adult mini-pigs and delivered doses from 22.5 to 40 Gy in single fractions (Bode et al. 2016). The animals subsequently underwent electrophysiological and histological examinations 6 months following treatment. They found that reduction in pulmonary vein electrogram amplitudes was dose dependent with a mean interaction effect of −5.8%/Gy. Similar to the previous study, histological examination revealed transmural scarring at the target with doses of >30 Gy; however complete AV conduction block with complete circumferential scarring only occurred at 40 Gy. This suggests that quite high doses may be required for AF treatment, which may present a significant challenge in the use of SBRT for therapeutic effect in humans. A further animal study conducted to perform in vivo measurements of actual dose delivered during cardiac SBRT irradiated the pulmonary vein ostia of four animals with CyberKnife® to 20–35 Gy using 6MV photons to produce scarring that could prevent aberrant signals that cause AF (Moss et al. 2004). The Synchrony® (Accuray, Inc., Sunnyvale, CA) system was used to track respiratory motion of the heart, while the contractile motion was untracked. Thermoluminescent (TLD) and metal-oxide-semiconductor field-effect transistor (MOSFET) dosimeters were utilized and confirmed the actual radiation dose delivered and found that the dose measured on the epicardium with TLDs averaged 5% less than predicted for those locations. Doses in the coronary sinus measured with MOSFET dosimeters were 6% less than predicted on average, which in consideration of uncertainties associated with dose measurement suggests that the delivered dose is reasonably close to the predicted dose, despite partly untracked cardiac motion. The doses to the esophagus however were less accurate and were 25% less than predicted.

In addition to the animal studies on cardiac SBRT there have also been two human case reports on the use of SBRT to treat VT. The first reported human treatment for VT showed positive early outcomes (Lo et al. 2013). The patient was a 71-year-old male who had a background history of coronary artery bypass grafting (CABG), and subsequent ICD insertion for VT that was refractory to medical management. Prior to treatment, he initially underwent insertion of a dummy lead with a single metal end for tracking purposes. 4D-CT and breath-hold CT were then performed while the patient was lying rolled 15° to the right so that the dummy lead could be identified via Synchrony® tracking. Cardiac motion with breath hold was recorded to be approximately 1 cm. A PTV was then created to incorporate cardiac motion. The target itself was contoured with the use of visualization and contouring software (CardioPlan™, CyberHeart™, Portola Valley, California, USA) incorporating an inferior LV VT circuit location. The patient received 25 Gy in a single fraction to the 75% isodose line using 175 nonzero beams. Patient setup required 30 min, and treatment time was 90 min including a patient-requested 30-min break period. There were no definite acute or late complications of SBRT. Follow-up ICD interrogations revealed a decrease from 562 VT episodes to 52 episodes per month on average, 2–9 months following treatment. PET/CT scans performed prior to and following treatment revealed mild extension of the inferior scar with a more complete perfusion defect at this site at 2.5 months posttreatment. There was no change in transthoracic echocardiography (TTE) findings at 1, 3, and 6 months posttreatment. The patient's overall health however declined in the months following SBRT, with multiple admissions for exacerbation of COPD, and the patient eventually passed away 9 months following treatment due to a COPD exacerbation and recurrent VT. His family declined autopsy.

Cvek et al. reported a case of a 72-year-old lady with recurrent VT, in whom an ICD was inserted, and catheter ablation was ineffective due to thickness of the myocardium (Cvek et al. 2014). She was not a candidate for cardiac surgery due to comorbidities. She initially underwent two electrophysiology (EP) studies with an electro-anatomic mapping system (CARTO, Biosense-Webster, Israel) to localize the source of the arrhythmia, which was at the base of the lateral wall of the left ventricle. Target localization was performed through indirect comparison of the images. The PTV consisted of the ectopic lesion during systole and diastole, with no additional margin. The LV electrode in the lateral branch of the coronary sinus was used as a fiducial marker for respiratory tracking using Synchrony®. Radiation was delivered through the use of CyberKnife®, using 105 beams, with a prescribed dose of 25 Gy in a single fraction to the 82% isodose line. The plan created could achieve 97% coverage and a conformity index of 1.27. In the 120 days after treatment, no malignant arrhythmia was detected. At 10 days posttreatment, there was a minimal rise in troponin T (0.024–0.033) and at 6 weeks no toxicities including radiation pneumonitis or pericardial effusion were detected.

Given the challenges presented by cardiac SBRT, planning studies are being performed to clarify the best method of delivering treatment to human patients. Blanck et al. performed a planning study to investigate various tracking methods by creating theoretical radiosurgery treatment plans on 24 patients (Blanck et al. 2016). In this study, the target contours covered the left atrial-venous wall, myocardium, and myocardial sleeves of the pulmonary veins (PV) transmural at the PV antrum, and were approximately 4–6 mm wide along the PV/LA and 2–4 mm deep based upon tissue thickness. CardioPlan® was used to assist with target contouring and a margin of only 3 mm was created for PTV (both right PTV and left PTV were created). OAR included the esophagus, bronchial tree, and aorta. As previously mentioned, there was particular concern regarding the esophagus, which is not uncommonly in direct contact with the target. The OAR constraints used were as shown in Table 9.

Table 9 Cardiac SBRT organ-at-risk constraints

OAR	Dose max	Volume
Esophagus		
≤ Grade 1	<14 Gy	V9 Gy < 1 cm³
≥ Grade 3	>19 Gy	V14.5 Gy > 5 cm³
Bronchial Tree		
≤ Grade 1	<14 Gy	V10 Gy < 1 cm³
≥ Grade 3	>22 Gy	V10.5 Gy > 4 cm³
Coronary Artery		
≤ Grade 1	<16 Gy	
≥ Grade 3	20 Gy Circumferential	No data
Major vessels		
≥ Grade 3	>37 Gy	V31 Gy > 10 cm³

Eighteen patients on the study were tracked using the CyberKnife® marker-less tracking system (XSight® Lung: Accuray, Sunnyvale, California, USA). The study found that through this system only 40% of patients could be treated safely due to inability to meet esophagus and bronchial tree constraints. Given the long treatment times associated with AF due to relatively large volumes compared to VT treatment, the regional dose rate was also analyzed, and the authors found that significant optimization was possible through delivering the dose sequentially to different parts of the target rather than delivering all beams in a predefined path. Four patients also underwent ultrasound tracking with beam blocking of the ultrasound probe and this was found to have no impact upon plan quality and given its real-time imaging capability was thought to be an exciting area for future research. Four patients also were investigated using a theoretical temporary fiducial marker at the right atrial septum, and, due to the large target area, found differential surrogate-target motion, particularly between the right atrial septum and left pulmonary vein, although it was possible to compensate for this using 4D planning.

Other tracking methods being investigated include noninvasive real-time image-guided AF treatment using an integrated MRI linear accelerator (Ipsen et al. 2014; Lowther 2016). Ipsen et al. reported on six healthy human subjects who underwent real-time cardiac MRI under free breathing conditions (Ipsen et al. 2014). The study found mean respiratory target motion to be 10.2 mm (superior-inferior), 2.4 mm (anterior-posterior), and 2 mm (left-right). A planning study was then conducted and found that increased margins to account for the untracked respiratory motion would lead to overlapping structures and necessitate compromise in either PTV coverage or OAR constraints. Therefore the study concluded that real-time tracking and motion compensation would be compulsory for any cardiac radiosurgery and proposed real-time tracking with MRI as a feasible noninvasive option to achieving this.

Cardiac SBRT for arrhythmias certainly presents an exciting and challenging frontier for radiation oncologists, inspiring us to continue to innovat and investigate methods of target localization in a noncancerous condition, as well as improve our ability to deliver increasingly precise high-dose radiotherapy in one of the most complex moving organs in the body. Although in its infancy stages, continued research into target delineation, appropriate dosing, OAR including cardiac toxicities, and motion management, as well as improvements in technology may allow SBRT to become a clinical reality in the armament against cardiac arrhythmias in the future.

10.2 Pediatrics

SBRT has proved to be an exciting additional treatment option within the adult population, with early and now more mature data showing positive clinical outcomes. This is particularly true for situations in which radiotherapy was previously thought to play a very limited role, such as in so-called "radioresistant" malignancies, and patients with oligometastatic disease. It is unsurprising therefore that interest in SBRT in the pediatric population in recent times is now emerging. Stereotactic radiosurgery has been used for pediatric patients with benign intracranial disorders, as well as in patients with recurrent CNS lesions with success (Stauder et al. 2012; Yen et al. 2010). There is also a strong rationale for SBRT in children. SBRT offers the possibility of biological dose escalation and hypofractionation, which may be invaluable in treating traditionally radioresistant cancers such as osteosarcoma, and nonrhabdomyosarcoma soft-tissue sarcomas in the pediatric population. Pediatric patients are often curable despite the presence of metastatic or oligometastatic disease; however these patients are often treated with surgery or chemotherapy, given concerns regarding the ability of radiotherapy to obtain adequate LC and its effect on normal tissues. Both these issues may possibly be overcome with the use of SBRT. In addition, SBRT may offer a salvage option in patients with treatment-resistant residual disease following primary treatment.

Pediatric radiotherapy is unique in that it requires attention to areas not typically considered in adults. Radiotherapy planning needs to account for growth and development of immature organs in children and minimizing dose to these structures, and/or ensuring symmetry in radiotherapy delivery to these areas. For example while osteonecrosis and fracture may be seen in both adults and children, an additional consideration in children is bone hypoplasia (Paulino et al. 2010). There is also concern regarding increased risk of late toxicities following survival of the initial cancer, as well as second cancer risk. The risk of secondary malignancy is relatively higher in children due to both their age and the fact that many children may have germline mutations associated with their primary malignancy. The effects of both volume of tissue receiving radiation need to be considered as well as how SBRT compares in this regard to other modalities such as 3DCRT and IMRT. Additionally, patients receiving SBRT need to be compliant and require excellent immobilization. This may be difficult in younger children. They may require sedation or general anesthetic for both simulation and treatment. By comparison, for children requiring anesthetic even with conventionally fractionated 3DCRT or IMRT, SBRT offers the opportunity to minimize the number of anesthetics required. This may be considered a particular advantage when considering utilizing single or short courses of SBRT as an alternative to fractionated palliative radiotherapy in children requiring repeated anesthetics for treatment delivery. Pediatric radiotherapy doses often differ from adults, as do OAR constraints, and further investigation will be required prior to applying adult SBRT data in children. Pediatric patients are also often treated concurrently with complex chemotherapy regimens, often used with the aim of decreasing the total radiotherapy dose required. Even in the adult population, there is a paucity of data regarding the use of SBRT with systemic agents, and certainly the role of SBRT in these settings requires further elucidation, with regard to both the effective tumor kill dose and limitations regarding normal tissue dose tolerances.

Given the unique issues facing children undergoing radiotherapy, the applicability of adult data to the pediatric population is uncertain; and while there is a growing volume of data for SBRT in adult patients, there are very few data in the pediatric population. There are now a handful of case reports and small retrospective series emerging. The largest retrospective series published to date is of 15 patients with 20 osseous lesions treated with SBRT between 2011 and 2015 at Memorial Sloan Kettering Cancer Center (Taunk et al. 2015). There were nine lesions secondary to neuroblastoma, seven with Ewing's sarcoma, two with rhabdomyosarcoma, one with osteosarcoma, and one with pheochromocytoma. Nineteen of the 20 lesions were metastatic. Twelve cases were treated for progression of previously irradiated disease, and eight cases were for oligometastatic disease from osteosarcoma or pheochromocytoma. The median age of patients was 17 years (range 4–31 years). Total SBRT dose ranged from 20 to 40 Gy in 3 to 5 fractions (median dose of 27 Gy in 3 fractions). Median follow-up post-SBRT was 22 months. LC for the group was 75% with four of the five failures occurring in patients that had had prior conventional radiotherapy. Common toxicities included grade 1 fatigue (40%) and dermatitis (45%). Crude grade 3 toxicity was 15%. One was of a 4-year-old patient with neuroblastoma who suffered from grade 3 myositis at 3 months following SBRT to 27 Gy in 3 fractions to the right scapula and left distal femur (Taunk et al. 2016). The authors postulated that the severe toxicity seen was secondary to a combination of the short interval between prior conventional radiotherapy (30 Gy in ten fractions, less than 4 months prior) and SBRT, the large volume treated, and the use of chemotherapy before and after SBRT. Another grade 3 toxicity reported was neuropathy in a patient with osteosarcoma that previously received 79.2 Cobalt Gray Equivalents (CGE) proton therapy to the sacrum 6 months prior with subsequent SBRT to 30 Gy in three fractions.

The second largest series is a retrospective study of patients with osteosarcoma or Ewing's sarcoma that received SBRT, including six patients less than 18 years old at the time of treatment, with ages ranging from 4.9 to 17.7 years (Brown et al. 2014). Five patients received "definitive" intent treatment to bony sites, including to the iliac wing, femoral head, iliac crest, sacrum, and T11. The doses for the "definitive" treatment included 50 Gy in five fractions ($n = 2$), 60 Gy in ten fractions ($n = 2$), and 30 Gy in five fractions ($n = 1$). No patients experienced local failure, with follow-up times ranging from 0.3 to 4 years. Minimal acute toxicity was seen. Three patients experienced late toxicity, which included grade 2 myonecrosis, grade 2 pain, grade 2 neuropathy, grade 2 avascular necrosis (AVN), grade 2 pathological fracture, and myelodysplastic syndrome. The grade 2 myonecrosis was seen in a patient receiving 50 Gy in five fractions to the right iliac wing with concurrent gemcitabine for osteosarcoma, 2 months after SBRT. The patient who was treated for extensive femoral head disease to 60 Gy in ten fractions experienced grade 2 AVN (8 months post-SRT) and pathological fracture (4 months post-SBRT), both of which were conservatively managed. In this case, dose constraints were not able to be met, and the patient had been counselled accordingly (Benedict et al. 2010). Two patients also received "palliative" intent treatment to bony sites including scapula, C7–T1, T4, and T7–9. The SBRT doses ranged from 16 to 21 Gy in a single fraction, and 24 Gy in three fractions. Three of these sites were treated for pain control and for two of these sites pain control was durable until death (0.04 and 0.2 years). No patients experienced any acute toxicity.

A few other case reports have also been published. Briefly this includes that of a 16-year-old female with relapsed Ewing's sarcoma with a single lung lesion following salvage chemotherapy, who was treated with SBRT to 30 Gy in five fractions, with a PET/CT showing complete resolution of the lesion at 2 months (Siddiqui et al. 2012); a 12-year-old male with WHO Grade 3 nasopharyngeal carcinoma with a single osseous metastasis treated with SBRT to 40 Gy in five fractions, with a bone scan at 3 years confirming LC, and follow-up at 4 years finding no acute or late toxicity (Farnia et al. 2014); and most recently a 10-year-old male with inoperable HCC metastatic to a celiac lymph node, complicated by central biliary obstruction and an elevated bilirubin receiving SBRT to 45 Gy to the primary and 35 Gy in five fractions to the nodal disease, with subsequent improvement in bilirubin, and a durable tumor response at 3–4 months (Hiniker et al. 2016).

At present there are no prospective data regarding SBRT in children. However, the evidence to date is suggestive that SBRT may potentially reduce treatment-related toxicity, improve local treatment efficacy, and (in the palliative setting) reduce the need for frequent visits and repetitive general anesthesia. Prospective clinical trials are now needed to validate these observations. To this effect, there is a phase II multicenter trial currently accruing at John Hopkins, Stanford, Mayo Clinic, and St Jude's Children's Research Hospital that will study the use of SBRT in oligometastatic disease in pediatric sarcoma patients (Clinical trials database: NCT01763970). This and hopefully future studies will provide high-level evidence to guide clinicians in the safe and effective use of this exciting technology in improving the outcomes and lives of children suffering from cancer.

References

Abelson JA, Murphy JD, Loo BW et al (2012) Esophageal tolerance to high-dose stereotactic ablative radiotherapy. Dis Esophagus 25(7):623–629

Abrams HL, Spiro R, Goldstein N (1950) Metastases in carcinoma; analysis of 1000 autopsied cases. Cancer 3(1):74–85

Abuodeh Y, Venkat P, Kim S et al (2016) Systematic review of case reports on the abscopal effect. Curr Probl Cancer 40(1):25–37

Ahmed KA, Barney BM, Macdonald OK et al (2013) Stereotactic body radiotherapy in the treatment of adrenal metastases. Am J Clin Oncol 36(5):509–513. doi:10.1097/COC.0b013e3182569189

Al-Omair A, Masucci L, Masson-Cote L et al (2013a) Surgical resection of epidural disease improves local control following postoperative spine stereotactic body radiotherapy. Neuro-Oncology 15(10):1413–1419

Al-Omair A, Smith R, Kiehl TR et al (2013b) Radiation-induced vertebral compression fracture following spine stereotactic radiosurgery: clinicopathological correlation: report of 2 cases. J Neurosurg Spine 18(5):430–435

Alongi F, Cozzi L, Arcangeli S, Iftode C et al (2013) Linac based SBRT for prostate cancer in 5 fractions with VMAT and flattening filter free beams: preliminary report of a phase II study. Radiat Oncol 8(1):171

Altoos B, Amini A, Yacoub M et al (2015) Local control rates of metastatic renal cell carcinoma (RCC) to thoracic, abdominal, and soft tissue lesions using stereotactic body radiotherapy (SBRT). Radiat Oncol 10(1):1

American Cancer Society (2016) Cancer Facts & Figures 2016. American Cancer Society, Atlanta

Amini A, Altoos B, Bourlon MT et al (2015) Local control rates of metastatic renal cell carcinoma (RCC) to the bone using stereotactic body radiation therapy: is RCC truly radioresistant? Pract Radiat Oncol 5(6):e589–e596

Ananthakrishnan A, Gogineni V, Saeian K (2006) Epidemiology of primary and secondary liver cancers. Semin Intervent Radiol 23(1):47–63

Andolino DL, Johnson CS, Maluccio M et al (2011) Stereotactic body radiotherapy for primary hepatocellular carcinoma. Int J Radiat Oncol Biol Phys 81(4):e447–e453

Arcangeli S, Strigari L, Gomellini S et al (2012) Updated results and patterns of failure in a randomized hypofractionation trial for high-risk prostate cancer. Int J Radiat Oncol Biol Phys 84(5):1172–1178

Ashworth AB, Senan S, Palma DA et al (2014) An individual patient data metaanalysis of outcomes and prognostic factors after treatment of oligometastatic non-small-cell lung cancer. Clin Lung Cancer 15(5):346–355

Bae SH, Kim MS, Cho CK et al (2012) Predictor of severe gastroduodenal toxicity after stereotactic body radiotherapy for abdominopelvic malignancies. Int J Radiat Oncol Biol Phys 84(4):e469–e474

Balagamwala EH, Angelov L, Koyfman SA et al (2012) Single-fraction stereotactic body radiotherapy for spinal metastases from renal cell carcinoma: clinical article. J Neurosurg 17(6):556–564

Barr A, Knox JJ, Wei AC et al (2016) Can stereotactic body radiotherapy effectively treat hepatocellular carcinoma? J Clin Oncol 34(5):404–408

Baumann P, Nyman J, Hoyer M et al (2009) Outcome in a prospective phase II trial of medically inoperable stage I non-small-cell lung cancer patients treated with stereotactic body radiotherapy. J Clin Oncol 27(20):3290–3296

Beddar AS, Briere TM, Balter P et al (2008) 4D-CT imaging with synchronized intravenous contrast injection to improve delineation of liver tumors for treatment planning. Radiother Oncol 87(3):445–448

Bekelman JE, Epstein AJ, Emanuel EJ (2013) Single- vs multiple-fraction radiotherapy for bone metastases from prostate cancer. JAMA 310(14):1501–1502

Benedict SH, Yenice KM, Followill D et al (2010) Stereotactic body radiation therapy: the report of AAPM task group 101. Med Phys 37(8):4078–4101

Berber B, Sanabria JR, Braun K et al (2013) Emerging role of stereotactic body radiotherapy in the treatment of pancreatic cancer. Expert Rev Anticancer Ther 13(4):481–487

Bezjak A, Paulus R, Gaspar L et al (2016) Primary study endpoint analysis for NRG oncology/RTOG 0813 trial of stereotactic body radiation therapy (SBRT) for centrally located non-small cell lung cancer (NSCLC). Int J Radiat Oncol Biol Phys 1(94):5–6

Bhatt N, Fogarty T, Maguire P (2016) Cardiac radiosurgery for the treatment of atrial fibrillation. World J Cardiovasc Dis 6(05):143

Bishop AJ, Tao R, Rebueno NC et al (2015) Outcomes for spine stereotactic body radiation therapy and an analysis of predictors of local recurrence. Int J Radiat Oncol Biol Phys 92(5):1016–1026

Blanck O, Bode F, Gebhard M et al (2014) Dose-escalation study for cardiac radiosurgery in a porcine model. Int J Radiat Oncol Biol Phys 89(3):590–598

Blanck O, Ipsen S, Chan MK et al (2016) Treatment planning considerations for robotic guided cardiac radiosurgery for atrial fibrillation. Cureus 8(7):e705

Bode F, Blanck O, Gebhard M et al (2016) Pulmonary vein isolation by radiosurgery: implications for non-invasive treatment of atrial fibrillation. Europace 17(12):1868

Boike TP, Lotan Y, Cho LC et al (2011) Phase I dose-escalation study of stereotactic body radiation therapy for low- and intermediate-risk prostate cancer. J Clin Oncol 29(15):2020–2026

Bolzicco G, Favretto MS, Scremin E et al (2010) Image-guided stereotactic body radiation therapy for clinically localized prostate cancer: preliminary clinical results. Technol Cancer Res Treat 9(5):473–477

Bral S, Gevaert T, Linthout N et al (2011) Prospective, risk-adapted strategy of stereotactic body radiotherapy for early-stage non-small-cell lung cancer: results of a phase II trial. Int J Radiat Oncol Biol Phys 80(5):1343–1349

Brenner DJ, Hall EJ (1999) Fractionation and protraction for radiotherapy of prostate carcinoma. Int J Radiat Oncol Biol Phys 43(5):1095–1101

Brock KK (2011) Imaging and image-guided radiation therapy in liver cancer. Semin Radiat Oncol 21(4):247–255

Brown JM, Carlson DJ, Brenner DJ (2014) The tumor radiobiology of SRS and SBRT: are more than the 5 Rs involved? Int J Radiat Oncol Biol Phys 88(2):254–262

Brunner TB, Nestle U, Grosu AL et al (2015) SBRT in pancreatic cancer: what is the therapeutic window? Radiother Oncol 114(1):109–116

Bujold A, Massey CA, Kim JJ et al (2013) Sequential phase I and II trials of stereotactic body radiotherapy for locally advanced hepatocellular carcinoma. J Clin Oncol 31(13):1631–1639

Calkins H, Kuck KH, Cappato R et al (2012) 2012 HRS/EHRA/ECAS expert consensus statement on catheter and surgical ablation of atrial fibrillation: recommendations for patient selection, procedural techniques, patient management and follow-up, definitions, endpoints, and research trial design. Europace 14(4):528

Camm J (2005) Atrial fibrillation—an end to the epidemic? Circulation 112(8):iii

Cardenes HR, Price TR, Perkins SM et al (2010) Phase I feasibility trial of stereotactic body radiation therapy for primary hepatocellular carcinoma. Clin Transl Oncol 12(3):218–225

Casamassima F, Livi L, Masciullo S et al (2012) Stereotactic radiotherapy for adrenal gland metastases: University of Florence experience. Int J Radiat Oncol Biol Phys 82(2):919–923

Cengiz M, Ozyigit G, Yazici G et al (2011) Salvage reirradiaton with stereotactic body radiotherapy for locally recurrent head-and-neck tumors. Int J Radiat Oncol Biol Phys 81(1):104–109

Chan MW, Thibault I, Atenafu EG et al (2016) Patterns of epidural progression following postoperative spine stereotactic body radiotherapy: implications for clinical target volume delineation. J Neurosurg Spine 24(4):652–659

Chang EL, Shiu AS, Mendel E et al (2007) Phase I/II study of stereotactic body radiotherapy for spinal metastasis and its pattern of failure. J Neurosurg Spine 7(2):151–160

Chang DT, Schellenberg D, Shen J et al (2009) Stereotactic radiotherapy for unresectable adenocarcinoma of the pancreas. Cancer 115(3):665–672

Chang J, Liu H, Zhang X et al (2011a) Four-dimensional CT-and on-board volumetric image-guided stereotactic ablative radiotherapy (SABR) for stage I non-small cell lung cancer. Int J Radiat Oncol Biol Phys 81(2):S623

Chang DT, Swaminath A, Kozak M et al (2011b) Stereotactic body radiotherapy for colorectal liver metastases: a pooled analysis. Cancer 117(17):4060–4069

Chang UK, Cho WI, Lee DH et al (2012) Stereotactic radiosurgery for primary and metastatic sarcomas involving the spine. J Neuro-Oncol 107(3):551–557

Chang JY, Li Q-Q, Xu Q-Y et al (2014a) Stereotactic ablative radiation therapy for centrally located early stage or isolated parenchymal recurrences of non-small cell lung cancer: how to fly in a "no fly zone". Int J Radiat Oncol Biol Phys 88(5):1120–1128

Chang UK, Lee DH, Kim MS (2014b) Stereotactic radiosurgery for primary malignant spinal tumors. Neurol Res 36(6):597–606

Chang JY, Senan S, Paul MA et al (2015) Stereotactic ablative radiotherapy versus lobectomy for operable stage I non-small-cell lung cancer: a pooled analysis of two randomised trials. Lancet Oncol 16(6):630–637

Chang JH, Cheung P, Erler D et al (2016) Stereotactic ablative body radiotherapy for primary renal cell carcinoma in non-surgical candidates: initial clinical experience. Clin Oncol (R Coll Radiol) 28(9):109–114

Chao ST, Koyfman SA, Woody N et al (2012) Recursive partitioning analysis index is predictive for overall survival in patients undergoing spine stereotactic body radiation therapy for spinal metastases. Int J Radiat Oncol Biol Phys 82(5):1738–1743

Chen HH, Tsai ST, Wang MS et al (2006) Experience in fractionated stereotactic body radiation therapy boost for newly diagnosed nasopharyngeal carcinoma. Int J Radiat Oncol Biol Phys 66(5):1408–1414

Chiang A, Zeng L, Zhang L et al (2013) Pain flare is a common adverse event in steroid-naive patients after spine stereotactic body radiation therapy: a prospective clinical trial. Int J Radiat Oncol Biol Phys 86(4):638–642

Choi CY, Adler JR, Gibbs IC et al (2010) Stereotactic radiosurgery for treatment of spinal metastases recurring in close proximity to previously irradiated spinal cord. Int J Radiat Oncol Biol Phys 78(2):499–506

Chow E, Harris K, Fan G, Tsao M et al (2007) Palliative radiotherapy trials for bone metastases: a systematic review. J Clin Oncol 25(11):1423–1436

Chow E, van der Linden YM, Roos D et al (2014) Single versus multiple fractions of repeat radiation for painful bone metastases: a randomised, controlled, non-inferiority trial. Lancet Oncol 15(2):164–171

Chuang C, Sahgal A, Lee L et al (2007) Effects of residual target motion for image-tracked spine radiosurgery. Med Phys 34(11):4484–4490

Chuong MD, Springett GM, Freilich JM et al (2013) Stereotactic body radiation therapy for locally advanced and borderline resectable pancreatic cancer is effective and well tolerated. Int J Radiat Oncol Biol Phys 86(3):516–522

Corbin KS, Hellman S, Weichselbaum RR (2013) Extracranial oligometastases: a subset of metastases curable with stereotactic radiotherapy. J Clin Oncol 31(11):1384–1390

Correa RJ, Rodrigues GB, Chen H et al (2016) Stereotactic ablative radiotherapy (SABR) for large renal tumors: a retrospective case series evaluating clinical outcomes, toxicity, and technical considerations. Am J Clin Oncol. doi:10.1097/COC.0000000000000329

Cox BW, Spratt DE, Lovelock M et al (2012a) International spine radiosurgery consortium consensus guidelines for target volume definition in spinal stereotactic radiosurgery. Int J Radiat Oncol Biol Phys 83(5):e597–e605

Cox BW, Jackson A, Hunt M et al (2012b) Esophageal toxicity from high-dose, single-fraction paraspinal stereotactic radiosurgery. Int J Radiat Oncol Biol Phys 83(5):e661–e667

Cvek J, Neuwirth R, Knybel L et al (2014) Cardiac radiosurgery for malignant ventricular tachycardia. Cureus 6(7):e190

Dahele M, Palma D, Lagerwaard F et al (2011) Radiological changes after stereotactic radiotherapy for stage I lung cancer. J Thorac Oncol 6(7):1221–1228

Dahele M, Verbakel W, Cuijpers J et al (2012) An analysis of patient positioning during stereotactic lung radiotherapy performed without rigid external immobilization. Radiother Oncol 104(1):28–32

Dalah E, Moraru I, Paulson E et al (2014) Variability of target and normal structure delineation using multimodality imaging for radiation therapy of pancreatic cancer. Int J Radiat Oncol Biol Phys 89(3):633–640

Daliani DD, Tannir NM, Papandreou CN et al (2009) Prospective assessment of systemic therapy followed by surgical removal of metastases in selected patients with renal cell carcinoma. BJU Int 104(4):456–460

Daly ME, Luxton G, Choi CY et al (2012) Normal tissue complication probability estimation by the Lyman-Kutcher-Burman method does not accurately predict spinal cord tolerance to stereotactic radiosurgery. Int J Radiat Oncol Biol Phys 82(5):2025–2032

Darby SC, Cutter DJ, Boerma M et al (2010) Radiation-related heart disease: current knowledge and future prospects. Int J Radiat Oncol Biol Phys 76(3):656–665

Dasu A (2007) Is the alpha/beta value for prostate tumours low enough to be safely used in clinical trials? Clin Oncol (R Coll Radiol) 19(5):289–301

Dawson LA, Normolle D, Balter JM et al (2002) Analysis of radiation-induced liver disease using the Lyman NTCP model. Int J Radiat Oncol Biol Phys 53(4):810–821

Dawson LA, Eccles C, Craig T (2006) Individualized image guided iso-NTCP based liver cancer SBRT. Acta Oncol 45(7):856–864

Dawson LA, Toronto O, Zhu A et al (2013) RTOG 1112 randomized phase III study of Sorafenib versus stereotactic bosy radiation therapy follwoed by sorafenib in hepatocelluar carcinoma. (www.RTOG.org)

De Meerleer G, Khoo V, Escudier B et al (2014) Radiotherapy for renal-cell carcinoma. Lancet Oncol 15(4):e170–e177

Desai A, Rai H, Haas J et al (2015) A retrospective review of CyberKnife stereotactic body radiotherapy for adrenal tumors (primary and metastatic): Winthrop University Hospital experience. Front Oncol 5:185

Deschavanne PJ, Fertil B (1996) A review of human cell radiosensitivity in vitro. Int J Radiat Oncol Biol Phys 34(1):251–266

Deshmukh A, Patel NJ, Pant S et al. (2013) Inhospital complications associated with catheter ablation of atrial fibrillation in the united states between 2000–2010: analysis of 93,801 procedures. Circulation; CIRCULATIONAHA. 113.003862

Donat SM, Diaz M, Bishoff JT et al (2013) Follow-up for clinically localized renal neoplasms: AUA guideline. J Urol 190(2):407–416

van Dongen JA, van Slooten EA (1978) The surgical treatment of pulmonary metastases. Cancer Treat Rev 5(1):29–48

Eccles CL, Patel R, Simeonov AK et al (2011) Comparison of liver tumor motion with and without abdominal compression using cine-magnetic resonance imaging. Int J Radiat Oncol Biol Phys 79(2):602–608

Edwards BK, Howe HL, Ries LA et al (2002) Annual report to the nation on the status of cancer, 1973–1999, featuring implications of age and aging on US cancer burden. Cancer 94(10):2766–2792

Emami B, Lyman J, Brown A et al (1991) Tolerance of normal tissue to therapeutic irradiation. Int J Radiat Oncol Biol Phys 21(1):109–122

Fakiris AJ, McGarry RC, Yiannoutsos CT et al (2009) Stereotactic body radiation therapy for early-stage non-small-cell lung carcinoma: four-year results of a prospective phase II study. Int J Radiat Oncol Biol Phys 75(3):677–682

Falcoz PE, Conti M, Brouchet L et al (2007) The thoracic surgery scoring system (Thoracoscore): risk model for in-hospital death in 15,183 patients requiring thoracic surgery. J Thorac Cardiovasc Surg 133(2):325–332

Farnia B, Louis CU, Teh BS et al (2014) Stereotactic body radiation therapy (SBRT) for an isolated bone metastasis in an adolescent male with nasopharyngeal carcinoma. Pediatr Blood Cancer 61(8):1520

Farrag A, Voordeckers M, Tournel K et al (2010) Pattern of failure after helical tomotherapy in head and neck cancer. Strahlenther Onkol 186(9):511–516

Ferlay J, Shin HR, Bray F et al (2010) Estimates of worldwide burden of cancer in 2008: GLOBOCAN 2008. Int J Cancer 127(12):2893–2917

Ferlay J, Soerjomataram I, Ervik M et al. (2015) GLOBOCAN 2012 v1. 1, Cancer Incidence and Mortality Worldwide: IARC CancerBase No. 11 [Internet]. Lyon, France: International Agency for Research on Cancer; 2013. http://globocan.iarc.fr

Finnigan R, Lamprecht B, Barry T et al (2016) Inter-and intra-fraction motion in stereotactic body radiotherapy for spinal and paraspinal tumours using cone-beam CT and positional correction in six degrees of freedom. J Med Imag Radiat Oncol 60(1):112–118

Flanigan RC, Mickisch G, Sylvester R et al (2004) Cytoreductive nephrectomy in patients with metastatic renal cancer: a combined analysis. J Urol 171(3):1071–1076

Folkert MR, Bilsky MH, Tom AK et al (2014) Outcomes and toxicity for hypofractionated and single-fraction image-guided stereotactic radiosurgery for sarcomas metastasizing to the spine. Int J Radiat Oncol Biol Phys 88(5):1085–1091

Foote M, Letourneau D, Hyde D et al (2011) Technique for stereotactic body radiotherapy for spinal metastases. J Clin Neurosci 18(2):276–279

Foote M, Bailey M, Smith L et al (2015) Guidelines for safe practice of stereotactic body (ablative) radiation therapy. J Med Imaging Radiat Oncol 59(5):646–653

Formenti SC (2015) Is classical stereotactic radiotherapy the optimal partner for immunotherapy? Oncology 29(5):211305

Franzese C, Franceschini D, Cozzi L et al (2017) Minimally invasive stereotactical radio-ablation of adrenal metastases as an alternative to surgery. Cancer Res Treat 49(1):20–28

Fuks Z, Kolesnick R (2005) Engaging the vascular component of the tumor response. Cancer Cell 8(2):89–91

Garcia-Barros M, Paris F, Cordon-Cardo C et al (2003) Tumor response to radiotherapy regulated by endothelial cell apoptosis. Science 300(5622):1155–1159

Gardner EA, Sumanaweera TS, Blanck O et al (2012) In vivo dose measurement using TLDs and MOSFET dosimeters for cardiac radiosurgery. J App Clin Med Phys 13(3):3745

Garg AK, Wang XS, Shiu AS et al (2011) Prospective evaluation of spinal reirradiation by using stereotactic body radiation therapy. Cancer 117(15):3509–3516

Gerszten PC, Burton SA, Ozhasoglu C et al (2005) Stereotactic radiosurgery for spinal metastases from renal cell carcinoma. J Neurosurg Spine 3(4):288–295

Gerszten PC, Sahgal A, Sheehan JP et al (2013) A multinational report on methods for institutional credentialing for spine radiosurgery. Radiat Oncol 8(1):158

Ghia AJ, Chang EL, Bishop AJ et al (2016) Single-fraction versus multifraction spinal stereotactic radiosurgery for spinal metastases from renal cell carcinoma: secondary analysis of phase I/II trials. J Neurosurg Spine 24(5):829–836

Gill B, Oermann E, Ju A et al (2012) Fiducial-free CyberKnife stereotactic body radiation therapy (SBRT) for single vertebral body metastases: acceptable local control and normal tissue tolerance with 5 fraction approach. Front Oncol 2:39

Gilson B, Lederman G, Qian G et al (2006) 2249: hypofractionated stereotactic extra-cranial radiosurgery (HFSR) for primary and metastatic renal cell carcinoma. Int J Radiat Oncol Biol Phys 66(3):S349

Goldstein SD, Ford EC, Duhon M et al (2010) Use of respiratory-correlated four-dimensional computed tomography to determine acceptable treatment margins for locally advanced pancreatic adenocarcinoma. Int J Radiat Oncol Biol Phys 76(2):597–602

Gorayski P, Burmeister B, Foote M (2015) Radiotherapy for cutaneous melanoma: current and future applications. Future Oncol 11(3):525–534

Goyal K, Einstein D, Ibarra RA et al (2012) Stereotactic body radiation therapy for nonresectable tumors of the pancreas. J Surg Res 174(2):319–325

Griffioen GH, Lagerwaard FJ, Haasbeek CJ et al (2014) A brief report on outcomes of stereotactic ablative radiotherapy for a second primary lung cancer: evidence in support of routine CT surveillance. J Thorac Oncol 9(8):1222–1225

Guckenberger M, Sweeney RA, Flickinger JC et al (2011) Clinical practice of image-guided spine radiosurgery—results from an international research consortium. Radiat Oncol 6(1):172

Guckenberger M, Klement RJ, Allgauer M et al (2013a) Applicability of the linear-quadratic formalism for modeling local tumor control probability in high dose per fraction stereotactic body radiotherapy for early stage non-small cell lung cancer. Radiother Oncol 109(1):13–20

Guckenberger M, Allgauer M, Appold S et al (2013b) Safety and efficacy of stereotactic body radiotherapy for stage 1 non-small-cell lung cancer in routine clinical practice: a patterns-of-care and outcome analysis. J Thorac Oncol 8(8):1050–1058

Guckenberger M, Mantel F, Gerszten PC et al (2014) Safety and efficacy of stereotactic body radiotherapy as primary treatment for vertebral metastases: a multi-institutional analysis. Radiat Oncol 9:226

Guckenberger M, Klement RJ, Allgauer M et al (2016) Local tumor control probability modeling of primary and secondary lung tumors in stereotactic body radiotherapy. Radiother Oncol 118(3):485–491

Guiou M, Mayr NA, Kim EY et al (2012) Stereotactic body radiotherapy for adrenal metastases from lung cancer. J Radiat Oncol 1(2):155–163

Gunjur A, Duong C, Ball D et al (2014) Surgical and ablative therapies for the management of adrenal 'oligometastases'—a systematic review. Cancer Treat Rev 40(7):838–846

Gurka MK, Collins SP, Slack R et al (2013) Stereotactic body radiation therapy with concurrent full-dose gemcitabine for locally advanced pancreatic cancer: a pilot trial demonstrating safety. Radiat Oncol 8(1):44

Haasbeek CJ, Lagerwaard FJ, Antonisse ME et al (2010) Stage I nonsmall cell lung cancer in patients aged > or =75 years: outcomes after stereotactic radiotherapy. Cancer 116(2):406–414

Haasbeek CJ, Palma D, Visser O et al (2012) Early-stage lung cancer in elderly patients: a population-based study of changes in treatment patterns and survival in the Netherlands. Ann Oncol 23(10):2743–2747

Hannan R, Ishihara D, Louder K et al (2016) Phase II trial of high-dose interleukin-2 (IL-2) and stereotactic radiation therapy (SABR) for metastatic clear cell renal cell carcinoma (ccRCC): interim analysis, ASCO annual meeting proceedings

Hara W, Loo BW, Goffinet DR et al (2008) Excellent local control with stereotactic radiotherapy boost after external beam radiotherapy in patients with nasopharyngeal carcinoma. Int J Radiat Oncol Biol Phys 71(2):393–400

Haseltine JM, Rimner A, Gelblum DY et al (2016) Fatal complications after stereotactic body radiation therapy for central lung tumors abutting the proximal bronchial tree. Pract Radiat Oncol 6(2):e27–e33

Hashmi A, Guckenberger M, Kersh R et al (2016) Re-irradiation stereotactic body radiotherapy for spinal metastases: a multi-institutional outcome analysis. J Neurosurg Spine 25(5):646–653

Heerkens HD, van Vulpen M, van den Berg CA et al (2014) MRI-based tumor motion characterization and gating schemes for radiation therapy of pancreatic cancer. Radiother Oncol 111(2):252–257

Helena AY, Sima CS, Huang J et al (2013) Local therapy with continued EGFR tyrosine kinase inhibitor therapy as a treatment strategy in EGFR-mutant advanced lung cancers that have developed acquired resistance to EGFR tyrosine kinase inhibitors. J Thorac Oncol 8(3):346–351

Hellman S, Weichselbaum RR (1995) Oligometastases. J Clin Oncol 13(1):8–10

Herder GJ, van Tinteren H, Golding RP et al (2005) Clinical prediction model to characterize pulmonary nodules: validation and added value of 18F-fluorodeoxyglucose positron emission tomography. Chest 128(4):2490–2496

Herfarth KK, Hof H, Bahner ML et al (2003) Assessment of focal liver reaction by multiphasic CT after stereotactic single-dose radiotherapy of liver tumors. Int J Radiat Oncol Biol Phys 57(2):444–451

Herman JM, Chang DT, Goodman KA et al (2015) Phase 2 multi-institutional trial evaluating gemcitabine and stereotactic body radiotherapy for patients with locally advanced unresectable pancreatic adenocarcinoma. Cancer 121(7):1128–1137

Heron DE, Ferris RL, Karamouzis M et al (2009) Stereotactic body radiotherapy for recurrent squamous cell carcinoma of the head and neck: results of a phase I dose-escalation trial. Int J Radiat Oncol Biol Phys 75(5):1493–1500

Heron DE, Rajagopalan MS, Stone B et al (2012) Single-session and multisession CyberKnife radiosurgery for spine metastases—University of Pittsburgh and Georgetown University experience: clinical article. J Neurosurg Spine 17(1):11–18

Higton AM, Monach J, Congleton J (2010) Investigation and management of lung cancer in older adults. Lung Cancer 69(2):209–212

Hiniker SM, Rangaswami A, Lungren MP et al (2016) Stereotactic body radiotherapy for pediatric hepatocellular carcinoma with central biliary obstruction. Pediatr Blood Cancer. doi:10.1002/pbc.26330

Hodges JC, Lotan Y, Boike TP et al (2012) Cost-effectiveness analysis of stereotactic body radiation therapy versus intensity-modulated radiation therapy: an emerging initial radiation treatment option for organ-confined prostate cancer. J Oncol Pract 8(3S):e31s–e37s

Hoopes DJ, Tann M, Fletcher JW et al (2007) FDG-PET and stereotactic body radiotherapy (SBRT) for stage I non-small-cell lung cancer. Lung Cancer 56(2):229–234

Hoyer M, Roed H, Sengelov L et al (2005) Phase-II study on stereotactic radiotherapy of locally advanced pancreatic carcinoma. Radiother Oncol 76(1):48–53

Hoyer M, Swaminath A, Bydder S et al (2012) Radiotherapy for liver metastases: a review of evidence. Int J Radiat Oncol Biol Phys 82(3):1047–1057

Huang K, Dahele M, Senan S et al (2012) Radiographic changes after lung stereotactic ablative radiotherapy (SABR)–can we distinguish recurrence from fibrosis? A systematic review of the literature. Radiother Oncol 102(3):335–342

Huang K, Senthi S, Palma DA et al (2013) High-risk CT features for detection of local recurrence after stereotactic ablative radiotherapy for lung cancer. Radiother Oncol 109(1):51–57

Huguet F, Yorke ED, Davidson M et al (2015) Modeling pancreatic tumor motion using 4-dimensional computed tomography and surrogate markers. Int J Radiat Oncol* Biol* Phys 91(3):579–587

Hussain SM, Semelka RC (2005) Hepatic imaging: comparison of modalities. Radiol Clin N Am 43(5):929–947. ix

Hyde D, Lochray F, Korol R et al (2012) Spine stereotactic body radiotherapy utilizing cone-beam CT image-guidance with a robotic couch: intrafraction motion analysis accounting for all six degrees of freedom. Int J Radiat Oncol* Biol* Phys 82(3):e555–e562

Iannuccilli JD, Grand DJ, Dupuy DE et al (2014) Percutaneous ablation for small renal masses—imaging follow-up. Sem Intervent Radiol 31(1):50–63

Inoue T, Kinoshita H, Komai Y et al (2012) Two cases of gastrointestinal perforation after radiotherapy in patients receiving tyrosine kinase inhibitor for advanced renal cell carcinoma. World J Surg Oncol 10(1):167

Ipsen S, Blanck O, Oborn B et al (2014) Radiotherapy beyond cancer: target localization in real-time MRI and treatment planning for cardiac radiosurgery. Med Phys 41(12):120702

Jabbari S, Gerszten PC, Ruschin M et al (2016) Stereotactic body radiotherapy for spinal metastases: practice guidelines, outcomes, and risks. Cancer J 22(4):280–289

Jackson P, Foroudi F, Pham D et al (2014) Short communication: timeline of radiation-induced kidney function loss after stereotactic ablative body radiotherapy of renal cell carcinoma as evaluated by serial 99m Tc-DMSA SPECT/CT. Radiat Oncol 9(1):1

James ND, Sydes MR, Clarke NW et al (2016) Addition of docetaxel, zoledronic acid, or both to first-line long-term hormone therapy in prostate cancer (STAMPEDE): survival results from an adaptive, multiarm, mutistage, platform randomized controlled trial. Lancet 357(10024):1163–1177

Jarraya H, Borde P, Mirabel X et al (2015) Lobulated enhancement evaluation in the follow-up of liver metastases treated by stereotactic body radiation therapy. Int J Radiat Oncol Biol Phys 92(2):292–298

Jensen NK, Mulder D, Lock M et al (2014) Dynamic contrast enhanced CT aiding gross tumor volume delineation of liver tumors: an interobserver variability study. Radiother Oncol 111(1):153–157

Jeon TY, Kim CK, Kim J et al (2015) Assessment of early therapeutic response to sorafenib in renal cell carcinoma xenografts by dynamic contrast-enhanced and diffusion-weighted MR imaging. Br J Radiol 88(1053):20150163

Jhaveri PM, Teh BS, Paulino AC et al (2012) A dose-response relationship for time to bone pain resolution after stereotactic body radiotherapy (SBRT) for renal cell carcinoma (RCC) bony metastases. Acta Oncol 51(5):584–588

Jung J, Yoon SM, Kim SY et al (2013) Radiation-induced liver disease after stereotactic body radiotherapy for small hepatocellular carcinoma: clinical and dose-volumetric parameters. Radiat Oncol 8(1):249

Jung J, Yoon SM, Park HC et al (2016) Radiotherapy for adrenal metastasis from hepatocellular carcinoma: a multi-institutional retrospective study (KROG 13-05). PLoS One 11(3):e0152642

Juusela H, Malmio K, Alfthan O et al (1997) Preoperative irradiation in the treatment of renal adenocarcinoma. Scand J Urol Nephrol 11(3):277–281

Kaizu T, Karasawa K, Tanaka Y et al (1989) Radiotherapy for osseous metastases from hepatocellular carcinoma: a retrospective study of 57 patients. Am J Gastroenterol 93(11):2167–2171

Kang SK, Zhang A, Pandharipande PV et al (2015) DWI for renal mass characterization: systematic review and meta-analysis of diagnostic test performance. AJR Am J Roentgenol 205(2):317–324

Kao J, Packer S, Vu HL et al (2009) Phase 1 study of concurrent sunitinib and image-guided radiotherapy followed by maintenance sunitinib for patients with oligometastases: acute toxicity and preliminary response. Cancer 115(15):3571–3580

Kao J, Chen CT, Tong CC et al (2014) Concurrent sunitinib and stereotactic body radiotherapy for patients with oligometastases. Targeted Oncol 9(2):145–153

Karam I, Poon I, Lee J et al (2015) Stereotactic body radiotherapy for head and neck cancer: an addition to the armamentarium against head and neck cancer. Future Oncol (London, England) 11(21):2937–2947

Karamichalakis N, Letsas KP, Vlachos K et al (2015) Managing atrial fibrillation in the very elderly patient: challenges and solutions. Vasc Health Risk Manage 11:555

Kasibhatla M, Steinberg P, Meyer J et al (2007) Radiation therapy and sorafenib: clinical data and rationale for the combination in metastatic renal cell carcinoma. Clin Genitourin Cancer 5(4):291–294

Katoh N, Onimaru R, Sakuhara Y et al (2008) Real-time tumor-tracking radiotherapy for adrenal tumors. Radiother Oncol 87(3):418–424

Katz AJ, Kang J (2014a) Stereotactic body radiotherapy as treatment for organ confined low- and intermediate-risk prostate carcinoma, a 7-year study. Front Oncol 4:240

Katz A, Kang J (2014b) Stereotactic body radiotherapy with or without external beam radiation as treatment for organ confined high-risk prostate carcinoma: a six year study. Radiat Oncol 9(1):1

Katz AJ, Santoro M (2010) Quality of life and efficacy for stereotactic body radiotherapy for treatment of organ confined prostate cancer. Annual Meeting of the Association for Radiation Oncology, San Diego, CA

Katz AJ, Santoro M, Ashley R et al (2010) Stereotactic body radiotherapy for organ-confined prostate cancer. BMC Urol 10:1

Kawaguchi K, Sato K, Yamada H et al (2012) Stereotactic radiosurgery in combination with chemotherapy as primary treatment for head and neck cancer. J Oral Maxillofacial Surg 70(2):461–472

Keall PJ, Mageras GS, Balter JM et al (2006) The management of respiratory motion in radiation oncology report of AAPM task group 76a. Med Phys 33(10):3874–3900

Kelsey CR, Schefter T, Nash SR et al (2005) Retrospective clinicopathologic correlation of gross tumor size of hepatocellular carcinoma: implications for stereotactic body radiotherapy. Am J Clin Oncol 28(6):576–580

Kestin L, Grills I, Guckenberger M et al (2014) Dose-response relationship with clinical outcome for lung stereotactic body radiotherapy (SBRT) delivered via online image guidance. Radiother Oncol 110(3):499–504

Khan L, Chiang A, Zhang L et al (2015a) Prophylactic dexamethasone effectively reduces the incidence of pain flare following spine stereotactic body radiotherapy (SBRT): a prospective observational study. Support Care Cancer 23(10):2937–2943

Khan L, Tjong M, Raziee H et al (2015b) Role of stereotactic body radiotherapy for symptom control in head and neck cancer patients. Support Care Cancer 23(4):1099–1103

Kim MS, Keum KC, Cha JH et al (2013) Stereotactic body radiotherapy with helical tomotherapy for pain palliation in spine metastasis. Technol Cancer Res Treat 12(4):363–370

King CR, Brooks JD, Gill H et al (2012) Long-term outcomes from a prospective trial of stereotactic body radiotherapy for low-risk prostate cancer. Int J Radiat Oncol Biol Phys 82(2):877–882

King CR, Freema D, Kaplan I et al (2013a) Stereotactic body radiotherapy for localized prostate cancer: pooled analysis from a multi-institutional consortium of prospective phase II trials. Radiother Oncol 109(2):217–221

King CR, Collins S, Fuller D et al (2013b) Health-related quality of life after stereotactic body radiation therapy for localized prostate cancer: results from a multi-institutional consortium of prospective trials. Int J Radiat Oncol Biol Phys 87(5):939–945

Kirkbride P, Cooper T (2011) Stereotactic body radiotherapy. Guidelines for commissioners, providers and clinicians: a national report. Clin Oncol (R Coll Radiol) 23(3):163–164

Kleibeuker EA, Matthijs A, Verheul H et al (2015) Combining radiotherapy with sunitinib: lessons (to be) learned. Angiogenesis 18(4):385–395

Klein J, Korol R, Lo SS et al (2014) Stereotactic body radiotherapy: an effective local treatment modality for hepatocellular carcinoma. Future Oncol 10(14):2227–2241

Klekamp J, Samii H (1998) Surgical results for spinal metastases. Acta Neurochir 140(9):957–967

Kodani N, Yamazaki H, Tsubokura T et al (2011) Stereotactic body radiation therapy for head and neck tumor: disease control and morbidity outcomes. J Radiat Res 52(1):24–31

Koong AC, Le QT, Ho A et al (2004) Phase I study of stereotactic radiosurgery in patients with locally advanced pancreatic cancer. Int J Radiat Oncol Biol Phys 58(4):1017–1021

Koong AC, Christofferson E, Le QT et al (2005) Phase II study to assess the efficacy of conventionally fractionated radiotherapy followed by a stereotactic radiosurgery boost in patients with locally advanced pancreatic cancer. Int J Radiat Oncol Biol Phys 63(2):320–323

Kothari G, Foroudi F, Gill S et al (2015) Outcomes of stereotactic radiotherapy for cranial and extracranial metastatic renal cell carcinoma: a systematic review. Acta Oncol 54(2):148–157

Koto M, Takai Y, Ogawa Y et al (2007) A phase II study on stereotactic body radiotherapy for stage I non-small cell lung cancer. Radiother Oncol 85(3):429–434

Kry SF, Alvarez P, Molineu A et al (2013) Algorithms used in heterogeneous dose calculations show systematic differences as measured with the radiological physics Center's anthropomorphic thorax phantom used for RTOG credentialing. Int J Radiat Oncol Biol Phys 85(1):e95–e100

Kudo M (2015) Clinical practice guidelines for hepatocellular carcinoma differ between Japan, United States, and Europe. Liver Cancer 4:85–95

Kumar R, Xiu Y, Yu JQ et al (2004) 18F-FDG PET in evaluation of adrenal lesions in patients with lung cancer. J Nucl Med 45(12):2058–2062

Kunkle DA, Uzzo RG (2008) Cryoablation or radiofrequency ablation of the small renal mass: a meta-analysis. Cancer 113(10):2671–2680

Kupelian PA, Willoughby TR, Reddy CA et al (2007) Hypofractionated intensity-modulated radiotherapy (70 Gy at 2.5 Gy per fraction) for localized prostate cancer: cleveland clinic experience. Int J Radiat Oncol Biol Phys 68(5):1424–1430

Lagerwaard FJ, Haasbeek CJ, Smit EF et al (2008) Outcomes of risk-adapted fractionated stereotactic radiotherapy for stage I non-small-cell lung cancer. Int J Radiat Oncol Biol Phys 70(3):685–692

Lagerwaard FJ, Verstegen NE, Haasbeek CJ (2012) Outcomes of stereotactic ablative radiotherapy in patients with potentially operable stage I non-small cell lung cancer. Int J Radiat Oncol Biol Phys 83(1):348–353

Langen KM (2001) Jones DT (2001) organ motion and its management. Int J Radiat Oncol Biol Phys 50(1):265–278

Lartigau EF, Tresch E, Thariat J et al (2013) Multi institutional phase II study of concomitant stereotactic reirradiation and cetuximab for recurrent head and neck cancer. Radiother Oncol 109(2):281–285

Lau W-Y, Sangro B, Chen P-J et al (2013) Treatment for hepatocellular carcinoma with portal vein tumor thrombosis: the emerging role for radioembolization using yttrium-90. Oncology 84(5):311–318

Laufer I, Iorgulescu JB, Chapman T et al (2013) Local disease control for spinal metastases following "separation surgery" and adjuvant hypofractionated or high-dose single-fraction stereotactic radiosurgery: outcome analysis in 186 patients: clinical article. J Neurosurg Spine 18(3):207–214

Lausch A, Sinclair K, Lock M et al (2013) Determination and comparison of radiotherapy dose responses for hepatocellular carcinoma and metastatic colorectal liver tumours. Br J Radiol 86(1027):20130147

Lawrence TS, Robertson JM, Anscher MS et al (1995) Hepatic toxicity resulting from cancer treatment. Int J Radiat Oncol Biol Phys 31(5):1237–1248

Le QT, Tate D, Koong A et al (2003) Improved local control with stereotactic radiosurgical boost in patients with nasopharyngeal carcinoma. Int J Radiat Oncol Biol Phys 56(4):1046–1054

Lee Y, Auh SL, Wang Y et al (2009a) Therapeutic effects of ablative radiation on local tumor require CD8+ T cells: changing strategies for cancer treatment. Blood 114(3):589–595

Lee MT, Kim JJ, Dinniwell R et al (2009b) Phase I study of individualized stereotactic body radiotherapy of liver metastases. J Clin Oncol 27(10):1585–1591

Lee DS, Kim YS, Cheon JS et al (2012) Long-term outcome and toxicity of hypofractionated stereotactic body radiotherapy as a boost treatment for head and neck cancer: the importance of boost volume assessment. Radiat Oncol (London, England) 7:85-717X-7-85

Lee SH, Tatsui CE, Ghia AJ et al (2016) Can the spinal instability neoplastic score prior to spinal radiosurgery predict compression fractures following stereotactic spinal radiosurgery for metastatic spinal tumor?: a post hoc analysis of prospective phase II single-institution trials. J Neuro-Oncol 126(3):509–517

Lesurtel M, Müllhaupt B, Pestalozzi B et al (2006) Transarterial chemoembolization as a bridge to liver transplantation for hepatocellular carcinoma: an evidence-based analysis. Am J Transplant 6(11):2644–2650

Li J, Yu W, Tiwary R et al (2010) alpha-TEA-induced death receptor dependent apoptosis involves activation of acid sphingomyelinase and elevated ceramide-enriched cell surface membranes. Cancer Cell Int 10(1):40

Lin CS, Jen YM, Chiu SY et al (2006) Treatment of portal vein tumor thrombosis of hepatoma patients with either stereotactic radiotherapy or three-dimensional conformal radiotherapy. Jpn J Clin Oncol 36(4):212–217

Lindberg K, Nyman J, Riesenfeld Källskog V et al (2015) Long-term results of a prospective phase II trial of medically inoperable stage I NSCLC treated with SBRT–the Nordic experience. Acta Oncol 54(8):1096–1104

Ling DC, Vargo JA, Ferris RL et al (2016) Risk of severe toxicity according to site of recurrence in patients treated with stereotactic body radiation therapy for recurrent head and neck cancer. Int J Radiat Oncol* Biol* Phys 95(3):973–980

Livsey JE, Cowan RA, Wylie JP et al (2003) Hypofractionated conformal radiotherapy in carcinoma of the prostate: five-year outcome analysis. Int J Radiat Oncol Biol Phys 57(5):1254–1259

Llovet JM, Fuster J, Bruix J et al (2004) The Barcelona approach: diagnosis, staging, and treatment of hepatocellular carcinoma. Liver Transpl 10(2 Suppl 1):S115–SS20

Lo SS, Sahgal A, Wang JZ et al (2010) Stereotactic body radiation therapy for spinal metastases. Discov Med 9(47):289–296

Lo SS, Moffatt-Bruce SD, Dawson LA et al (2011) The role of local therapy in the management of lung and liver oligometastases. Nat Rev Clin Oncol 8(7):405–416

Lo A, Loo B, Maguire P et al (2013) SBRT for cardiac arrhythmia ablation. J Radiosurge & SBRT 2:15

Lo CH, Huang WY, Chao HL et al (2014) Novel application of stereotactic ablative radiotherapy using CyberKnife® for early-stage renal cell carcinoma in patients with pre-existing chronic kidney disease: initial clinical experiences. Oncol Lett 8(1):355–360

Lo SS, Foote M, Siva S et al (2016) Technical know-how in stereotactic ablative radiotherapy (SABR). J Med Radiat Sci 63(1):5–8

Loblaw D, Sethukavalan P, Cheung P et al (2013) Comparison of biochemical and toxicity outcomes from a contemporaneous cohort study of low-risk prostate cancer treated with different radiation techniques. Int J Radiat Oncol* Biol* Phys 87(2):S26

Lock MI, Hoyer M, Bydder SA et al (2012) An international survey on liver metastases radiotherapy. Acta Oncol 51(5):568–574

Lock M, Callan L, Gaede S et al (2014) Identification of patients with liver cancer that will not benefit from radiation. Int J Radiat Oncol Biol Phys 1(90):S594

Lock M, Malayeri AA, Mian OY et al (2016) Computed tomography imaging assessment of postexternal beam radiation changes of the liver. Future Oncol 12(23):2729–2739

Loehrer PJ, Feng Y, Cardenes H et al (2011) Gemcitabine alone versus gemcitabine plus radiotherapy in patients with locally advanced pancreatic cancer: an eastern cooperative oncology group trial. J Clin Oncol 29(31):4105–4112

Loganathan RS, Stover DE, Shi W et al (2006) Prevalence of COPD in women compared to men around the time of diagnosis of primary lung cancer. Chest 129(5):1305–1312

Lou F, Huang J, Sima CS et al (2013) Patterns of recurrence and second primary lung cancer in early-stage lung cancer survivors followed with routine computed tomography surveillance. J Thorac Cardiovasc Surg 145(1):75–81. discussion 81-2

Louie AV, van Werkhoven E, Chen H et al (2015) Patient reported outcomes following stereotactic ablative radiotherapy or surgery for stage IA non-small-cell lung cancer: results of the ROSEL multicenter randomized trial. Radiother Oncol 117(1):44–48

Lowther NJ (2016) Non-invasive cardiac radiosurgery with MRI guidance: a ground-truth for real-time target localisation using the XCAT phantom, University of Canterbury

Luketich JD, Burt ME (1996) Does resection of adrenal metastases from non-small cell lung cancer improve survival? Ann Thorac Surg 62(6):1614–1616

Lukka H, Hayter C, Julian JA et al (2005) Randomized trial comparing two fractionation schedules for patients with localized prostate cancer. J Clin Oncol 23(25):6132–6138

Lutz S, Berk L, Chang E, Chow E et al (2011) Palliative radiotherapy for bone metastases: an ASTRO evidence-based guideline. Int J Radiat Oncol Biol Phys 79(4):965–976

Mageras GS, Yorke E (2004) Deep inspiration breath hold and respiratory gating strategies for reducing organ motion in radiation treatment. Semin Radiat Oncol 14(1):65–75

Maguire PJ, Gardner E, Jack AB et al (2011) Cardiac radiosurgery (CyberHeart™) for treatment of arrhythmia: physiologic and histopathologic correlation in the porcine model. Cureus 3(8):e32

Mahadevan A, Jain S, Goldstein M et al (2010) Stereotactic body radiotherapy and gemcitabine for locally advanced pancreatic cancer. Int J Radiat Oncol Biol Phys 78(3):735–742

Majewski W, Tabor M, Banaszek P et al (2016) The efficacy of stereotactic radiotherapy for metastases from renal cell carcinoma. Neoplasma 63(1):99–106

Mantz CA, Fernandez E et al (2013) Real-time target tracking prostate SBRT and the real-time tracking system 4D localization system: 5-year quality of life and disease outcomes. Int J Radiat Oncol* Biol* Phys 87(2):S393

McBride SM, Wong DS, Dombrowski JJ et al (2012) Hypofractionated stereotactic body radiotherapy in low-risk prostate adenocarcinoma. Cancer 118(15): 3681–3690

McBride S, Wagner A, Kaplan I (2013) A phase 1 dose-escalation study of robotic radiosurgery in inoperable primary renal cell carcinoma. Int J Radiat Oncol Biol Phys 87(2):S84

McCammon R, Schefter TE, Gaspar LE et al (2009) Observation of a dose–control relationship for lung and liver tumors after stereotactic body radiation therapy. Int J Radiat Oncol Biol Phys 73(1):112–118

McDonald MW, Lawson J, Garg MK et al (2011) ACR appropriateness criteria retreatment of recurrent head and neck cancer after prior definitive radiation expert panel on radiation oncology-head and neck cancer. Int J Radiat Oncol Biol Phys 80(5):1292–1298

McDonald MW, Moore MG, Johnstone PA (2012) Risk of carotid blowout after reirradiation of the head and neck: a systematic review. Int J Radiat Oncol Biol Phys 82(3):1083–1089

McGarry RC, Papiez L, Williams M et al (2005) Stereotactic body radiation therapy of early-stage non-small-cell lung carcinoma: phase I study. Int J Radiat Oncol Biol Phys 63(4):1010–1015

McGinn CJ, Ten Haken RK, Ensminger WD et al (1998) Treatment of intrahepatic cancers with radiation doses based on a normal tissue complication probability model. J Clin Oncol 16(6):2246–2252

Meier R (2015) Dose-escalated robotic SBRT for stage I–II prostate cancer. Front Oncol 5:48

Mellon EA, Hoffe SE, Springett GM et al (2015) Long-term outcomes of induction chemotherapy and neoadjuvant stereotactic body radiotherapy for borderline resectable and locally advanced pancreatic adenocarcinoma. Acta Oncol 54(7):979–985

Mendez Romero A, Wunderink W, Hussain SM et al (2006) Stereotactic body radiation therapy for primary and metastatic liver tumors: a single institution phase i-ii study. Acta Oncol 45(7):831–837

Miller JA, Balagamwala EH, Angelov L et al (2016) Stereotactic radiosurgery for the treatment of primary and metastatic spinal sarcomas. Technol Cancer Res Treat. doi:10.1177/1533034616643221

Minn AY, Schellenberg D, Maxim P et al (2009) Pancreatic tumor motion on a single planning 4D-CT does not correlate with intrafraction tumor motion during treatment. Am J Clin Oncol 32(4):364–368

Mitchell IC, Nwariaku FE (2007) Adrenal masses in the cancer patient: surveillance or excision. Oncologist 12(2):168–174

Mittal S, El-Serag HB (2013) Epidemiology of HCC: consider the population. J Clin Gastroenterol 47:S2

Mittendorf EA, Lim SJ, Schacherer CW et al (2008) Melanoma adrenal metastasis: natural history and surgical management. Am J Surg 195(3):363–368. discussion 368-9

Mole R (1953) Whole body irradiation—radiobiology or medicine? Br J Radiol 26(305):234–241

Moningi S, Dholakia AS, Raman SP et al (2015) The role of stereotactic body radiation therapy for pancreatic cancer: a single-institution experience. Ann Surg Oncol 22(7):2352–2358

Moss AJ, Greenberg H, Case RB et al (2004) Long-term clinical course of patients after termination of ventricular tachyarrhythmia by an implanted defibrillator. Circulation 110(25):3760–3765

Motzer RJ, Bander NH, Nanus DM (1996) Renal-cell carcinoma. N Engl J Med 335(12):865–875

Motzer RJ, Hutson TE, Tomczak P et al (2009) Overall survival and updated results for sunitinib compared with interferon alfa in patients with metastatic renal cell carcinoma. J Clin Oncol 27(22):3584–3590

Motzer RJ, Escudier B, McDermott DF et al (2015a) Nivolumab versus Everolimus in advanced renal-cell carcinoma. N Engl J Med 373(19):1803–1813

Motzer RJ, Rini BI, McDermott DF et al (2015b) Nivolumab for metastatic renal cell carcinoma: results of a randomized phase II trial. J Clin Oncol 33(13):1430–1437

Muth A, Persson F, Jansson S et al (2010) Prognostic factors for survival aftyer surgery for adrenal metastasis. Eur J Surg Oncol 36(7):699–704

Naderi S, Wang Y, Miller AL et al (2014) The impact of age on the epidemiology of atrial fibrillation hospitalizations. Am J Med 127(2):158 e1–158 e7

Nagata Y, Takayama K, Matsuo Y et al (2005) Clinical outcomes of a phase I/II study of 48 Gy of stereotactic body radiotherapy in 4 fractions for primary lung cancer using a stereotactic body frame. Int J Radiat Oncol* Biol* Phys 63(5):1427–1431

Nagata Y, Hiraoka M, Shibata T et al (2015) Prospective trial of stereotactic body radiation therapy for both operable and inoperable T1N0M0 non-small cell lung cancer: Japan Clinical Oncology Group Study JCOG0403. Int J Radiat Oncol* Biol* Phys 93(5):989–996

Nair VJ, Szanto J, Vandervoort E et al (2013) CyberKnife for inoperable renal tumors: Canadian pioneering experience. Can J Urol 20(5):6944–6949

Nguyen Q-N, Shiu AS, Rhines LD et al (2010) Management of spinal metastases from renal cell carcinoma using stereotactic body radiotherapy. Int J Radiat Oncol* Biol* Phys 76(4):1185–1192

Ning S, Trisler K, Wessels BW et al (1997) Radiobiologic studies of radioimmunotherapy and external beam radiotherapy in vitro and in vivo in human renal cell carcinoma xenografts. Cancer 80(12 Suppl):2519–2528

Nomiya T, Tsuji H, Hirasawa N et al (2008) Carbon ion radiation therapy for primary renal cell carcinoma: initial clinical experience. Int J Radiat Oncol Biol Phys 72(3):828–833

Nyman J, Hallqvist A, Lund JA et al (2016) SPACE—a randomized study of SBRT vs conventional fractionated radiotherapy in medically inoperable stage I NSCLC. Radiother Oncol 121(1):1–8

O'Sullivan B, Huang SH, Siu LL et al (2013) Deintensification candidate subgroups in human papillomavirus-related oropharyngeal cancer according to minimal risk of distant metastasis. J Clin Oncol 31(5):543–550

Oliveri RS, Wetterslev J, Gluud C (2011) Transarterial (chemo)embolisation for unresectable hepatocellular carcinoma. Cochrane Database Syst Rev 3:CD004787

Onishi H, Shirato H, Nagata Y, Hiraoka M et al (2007) Hypofractionated stereotactic radiotherapy (HypoFXSRT) for stage I non-small cell lung cancer: updated results of 257 patients in a Japanese multi-institutional study. J Thorac Oncol 2(7 Suppl 3):S94–S100

Onishi H, Ozaki M, Kuriyama K et al (2012) Serious gastric ulcer event after stereotactic body radiotherapy (SBRT) delivered with concomitant vinorelbine in a patient with left adrenal metastasis of lung cancer. Acta Oncol 51(5):624–628

Oshiro Y, Takeda Y, Hirano S, Ito H et al (2011) Role of radiotherapy for local control of asymptomatic adrenal metastasis from lung cancer. Am J Clin Oncol 34(3):249–253

Ost P, Jereczek-Fossa BA, As NV et al (2016) Progression-free survival following stereotactic body radiotherapy for oligometastatic prostate cancer treatment-naive recurrence: a multi-institutional analysis. Eur Urol 69(1):9–12

Owen D, Iqbal F, Pollock BE et al (2015) Long-term follow-up of stereotactic radiosurgery for head and neck malignancies. Head Neck 37(11):1557–1562

Ozyigit G, Cengiz M, Yazici G et al (2011) A retrospective comparison of robotic stereotactic body radiotherapy and three-dimensional conformal radiotherapy for the reirradiation of locally recurrent nasopharyngeal carcinoma. Int J Radiat Oncol Biol Phys 81(4):e263–e268

Palma D, Lagerwaard F (2012) Rodrigues et al. curative treatment of stage I non-small-cell lung cancer in patients with severe COPD: stereotactic radiotherapy outcomes and systematic review. Int J Radiat Oncol Biol Phys 82(3):1149–1156

Pan H, Simpson DR, Mell LK et al (2011) A survey of stereotactic body radiotherapy use in the United States. Cancer 117(19):4566–4572

Parameswaran B, Lau E, Bergen N et al (2013) Dynamic contrast enhanced MR evaluation of inoperable renal tumours treated with stereotactic radiation: preliminary results: daunting but worthwhile? J Med Imag Radiat Oncol 57(Suppl 1):156

Park C, Papiez L, Zhang S et al (2008) Universal survival curve and single fraction equivalent dose: useful tools in understanding potency of ablative radiotherapy. Int J Radiat Oncol Biol Phys 70(3):847–852

Pastorino U, Buyse M, Friedel G et al (1997) Long-term results of lung metastasectomy: prognostic analyses based on 5206 cases. J Thorac Cardiovasc Surg 113(1):37–49

Paulino AC, Constine LS, Rubin P et al (2010) Normal tissue development, homeostasis, senescence, and the sensitivity to radiation injury across the age spectrum. Semin Radiat Oncol 20(1):12–20

Pham D, Kron T, Foroudi F et al (2014a) A review of kidney motion under free, deep and forced-shallow breathing conditions: implications for stereotactic ablative body radiotherapy treatment. Technol Cancer Res Treat 13(4):315–323

Pham D, Thompson A, Kron T et al (2014b) Stereotactic ablative body radiation therapy for primary kidney cancer: a 3-dimensional conformal technique associated with low rates of early toxicity. Int J Radiat Oncol Biol Phys 90(5):1061–1068

Pham D, Kron T, Styles C et al (2015) The use of dual vacuum stabilization device to reduce kidney motion for stereotactic radiotherapy planning. Technol Cancer Res Treat 14(2):149–157

Pollom EL, Alagappan M, von Eyben R et al (2014) Single- versus multifraction stereotactic body radiation therapy for pancreatic adenocarcinoma: outcomes and toxicity. Int J Radiat Oncol Biol Phys 90(4):918–925

Pompili M, Francica G, Ponziani FR et al (2013) Bridging and downstaging treatments for hepatocellular carcinoma in patients on the waiting list for liver transplantation. World J Gastroenterol 19(43):7515–7530

Ponsky L, Lo SS, Zhang Y et al (2015) Phase I dose-escalation study of stereotactic body radiotherapy (SBRT) for poor surgical candidates with localized renal cell carcinoma. Radiother Oncol 117(1):183–187

Potters L, Gaspar LE, Kavanagh B et al (2010) American Society for Therapeutic Radiology and Oncology (ASTRO) and American College of Radiology (ACR) practice guidelines for image-guided radiation therapy (IGRT). Int J Radiat Oncol Biol Phys 76(2):319–325

Qian G, Lowry J, Silverman P et al (2003) Stereotactic extra-cranial radiosurgery for renal cell carcinoma. Int J Radiat Oncol* Biol* Phys 57(2):S283

Quirk M, Kim YH, Saab S et al (2015) Management of hepatocellular carcinoma with portal vein thrombosis. World J Gastroenterol 21(12):3462–3471

Rajagopalan MS, Heron DE, Wegner RE et al (2013) Pathologic response with neoadjuvant chemotherapy and stereotactic body radiotherapy for borderline resectable and locally-advanced pancreatic cancer. Radiat Oncol 8(1):254

Rami-Porta R, Crowley JJ, Goldstraw P (2009) Review the revised TNM staging system for lung cancer. Ann Thorac Cardiovasc Surg 15(1):5

Ranck MC et al (2013) Stereotactic body radiotherapy for the treatment of oligometastatic renal cell carcinoma. Am J Clin Oncol 36(6):589–595

Ranck MC, Golden DW, Corbin KS et al (2013) Stereotactic body radiotherapy for the treatment of oligometastatic renal cell carcinoma. Am J Clin Oncol 36(6):589–595

Raz DJ, Zell JA, Ou SH et al (2007) Natural history of stage I non-small cell lung cancer: implications for early detection. Chest 132(1):193–199

Redmond KJ, Lo SS, Fisher C et al (2016) Post-operative spine stereotactic body radiotherapy (SBRT): a critical review to guide practice. Int J Radiat Oncol* Biol* Phys 95(5):1414–1428

Reynders K, Illidge T, Siva S et al (2015) The abscopal effect of local radiotherapy: using immunotherapy to make a rare event clinically relevant. Cancer Treat Rev 41(6):503–510

Ricardi U, Filippi AR, Guarneri A et al (2010) Stereotactic body radiation therapy for early stage non-small cell lung cancer: results of a prospective trial. Lung Cancer 68(1):72–77

Roh KW, Jang JS, Kim MS et al (2009) Fractionated stereotactic radiotherapy as reirradiation for locally recurrent head and neck cancer. Int J Radiat Oncol Biol Phys 74(5):1348–1355

Rose PS, Laufer I, Boland PJ et al (2009) Risk of fracture after single fraction image-guided intensity-modulated radiation therapy to spinal metastases. J Clin Oncol 27(30):5075–5079

Rose SC, Kikolski SG, Gish RG et al (2013) Society of Interventional Radiology critique and commentary on the Cochrane report on transarterial chemoembolization. Hepatology 57(4):1675–1676

Rowell NP, Williams C et al (2003) Radical radiotherapy for stage I/II non-small cell lung cancer in patients not sufficiently fit for or declining surgery (medically inoperable). The Cochrane Library

Ruhl R, Ludemann L, Czarnecka A et al (2010) Radiobiological restrictions and tolerance doses of repeated single-fraction hdr-irradiation of intersecting small liver volumes for recurrent hepatic metastases. Radiat Oncol 5(1):44

Rule W, Timmerman R, Tong L et al (2011) Phase I dose-escalation study of stereotactic body radiotherapy in patients with hepatic metastases. Ann Surg Oncol 18(4):1081–1087

Rwigema JC, Heron DE, Ferris RL et al (2011) The impact of tumor volume and radiotherapy dose on outcome in previously irradiated recurrent squamous cell carcinoma of the head and neck treated with stereotactic body radiation therapy. Am J Clin Oncol 34(4):372–379

Rwigema JC, Heron DE, Parikh SD et al (2012) Adjuvant stereotactic body radiotherapy for resected pancreatic adenocarcinoma with close or positive margins. J Gastrointest Cancer 43(1):70–76

Ryu S, Fang YF, Rock J et al (2003) Image-guided and intensity-modulated radiosurgery for patients with spinal metastasis. Cancer 97(8):2013–2018

Sahgal A, Ames C, Chou D et al (2009) Stereotactic body radiotherapy is effective salvage therapy for patients with prior radiation of spinal metastases. Int J Radiat Oncol* Biol* Phys 74(3):723–731

Sahgal A, Bilsky M, Chang EL et al (2011) Stereotactic body radiotherapy for spinal metastases: current status, with a focus on its application in the postoperative patient: a review. J Neurosurg Spine 14(2):151–166

Sahgal A, Roberge D, Schellenberg D et al (2012a) The Canadian association of radiation oncology scope of practice guidelines for lung, liver and spine stereotactic body radiotherapy. Clin Oncol (R Coll Radiol) 24(9):629–639

Sahgal A, Ma L, Weinberg V et al (2012b) Reirradiation human spinal cord tolerance for stereotactic body radiotherapy. Int J Radiat Oncol Biol Phys 82(1):107–116

Sahgal A, Weinberg V, Ma L et al (2013a) Probabilities of radiation myelopathy specific to stereotactic body radiation therapy to guide safe practice. Int J Radiat Oncol Biol Phys 85(2):341–347

Sahgal A, Atenafu EG, Chao S et al (2013b) Vertebral compression fracture after spine stereotactic body radiotherapy: a multi-institutional analysis with a focus on radiation dose and the spinal instability neoplastic score. J Clin Oncol 31(27):3426–3431

Sathishkumar S, Boyanovsky B, Karakashian AA et al (2005) Elevated sphingomyelinase activity and ceramide concentration in serum of patients undergoing high dose spatially fractionated radiation treatment: implications for endothelial apoptosis. Cancer Biol Ther 4(9):979–986

Schanne DH, Nestle U, Allgauer M et al (2015) Stereotactic body radiotherapy for centrally located stage I NSCLC: a multicenter analysis. Strahlenther Onkol 191(2):125–132

Schellenberg D, Kim J, Christman-Skieller C et al (2011) Single-fraction stereotactic body radiation therapy and sequential gemcitabine for the treatment of locally advanced pancreatic cancer. Int J Radiat Oncol Biol Phys 81(1):181–188

Schueneman AJ, Himmelfarb E, Geng L et al (2003) SU11248 maintenance therapy prevents tumor regrowth after fractionated irradiation of murine tumor models. Cancer Res 63(14):4009–4016

Sciubba DM, Gokaslan ZL (2006) Diagnosis and management of metastatic spine disease. Surg Oncol 15(3):141–151

Scorsetti M, Mancosu P, Navarria P et al (2011) Stereotactic body radiation therapy (SBRT) for adrenal metastases: a feasibility study of advanced techniques with modulated photons and protons. Strahlenther Onkol 187(4):238–244. doi:10.1007/s00066-011-2207-9. Epub 2011 Mar 25

Senthi S, Lagerwaard FJ, Haasbeek CJ et al (2012) Patterns of disease recurrence after stereotactic ablative radiotherapy for early stage non-small-cell lung cancer: a retrospective analysis. Lancet Oncol 13(8):802–809

Senthi S, Haasbeek CJ, Slotman BJ et al (2013) Outcomes of stereotactic ablative radiotherapy for central lung tumours: a systematic review. Radiother Oncol 106(3):276–282

Seo Y, Kim MS, Yoo S et al (2009) Stereotactic body radiation therapy boost in locally advanced pancreatic cancer. Int J Radiat Oncol Biol Phys 75(5):1456–1461

Seong J, Koom WS, Park HC (2005) Radiotherapy for painful bone metastases from hepatocellular carcinoma. Liver Int 25(2):261–265

Seong J, Lee IJ, Shim SJ et al (2009) A multicenter retrospective cohort study of practice patterns and clinical outcome on radiotherapy for hepatocellular carcinoma in Korea. Liver Int 29(2):147–152

Seung SK, Curti BD, Crittenden M et al (2012) Phase 1 study of stereotactic body radiotherapy and interleukin-2-tumor and immunological responses. Sci Transl Med 4(137):137ra74

Sharabi AB, Tran PT, Lim M et al (2015) Stereotactic radiation therapy combined with immunotherapy: augmenting the role of radiation in local and systemic treatment. Oncology 29(5):211304

Sharma A, Wong D, Weidlich G et al (2010) Noninvasive stereotactic radiosurgery (CyberHeart) for creation of ablation lesions in the atrium. Heart Rhythm 7(6):802–810

Shibamoto Y, Hashizume C, Baba F et al (2015) Stereotactic body radiotherapy using a radiobiology-based regimen for stage I non-small-cell lung cancer: five-year mature results. J Thorac Oncol 10(6):960–964

Shim SJ, Seong J, Han KH et al (2005) Local radiotherapy as a complement to incomplete transcatheter arterial chemoembolization in locally advanced hepatocellular carcinoma. Liver Int 25(6):1189–1196

Shirvani SM, Jiang J, Chang JY et al (2012) Comparative effectiveness of 5 treatment strategies for early-stage non-small cell lung cancer in the elderly. Int J Radiat Oncol Biol Phys 84(5):1060–1070

Siddiqui F, Patel M, Khan M et al (2009) Stereotactic body radiation therapy for primary, recurrent, and metastatic tumors in the head-and-neck region. Int J Radiat Oncol Biol Phys 74(4):1047–1053

Siddiqui F, Kunos CA, Paulino AC (2012) Stereotactic body radiation therapy in head and neck, gynecologic, and pediatric malignancies. J Radiat Oncol 1(1):31–42

Siegel RL, Miller KD, Jemal A (2015) Cancer statistics, 2015. CA: A Cancer J Clinicians 65(1):5–29

Siegel RL, Miller KD, Jemal A (2016) Cancer statistics, 2016. CA Cancer J Clin 66(1):7–30

Simpson J, Drzymala R, Rich K (2006) Stereotactic radiosurgery and radiotherapy. Technical basis of radiation therapy, pp 233–253

Siva S et al (2012) A systematic review of stereotactic radiotherapy ablation for primary renal cell carcinoma. BJU Int 110(11 Pt B): E737–743.

Siva S, MacManus M, Ball D (2010) Stereotactic radiotherapy for pulmonary oligometastases: a systematic review. J Thorac Oncol 5(7):1091–1099

Siva S, MacManus MP, Martin RF et al (2015) Abscopal effects of radiation therapy: a clinical review for the radiobiologist. Cancer Lett 356(1):82–90

Siva S, Jackson P, Kron T et al (2016a) Impact of stereotactic radiotherapy on kidney function in primary renal cell carcinoma: establishing a dose-response relationship. Radiother Oncol 118(3):540–546

Siva S, Daniels CP, Ellis RJ et al (2016b) Stereotactic ablative body radiotherapy for primary kidney cancer: what have we learned from prospective trials and what does the future hold? Future Oncol 12(5):601–606

Siva S, Ellis RJ, Ponsky L et al (2016c) Consensus statement from the international radiosurgery oncology consortium for kidney for primary renal cell carcinoma. Future Oncol 12(5):637–645

Soffen EM, Solin LJ, Rubenstein JH et al (1990) Palliative radiotherapy for symptomatic adrenal metastases. Cancer 65(6):1318–1320

Soltys SG, Kalani MY, Cheshier SH et al (2008) Stereotactic radiosurgery for a cardiac sarcoma: a case report. Technol Cancer Res Treat 7(5):363–368

Song SY, Choi W, Shin SS et al (2009) Fractionated stereotactic body radiation therapy for medically inoperable stage I lung cancer adjacent to central large bronchus. Lung Cancer 66(1):89–93

Song CW, Kim MS, Cho LC et al (2014) Radiobiological basis of SBRT and SRS. Int J Clin Oncol 19(4):570–578

Staehler M, Haseke N, Nuhn P et al (2011) Simultaneous anti-angiogenic therapy and single-fraction radiosurgery in clinically relevant metastases from renal cell carcinoma. BJU Int 108(5):673–678

Staehler M, Bader M, Schlenker B et al (2015) Single fraction radiosurgery for the treatment of renal tumors. J Urol 193(3):771–775

Stauder MC, Ni Laack N, Ahmed KA et al (2012) Stereotactic radiosurgery for patients with recurrent intracranial ependymomas. J Neuro-Oncol 108(3):507–512

Svedman C, Sandström P, Pisa P et al (2006) A prospective phase II trial of using extracranial stereotactic radiotherapy in primary and metastatic renal cell carcinoma. Acta Oncol 45(7):870–875

Svedman C, Karlsson K, Rutkowska E et al (2008) Stereotactic body radiotherapy of primary and metastatic renal lesions for patients with only one functioning kidney. Acta Oncol 47(8):1578–1583

Swaminath A, Chu W (2015) Stereotactic body radiotherapy for the treatment of medically inoperable primary renal cell carcinoma: current evidence and future directions. Can Urol Assoc J 9(7–8):275–280

Takeda A, Kunieda E, Fujii H et al (2013) Evaluation for local failure by 18 F-FDG PET/CT in comparison with CT findings after stereotactic body radiotherapy (SBRT) for localized non-small-cell lung cancer. Lung Cancer 79(3):248–253

Takiar V, Garden AS, Ma D et al (2016) Reirradiation of head and neck cancers with intensity modulated radiation therapy: outcomes and analyses. Int J Radiat Oncol Biol Phys 95(4):1117–1131

Takigawa M, Takahashi A, Kuwahara T et al (2014) Long-term follow-up after catheter ablation of paroxysmal atrial fibrillation: the incidence of recurrence and progression of atrial fibrillation. Circ Arrhythm Electrophysiol 7(2):267–273

Tang C, Hess K, Bishop AJ et al (2015) Creation of a prognostic index for spine metastasis to stratify survival in patients treated with spinal stereotactic radiosurgery: secondary analysis of mature prospective trials. Int J Radiat Oncol Biol Phys 93(1):118–125

Tanguturi SK, Wo JY, Zhu AX et al (2014) Radiation therapy for liver tumors: ready for inclusion in guidelines? Oncologist 19(8):868–879

Tanvetyanon T, Robinson LA, Schell MJ et al (2008) Outcomes of adrenalectomy for isolated synchronous versus metachronous adrenal metastases in non-small-cell lung cancer: a systematic review and pooled analysis. J Clin Oncol 26(7):1142–1147

Tate DJ, Adler JR Jr, Chang SD et al (1999) Stereotactic radiosurgical boost following radiotherapy in primary nasopharyngeal carcinoma: impact on local control. Int J Radiat Oncol Biol Phys 45(4):915–921

Taunk NK, Spratt DE, Bilsky M et al (2015) Spine radiosurgery in the management of renal cell carcinoma metastases. J Natl Compr Cancer Netw 13(6):801–809. quiz 809

Taunk NK, Kushner B, Ibanez K et al (2016) Short-interval retreatment with stereotactic body radiotherapy (SBRT) for pediatric neuroblastoma resulting in severe myositis. Pediatr Blood Cancer 63(4):731–733

Teh B, Bloch C, Galli-Guevara M et al (2007) The treatment of primary and metastatic renal cell carcinoma (RCC) with image-guided stereotactic body radiation therapy (SBRT). Biomed Imaging Interv J 3(1):e6

Tekatli H, Haasbeek N, Dahele M et al (2016) Outcomes of hypofractionated high-dose radiotherapy in poor-risk patients with "ultracentral" non-small cell lung cancer. J Thorac Oncol 11(7):1081–1089

Ten Haken RK, Martel MK, Kessler ML et al (1993) Use of Veff and iso-NTCP in the implementation of dose escalation protocols. Int J Radiat Oncol* Biol* Phys 27(3):689–695

Thariat J, Marcy PY, Lacout A et al (2011) Benefit of optimizing the dose to the carotid in hypofractionated stereotactic body reirradiation? Int J Radiat Oncol Biol Phys 81(5):1593–1594

Thibault I, Al-Omair A, Masucci GL et al (2014) Spine stereotactic body radiotherapy for renal cell cancer spinal metastases: analysis of outcomes and risk of vertebral compression fracture: clinical article. J Neurosurg Spine 21(5):711–718

Thibault I, Chang EL, Sheehan J et al (2015) Response assessment after stereotactic body radiotherapy for spinal metastasis: a report from the SPIne response assessment in Neuro-oncology (SPINO) group. Lancet Oncol 16(16):e595–e603

Thomas TO, Hasan S, Small W et al (2014) The tolerance of gastrointestinal organs to stereotactic body radiation therapy: what do we know so far? J Gastrointest Oncol 5(3):236

Timmerman R, Papiez L, McGarry R et al (2003) Extracranial stereotactic radioablation: results of a phase I study in medically inoperable stage I non-small cell lung cancer. Chest 124(5):1946–1955

Timmerman R, McGarry R, Yiannoutsos C et al (2006) Excessive toxicity when treating central tumors in a phase II study of stereotactic body radiation therapy for medically inoperable early-stage lung cancer. J Clin Oncol 24(30):4833–4839

Timmerman RD, Kavanagh BD, Cho LC et al (2007) Stereotactic body radiation therapy in multiple organ sites. J Clin Oncol 25(8):947–952

Timmerman R, Paulus R, Galvin J et al (2010) Stereotactic body radiation therapy for inoperable early stage lung cancer. JAMA 303(11):1070–1076

Tinkle CL, Shiao SL, Weinberg VK et al (2015) Comparison of stereotactic body radiotherapy and conventional external beam radiotherapy in renal cell carcinoma. ASCO annual meeting proceedings

Tomiyama N, Yasuhara Y, Nakajima Y et al (2006) CT-guided needle biopsy of lung lesions: a survey of severe complication based on 9783 biopsies in Japan. Eur J Radiol 59(1):60–64

Tong CC, Ko EC, Sung MW et al (2012) Phase II trial of concurrent sunitinib and image-guided radiotherapy for oligometastases. PLoS One 7(6):e36979

Torre LA, Bray F, Siegel RL et al (2015) Global cancer statistics, 2012. Cancer J Clin 65(2):87–108

Tree AC, Khoo VS, Eeles RA et al (2013) Stereotactic body radiotherapy for oligometastases. Lancet Oncol 14(1):e28–e37

Truman JP, García-Barros M, Kaag M et al (2010) Endothelial membrane remodeling is obligate for anti-angiogenic radiosensitization during tumor radiosurgery. PLoS One 5(8):e12310

Tse RV, Hawkins M, Lockwood G et al (2008) Phase I study of individualized stereotactic body radiotherapy for hepatocellular carcinoma and intrahepatic cholangiocarcinoma. J Clin Oncol 26(4):657–664

Tunio MA, Hashmi A, Rafi M et al (2010) Need for a new trial to evaluate postoperative radiotherapy in renal cell carcinoma: a meta-analysis of randomized controlled trials. Ann Oncol 21(9):1839–1845

Unger KR, Lominska CE, Deeken JF et al (2010) Fractionated stereotactic radiosurgery for reirradiation of head-and-neck cancer. Int J Radiat Oncol Biol Phys 77(5):1411–1419

Vansteenkiste J, De Ruysscher D, Eberhardt WE et al (2013) Early and locally advanced non-small-cell lung cancer (NSCLC): ESMO Clinical Practice Guidelines for diagnosis, treatment and follow-up. Ann Oncol 24(Suppl 6):vi89–vi98

Vansteenkiste J, Crino L, Dooms C et al (2014) 2nd ESMO consensus conference on lung cancer: early-stage non-small-cell lung cancer consensus on diagnosis, treatment and follow-up. Ann Oncol 25(8):1462–1474

Vargo JA, Wegner RE, Heron DE et al (2012) Stereotactic body radiation therapy for locally recurrent, previously irradiated nonsquamous cell cancers of the head and neck. Head Neck 34(8):1153–1161

Vargo JA, Ferris RL, Clump DA et al (2014a) Stereotactic body radiotherapy as primary treatment for elderly patients with medically inoperable head and neck cancer. Front Oncol 4:214

Vargo JA, Heron D, Ferris RL et al (2014b) Examining tumor control and toxicity after stereotactic body radiotherapy in locally recurrent previously irradiated head and neck cancers: implications of treatment duration and tumor volume. Head Neck 36(9):1349–1355

Vargo JA, Ferris RL, Ohr J et al (2015) A prospective phase 2 trial of reirradiation with stereotactic body radiation therapy plus cetuximab in patients with previously irradiated recurrent squamous cell carcinoma of the head and neck. Int J Radiat Oncol Biol Phys 91(3):480–488

Vedam SS, Keall PJ, Kini VR et al (2001) Determining parameters for respiration-gated radiotherapy. Med Phys 28(10):2139–2146

Vedam SS, Kini VR, Keall PJ et al (2003) Quantifying the predictability of diaphragm motion during respiration with a noninvasive external marker. Med Phys 30(4):505–513

Verstegen NE, Lagerwaard FJ, Haasbeek CJ et al (2011) Outcomes of stereotactic ablative radiotherapy following a clinical diagnosis of stage I NSCLC: comparison with a contemporaneous cohort with pathologically proven disease. Radiother Oncol 101(2):250–254

Verstegen N, Oosterhuis J, Palma D et al (2013) Stage I–II non-small-cell lung cancer treated using either stereotactic ablative radiotherapy (SABR) or lobectomy by video-assisted thoracoscopic surgery (VATS): outcomes of a propensity score-matched analysis. Ann Oncol 24(6):1543–1548

Viani GA, Stefano EJ, Afonso SL (2009) Higher-than-conventional radiation doses in localized prostate cancer treatment: a meta-analysis of randomized, controlled trials. Int J Radiat Oncol Biol Phys 74(5):1405–1418

Vickress J, Lock M, Lo S et al (2017) A multivariable model to predict survival for patients with hepatic carcinoma or liver metastasis receiving radiotherapy. Future Oncol 13(1):19–30

Voynov G, Heron DE, Burton S et al (2006) Frameless stereotactic radiosurgery for recurrent head and neck carcinoma. Technol Cancer Res Treat 5(5):529–535

Wahidi MM, Govert JA, Goudar RK et al (2007) Evidence for the treatment of patients with pulmonary nodules: when is it lung cancer?: ACCP evidence-based clinical practice guidelines. Chest J 132(3_suppl):94S–107S

Walsh L, Stanfield JL, Cho LC et al (2006) Efficacy of ablative high-dose-per-fraction radiation for implanted human renal cell cancer in a nude mouse model. Eur Urol 50(4):795–800. discussion 800

Wang XS, Rhines LD, Shiu AS et al (2012) Stereotactic body radiation therapy for management of spinal metastases in patients without spinal cord compression: a phase 1-2 trial. Lancet Oncol 13(4):395–402

Wang K, Heron DE, Clump DA et al (2013) Target delineation in stereotactic body radiation therapy for recurrent head and neck cancer: a retrospective analysis of the impact of margins and automated PET-CT segmentation. Radiother Oncol 106(1):90–95

Wang YJ, Han TT, Xue JX et al (2014) Stereotactic gamma-ray body radiation therapy for asynchronous bilateral renal cell carcinoma. Radiol Med 119(11):878–883

Wang CJ, Cai X, Kim DW et al (2016) The effect of stereotactic ablative radiotherapy on time to change of systemic therapy in extra-cranial renal cell carcinoma metastases. J Clin Oncol (Meeting Abstracts) 34(2 suppl):533

van der Werf-Messing B (1973) Proceedings: carcinoma of the kidney. Cancer 32(5):1056–1061

Wersall PJ, Blomgren H, Lax I et al (2005) Extracranial stereotactic radiotherapy for primary and metastatic renal cell carcinoma. Radiother Oncol 77(1):88–95

Winter JD, Wong R, Swaminath A et al (2015) Accuracy of robotic radiosurgical liver treatment throughout the respiratory cycle. Int J Radiat Oncol Biol Phys 93(4):916–924

Wong P, Houghton P, Kirsch DG et al. Combining targeted agents with modern radiotherapy in soft tissue sarcomas. J Natl Cancer Inst 2014; 106(11): doi:10.1093/jnci/dju329.

Yamada Y, Laufer I, Cox BW et al (2013) Preliminary results of high-dose single-fraction radiotherapy for the management of chordomas of the spine and sacrum. Neurosurgery 73(4):673–680. discussion 680

Yamamoto T et al (2016) Renal atrophy after stereotactic body radiotherapy for renal cell carcinoma. Radiat Oncol 11(1):72

Yamazaki H, Ogita M, Himei K et al (2015) Carotid blowout syndrome in pharyngeal cancer patients treated by hypofractionated stereotactic re-irradiation using CyberKnife: a multi-institutional matched-cohort analysis. Radiother Oncol 115(1):67–71

Yang JC, Sherry RM, Steinberg SM et al (2003) Randomized study of high-dose and low-dose interleukin-2 in patients with metastatic renal cancer. J Clin Oncol 21(16):3127–3132

Yang W, Fraass BA, Reznik R et al (2014) Adequacy of inhale/exhale breathhold CT based ITV margins and image-guided registration for free-breathing pancreas and liver SBRT. Radiat Oncol 9(1):11

Yao HH, Hong MK, Corcoran NM et al (2014) Advances in local and ablative treatment of oligometastasis in prostate cancer. Asia Pac J Clin Oncol 10(4):308–321

Yazici G, Sanli TY, Cengiz M et al (2013) A simple strategy to decrease fatal carotid blowout syndrome after stereotactic body reirradiaton for recurrent head and neck cancers. Radiat Oncol (London, England) 8:242-717X-8-242

Yen CP, Monteith SJ, Nguyen JH et al (2010) Gamma knife surgery for arteriovenous malformations in children: clinical article. J Neurosurg 6(5):426–434

Yeoh EE, Botten RJ, Butters J et al (2011) Hypofractionated versus conventionally fractionated radiotherapy for prostate carcinoma: final results of phase III randomized trial. Int J Radiat Oncol Biol Phys 81(5):1271–1278

Yoon SM, Lim YS, Won HJ et al (2012) Radiotherapy plus transarterial chemoembolization for hepatocellular carcinoma invading the portal vein: long-term patient outcomes. Int J Radiat Oncol Biol Phys 82(5):2004–2011

Yu JB, Cramer LD, Herrin J et al (2014) Stereotactic body radiation therapy versus intensity-modulated radiation therapy for prostate cancer: comparison of toxicity. J Clin Oncol 32(12):1195–1201

Zelefsky MJ, Greco C, Motzer R et al (2012) Tumor control outcomes after hypofractionated and single-dose stereotactic image-guided intensity-modulated radiotherapy for extracranial metastases from renal cell carcinoma. Int J Radiat Oncol Biol Phys 82(5):1744–1748

Zeng ZC, Tang ZY, Fan J et al (2005) Radiation therapy for adrenal gland metastases from hepatocellular carcinoma. Jpn J Clin Oncol 35(2):61–67

Zhang HP, Takayama K, Su B et al (2011) Effect of sunitinib combined with ionizing radiation on endothelial cells. J Radiat Res 52(1):1–8

Zimetbaum P (2012) Antiarrhythmic drug therapy for atrial fibrillation. Circulation 125(2):381–389

Altered Fraction Radiotherapy in Palliation

Srinivas Raman, Natalie Logie, Joshua Jones, Eric Chang, Steven Lutz, and Edward Chow

Contents

1 Introduction

The skeletal system and central nervous system are two common sites of metastatic spread in solid tumors. Radiotherapy is a highly effective treatment modality for these sites of metastatic disease. Given that the intent of treatment is not curative, the goals in palliative radiotherapy are centered on symptom management and quality of life. Therefore, the decisions around dose fractionation and radiotherapy technique in palliative therapy can be complex, taking into account patient performance status, prognosis, and goals of therapy. There is increasing interest in the use of hypo-fractionated and stereotactic radiotherapy in the treatment of skeletal and brain metastases due to the convenience of shorter treatments, high rates of local control, and low toxicity rates. This chapter discusses the role for alternate fractionation in palliative radiotherapy to bone metastases, spinal cord compression, and brain metastases.

S. Raman • E. Chow (✉)
University of Toronto, Toronto, ON, Canada
e-mail: srinivas.raman@sunnybrook.ca;
edward.chow@sunnybrook.ca

N. Logie
University of Alberta, Edmonton, AB, Canada
e-mail: logie@ualberta.ca

J. Jones
University of Pennsylvania, Philadelphia, PA, USA
e-mail: joshua.jones@uphs.upenn.edu

E. Chang
University of Southern California,
Los Angeles, CA, USA
e-mail: Eric.Chang@health.usc.edu

S. Lutz
Blanchard Valley Health System, Findlay, OH, USA
e-mail: slutz@bvhealthsystem.org

Med Radiol Radiat Oncol (2017)
DOI 10.1007/174_2017_41, © Springer International Publishing AG
Published Online: 14 June 2017

2   Site-Specific Characteristics and Management at Diagnosis

2.1   Bone Metastases

Bone metastases are an important source of morbidity and can significantly affect patient quality of life and function. The clinical presentation of patients with bone metastases is variable. If symptomatic, patients usually present with pain, sometimes with hypercalcemia, fracture, or neurological symptoms, depending on the site of metastases. The most common location of bone metastases is in the spinal column, followed by the pelvis and proximal femora (Tubiana-Hulin 1991; Choi and Raghavan 2012). Tumors that are most likely to metastasize to the bone include breast, prostate, and lung primary malignancies (Mundy 2002).

The diagnosis of bone metastases is usually made by imaging and the choice of imaging modality is dependent on the presenting clinical scenario. Bone scans are a highly sensitive modality for detecting osteoblastic bone metastases in solid tumors and are particularly useful for evaluating the entire skeletal system. Other imaging modalities such as plain film X-ray, computed tomography (CT), magnetic resonance imaging (MRI), and positron emission tomography (PET) may also be used as clinically indicated for detailed local evaluation or assessment of other structures.

2.2   Spinal Cord Compression

Malignant spinal cord compression (MSCC) is a feared complication in advanced cancer that can have devastating consequences on neurologic function and quality of life. One definition of MSCC is the "compression of the dural sac and its contents (spinal cord and/or cauda equina) by an extradural tumor mass. The minimum radiologic evidence for cord compression is indentation of the theca at the level of clinical features" (Loblaw et al. 2005). MSCC most often arises from breast, prostate, and lung primary malignancies. Other

common sources include renal cell carcinoma, lymphoma, and multiple myeloma (Cole and Patchell 2008). The origin of most spinal cord compressions is extramedullary in the epidural space, resulting from malignant involvement of the anterior vertebral column (Cole and Patchell 2008). Less commonly, the origin is from the leptomeningeal and intramedullary regions. The thoracic spine is most commonly affected (60%), followed by the lumbosacral spine (30%) and cervical spine (10%).

Patients usually present with a history of back pain, which usually precedes neurologic symptoms by weeks to months (Cole and Patchell 2008). Neurological symptoms can include radicular pain, weakness/paralysis, sensory deficits, gait ataxia, and bowel or bladder dysfunction. Patients with signs or symptoms suggestive of MSCC must be promptly investigated and treated to prevent further neurologic compromise which can be permanent. The diagnosis of cord compression is usually made based on the results of MRI, which is the preferred imaging modality in most centers. Alternatively, myelography ± CT can also identify cord compression with similar specificity and sensitivity to MRI (Hagenau et al. 1987; Godersky et al. 1987).

2.3   Brain Metastases

Patients with brain metastases are a heterogeneous population. Metastases occur primarily from lung, breast, and melanoma and affected patients can present with headaches, focal neurologic deficits, cognitive disturbance, seizures, and stroke (Posner 1996). Typically, brain metastases occur at the junction of the gray matter and white matter, and the terminal "watershed areas" of arterial circulation (Delattre et al. 1988). Approximately 80% of brain metastases occur in the cerebral hemispheres, with the remaining in the cerebellum (15%) and the brainstem (5%). Approximately half of patients present with multiple brain metastases (Nussbaum et al. 1996). The diagnosis of brain metastases is often made on imaging, although in patients with a single/

solitary metastasis, biopsy may be required to make a definitive diagnosis. Gadolinium contrast-enhanced MRI is the preferred imaging modality with a high sensitivity; although nonenhanced MRI and contrast-enhanced CT are reasonable alternatives in patients with MRI contrast agent contraindications (Schaefer et al. 1996).

3 Indications for Palliative Radiotherapy

3.1 Bone Metastases

Most patients with painful, uncomplicated bone metastases will benefit from radiation therapy as a therapeutic intervention (Chow et al. 2007). This includes patients with previous radiation therapy to the involved bone metastases, older patients, and patients with a short life expectancy (Huisman et al. 2012; Campos et al. 2010; Meeuse et al. 2010). The definition of uncomplicated bone metastases varies but usually excludes patients with cauda equina or spinal cord compression and impending or existing fracture, as these patients may benefit from surgical management as part of their treatment (Cheon et al. 2015). Other strategies for bone metastases include osteoclast inhibitors, analgesics/anti-inflammatory agents, radiopharmaceuticals, focused ultrasound therapy, and systemic therapy.

Patients with a pathologic fracture or impending fracture in long bones or weight-bearing bones may benefit from surgical stabilization to improve pain, decrease morbidity, maximize functional outcomes, and provide durable skeletal integrity (Damron and Sim 1999; Nielsen et al. 1991). Operative options include endoprosthetic reconstruction, intramedullary nailing, and plate/screw fixation devices. After surgical stabilization, a course of fractionated postoperative radiotherapy (PORT) is recommended (Lutz et al. 2011). The rationale for PORT is to reduce or destroy residual tumor, promote remineralization and bone healing, decrease pain, and control residual metastatic disease to reduce the risk of subsequent fracture or loss of fixation.

Surgical options may also be considered for patients with fractures for the well-selected patient with spine metastases and painful vertebral compression fractures (good performance status, no evidence of spinal cord compression or mechanical instability) in conjunction with radiotherapy (RT) (Mundy 2002). Randomized controlled trials have compared conservative treatment options (including RT) to kyphoplasty (KP) and vertebroplasty (VP) with mixed results. As such, a meta-analysis of the available data compared KP to VP to conservative management (Papanastassiou et al. 2012). The authors concluded that KP and VP resulted in reduced pain and subsequent fractures and that KP resulted in an overall higher quality of life (Papanastassiou et al. 2012).

Recently, stereotactic body radiotherapy (SBRT) has emerged as an attractive alternative to conventional external beam radiotherapy (EBRT) and is increasingly being used in North America (Pan et al. 2011). Potential advantages of SBRT for bone metastases include faster and more durable pain relief, better local control and efficacy (particularly in radioresistant histologic tumor types), and avoidance of critical structures during reirradiation (Bhattacharya and Hoskin 2015; Chang et al. 2012). Disadvantages of SBRT include cost, treatment complexity, increased toxicity/fracture risk, and uncertainty of whether ablative doses to bone metastases alter the natural course of the malignancy. SBRT has been most extensively studied in the setting of spine metastases. Spinal SBRT was initially utilized for patients who had failed EBRT as a salvage technique or for patients where surgery or EBRT was not appropriate (Gerszten et al. 2007). More recently it has been investigated as an up-front treatment. The RTOG 0631 phase III randomized trial is under way accruing to compare the efficacy of single-fraction palliative spine EBRT (8 Gy/1) to spine SBRT (either 16 Gy/1 or 18 Gy/1) (Ryu et al. 2014).

Until randomized data comparing EBRT to SBRT for spinal metastases is available, the clinical selection process to determine appropriate patients for SBRT is not well defined. RTOG 0631 includes ECOG 0–2 patients with up to three sites of disease and up to two contiguous spinal levels with a pain score of ≥5/10 on the numerical rating pain scale while excluding patients with spinal instability due to fracture, fracture with retropulsion, and/or frank spinal cord compression (Ryu et al. 2014). Other sources tend to agree that high-grade spinal cord compression or instability is a contraindication while tumor size >5 cm and involvement of multiple vertebral levels may also be contraindications. A recursive partitioning analysis (RPA) was developed by Chao et al. utilizing KPS <70 vs. KPS ≥70 and time from primary diagnosis (TPD) ≤30 months vs. TPD >30 months to predict overall survival (OS) for patients receiving spinal SBRT (Chao et al. 2012) (Table 1). Another framework for deciding about optimal treatment for patients with spinal metastases was developed at Memorial Sloan Kettering

and is based on neurologic, oncologic, mechanical, and systematic parameters (NOMS) (Laufer et al. 2013a) (Table 2).

There are no well-defined indications for the routine use of SBRT for nonspine bone metastases and clinical data from spine metastases trials may guide future directions in this area. For now, the use of SBRT for nonspine bone metastases must be individualized, taking into account the potential advantages and disadvantages listed above.

3.2 Spinal Cord Compression

MSCC can be treated with surgical decompression and/or radiation therapy. Occasionally, chemosensitive malignancies such as lymphoma, neuroblastoma, and germ cell neoplasms can be treated with chemotherapy alone. The choice of decompressive surgery vs. radiation therapy as up-front management can be complex and must ideally be made in a multidisciplinary setting with input from both radiation oncologists and spinal surgeons. The ASTRO evidence-based guideline recommends that a number of radiographic, patient, tumor, and treatment factors be taken into consideration in the decision-making process (Lutz et al. 2011) (Table 3). If decompressive

Table 1 RPA for predicting MS for patients receiving spine SBRT

Characteristics	RPA group	MS (months)
Time from primary diagnosis >30 months AND KPS ≥70	Group 1	21.1
Does not meet group 1 or group 3 criteria	Group 2	8.7
Time from primary diagnosis ≤30 months AND age ≥70	Group 3	2.4

Table 2 The NOMS framework for patients with spinal metastases

Neurologic	Oncologic	Mechanical	Systemic	Decision
Grade 0–1 ESCC AND no myelopathy	Radiosensitive	Stable		EBRT
	Radiosensitive	Unstable		Stabilization followed by EBRT
	Radioresistant	Stable		SBRT
	Radioresistant	Unstable		Stabilization followed by SBRT
Grade 2–3 ESCC OR myelopathy	Radiosensitive	Stable		EBRT
	Radiosensitive	Unstable		Stabilization followed by EBRT
	Radioresistant	Stable	Able to tolerate surgery	Decompression/stabilization followed by SBRT
	Radioresistant	Stable	Unable to tolerate surgery	EBRT
	Radioresistant	Unstable	Able to tolerate surgery	Decompression/stabilization followed by SBRT
	Radioresistant	Unstable	Unable to tolerate surgery	Stabilization followed by EBRT

Note: Stabilization options include percutaneous cement augmentation, percutaneous pedicle screw instrumentation, and open instrumentation

ESCC epidural spinal cord compression as defined on Spine Oncology Group scoring system

Table 3 ASTRO evidence-based guideline for selecting patients considered for surgical intervention for spinal cord decompression

Characteristics	Factors favoring surgical decompression plus radiation therapy
Radiographic	1. Solitary site of tumor progression
	2. Absence of visceral or brain metastases
	3. Spinal instability
Patient	1. Age <65 years
	2. KPS ≥70
	3. Projected survival >3 months
	4. Slow progression of neurologic symptoms
	5. Maintained ambulation
	6. Non-ambulatory <48 h
Tumor	1. Relatively radio-resistant tumor histologic type (i.e., melanoma)
	2. Site of origin suggesting relatively indolent course (i.e., prostate, breast, kidney)
Treatment	1. Previous EBRT failed

surgery is performed, this is usually followed by a course of EBRT to treat and eradicate microscopic residual disease (Lutz et al. 2011).

Although there are some data for the efficacy and safety of spine stereotactic body radiotherapy (SBRT) in low-grade MSCC (Ryu et al. 2010), most sources agree that high-grade MSCC is a contraindication to up-front management with SBRT (Lutz et al. 2011). Another option for patients with high-grade MSCC is to perform a "separation surgery" followed by high-dose spine radiosurgery or hypo-fractionated radiotherapy (Laufer et al. 2013b). Separation surgery refers to posterolateral resection of the epidural tumor and posterior segmental fixation without vertebral body or paraspinal tumor resection or reconstruction. This is a particularly attractive approach for patients with high-grade MSCC, medical comorbidities, and/or radioresistant histology. The rationale for this approach is to perform a less invasive surgery to provide a physical gap between the epidural disease and spinal cord. Since the limiting factor for adequate dose coverage to the epidural disease is usually proximity to the spinal cord, this separation procedure allows

the patient to receive a higher radiation dose to the residual disease, leading to excellent and durable local control (Laufer et al. 2013b; Sahgal et al. 2011; Al-Omair et al. 2013).

3.3 Brain Metastases

Treatment options for brain metastases broadly include surgical resection, radiotherapy, systemic therapy, or best practice supportive care. Generally the use of systemic therapy is reserved for patients with asymptomatic brain metastases and/or the use of agents that can penetrate the blood-brain barrier. Radiotherapy to the whole brain (WBRT), stereotactic radiosurgery (SRS), and surgical resection are the mainstays of active management in most patients. The optimal strategy for management must take into account many factors including size/number of brain metastases, total intracranial tumor volume, tumor radiosensitivity, prognosis, functional status, prior treatment, and surgical resectability. The general paradigm is that patients with limited brain metastases and favorable prognosis may benefit from more aggressive local treatment such as surgical resection and/or SRS. Other patients without these characteristics may be better suited for WBRT or best practice supportive care. The mean survival (MS) for patients with symptomatic brain metastases treated conservatively with supportive management is approximately 1–2 months (Markesbery et al. 1978). WBRT may be associated with improvement in neurological symptoms, MS, and quality of life compared to best practice supportive care (Borgelt et al. 1980; Wong et al. 2008). Randomized evidence comparing WBRT (20 Gy in five fractions) to optimal supportive care (OSC) is available comparing patients with brain metastases from NSCLC unsuitable for surgery or SRS (inclusive of KPS 30–100). This noninferiority trial did not find a significant difference in more than 7 QALY (quality-adjusted life-year) days between treatment arms in addition to having a nonsignificant difference in survival (9.2 weeks vs. 8.5 weeks, $p = 0.8084$) and quality of life comparing WBRT to OSC (Mulvenna et al. 2016). Subgroup analysis demonstrated a significant difference in survival for patients age <60 according to treatment arm, and the authors concluded that for patients age <60, WBRT should be considered (Mulvenna et al. 2016).

To assist in clinical decision making, prognostic scoring systems have been developed and validated to predict survival in patients with brain metastases. The Recursive Partitioning Analysis (RPA) score was developed from a database of 1200 patients with brain metastases included in three consecutive RTOG trials and was first utilized to classify patients into three performance groups that correlated with OS (Gaspar et al. 1997, 2000) (Table 4). The Graded Prognostic Assessment (GPA), which is specific to the

primary tumor, was later developed and validated as well (Sperduto et al. 2010; Berkey et al. 2008) (Table 5). These scoring systems with or without consideration of other patient/disease-specific factors may be utilized by clinicians to determine treatment strategies.

For patients with a single brain metastasis and favorable prognosis, surgical resection is considered the standard of care when possible. There have been no reported trials comparing SRS with surgical resection of a single brain metastasis. Surgical resection has been compared to WBRT in three randomized clinical trials (RCT), all of which compared surgical resection with WBRT to WBRT alone (Patchell et al. 1990; Vecht et al. 1993; Mink et al. 1996). Two of the trials showed a survival advantage for those randomized to receive surgical resection followed by WBRT compared to WBRT alone (Berkey et al. 2008; Patchell et al. 1990). The third trial failed to show a difference between the groups, although this trial had a greater proportion of patients with uncontrolled extracranial disease (Mink et al. 1996). Surgical resection may be followed by WBRT as this approach has been shown to

Table 4 RPA prognostic scoring system and resulting MS

Criteria	RPA class	MS (months)
KPS ≥70, primary malignancy controlled, absent extracranial disease, and age <65	Class 1	7.1
KPS ≥70 but does not meet class 1 criteria	Class 2	4.2
KPS <70	Class 3	2.3

Table 5 Diagnosis-specific GPA prognostic scoring with survival grouping scored by primary histology classification

Primary	Criteria	GPA scoring points				
NSCLC/SCLC	Points	0	0.5	1		
	Age	>60	50–60	<50		
	KPS	<70	70–80	90–100		
	Number of BM	>3	2–3	1		
	Extracranial metastases	Present	–	Absent		
	Final score	0–1	1.5–2.5	3	3.5–4	
	NSCLC MS (months)	3.0	6.5	11.3	14.8	
	SCLC MS (months)	2.8	5.3	9.6	17.1	
Melanoma/renal cell	Points	0	1	2		
	KPS	<70	70–80	90–100		
	Number of BM	>3	2–3	1		
	Final score	0–1	1.5–2.5	3	3.5–4	
	Melanoma MS (months)	3.4	4.7	8.8	13.2	
	Renal cell MS (months)	3.3	7.3	11.3	14.8	
Breast/GI cancer	Points	0	1	2	3	4
	KPS	<70	70	80	90	100
	Final score	0–1	1.5–2.5	3	3.5–4	
	Breast MS (months)	6.1	9.4	16.9	18.7	
	GI cancer MS (months)	3.1	4.4	6.9	13.5	

improve intracranial control, but there has been no demonstrated overall survival benefit (Patchell et al. 1998). Postoperative SRS may also be utilized in patients wishing to avoid WBRT; however there is no randomized evidence yet to support or refute this approach.

In patients with multiple brain metastases or a less favorable prognosis, radiotherapy techniques include WBRT, SRS, or a combination of both. There is no randomized evidence comparing WBRT and SRS directly. However, RTOG 9508 investigated patients with 1–3 brain metastases randomized to receive WBRT or WBRT followed by SRS boost (Andrews et al. 2004). MS was significantly higher for patients with a single brain metastasis receiving SRS boost; however there was no survival advantage seen for patients with multiple brain metastases. Four randomized control trials have investigated SRS alone vs. SRS with WBRT for patients with limited brain metastases (Chang et al. 2009; Kocher et al. 2011; Aoyama et al. 2006; Brown et al. 2016). Only the trial by Chang et al. showed a survival difference favoring SRS alone (Chang et al. 2009); the other three trials demonstrated a significantly higher rate of intracranial progression and utilization of salvage therapies in the SRS-alone arm (Kocher et al. 2011; Aoyama et al. 2006; Brown et al. 2016). Additionally, Kocher et al. found a significantly higher rate of neurologic death in the SRS-alone arm (Kocher et al. 2011). Two of the trials which measured neurocognitive outcomes using sensitive psychological instruments showed a significant difference favoring SRS alone and the trial by Chang et al. was stopped early as a result of this (Chang et al. 2009; Brown et al. 2016). A meta-analysis of the earlier three trials (Chang et al. 2009; Kocher et al. 2011; Aoyama et al. 2006) found that the addition of WBRT had significantly greater local control; however, patients with a single brain metastasis had a significantly lower rate of distant brain failure (Sahgal et al. 2015). The meta-analysis also suggested that patients under 50 years had a survival benefit when treated with SRS alone.

Randomized clinical trials for SRS have typically limited the treatment of patients receiving SRS to 1–4 lesions. Prospective trials have reviewed utilizing SRS to treat 1–10 lesions finding no survival difference between patients with 2–4 lesions and patients with 5–10 lesions and no difference in SRS-induced adverse events (Yamamoto et al. 2014). Therefore, the use of SRS for patients with 5–10 lesions may be an appropriate treatment strategy and patient- or treatment-related factors may be more practical limitations for treating patients with >4 lesions with SRS.

In conclusion, for patients with a single brain metastasis, surgical resection ± postoperative radiotherapy may be considered. For patients with multiple brain metastases, treatment options may include SRS ± WBRT, WBRT ± SRS, or best practice supportive care. The utilization of either the RPA or the GPA may help to select appropriate treatment modalities for patients.

4 Techniques

4.1 Bone Metastases

For conventional EBRT to bone metastases, there are many possible fractionation schemes including 30 Gy in ten fractions, 24 Gy/6, 20 Gy/5, and 8 Gy/1 (Lutz et al. 2011). There are data from multiple randomized trials and a meta-analysis to support the use of single-fraction radiotherapy for uncomplicated bone metastases (Lutz et al. 2011). The data for retreatment fractionation schemes are less well established; however both 8 Gy in one fraction and 20 Gy in multiple fractions seem to be equally efficacious (Chow et al. 2014). The treatment technique is dependent on the location of bone metastases. A simple two-photon beam AP/PA arrangement with energy of 6–18 MV is adequate in most cases. For rib lesions, opposed tangents or an electron beam arrangement may be used depending on the location and depth of the lesion being treated. The gross tumor volume (GTV) is defined by visualized/symptomatic disease on imaging. A 0.5 cm expansion may be applied to cover the clinical target volume (CTV) and a further 0.5 cm margin can be applied for the planning target volume

(PTV). For rib and sternal lesions, the PTV margin may be increased to 1 cm to account for increased motion from breathing.

For metastases in the thoracic spine/lumbar spine/sacral region, the beam arrangement could be a parallel opposed field setup (prescribed to mid-plane) or direct posterior field alone (prescribed to the posterior edge of the vertebral body) (Roos et al. 2005; Jeremic et al. 1998; Sande et al. 2009) while cervical spine metastases may be treated with lateral opposing fields to avoid treatment of the oral cavity. Classically, the radiation portal includes the entire area of visible disease and 1–2 uninvolved vertebral bodies above, below, and above the gross tumor. However, with low rates of failure in the adjacent vertebral body and efficacy of salvage SBRT, this strategy has come into question (Klish et al. 2011). Cumulative doses to the spinal cord less than 120 Gy2 BED are thought to be safe, as no cases of spinal cord myelopathy have been reported below this threshold (Rades et al. 2008a; Nieder et al. 2006). Increasing the cumulative dose to 130–150 Gy2 BED may be necessary in some cases but is associated with a small risk of spinal cord myelopathy (Nieder et al. 2006). Conventional EBRT dose constraints for other organs are discussed in other chapters.

For SBRT to spine metastases, a wide range of prescription doses have been reported including 16–24 Gy in a single fraction, 24 Gy/2, 21–27 Gy/3, and 30–35 Gy/5. There is no established superiority of one prescription dose over another. A stable setup position can be achieved with a patient supine immobilized using a vacuum bag (Bhattacharya and Hoskin 2015). CT simulation should use ≤3 mm slice thickness fused with a planning MRI including both T1 postcontrast and T2 sequences. Consensus guidelines are available to help delineate the GTV and CTV (Cox et al. 2012). The GTV should be defined as per all imaging available and includes paravertebral or epidural tumor extension. The CTV typically includes the entire vertebral body including superior and inferior end plates but excluding discs (Cox et al. 2012) and should include the right and the left lateral pedicles (Ryu et al. 2014). The CTV should also include any abnormal marrow signal seen; however the posterior elements are typically not included unless clinically involved to prevent completely encircling the cord (Cox et al. 2012). The PTV is a uniform CTV expansion ≤3 mm and should never overlap the cord (Cox et al. 2012). As per RTOG 0631, up to two contiguous vertebral bodies may be treated and image-guided treatment was performed with no greater than a 2 mm difference allowable between simulation, localization, and end of treatment (Ryu et al. 2014). Including vertebral bodies above and below the affected vertebrae is not required as failure rates are low in these regions (Klish et al. 2011).

The treatment technique for SBRT to nonspine bone metastases is dependent on the location of the metastases. For rib and sternal metastases, a 4-D CT should be used to account for breathing motion. For lesions superior to the T3 vertebral body, immobilization should be performed with an immobilization mask. For other regions, immobilization may be performed with commercially available systems such as BodyFix (Electa AB, Stockholm, Sweden) or Vac-Q-Fix (Varian, Palo Alto, California, USA). The optimal prescription dose is not known. From a published series by Mayo Clinic, commonly used doses include 24 Gy in a single fraction, 18 Gy/1 and 30 Gy/3 (Owen et al. 2014). The GTV includes all visualized disease on imaging and an MRI scan is often helpful in delineating the full extent of disease. A CTV margin may be added to include subclinical disease. If 4-D CT is used, the internal target volume (ITV) is the sum of the CTV from the inhale, exhale, and average scans. Daily image guidance with cone-beam CT is strongly recommended. With appropriate immobilization and daily image guidance, the PTV expansion can be reduced to <5 mm and is determined by institutional experience with setup and imaging uncertainty. Both intensity-modulated radiation therapy (IMRT) and volumetric modulated arc therapy (VMAT) techniques may be utilized to achieve the required dose conformity. The report of the American Association of Physicists in Medicine (AAPM) Task Group 101 can guide the normal tissue dose constraints for different SBRT fractionation schemes (Benedict et al. 2010).

4.2 Spinal Cord Compression

A number of conventional EBRT fractionation schemes for cord MSCC have been reported such as 40 Gy in 20 fractions, 30 Gy/10, 20 Gy/5, and 8 Gy/1 (Loblaw et al. 2005; Lutz et al. 2011). For patients with a short life expectancy (<3–6 months), a single 8 Gy fraction is appropriate; however, for patients with a more favorable prognosis, a protracted course of radiation may provide more durable local control (Loblaw et al. 2005). In the case of postoperative radiotherapy, there are no guidelines for the optimal fractionation schedule; however the majority of published reports use a fractionated course of radiotherapy (Lutz et al. 2011). For MSCC, an MRI or a CT myelogram may be required to identify the location and extent of disease; otherwise the treatment technique is identical to spine metastases as described above.

As mentioned above, the use of SBRT is contraindicated in high-grade cord compression. The concept of "separation surgery" followed by high-dose spine radiosurgery or hypo-fractionated radiotherapy is an evolving paradigm and the treatment planning and delivery follow similar principles as spine radiosurgery/SBRT for de novo spine metastases. Patients undergo a preoperative MRI to help delineate the preoperative GTV which includes the osseous, epidural, and paraspinal regions of the tumor and a postoperative CT myelogram can be helpful in defining the dural margin in the presence of spinal instrumentation (Ryu et al. 2010).

4.3 Brain Metastases

When planning for WBRT, patients may be planned with a CT simulation or via clinical setup. Head immobilization typically includes a thermoplastic mask. A pair of opposing lateral fields to cover the brain, meninges, and foramen magnum is designed (Vecht et al. 1993). Radiotherapy is typically prescribed to the midplane (Chang et al. 2009). The most commonly used prescription dose is 30 Gy in ten fractions; however, other commonly used dose schedules include 20 Gy/5 and 40 Gy/20. For hippocampal dose-sparing techniques (thought to reduce neurocognitive loss), the CT simulation should be fused with a T1 contrast-enhanced MRI using ≤1.5 mm slice thickness (Oehlke et al. 2015). The hippocampal region should be defined on the MRI with a 3-D expansion of 5–7 mm to define the dose avoidance structure (Oehlke et al. 2015; Gondi et al. 2014). The PTV is defined as the entire brain with a 0–3 mm margin and the hippocampal region subtracted (Oehlke et al. 2015; Gondi et al. 2014). The dose to the D_{min} (minimum dose) of the hippocampus should be limited to less than 9 Gy with a point maximum (D_{max}) of 16 Gy (Gondi et al. 2014).

For stereotactic radiotherapy, the prescription dose and fractionation can depend on the size of the treated lesion (Shaw et al. 2000). For lesions <2 cm in diameter, single-fraction doses as high as 20–24 Gy may be prescribed. For lesions between 2 and 3 cm, the dose should be deescalated to <18 Gy to reduce the risk of radionecrosis. For lesions >3 cm, the dose should be further deescalated to <18 Gy if possible, or fractionated stereotactic radiotherapy should be considered. Patients planned for SRS should be simulated with a CT scan fused with a contrast-enhanced T1-weighted MRI in the treatment position. Rigid head immobilization is required and may include a stereotactic frame which may be attached to the skull under local anesthesia or frameless techniques using a thermoplastic mask with bite block positioned against the upper dentition with CT localization (Suh 2010). When defining tumor volumes, GTV tumor volume should be defined as the enhancing region on MRI slices with a thickness of 1–1.5 mm (Noël et al. 2003; Kirkpatrick et al. 2015). Noel et al. found that when adding a 1 mm CTV to the GTV where 20 Gy was prescribed to the isocenter and 14 Gy to the CTV margin, the mean dose to the GTV was significantly greater (16.8 Gy vs. 14.6 Gy, $p < 0.001$) and 2-year local control rates were significantly higher (Noël et al. 2003). Similarly, Kirkpatrick et al. investigated GTV to PTV expansion of 1–3 mm concluding that a 1 mm expansion offered high rates of local control with low rates of morbidity (Kirkpatrick et al. 2015).

The dose is typically prescribed to 50–90% of the target volume (Patchell et al. 1998; Shaw et al. 2000). For fractionated SRS, volume and prescription parameters are similar but in some cases were prescribed to 95% of the PTV (Wegner et al. 2015).

5 Results

5.1 Bone Metastases

5.1.1 Conventional EBRT

Radiotherapy is a highly effective treatment for the treatment of painful bone metastases; 50–90% of patients will attain some relief of their pain and up to 1/3 of patients will complete resolution of their pain (Lutz et al. 2011). There is evidence from at least three large RCT and a meta-analysis which show that single-fraction and multiple-fraction regimens have shown to have equivalent rates and magnitude of pain relief (Chow et al. 2007; Steenland et al. 1999; Hartsell et al. 2005; Yarnold 1999).

In the Dutch Bone Metastasis Study, 1171 patients with painful bone metastases were randomized to receive 8 Gy in a single fraction or 24 Gy/6 (Steenland et al. 1999). The overall pain relief, time to response, and toxicity rates were similar in both arms. The single-fraction arm had a higher rate of retreatment (25%) in comparison to the multiple-fraction arm (7%). In the RTOG 9714 trial, 898 patients with breast or prostate cancer and painful bone metastases were randomized to receive 8 Gy in a single fraction or 30 Gy/10 (Hartsell et al. 2005). The complete and partial pain relief, narcotic use rate, and pathologic fracture were similar in both arms. There was a higher rate of acute toxicity in the multiple-fraction arm (17%) in comparison to the single-fraction arm (10%). Also, the single-fraction arm had a higher rate of retreatment (18%) in comparison to the multiple-fraction arm (9%). In the Bone Pain Trial Working Party study, 765 patients with painful bone metastases were randomized to receive 8 Gy in a single fraction, 20 Gy/5 or 30 Gy/10 (Yarnold 1999). The overall pain response rate and time to response were similar in all three arms. The single-fraction arm had a higher rate of retreatment (23%) in comparison to the multiple-fraction arm (10%).

The findings of these three RCT were confirmed in a meta-analysis by Chow et al., which included data from 16 RCT (Chow et al. 2007). There were no differences in overall pain response rate, acute toxicities, pathologic fracture rate, or spinal cord compression rate between single-fraction and multiple-fraction treatment. Single-fraction treatment was associated with a higher rate of retreatment (20%) in comparison to multiple-fraction treatment (8%). Regarding the optimal single-fraction dose, results from another systematic review by Dennis et al. suggest that doses below 8 Gy have inferior response rates and higher rates of retreatment (Dennis et al. 2013).

Since many of the randomized bone metastasis fractionation studies included patients with spinal metastases, it is reasonable to also consider single-fraction RT for patients with spine metastases. The clinical outcomes for spine and nonspine bone metastases appear to be similar in terms of survival and response rates (Roos et al. 2005). However, Roos et al. reported a statistically significant difference in time to treatment failure (3.5 months vs. 2.2 months) favoring spine bone metastases vs. nonspine bone metastases receiving radiotherapy (Roos et al. 2005).

It is also important to note that the randomized bone metastasis fractionation studies excluded patients with complicated bone metastases. While the literature has not maintained a unified definition of the term "complicated," this category has often included metastases associated with impeding/existing pathologic fracture or existing spinal cord or cauda equina compression (Cheon et al. 2015). It is unclear if single- and multiple-fraction treatments are equivalent in patients with impending cord compression, pathologic fracture, or neuropathic pain. For example, in patients with uncomplicated bone metastases, spinal cord compression rates after multi-fraction RT have been reported as 5.7% vs. 4.1% for single fraction (OR = 1.40, 95% CI = 0.73–2.67) (Chow et al. 2012). For patients with neuropathic pain, fractionated RT may be preferred due to a trend towards decreased time to treatment failure: 3.7 months vs. 2.4 months ($p = 0.056$) (Roos et al. 2005).

5.1.2 Retreatment

Retreatment of bone metastases is a feasible and effective approach for recurrent pain or progressive disease. In a meta-analysis of 2694 patients undergoing reirradiation, Huisman et al. demonstrated an overall pain response rate of 58% (Huisman et al. 2012). The National Cancer Institute of Canada (NCIC) SC-20 study, a noninferiority phase III RCT, investigated the optimal prescription dose for patients requiring retreatment (Chow et al. 2014). Eight-hundred and fifty patients with painful bone metastases were randomized to receive retreatment with 8 Gy in a single fraction or 20 Gy in multiple fractions. For the 20 Gy arm, the treatment was given over eight fractions if the metastasis was in the spine or pelvis and patients previously received multiple-fraction treatment to this area. Otherwise the 20 Gy was delivered over five fractions. Overall, 48% of patients who received their assigned treatment had reduced pain at the site of repeat radiation or reduced need for opioid analgesia. There was no statistically significant difference in the rate of pain relief on intention-to-treat analysis (28% for 8 Gy vs. 32% for 20 Gy) or per-protocol analysis (45% for 8 Gy vs. 51% for 20 Gy). However the findings were not robust on per-protocol analysis, as the upper limit of the 95% CI was greater than the prespecified noninferiority margin. Also, there was a higher rate of acute toxicity in the 20 Gy arm in comparison to the 8 Gy arm. The overall conclusion of the trial was that retreatment with 8 Gy in a single fraction seems to be noninferior and less toxic than 20 Gy/5. However, given that the findings were not robust on the per-protocol analysis, the authors acknowledge that a small percentage of patients may benefit from repeat treatment with multiple fractions.

5.1.3 Postoperative radiotherapy

Regarding pathologic or impending fractures, there is a paucity of literature to guide the use of postoperative radiotherapy. In a retrospective review of 64 surgical stabilization cases from the University of Kansas, the use of PORT was associated with better functional outcomes on multivariate analysis (Townsend et al. 1995). The patients who received radiation were at lower risk of requiring a second orthopedic procedure (15% vs. 2%) and had a better likelihood of regaining normal function (53% vs. 11.5%). Also the median survival in the cohort receiving surgery and radiation (12.4 months) was higher than the surgery-alone arm (3.2 months). However the results of the study need to be interpreted with caution due to the small sample size, retrospective study design, and potential selection biases.

In a more recent review of 82 postoperative radiotherapy cases, the patterns of local failure were investigated (Epstein-Peterson et al. 2015). The median BED was 39 Gy in ten fractions and the radiation fields covered an average of 71% of the hardware. On multivariate analysis, decreased coverage of surgical hardware and greater time between surgery and EBRT were statistically significant predictors for increased risk of local failure. The optimal dose fractionation for PORT is unknown. From a prospective RCT of 107 patients with bone metastases, patients who received 30 Gy in ten fractions had better remineralization as measured on CT in comparison to patients who received 8 Gy/1 (Koswig and Budach 1999). It is unknown whether the degree of remineralization is associated with better clinical outcomes. In the absence of the high-quality data, we recommend a course of fractionated treatment for PORT to optimize functional outcomes and decrease the risk of local failure.

5.1.4 SBRT

With regard to SBRT, the majority of published reports mainly include data from treatment to spine metastases (Bhattacharya and Hoskin 2015). The available data are heterogeneous and include retrospective reviews and phase I/II data with a phase III trial under way (De Bari et al. 2016). Symptomatic improvement/control is reported in the range of 80–90% (De Bari et al. 2016) with the largest retrospective review ($n = 393$) reporting long-term pain improvement in 86% of cases (Gerszten et al. 2007). Radiographic improvement/control at 1 year is reported in the range of 70–90% (De Bari et al.

2016) with phase I/II data reporting 1-year free-dom from imaging-documented failure of 84% (Chang et al. 2007). Of the recurrences after SBRT, approximately half were documented in the epidural space likely due to underdosing of the tumor secondary to spinal cord constraints. However, 17.9% of recurrences were seen in the pedicles and posterior elements of the spine (areas often included within EBRT but not SBRT) (Chang et al. 2007). Reported median survival for patients receiving spine SBRT from phase I/II trials was 30 months (Garg et al. 2012). While this number is significantly higher than seen with EBRT, these patients are often highly selected.

Spinal SBRT may be delivered as single-fraction or multiple-fraction regimens including 16–24 Gy in a single fraction, 21–27 Gy/3, or 30–35 Gy/5 (Lutz et al. 2012). While there are no RCT comparing dose fractionation in spinal SBRT, one multicenter retrospective review com-pared results for single-fraction and multiple-fraction spinal SBRT. For single-fraction spinal SBRT, higher rates of pain control were seen (100% vs. 88%, $p = 0.003$) (Heron et al. 2012). However, multiple-fraction spinal SBRT had lower rates of retreatment (1% vs. 13%, $p < 0.001$), higher 2-year local control (96% vs. 70%, $p = 0.001$), and greater 1-year OS (63% vs. 46%, $p = 0.002$) (Heron et al. 2012). Rates of toxicity in this review were similar for both single- and mul-tiple-fraction SBRT. The authors concluded that, given the retrospective nature of this study and dif-ferences in tumor histology between single-frac-tion and multiple-fraction group, no fractionation schedule could be recommended over another (Heron et al. 2012). In the largest retrospective review of spinal SBRT using single-fraction RT with a maximum tumor dose of 15–22.5 Gy, the authors concluded that maximum tumor dose of 20 Gy or 16 Gy to the tumor margin provides good tumor control (Gerszten et al. 2007).

In one series of 74 patients with oligometastatic disease, 85 nonspine bone metastases were treated with SBRT (Owen et al. 2014). The series con-tained a range of prescription doses; the most com-mon regimens were 24 Gy in one fraction, 18 Gy in one fraction, or 30 Gy in three fractions. The local control rate at 1 year was 92% with a median time to local failure of 2.8 months. At a median follow-up of 7.6 months, the median SBRT-specific over-all survival and progression-free survival were 9.3 months and 9.7 months, respectively. Eighteen patients developed acute toxicities, mainly grade 1/2 fatigue and pain flare, and nine patients devel-oped late grade 1/2 toxicities. There were no late grade 3/4 toxicities reported. Two patients devel-oped asymptomatic pathologic fractures.

5.2 Spinal Cord Compression

Radiation therapy is a highly effective treatment for MSCC. Approximately 60–80% of patients will have an improvement in back pain and the majority of patients maintain/improve ambula-tory function (Maranzano and Latini 1995; Maranzano et al. 2005). For patients who are ambulatory pretreatment, approximately 80% of patients will maintain their ambulatory function, whereas in patients who are not ambulatory prior to treatment, only one-third of patients are able to regain their ambulatory status (Maranzano and Latini 1995). Tumor type, interval between tumor diagnosis and MSCC, presence of visceral metas-tases, pre-RT motor function, and time of devel-oping motor deficits before RT have all found to be predictive for posttreatment ambulatory func-tion (Rades et al. 2008b, 2011a).

In the landmark trial comparing decompres-sive surgery and radiotherapy vs. radiotherapy alone from Patchell et al., the interim analysis showed that the clinical outcomes in the decom-pressive surgery and radiotherapy arm were bet-ter and the study was closed early (Patchell et al. 2005). In 101 patients, ambulatory rate, duration of ambulatory status, and survival were better in the arm treated with surgery and radiotherapy. This trial included patients with an expected life expectancy >3 months and excluded patients with paraplegia of >48 h and patients with radio-sensitive tumors. Due to the small sample size of the trial and issues with the trial design, a recent matched pair analysis was performed by Rades et al. (2010a). Surgery and radiation in 108 patients were compared with radiation alone in 216 patients. There were no differences in ambulatory outcomes, local control, or survival between the two arms. The results of this matched pair study support the use of radiotherapy alone as an alternative to combination treatment with surgery and radiotherapy, particularly for nonradioresistant histology.

The median survival of all patients presenting with MSCC is 3–6 months (Cole and Patchell 2008). To better predict life expectancy in patients with MSCC, Rades et al. proposed a scoring system based on six clinical factors found to be prognostic on multivariate analysis (Rades et al. 2006a, 2008c): primary tumor type, presence of other bone metastases, presence of visceral metastases, interval from tumor diagnosis to MSCC, ambulatory status before radiotherapy, and time to develop motor deficits before radiotherapy (see Table 6). The scoring system was externally validated and simplified to include three prognostic categories (Rades et al. 2010b): 20–30 points (14% 6-month survival), 31–35 points (56% 6-month survival), and 36–45 points (80% 6-month survival).

Table 6 MSCC prognostic scoring criteria

Factors	Score
Type of primary tumor	
Breast cancer	8
Prostate cancer	7
Myeloma/lymphoma	9
Lung cancer	3
Other tumors	4
Other bone metastases at the time of RT	
Yes	5
No	7
Visceral metastases at the time of RT	
Yes	2
No	8
Interval from tumor diagnosis to MSCC	
≤15 months	4
>15 months	7
Ambulatory status before RT	
Ambulatory	7
Nonambulatory	3
Time to develop motor deficits before RT	
1–7 days	3
8–14 days	6
>14 days	8

For conventional EBRT, there is evidence to suggest that the choice of fractionation can by guided by the life expectancy of the patient. For patients with a poor prognosis, shorted fractionation regimens may produce equivalent results to protracted fractionation schemes. At least three phase III RCT have addressed this question. Maranzano et al. compared a single 8 Gy treatment vs. 16 Gy/2 for treating MSCC in 327 patients with expected prognosis ≤3 months (Maranzano et al. 2009). Both schedules were found to be equally effective in terms of duration of response and median overall survival. In another similar trial, Maranzano et al. compared short-course RT (16 Gy/2) vs. split-course RT (30 Gy in 8 fractions; 5 Gy × 3 + 3 Gy × 5) for treating MSCC in 300 patients with expected prognosis ≤6 months (Maranzano et al. 2005). Both schedules were found to be equally effective in terms of response rate, duration of response, ambulatory rate, survival, or toxicities. In another third trial, Rades et al. compared 20 Gy/5 vs. 30 Gy/10 for treating MSCC in 203 patients in patients with ≤35 points on the MSCC life expectancy model (Rades et al. 2016); the median survival of patients in the trial was 3.2 months. There was no difference in response rates, ambulatory outcomes, progression-free survival, or overall survival between the two arms.

Conversely there is a smaller body of evidence to suggest that patients with a favorable prognosis may benefit from a longer course of radiotherapy (at least 30 Gy in ten fractions). For example, in a prospective, nonrandomized trial of 265 patients treated with radiotherapy alone for MSCC, longer course radiotherapy was associated with a 1-year local control of 81% in comparison to 61% for short-course radiotherapy (Rades et al. 2011b). In a retrospective case-matched analysis of 382 patients with a favorable prognosis, dose escalation beyond 30 Gy in ten fractions to 37.5 Gy/15 or 40 Gy/20 was associated with improved local control, progression-free survival, and overall survival (Rades et al. 2011c). Also from other retrospective data, patients with a favorable prognosis (Rades prognostic score >36) or oligometastatic disease seemed to have a survival benefit with longer course radiotherapy (Rades et al. 2008c, 2006b).

5.3 Brain Metastases

The MS for patients with brain metastases receiving WBRT is estimated between 3 and 6 months (Priestman et al. 1996; Graham et al. 2010). Survival for patients undergoing WBRT has been reviewed in the context of dose and fractionation with a range treatment options available. A meta-analysis of three RCT (Priestman et al. 1996; Chatani et al. 1994; Harwood and Simpson 1977) compared BED10 <39 Gy (20 Gy/5, 10 Gy/1, or 12 Gy/2) to BED10 = 39 Gy (30 Gy/10) demonstrating a significant improvement in OS (HR = 1.21, 95% CI = 1.04–1.40, p = 0.001) favoring the BED10 = 39 Gy arm (Tsao et al. 2012). One of the included RCT did not conclude a statistical improvement in MS with higher BED10 (132 days vs. 121 days (30 Gy/10 vs. 10 Gy/1), p = 0.082) (Harwood and Simpson 1977), while another concluded that the main benefit was seen for patients patients with favorable disease biology (88 days vs. 72 days) (30 Gy/10 vs. 12 Gy/2; p = 0.04) (Priestman et al. 1996). Two seminal phase III studies, RTOG 6901 and RTOG 7361, examined dose escalation for palliative WBRT (40 Gy/20, 40 Gy/15, 30 Gy/15, 20 Gy/10 and 40 Gy/20, 30 Gy/10, 20 Gy/5, respectively) concluding no overall survival advantage for any of the dose fractionation groups compared (Harwood and Simpson 1977). Two more recent RCT comparing 40 Gy in 20 fractions BID vs. 20 Gy/4–5 did not show a statistically significant difference in MS (6.1 months vs. 6.6 months; p = 0.65) (Graham et al. 2010) and (19.1 weeks vs. 19.1 weeks; p = 0.418) (Davey et al. 2008).

Significant clinical response to WBRT occurs in 60–90% of patients (Markesbery et al. 1978). However, it is estimated that 57% of patients receiving WBRT will experience intracranial progression (Lagerwaard et al. 1999). Dose and fractionation may impact both time to progression and the rate of in-brain recurrence.

Comparing 40 Gy in 20 fractions BID vs. 20 Gy/5, intracranial progression was 44% vs. 64% (p = 0.03) and death attributed to CNS progression was 32% vs. 52% (p = 0.03) (Graham et al. 2010). Similarly, the time to retreatment for intracranial relapse was 32 weeks for patients treated with 40 Gy/20 BID compared to 14 weeks for patients treated with 20 Gy/5 (p = 0.03) (Davey et al. 2008).

Overall, patients with well-controlled or absent extracranial disease, good performance status, and favorable disease biology, higher dose, and fractionation schedules (ex. 30 Gy/10, 40 Gy/20 BID) should be considered to reduce rates of intracranial progression and time to intracranial progression.

Typically SRS is delivered as a single fraction, although the treatment may be fractionated. The RTOG 9005 trial investigated the safety of single-fraction SRS for patients with recurrent brain tumors (including both metastases and primary brain tumors). Similarly RTOG 9508 utilized a similar treatment schedule for patients receiving an SRS boost (in addition to 37.5 Gy/15 WBRT) (Patchell et al. 1998). Doses were compared for BM and OS and found similar for all three. However, those receiving 24 Gy had a significantly lower rate of local failure (Vogelbaum et al. 2006). The authors concluded that for patients with lesions ≤2 cm, local control (LC) was significantly better. They also noted that the dose limit for treating lesions >2 cm should be weighed carefully (Vogelbaum et al. 2006). A systematic review of 11 trials including both single- and multi-fractionated SRS for BM concluded that a BED12 of ≥40 Gy (20 Gy/1, 23.2 Gy/2, 25.5 Gy/3) should be preferentially applied to achieve a higher rate of 1-year LC (Wiggenraad et al. 2011). Recognizing limitations with retrospective review and prescription preferences (which may be related to lesion size), adjusted linear quadratic modeling, and isodose specifications (gamma knife dose is typically specified to the 50% isodose whereas linear accelerator series to 80–100%), 1-year LC was excellent (80%) for SRS dose >20 Gy but <50% for SRS dose ≤15 Gy (Wiggenraad et al. 2011). Isodose prescription points may play an important role in local control as seen in RTOG 9005 where patients treated on a linear accelerator were 2.84 more times likely to have local failure (LF) compared to patients treated with a gamma knife (Shaw et al. 2000). Overall survival for patients did not appear to be influenced by dose or treatment delivery system (isodose prescription point) (Andrews et al. 2004).

Lesions >3–4 cm have represented a treatment challenge for SRS. In RTOG 9005 lesions >4 cm were not treated due to concerns of unacceptable toxicity (Shaw et al. 2000). Two retrospective reviews concluded that for larger lesions or lesions in eloquent areas, fractionated SRS was well tolerated (Wegner et al. 2015; Kim et al. 2011). Wegner et al. found that the median prescription dose was 24 Gy/2–5 with a 1-year PFS of 63% with no patients experiencing acute or late toxicity associated with SRS (Wegner et al. 2015). Kim et al. found a 1-year PFS of 69% utilizing fractionated SRS (36 Gy in six fractions) with a 5% rate of toxicity (significantly lower than the group eligible for single-fraction SRS (17%, $p = 0.05$) (Kim et al. 2011).

In summary, single-fraction SRS doses >20 Gy may be associated with a higher rate of LC, although treatment of lesions >2 cm may be limited by toxicity concerns. Treatment for lesions 2–3 cm may be treated with single-fraction SRS while tumors >3 cm may be considered for fractionated SRS or surgery to reduce toxicity concerns.

6 Complications and Management

6.1 Bone Metastases

Toxicities after conventional palliative EBRT vary depending on the site of metastases but can commonly include side effects such as pain flare, fatigue, loss of appetite, nausea, esophagitis, diarrhea, radiation dermatitis, and pathologic fracture. Most of the reported acute side effects are mild (grade 1/2) and are managed expectantly. For example, Roos et al. documented toxicity for 87% of evaluable patients with both grade 3 GI toxicity and grade 3 pulmonary toxicity seen in approximately 1% of patients (Roos et al. 2005). Pain flare refers to the temporary worsening of pain at the treated site and usually occurs within 10 days of completing radiotherapy (Hird et al. 2009). The reported incidence of pain flare ranges from 2 to 44% after conventional EBRT and 10 to 68% for SBRT (McDonald et al. 2014). A recent phase III RCT showed that in patients receiving single-fraction palliative radiotherapy to painful bone metastases, the use of dexamethasone 8 mg/day for 5 days reduced the rate of pain flare from 35 to 26% (Chow et al. 2015). Therefore dexamethasone seems to be an effective prophylaxis for the prevention of pain flare.

The development of late toxicities is rare and usually is a consequence of overlapping, prior radiation treatment. Although the RTOG 9714 trial showed a higher rate of acute toxicity with multiple-fraction treatment, the meta-analysis by Chow et al. did not suggest that there was a difference between single-fraction and multiple-fraction radiotherapy (Chow et al. 2007; Hartsell et al. 2005). In the retreatment setting, the use of the multiple fractions is associated with a high rate of acute toxicity based on the results of the NCIC SC20 trial (Chow et al. 2014).

With higher biological doses used in SBRT, there is also a higher risk of potentially serious complications such as vertebral fracture and radiation myelopathy after treatment to the spine (De Bari et al. 2016). The possible mechanism of vertebral fracture postradiotherapy is proposed to be related to osteoradionecrosis (Sahgal et al. 2013a). A multi-institutional analysis found the incidence to be 14% (47% new fractures and 53% were fracture progression) with median time to presentation being 2.46 months and risk of fracture associated with radiation doses ≥20 Gy/1 fraction (Sahgal et al. 2013b). The spinal instability neoplastic scoring (SINS), as detailed in Table 7, may be utilized to predict patients at highest risk of vertebral compression fracture postspinal SBRT (Sahgal et al. 2013b; Fisher et al. 2010). Percutaneous cement augmentation may be considered prior to spinal

Table 7 Spine Instability Neoplastic Score (SINS)

SINS component	Score
Location	
Junctional (occiput—C2, C7-T2, T11-L1, L5-S1	3
Mobile spine (C3-C6, L2-L4)	2
Semirigid (T3-T10)	1
Rigid (S2-S5)	0
Pain	
Yes	3
Occasional pain but not mechanical	1
Pain-free lesion	0
Bone lesion	
Lytic	2
Mixed (lytic/blastic)	1
Blastic	0
Radiographic spinal alignment	
Subluxation/translation present	4
De novo deformity (kyphosis/scoliosis)	2
Normal alignment	0
Vertebral body collapse	
>50% collapse	3
<50% collapse	2
No collapse with >50% body involved	1
None of the above	0
Posterolateral involvement of spinal elements	
Bilateral	3
Unilateral	1
None of the above	0

SBRT for patients at high risk of compression fracture (Jawad et al. 2016).

Phase I/II data have reported fairly low rates of radiation myelopathy. Ryu et al. reported no incidence of radiation myelopathy in 44 treated patients while Garg et al. reported two cases in 66 treated patients (Ryu et al. 2014; Garg et al. 2012). Of the patients experiencing radiation myelopathy, one patient was prescribed 24 Gy and had a maximum nerve root dose of 14.67 Gy while another was prescribed 18 Gy and had a maximum cord dose of 12.67 Gy (Garg et al. 2012). The American Association of Physicists in Medicine (AAPM) recommends limiting the dose for single-fraction spinal SBRT to <0.35 cc to a threshold dose of 10 Gy (14 Gy point max); or for three-fraction SBRT, a threshold dose of 18 Gy (23.4 Gy point max); or for five fractions

of SBRT a threshold dose of 23 Gy (31 Gy point max) (Benedict et al. 2010).

The rate of pain flare with SBRT may be higher than reported with EBRT. For example, Chiang et al. reported a rate of pain flare of 68.3% of 41 patients investigated, with 85% of these patients experiencing improvement in symptoms when initiated on dexamethasone (4 mg daily while on RT and 5 days thereafter) (Chiang et al. 2013). Prophylactic dexamethasone for patients receiving spinal SBRT was investigated in a single-center prospective trial. The total incidence of reported pain flare was 19% and the authors recommend considering prophylaxis for patients receiving spinal SBRT (Khan et al. 2015).

6.2 Spinal Cord Compression

EBRT for MSCC is usually well tolerated and the side effect profile is dependent on the location of the spine that is being irradiated. If the esophagus or pharynx is in the radiation field, patients may develop acute esophagitis or pharyngitis. If the stomach or small bowel is in the radiation field, transient nausea/vomiting may occur. If the large bowel or rectum is in the radiation field, diarrhea may occur. Cumulative doses to the spinal cord above 120 Gy2 BED increase the risk of spinal cord myelopathy (Nieder et al. 2006). Results from the recent SCORE-2 RCT do not report any acute grade 3/4 toxicity or late complications in patients undergoing a fractionated course of RT for MSCC (Rades et al. 2016). Results from a previous RCT by Maranzano et al. showed a 1.5% rate of grade 3 esophagitis or pharyngitis, a 1.5% rate of grade 3 diarrhea, and a 6% rate of vomiting or nausea (Maranzano et al. 2005). No late toxicities were observed in this study as well.

6.3 Brain Metastases

General acute toxicities seen for BM patients receiving WBRT include hair loss, headaches, nausea, fatigue, and worsening neurological symptoms (Mulvenna et al. 2016). Long term, neurocognition after radiotherapy is of concern. Radiotherapy may impact memory and learning on standardized cognitive tests (Chang et al. 2009) and patient reported reduced outcomes in domains of attention and motivation (Cole et al. 2013). However, it should be noted that progressive intracranial lesions are associated with high morbidity and mortality. The Mini-Mental State Examination (MMSE) score for patients receiving WBRT overall may demonstrate a significant decline at 3 months after completing radiotherapy (MMSE drop of 0.5 vs. 6.3, $p = 0.02$) (Regine et al. 2001).

Neurocognitive decline has been investigated in the setting of different radiotherapy schedules and techniques. Comparing patients receiving 30 Gy in ten fractions vs. 54.4 Gy/34 BID, there was no significant difference in MMSE drop 3 months after WBRT (1.1 vs. 1.3) (Cole et al. 2013). Similarly, in a meta-analysis comparing relative biologic effect (RBE) of equivalent doses >39 Gy vs. RBE = 39 Gy, there was no significant difference in neurological function after WBRT (OR = 1.14, 95% CI 0.92–1.42, $p = 0.23$). However, when comparing BED10 = 39 Gy (30 Gy/10) vs. BED10 <39 Gy there was a statistically significant improvement in neurological function favoring 30 Gy/10 (OR = 1.74, 95% CI 1.06–2.84, $p = 0.03$) (Tsao et al. 2012).

Stereotactic radiosurgery is associated with less deterioration in domains of memory and learning on standardized neurocognitive testing compared to patients receiving WBRT. The Hopkins Verbal Learning Test-Revised (HVLT-R) was utilized to compare patients randomized to either SRS alone or SRS and WBRT (Chang et al. 2009). At 4 months, total recall decline in function was higher in the WBRT group with mean posterior probability of decline of 52% compared to 24% in the group receiving SRS alone. Patient factors and preferences in the context of these results should be considered when discussing treatment options.

Hippocampal radiotherapy-sparing techniques have been of recent interest in an attempt to preserve cognitive functioning for patients receiving WBRT. Results from RTOG 0933, a phase II trial on hippocampal dose sparing in WBRT, demonstrated that, at 4 months post-WBRT on the HVLT-R, there was a mean relative decline in recall of 7.0% (95% CI = −4.7–18.7%), significantly lower than historical controls (Gondi et al. 2014). However, in a review of 20 BM patients treated with hippocampal dose sparing, 2 patients had developed new metastases in the area of sparing (Oehlke et al. 2015).

Radionecrosis is a debilitating concern with RT seen more frequently with single-fraction SRS. The rate of radionecrosis reported in RTOG 9005 had an increasing incidence over time with rates of 5%, 8%, 9%, and 11% at 6, 12, 18, and 24 months, respectively (Shaw et al. 2000). Rates of reported radionecrosis are variable. Minniti et al. reported an incidence of symptomatic necrosis as 10% and asymptomatic necrosis as 14% with median time to presentation at 10–11 months (Minniti et al. 2011). The authors found a correlation of dose and volume where lesions with V12 Gy >8.5 cm^3 had a significantly higher rate of necrosis (Minniti et al. 2011).

Recognition and management of radionecrosis presents a clinical challenge. It can be difficult to discern between tumor progression and radionecrosis both clinically and on imaging. Patients may present with generalized neurologic deficits due to mass effect and edema such as headache and somnolence or focal neurological deficits (Fink et al. 2012). Both radionecrosis and tumor progression may manifest as a ring-enhancing mass and edema on T2-weighted MRI (Chao et al. 2013). The use of T1/T2 mismatch MRI sequences may be helpful to differentiate recurrence from necrosis. Other potential emerging technologies for diagnosing radionecrosis include PET, thallium-201 SPECT, and MRS (Chao et al. 2013). The clinical course of radionecrosis may be irreversible and progress over time to destructive necrosis, small vessel arteriopathy, and stroke (Fink et al. 2012). Management options include steroids, antiplatelet agents, anticoagulant agents, hyperbaric oxygen, surgical resection, or bevacizumab (Giglio and Gilbert 2003; Gonzalez et al. 2007). Steroids remain the standard of care to control edema but side effects need to be considered (Gonzalez et al. 2007). In a review of 11 patients with BM treated with bevacizumab (7.5–15 mg/kg q2–6 weeks), 64% of patients had improvement in symptoms and all patients were able to clinically taper steroids. No patients experienced an intratumoral bleed (a severe adverse event potentially associated with bevacizumab) (Boothe et al. 2013).

7 Summary

Alternate fractionation is a particularly attractive option in advanced cancer patients due to the convenience of shorter treatments and less disruption of patient life. Hypo-fractionated radiotherapy can be given using standard techniques and conventional prescription doses, or the radiotherapy can be delivered in high dose per fraction using precise, "stereotactic" techniques. In this chapter we reviewed the evidence, indications, and technique for both paradigms of hypofractionation in palliative radiotherapy to brain metastases, spinal cord compression, and skeletal metastases.

References

Al-Omair A, Masucci L, Masson-Cote L et al (2013) Surgical resection of epidural disease improves local control following postoperative spine stereotactic body radiotherapy. Neuro-oncol 15(10):1413–1419

Andrews DW, Scott CB, Sperduto PW et al (2004) Whole brain radiation therapy with or without stereotactic radiosurgery boost for patients with one to three brain metastases: phase III results of the RTOG 9508 randomised trial. Lancet 363(9422):1665–1672

Aoyama H, Shirato H, Tago M, et al. Stereotactic radiosurgery plus whole-brain radiation therapy vs stereotactic radiosurgery alone for treatment of brain metastases: a randomized controlled trial. JAMA 2006;295(21):2483–2491.

Benedict SH, Yenice KM, Followill D et al (2010) Stereotactic body radiation therapy: the report of AAPM Task Group 101. Med Phys 37(8):4078–4101

Bhattacharya I, Hoskin P (2015) Stereotactic body radiotherapy for spinal and bone metastases. Clin Oncol 27(5):298–306

Boothe D, Young R, Yamada Y et al (2013) Bevacizumab as a treatment for radiation necrosis of brain metastases post stereotactic radiosurgery. Neuro-oncol 15(9):1257–1263

Borgelt B, Gelber R, Kramer S et al (1980) The palliation of brain metastases: final results of the first two studies by the Radiation Therapy Oncology Group. Int J Radiat Oncol Biol Phys 6(1):1–9

Brown PD, Jaeckle K, Ballman KV et al (2016) Effect of radiosurgery alone vs radiosurgery with whole brain radiation therapy on cognitive function in patients with 1 to 3 brain metastases: a randomized clinical trial. JAMA 316(4):401–409

Campos S, Presutti R, Zhang L et al (2010) Elderly patients with painful bone metastases should be offered palliative radiotherapy. Int J Radiat Oncol Biol Phys 76(5):1500–1506

Chang EL, Shiu AS, Mendel E et al (2007) Phase I/II study of stereotactic body radiotherapy for spinal metastasis and its pattern of failure. J Neurosurg Spine 2:151–160

Chang EL, Wefel JS, Hess KR et al (2009) Neurocognition in patients with brain metastases treated with radiosurgery or radiosurgery plus whole-brain irradiation: a randomised controlled trial. Lancet Oncol 10(11):1037–1044

Chang U-K, Cho W-I, Kim M-S et al (2012) Local tumor control after retreatment of spinal metastasis using stereotactic body radiotherapy: comparison with initial treatment group. Acta Oncol 51(5):589–595

Chao ST, Koyfman SA, Woody N et al (2012) Recursive partitioning analysis index is predictive for overall survival in patients undergoing spine stereotactic body radiation therapy for spinal metastases. Int J Radiat Oncol Biol Phys 82(5):1738–1743

Chao ST, Ahluwalia MS, Barnett GH et al (2013) Challenges with the diagnosis and treatment of cerebral radiation necrosis. Int J Radiat Oncol Biol Phys 87(3):449–457

Chatani M, Matayoshi Y, Masaki N et al (1994) Radiation therapy for brain metastases from lung carcinoma. Prospective randomized trial according to the level of lactate dehydrogenase. Strahlenther Onkol 170(3):155–161

Cheon PM, Wong E, Thavarajah N et al (2015) A definition of "uncomplicated bone metastases" based on previous bone metastases radiation trials comparing single-fraction and multi-fraction radiation therapy. J Bone Oncol 4(1):13–17

Chiang A, Zeng L, Zhang L et al (2013) Pain flare is a common adverse event in steroid-naive patients after spine stereotactic body radiation therapy: a prospective clinical trial. Int J Radiat Oncol Biol Phys 86(4):638–642

Choi J, Raghavan M (2012) Diagnostic imaging and image-guided therapy of skeletal metastases. Cancer Control. 19(2):102–112

Chow E, Harris K, Fan G et al (2007) Palliative radiotherapy trials for bone metastases: a systematic review. J Clin Oncol 25(11):1423–1436

Chow E, Zeng L, Salvo N et al (2012) Update on the systematic review of palliative radiotherapy trials for bone metastases. J Clin Oncol 24(2):112–124

Chow E, van der Linden YM, Roos D et al (2014) Single versus multiple fractions of repeat radiation for painful bone metastases: a randomised, controlled, noninferiority trial. Lancet Oncol 15(2):164–171

Chow E, Meyer RM, Ding K et al (2015) Dexamethasone in the prophylaxis of radiation-induced pain flare after palliative radiotherapy for bone metastases: a double-blind, randomised placebo-controlled, phase 3 trial. Lancet Oncol 16(15):1463–1472

Cole JS, Patchell RA (2008) Metastatic epidural spinal cord compression. Lancet Neurol 7(5):459–466

Cole AM, Scherwath A, Ernst G et al (2013) Self-reported cognitive outcomes in patients with brain metastases before and after radiation therapy. Int J Radiat Oncol Biol Phys 87(4):705–712

Cox BW, Spratt DE, Lovelock M et al (2012) International Spine Radiosurgery Consortium consensus guidelines for target volume definition in spinal stereotactic radiosurgery. Int J Radiat Oncol Biol Phys 83(5):e597–e605

Damron T, Sim F (1999) Surgical treatment for metastatic disease of the pelvis and the proximal end of the femur. Instruct Course Lect 49:461–470

Davey P, Hoegler D, Ennis M et al (2008) A phase III study of accelerated versus conventional hypofractionated whole brain irradiation in patients of good performance status with brain metastases not suitable for surgical excision. Radiother Oncol 88(2):173–176

De Bari B, Alongi F, Mortellaro G et al (2016) Spinal metastases: Is stereotactic body radiation therapy supported by evidences? Crit Rev Oncol Hematol 98:147–158

Delattre JY, Krol G, Thaler HT, Posner JB (1988) Distribution of brain metastases. Arch Neurol 45(7):741–744

Dennis K, Makhani L, Zeng L et al (2013) Single fraction conventional external beam radiation therapy for bone metastases: a systematic review of randomised controlled trials. Radiother Oncol 106(1):5–14

Epstein-Peterson ZD, Sullivan A, Krishnan M et al (2015) Postoperative radiation therapy for osseous metastasis: outcomes and predictors of local failure. Pract Radiat Oncol 5(5):e531–e5e6

Fink J, Born D, Chamberlain MC (2012) Radiation necrosis: relevance with respect to treatment of primary and secondary brain tumors. Cur Neurol Neurosci Rep 12(3):276–285

Fisher CG, DiPaola CP, Ryken TC et al (2010) A novel classification system for spinal instability in neoplastic disease: an evidence-based approach and expert consensus from the Spine Oncology Study Group. Spine 35(22):E1221–E1229

Garg AK, Shiu AS, Yang J et al (2012) Phase 1/2 trial of single-session stereotactic body radiotherapy for previously unirradiated spinal metastases. Cancer 118(20):5069–5077

Gaspar L, Scott C, Rotman M et al (1997) Recursive partitioning analysis (RPA) of prognostic factors in three Radiation Therapy Oncology Group (RTOG) brain metastases trials. Int J Radiat Oncol Biol Phys 37(4):745–751

Gaspar LE, Scott C, Murray K, Curran W (2000) Validation of the RTOG recursive partitioning analysis (RPA) classification for brain metastases. Int J Radiat Oncol Biol Phys 47(4):1001–1006

Gerszten PC, Burton SA, Ozhasoglu C et al (2007) Radiosurgery for spinal metastases: clinical experience in 500 cases from a single institution. Spine 32(2):193–199

Giglio P, Gilbert MR (2003) Cerebral radiation necrosis. Neurologist 9(4):180–188

Godersky JC, Smoker WR, Knutzon R (1987) Use of magnetic resonance imaging in the evaluation of metastatic spinal disease. Neurosurgery 21(5):676–680

Gondi V, Pugh SL, Tome WA et al (2014) Preservation of memory with conformal avoidance of the hippocampal neural stem-cell compartment during whole-brain radiotherapy for brain metastases (RTOG 0933): a phase II multi-institutional trial. J Clin Oncol 32(34):3810–3816

Gonzalez J, Kumar AJ, Conrad CA et al (2007) Effect of bevacizumab on radiation necrosis of the brain. Int J Radiat Oncol Biol Phys 67(2):323–326

Graham P, Bucci J, Browne L (2010) Randomized comparison of whole brain radiotherapy, 20 Gy in four daily fractions versus 40 Gy in 20 twice-daily fractions, for brain metastases. Int J Radiat Oncol Biol Phys 77(3):648–654

Hagenau C, Grosh W, Currie M et al (1987) Comparison of spinal magnetic resonance imaging and myelography in cancer patients. J Clin Oncol 5(10):1663–1669

Hartsell WF, Scott CB, Bruner DW, Scarantino CW, Ivker RA, Roach M et al (2005) Randomized trial of short-versus long-course radiotherapy for palliation of painful bone metastases. J Natl Cancer Inst 97(11):798–804

Harwood AR, Simpson WJ (1977) Radiation therapy of cerebral metastases: a randomized prospective clinical trial. Int J Radiat Oncol Biol Phys 2(11):1091–1094

Heron DE, Rajagopalan MS, Stone B et al (2012) Single-session and multisession CyberKnife radiosurgery for spine metastases—University of Pittsburgh and Georgetown University experience: clinical article. J Neurosurg Spine 17(1):11–18

Hird A, Chow E, Zhang L et al (2009) Determining the incidence of pain flare following palliative radiotherapy for symptomatic bone metastases: results from three Canadian cancer centers. Int J Radiat Oncol Biol Phys 75(1):193–197

Huisman M, van den Bosch MA, Wijlemans JW et al (2012) Effectiveness of reirradiation for painful bone metastases: a systematic review and meta-analysis. Int J Radiat Oncol Biol Phys 84(1):8–14

Jawad MS, Fahim DK, Gerszten PC et al (2016) Vertebral compression fractures after stereotactic body radiation therapy: a large, multi-institutional, multinational evaluation. J Neurosurg Spine 24(6):928–936

Jeremic B, Shibamoto Y, Acimovic L et al (1998) A randomized trial of three single-dose radiation therapy regimens in the treatment of metastatic bone pain. Int J Radiat Oncol Biol Phys 42(1):161–167

Khan L, Chiang A, Zhang L et al (2015) Prophylactic dexamethasone effectively reduces the incidence of pain flare following spine stereotactic body radiotherapy (SBRT): a prospective observational study. Sup Care Cancer 23(10):2937–2943

Kim Y-J, Cho KH, Kim J-Y et al (2011) Single-dose versus fractionated stereotactic radiotherapy for brain metastases. Int J Radiat Oncol Biol Phys 81(2):483–489

Kirkpatrick JP, Wang Z, Sampson JH et al (2015) Defining the optimal planning target volume in image-guided stereotactic radiosurgery of brain metastases: results of a randomized trial. Int J Radiat Oncol Biol Phys 91(1):100–108

Klish DS, Grossman P, Allen PK et al (2011) Irradiation of spinal metastases: should we continue to include one uninvolved vertebral body above and below in the radiation field? Int J Radiat Oncol Biol Phys 81(5):1495–1499

Kocher M, Soffietti R, Abacioglu U et al (2011) Adjuvant whole-brain radiotherapy versus observation after radiosurgery or surgical resection of one to three cerebral metastases: results of the EORTC 22952-26001 study. J Clin Oncol 29(2):134–141

Koswig S, Budach V (1999) Remineralization and pain relief in bone metastases after after different radiotherapy fractions (10 times 3 Gy vs. 1 time 8 Gy). A prospective study. Strahlenther Onkol 175(10):500–508

Lagerwaard F, Levendag P, Nowak PC et al (1999) Identification of prognostic factors in patients with brain metastases: a review of 1292 patients. Int J Radiat Oncol Biol Phys 43(4):795–803

Laufer I, Rubin DG, Lis E et al (2013a) The NOMS framework: approach to the treatment of spinal metastatic tumors. Oncologist 18(6):744–751

Laufer I, Iorgulescu JB, Chapman T et al (2013b) Local disease control for spinal metastases following "separation surgery" and adjuvant hypofractionated or high-dose single-fraction stereotactic radiosurgery: outcome analysis in 186 patients: clinical article. J Neurosurg Spine 18(3):207–214

Loblaw DA, Perry J, Chambers A et al (2005) Systematic review of the diagnosis and management of malignant extradural spinal cord compression: the Cancer Care Ontario Practice Guidelines Initiative's Neuro-Oncology Disease Site Group. J Clin Oncol 23(9):2028–2037

Lutz S, Berk L, Chang E et al (2011) Palliative radiotherapy for bone metastases: an ASTRO evidence-based guideline. Int J Radiat Oncol Biol Phys 79(4):965–976

Lutz S-M, Lo SS-M, Chang EL et al (2012) ACR Appropriateness Criteria® non-spine bone metastases. J Pallat Med 15(5):521–526

Maranzano E, Latini P (1995) Effectiveness of radiation therapy without surgery in metastatic spinal cord compression: final results from a prospective trial. Int J Radiat Oncol Biol Phys 32(4):959–967

Maranzano E, Bellavita R, Rossi R et al (2005) Short-course versus split-course radiotherapy in metastatic spinal cord compression: results of a phase III, randomized, multicenter trial. J Clin Oncol 23(15):3358–3365

Maranzano E, Trippa F, Casale M et al (2009) 8Gy single-dose radiotherapy is effective in metastatic spinal cord compression: results of a phase III randomized multicentre Italian trial. Radiother Oncol 93(2):174–179

Markesbery WR, Brooks WH, Gupta GD et al (1978) Treatment for patients with cerebral metastases. Arch Neurol 35(11):754–756

McDonald R, Chow E, Rowbottom L et al (2014) Incidence of pain flare in radiation treatment of bone metastases: a literature review. J Bone Oncol 3(3):84–89

Meeuse JJ, van der Linden YM, van Tienhoven G et al (2010) Efficacy of radiotherapy for painful bone metastases during the last 12 weeks of life. Cancer 116(11):2716–2725

Mink AH, Kestle J, Rathbone MP et al (1996) A randomized trial to assess the efficacy of surgery in addition to radiotherapy in patients with a single cerebral metastasis. Cancer 78(7):1470–1476

Minniti G, Clarke E, Lanzetta G et al (2011) Stereotactic radiosurgery for brain metastases: analysis of outcome and risk of brain radionecrosis. Radiat Oncol 6(1):1

Mulvenna P, Nankivell M, Barton R (2016) Dexamethasone and supportive care with or without whole brain radiotherapy in treating patients with non-small cell lung cancer with brain metastases unsuitable for resection or stereotactic radiotherapy (QUARTZ): results from a phase 3, non-inferiority, randomised trial. Lancet 388(10055):2004–2014

Mundy GR (2002) Metastasis: metastasis to bone: Causes, consequences and therapeutic opportunities. Nat Rev Cancer 2(8):584–593

Nieder C, Grosu AL, Andratschke NH et al (2006) Update of human spinal cord reirradiation tolerance based on additional data from 38 patients. Int J Radiat Oncol Biol Phys 66(5):1446–1449

Nielsen OS, Munro A, Tannock I (1991) Bone metastases: pathophysiology and management policy. J Clin Oncol 9(3):509–524

Noël G, Simon JM, Valery C-A et al (2003) Radiosurgery for brain metastasis: impact of CTV on local control. Radiother Oncol 68(1):15–21

Nussbaum ES, Djalilian HR, Cho KH et al (1996) Brain metastases: histology, multiplicity, surgery, and survival. Cancer 78(8):1781–1788

Oehlke O, Wucherpfennig D, Fels F et al (2015) Whole brain irradiation with hippocampal sparing and dose escalation on multiple brain metastases. Strahlenther Onkol 191(6):461–469

Owen D, Laack NN, Mayo CS et al (2014) Outcomes and toxicities of stereotactic body radiation therapy for non-spine bone oligometastases. Pract Radiat Oncol 4(2):e143–e1e9

Pan H, Simpson DR, Mell LK et al (2011) A survey of stereotactic body radiotherapy use in the United States. Cancer 117(19):4566–4572

Papanastassiou ID, Phillips FM, Van Meirhaeghe J et al (2012) Comparing effects of kyphoplasty, vertebroplasty, and non-surgical management in a systematic review of randomized and non-randomized controlled studies. Eur Spine J 21(9):1826–1843

Patchell RA, Tibbs PA, Walsh JW et al (1990) A randomized trial of surgery in the treatment of single metastases to the brain. N Engl J Med 322(8):494–500

Patchell RA, Tibbs PA, Regine WF et al (1998) Postoperative radiotherapy in the treatment of single metastases to the brain: a randomized trial. JAMA 280(17):1485–1489

Patchell RA, Tibbs PA, Regine WF et al (2005) Direct decompressive surgical resection in the treatment of spinal cord compression caused by metastatic cancer: a randomised trial. Lancet 366(9486):643–648

Posner JB (1996) Brain metastases: 1995. A brief review. J Neuro-oncol 27(3):287–293

Priestman T, Dunn J, Brada M et al (1996) Final results of the Royal College of Radiologists' trial comparing two different radiotherapy schedules in the treatment of cerebral metastases. Clin Oncol 8(5):308–315

Rades D, Fehlauer F, Schulte R et al (2006a) Prognostic factors for local control and survival after radiotherapy of metastatic spinal cord compression. J Clin Oncol 24(21):3388–3393

Rades D, Veninga T, Stalpers LJ et al (2006b) Outcome after radiotherapy alone for metastatic spinal cord compression in patients with oligometastases. J Clin Oncol 25(1):50–56

Rades D, Rudat V, Veninga T et al (2008a) Prognostic factors for functional outcome and survival after reirradiation for in-field recurrences of metastatic spinal cord compression. Cancer 113(5):1090–1096

Rades D, Rudat V, Veninga T et al (2008b) A score predicting posttreatment ambulatory status in patients irradiated for metastatic spinal cord compression. Int J Radiat Oncol Biol Phys 72(3):905–908

Rades D, Dunst J, Schild SE (2008c) The first score predicting overall survival in patients with metastatic spinal cord compression. Cancer 112(1):157–161

Rades D, Huttenlocher S, Dunst J et al (2010a) Matched pair analysis comparing surgery followed by radiotherapy and radiotherapy alone for metastatic spinal cord compression. J Clin Oncol 28(22):3597–3604

Rades D, Douglas S, Veninga T et al (2010b) Validation and simplification of a score predicting survival in patients irradiated for metastatic spinal cord compression. Cancer 116(15):3670–3673

Rades D, Douglas S, Huttenlocher S et al (2011a) Validation of a score predicting post-treatment ambulatory status after radiotherapy for metastatic spinal cord compression. Int J Radiat Oncol Biol Phys 79(5):1503–1506

Rades D, Lange M, Veninga T et al (2011b) Final results of a prospective study comparing the local control of short-course and long-course radiotherapy for metastatic spinal cord compression. Int J Radiat Oncol Biol Phys 79(2):524–530

Rades D, Panzner A, Rudat V et al (2011c) Dose escalation of radiotherapy for metastatic spinal cord compression (MSCC) in patients with relatively favorable survival prognosis. Strahlenther Onkol 187(11):729–735

Rades D, Šegedin B, Conde-Moreno AJ et al (2016) Radiotherapy with 4 Gy× 5 versus 3 Gy× 10 for metastatic epidural spinal cord compression: final results of the SCORE-2 Trial (ARO 2009/01). J Clin Oncol 34(6):597–602

Regine W, Scott C, Murray K et al (2001) Neurocognitive outcome in brain metastases patients treated with accelerated-fractionation vs. accelerated-hyperfractionated radiotherapy: an analysis from Radiation Therapy Oncology Group Study 91-04. Int J Radiat Oncol Biol Phys 51(3):711–717

Roos DE, Turner SL, O'Brien PC et al (2005) Randomized trial of 8Gy in 1 versus 20Gy in 5 fractions of radiotherapy for neuropathic pain due to bone metastases (Trans-Tasman Radiation Oncology Group, TROG 96.05). Radiat Oncol 75(1):54–63

Ryu S, Rock J, Jain R et al (2010) Radiosurgical decompression of metastatic epidural compression. Cancer 116(9):2250–2257

Ryu S, Pugh SL, Gerszten PC et al (2014) RTOG 0631 phase 2/3 study of image guided stereotactic radiosurgery for localized (1-3) spine metastases: phase 2 results. Pract Radiat Oncol 4(2):76–81

Sahgal A, Bilsky M, Chang EL et al (2011) Stereotactic body radiotherapy for spinal metastases: current status, with a focus on its application in the postoperative patient: a review. J Neurosurg Spine 14(2):151–166

Sahgal A, Whyne CM, Ma L et al (2013a) Vertebral compression fracture after stereotactic body radiotherapy for spinal metastases. Lancet Oncol 14(8):e310–ee20

Sahgal A, Atenafu EG, Chao S et al (2013b) Vertebral compression fracture after spine stereotactic body radiotherapy: a multi-institutional analysis with a focus on radiation dose and the spinal instability neoplastic score. J Clin Oncol 31(27):3426–3431

Sahgal A, Aoyama H, Kocher M et al (2015) Phase 3 trials of stereotactic radiosurgery with or without whole-brain radiation therapy for 1 to 4 brain metastases: individual patient data meta-analysis. Int J Radiat Oncol Biol Phys 91(4):710–717

Sande TA, Ruenes R, Lund JA et al (2009) Long-term follow-up of cancer patients receiving radiotherapy for bone metastases: results from a randomised multicentre trial. Radiot Oncol 91(2):261–266

Schaefer P, Budzik R Jr, Gonzalez R (1996) Imaging of cerebral metastases. Neurosurg Clin N Am 7(3):393–423

Shaw E, Scott C, Souhami L et al (2000) Single dose radiosurgical treatment of recurrent previously irradiated primary brain tumors and brain metastases: final report of RTOG protocol 90-05. Int J Radiat Oncol Biol Phys 47(2):291–298

Sperduto PW, Berkey B, Gaspar LE et al (2008) A new prognostic index and comparison to three other indices for patients with brain metastases: an analysis of 1,960 patients in the RTOG database. Int J Radiat Oncol Biol Phys 70(2):510–514

Sperduto PW, Chao ST, Sneed PK et al (2010) Diagnosis-specific prognostic factors, indexes, and treatment outcomes for patients with newly diagnosed brain metastases: a multi-institutional analysis of 4,259 patients. Int J Radiat Oncol Biol Phys 77(3):655–661

Steenland E, Leer J, van Houwelingen H et al (1999) The effect of a single fraction compared to multiple fractions on painful bone metastases: a global analysis of the Dutch Bone Metastasis Study. Radiother Oncol 52(2):101–109

Suh JH (2010) Stereotactic radiosurgery for the management of brain metastases. N Engl J Med 362(12):1119–1127

Townsend PW, Smalley SR, Cozad SC et al (1995) Role of postoperative radiation therapy after stabilization of fractures caused by metastatic disease. Int J Radiat Oncol Biol Phys 31(1):43–49

Tsao MN, Lloyd N, Wong RK, et al 2012 Whole brain radiotherapy for the treatment of newly diagnosed multiple brain metastases. The Cochrane Library

Tubiana-Hulin M (1991) Incidence, prevalence and distribution of bone metastases. Bone 12:S9–S10

Vecht CJ, Haaxma-Reiche H, Noordijk EM et al (1993) Treatment of single brain metastasis: radiotherapy alone or combined with neurosurgery. Ann Neurol 33(6):583–590

Vogelbaum MA, Angelov L, Lee S-Y et al (2006) Local control of brain metastases by stereotactic radiosurgery in relation to dose to the tumor margin. J Neurosurg 104(6):907–912

Wegner RE, Leeman JE, Kabolizadeh P et al (2015) Fractionated stereotactic radiosurgery for large brain metastases. Am J Clin Oncol 38(2):135–139

Wiggenraad R, Verbeek-de Kanter A, Kal HB et al (2011) Dose–effect relation in stereotactic radiotherapy for brain metastases. A systematic review. Radiother Oncol 98(3):292–297

Wong JJ-W, Hird A, Kirou-Mauro A et al (2008) Quality of life in brain metastases radiation trials: a literature review. Curr Oncol 15(5):25–45

Yamamoto M, Serizawa T, Shuto T et al (2014) Stereotactic radiosurgery for patients with multiple brain metastases (JLGK0901): a multi-institutional prospective observational study. Lancet Oncol 15(4):387–395

Yarnold J (1999) 8 Gy single fraction radiotherapy for the treatment of metastatic skeletal pain: randomised comparison with a multifraction schedule over 12 months of patient follow-up. On behalf of the Bone Pain Trial Working Party. Radiother Oncol 52(2):111–121

Erratum to: The Radiobiological Aspects of Altered Fractionation

Alan E. Nahum and Richard P. Hill

Erratum to: Med Radiol Radiat Oncol
DOI 10.1007/174_2017_93

In section 9 (Is a Single Value of α/β for Tumors of a Given Type a Sound Concept for a Patient Population?) of this chapter, the text in the last line of the second paragraph was presented incorrectly.

It has been updated now as below,

When TCP $\approx$70% the constant-β TCP decreases with increasing numbers of fractions; when TCP $\approx$30% the constant-β TCP increases with increasing numbers of fractions.

The updated online version for this chapter can be found under DOI 10.1007/174_2017_93

A. E. Nahum (✉)
Physics Department, University of Liverpool,
Liverpool, UK
e-mail: alan_e_nahum@yahoo.co.uk

R. P. Hill
Princess Margaret Cancer Centre, Toronto,
Ontario, Canada

Med Radiol Radiat Oncol (2018)   419
DOI 10.1007/174_2018_174, © Springer International Publishing AG
Published Online: 26 April 2018

Index

Med Radiol Radiat Oncol (2018)
DOI 10.1007/978-3-319-51198-6, © Springer International Publishing AG, part of Springer Nature

Printed by Printforce, the Netherlands